WOMEN'S HEALTH ISSUES
ACROSS THE LIFE CYCLE

A Quality of Life Perspective

Angela Sammarco, PhD, RN
Associate Professor
College of Staten Island
City University of New York
Staten Island, New York

JONES & BARTLETT
LEARNING

World Headquarters
Jones & Bartlett Learning
5 Wall Street
Burlington, MA 01803
978-443-5000
info@jblearning.com
www.jblearning.com

Jones & Bartlett Learning books and products are available through most bookstores and online booksellers. To contact Jones & Bartlett Learning directly, call 800-832-0034, fax 978-443-8000, or visit our website, www.jblearning.com.

Production Credits
VP, Executive Publisher: David D. Cella
Executive Editor: Amanda Martin
Acquisitions Editor: Teresa Reilly
Editorial Assistant: Danielle Bessette
Production Editor: Vanessa Richards
Marketing Communications Manager: Katie Hennessy
VP, Manufacturing and Inventory Control: Therese Connell
Composition: Cenveo Publisher Services
Cover Design: Scott Moden
Rights & Media Specialist: Wes DeShano
Media Development Editor: Troy Liston
Cover Image: © Masson/Shutterstock
Printing and Binding: Edwards Brothers Malloy
Cover Printing: Edwards Brothers Malloy

Library of Congress Cataloging-in-Publication Data
Names: Sammarco, Angela, author.
Title: Women's health issues across the life cycle : a quality of life
   perspective / Angela Sammarco.
Description: Burlington, MA : Jones & Bartlett Learning, [2017]
Identifiers: LCCN 2015043494 | ISBN 9780763771614 (pbk.)
Subjects: | MESH: Women's Health. | Quality of Life.
Classification: LCC RA564.85 | NLM WA 309.1 | DDC 613/.04244—dc23
LC record available at http://lccn.loc.gov/2015043494

6048

Printed in the United States of America
20 19 18 17 16   10 9 8 7 6 5 4 3 2 1

This book is lovingly dedicated to my children,
Christine Angela McIntyre and Andrew Michael Sammarco.
I will always be with you.

Contents

Preface

Necessity is truly the mother of invention. The idea for writing *Women's Health Issues Across the Life Cycle: A Quality of Life Perspective* was inspired by the need to find a textbook that would be just right for a women's health course I was developing for baccalaureate nursing students. The foundation of this course centered on major theoretical concepts that emerged from my program of research. However, a textbook that strongly focused on women's health issues across the life cycle with a clear application of a quality of life theoretical framework was not to be found. Current textbooks in women's health, although likely suitable for other purposes, were insufficient to meet the learning needs of my students. Thus, this conundrum compelled me to write this book.

My program of research has focused on investigating the quality of life of breast cancer survivors across the life cycle. In my research, I noted how developmental stage and place in life strongly influenced women's perception of their quality of life. The traditional understanding of the developmental stage and place in life of women has shifted dramatically over the last century in response to physical, psychological, and emotional changes in women as well as external social, economic, and political changes in the world. The developmental stage and place in life of a woman creates unique quality of life needs. Moreover, at various points along the life cycle of women, certain health issues tend to arise and become predominant threats to life and well-being. These health issues can impact women's quality of life in dramatic ways that are often overlooked, misunderstood, or inadequately addressed. Quality of life has become an essential factor that affects healthcare decisions and outcomes. A discussion of women's health issues from a quality of life perspective is timely and essential in increasing the body of knowledge of women's health, as well as being influential in assisting healthcare providers in improving quality of life outcomes for women. Thus, this book presents a developmental perspective of the key life-stages of women, the overriding health issues of these life-stages that threaten life and well-being, and female-centered strategies and interventions that will best promote and maintain health and quality of life.

In addition to these theoretical concepts that form the conceptual core of this book, another major concept highlighted is the disparity between men and women that has long existed in health care and research. The health care of women has been influenced by historical and contemporary cultural attitudes and beliefs toward women as well as women's relationships with the healthcare system. Societal views and stereotypes of women have influenced policy decisions in medical research, insurance reimbursement, and protocols for diagnosis and treatment of diseases and health conditions. Until recently, medical research was conducted almost solely on men, except for conditions exclusive to women. Women were excluded from participating as subjects in most research studies since it was believed that gynecological and obstetrical factors would interfere with research outcomes. Moreover, it was erroneously assumed that there was little difference between male and female human responses and physiological functions. Disease presentation, progression, and response to treatment were believed to be similar in men and women. Research evidence has since shown these assumptions to be incorrect, as a clearer understanding of gender similarities and differences in physiology and disease experience has emerged. Laws now require that all research funded by the National Institutes of Health include women as subjects unless the research is investigating a condition exclusive to men. Legislation, the women's movement, and consumer movements have worked to reduce the gender disparity in health care, yet gaps remain. The discussion of current findings of women-centered research in this book helps to further narrow information gaps that continue to exist from previous male-centered inquiry into health care and treatment modalities.

Another major concept addressed in this book is the disparity in the health care of women of cultural and ethnic minorities. As seen with gender disparities, historical and contemporary cultural attitudes, stereotypes, and beliefs toward women of cultural and ethnic minorities as well as their relationships with the healthcare system have influenced healthcare disparities in minority women. Societal views and prejudices as well as issues of access to quality and affordable health care for women of cultural and ethnic minorities are addressed. Strategies and interventions of health promotion and maintenance to improve the well-being and quality of life of minority women are presented throughout.

Users of *Women's Health Issues Across the Life Cycle: A Quality of Life Perspective* should find its organization helpful. Chapters 1–4 are the foundational chapters that explain the core concepts of the book. Chapter 1 introduces the dimensions of women's health. Biological, cultural, historical, social, and political perspectives are presented to enable the user to develop a comprehensive understanding of the multifaceted aspects of women's health. Frequently these perspectives reveal gender disparities whereby discrimination and unequal treatment threatens the lives and well-being of women in various ways. A feminist voice is interwoven throughout the book, based on the position whereby women are entitled to the same political, economic, and social rights and opportunities as men. The feminist voice provides an essential viewpoint for the health and health care of women in promoting change in how health care is delivered to women as well as in achieving social transformation. The historical development of women's health is also presented. This perspective describes the many movements and waves of advocacy that have brought about dramatic changes that have spanned the 19th and 20th centuries and have produced the current level of health care that has nearly doubled the life span of women.

Chapter 2 presents the theoretical core of the book. The complex issues of women's health impact quality of life throughout the lifespan, and so must be acknowledged, explored, and kept in the mainstream of women's health care. This discussion addresses the dramatic changes in the life stages of women, the shifting social expectations of women throughout the lifespan, and how the crucial issues of illness superimposed upon the complicated role demands of women can profoundly influence quality of life. This discussion provides a formidable backdrop for the exploration of the construct of quality of life that follows. An in-depth discussion explores the conceptualization, definitions, and measures taken to establish conceptual clarity of the quality of life construct. The essential nature of quality of life in women's health is emphasized and provides an introduction of the Ferrans Conceptual Model of Quality of Life as the organizing framework of this book.

In Chapter 3, an exploration of the theoretical perspective of vulnerability in women, as well as various vulnerable populations of women, are presented. This discussion acknowledges that numerous individual and social factors inexorably shape the health of women. These factors often place women at greater risk for health problems and can increase their vulnerability to disease, injury, and psychological trauma. Although women in general may be considered vulnerable, many subgroups of women are at greater than average risk for developing health problems, and thus comprise vulnerable populations. This perspective includes a discussion of concepts particularly essential for the promotion of well-being and positive quality of life outcomes of vulnerable populations of women.

Chapter 4 explores the influence of the major public health concerns of stress, overweight/obesity, and physical inactivity on women's health, well-being, and quality of life. The essential roles of stress reduction, healthful diet, and regular exercise in the maintenance of health and well-being are emphasized. Also discussed are complementary and alternative therapeutic modalities that women commonly use to promote health, prevent disease, and enhance well-being and quality of life. It is estimated that nearly 40% of Americans use alternative or complementary healthcare approaches for specific conditions or to maintain overall well-being. In addition, more women than men use complementary or alternative health practices. The discussion of complementary and alternative health practices provides evidence-based information about of the nature, efficacy, and safety of these health practices so that intelligent choices by healthcare consumers may be made.

The next sections of the book present in-depth discussions of selected overriding health issues that commonly arise at particular life stages of women and threaten women's health, well-being, and quality of life. Chapters 5–8 address adolescent and young adult women's health issues, including discussions about eating disorders, bipolar disorder, substance abuse, and consequences of risky sexual behavior. Chapters 9–12 address adult women's health issues and includes discussions about violence, breast cancer, gynecologic cancers, and menopause. Chapters 13–16 address older women's health issues, including discussions about heart disease, stroke, osteoporosis/osteoarthritis, and Alzheimer's disease.

Women's Health Issues Across the Life Cycle: A Quality of Life Perspective does not answer every question that may arise regarding women's health but is intended to stimulate readers to think, critically analyze, ask more questions, and participate in a vibrant dialogue on women's health. This book is written for, but not limited to, baccalaureate and graduate students majoring in nursing or other healthcare professions, who desire a focus in women's health, as well as baccalaureate or graduate level students in women's health issues courses offered in women's studies curricula. It contributes to the dialogue in women's health begun ages ago by women who wanted better health, well-being, and quality of life for themselves and their families. This dialogue has been maintained by voices across the centuries that refused to be silenced, and has collectively brought about advances in women's health that were never thought possible. I invite readers to continue this dialogue in women's health.

Acknowledgments

It can accurately be stated that this book was written *come hell or high water*. On October 29, 2012, the flooding caused by Hurricane Sandy engulfed my home and claimed the life of my husband, Andrew P. Sammarco. In the ensuing chaos and aftermath following the hurricane, my children and I were fatherless, husbandless, homeless, and traumatized beyond belief. We were refugees. Indeed, we experienced firsthand some of the issues and concerns that I have written about in this book, especially with respect to quality of life. The love and support of family, friends, and colleagues were foremost in helping my children and me heal, recover, rebuild, and begin new lives. I mention this profound occurrence because the hell and high water of Hurricane Sandy almost prevented the completion of this book. Work on the manuscript had to be suspended for close to 18 months due to the overwhelming demands of recovery. Picking up the reins of this project after the events of Hurricane Sandy was indeed a challenge, and completing this book produced an exceptional sense of accomplishment. Special thanks are extended to my editors and production team at Jones & Bartlett Learning for their incredible patience and support during our recovery from these events, and for their faith in the value of this project.

It is with profound gratitude that I thank my friends and colleagues who helped during the journey to complete this book. Heartfelt thanks to my best friend and research partner, Lynda M. Konecny, MSN, RN, for her limitless caring, support, inspiration, and sense of humor, all of which kept my batteries charged and my feet on the right path to travel this journey to its end. Special thanks to my dear friends and colleagues, June Como, EdD, RN; Danna Curcio, PhD, RN; Dawn Fairlie, PhD, RN; and Marie Giordano, PhD, RN, for their support, insight, suggestions, and ability to cheer me on to the finish line.

Loving thanks are also extended to these very special people in my life: To my mom, brothers, sisters-in-law, and nieces for their constant love, caring, and support especially during this project. To my sister-in-law, Laraine Tursi, MA, medical librarian extraordinaire, special acknowledgment of her untiring assistance with gathering literature resources throughout the creation of this book. To Maeve A. Lowery, MD, and her intrepid team, who, at the darkest hour, made it possible for me to keep calm and carry on. To my dear friend and companion Eric R. Schwab, Esq., for his sustaining love and encouragement. Most of all, words cannot begin to express the loving gratitude I feel for my daughter, Christine Angela McIntyre; my son-in-law, Corey McIntyre; and my son, Andrew Michael Sammarco. You are truly the wind beneath my wings.

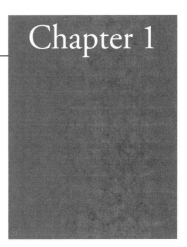

Chapter 1

The Dimensions of Women's Health

LEARNING OUTCOMES

On completion of this chapter, the learner will be able to:

1. Explain the multiple dimensions of women's health.
2. Analyze the diversity of women's health needs over the life cycle and how these needs reflect differences in race, class, ethnicity, culture, sexual preference, levels of education, and access to health care.
3. Explain the historical background of the women's health movement.
4. Describe the advances made in reproductive rights, women's health research, and the political dimensions of women's health.
5. Distinguish barriers to access of adequate healthcare services, providers, and health information encountered by women.
6. Discuss the economic, social, cultural, and political factors that influence women's health throughout the world.
7. Distinguish priority health issues on the global agenda of women's health.

Introduction

The paradigm of women's health is a multifaceted, complex area encompassing practice, education, and research. Women's health concentrates on the physical, psychosocial, political, and economical well-being of women. Women's health facilitates the prevention of illness and the maintenance of wellness through screening, diagnosing, and managing conditions that are unique to women, are more common in women, are more serious in women, and have manifestations, risk factors, or interventions that are different for women. In essence, women's health includes the values and knowledge of women and their own experiences of health and illness (Donoghue, 1996).

Women's health acknowledges the diversity of women's health needs over the life cycle and how these needs reflect differences in race, class, ethnicity, culture, sexual preference, levels of education, and access to health care (Donoghue, 1996). It emphasizes multidisciplinary team approaches to the health care of women and strives for the empowerment of women, as for all patients, to be informed participants in their own health care (Donoghue, 1996).

Women's health includes the study of disease as well as factors that enhance women's well-being and quality of life. It encompasses the entire body and brings to focus the simple recognition that men and women have some fundamentally different health needs and that women's health needs must be pursued in their own right (Office on Women's Health [OWH], 2002). Women's health is based on the study of biological characteristics distinctive to women, the most apparent being reproductive organs, but also differences in body structure, hormones, and brain chemistry. As such, women's health recognizes the importance of the study of gender differences as well as consideration of gender similarities.

Countless factors influence the ways women develop, sicken, recover, interact with others, reproduce, age, and receive health care. A variety of sociocultural issues impact women's health. Women's place in society influences the occurrence of sexual violence. Sociocultural issues affect women's entry into the workforce as well as the type of workplace they encounter. Women's ability to obtain and benefit from health care is also affected by sociocultural issues. Access to health care has emerged as an essential factor in women's health and an important priority in the research agenda. Access to health care includes physical accessibility to healthcare providers as well as the ability to trust providers, pay for health care, understand their health care, negotiate the healthcare system, and know if and when a health problem is developing. The issue of access to health care and healthcare decision making is especially important because women are more likely than men to make healthcare decisions for themselves and their families.

A full understanding of women's health requires biological, cultural, historical, social, and political perspectives. Frequently these perspectives uncover gender disparities whereby discrimination and unequal treatment threaten the lives and well-being of women in numerous ways. Feminism—the belief that women are entitled to the same political, economic, and social rights and opportunities as men—provides an essential viewpoint for the health and health care of women. The aim of a feminist viewpoint is to not only change how health care is delivered to women but to achieve social transformation. Social transformation involves attaining balance in provider–patient relationships, access to information, shared decision making, and striving for societal change (Andrist, 1997).

Historical Background of Women's Health

The 19th and 20th centuries were periods of extraordinary developments in women's health initiated by multiple waves of women's health movements. In order to understand the dramatic changes that have affected women's health throughout this stretch of time, it is essential to examine the social and cultural context that led up to and then underscored the resultant changes. The definition of women's health has evolved over time. Crucial to this evolution has been the shift of goals and perspectives of the advocates of women's health to reflect changing social mores and economic conditions. The dramatic changes in women's health that spanned the 19th and 20th centuries have produced a current level of health care that has nearly doubled the life span of women (OWH, 2002).

The Popular Health Movement

In the 19th century, industrialization brought changes in social and family structure that saw a decrease in the burden of women's work at home, increased access of women to obtaining an education, a decrease in birth rates, and an increase in life expectancy. Populations shifted to cities where workers were pulled outside the home for employment. Initially women and children joined the labor force outside the home but this trend decreased as women became increasingly excluded from the workforce and were economically dependent on men to provide basic goods. During this period, physicians took control of medicine and ushered in an age known as "Heroic Medicine." Throughout this era, physicians (nearly all male) steered medicine away from the services of midwives, homeopaths, herbalists, and traditional healers of the times (many of whom were women) and used a variety of painful and intrusive procedures such as bloodletting, purgatives, surgery, and blistering (Geary, 1995).

Between 1830 and 1870, the Popular Health Movement arose in backlash to heroic medicine and physicians' efforts to discredit traditional practitioners. Activist groups consisting of middle-class women and working-class radicals advocated for education on physiology, nutrition, hygiene, self-determination, hydrotherapy, and disease prevention (Geary, 1995). Healthy lifestyles were advanced in order to avoid disease and the need for physicians. Elimination of the corset and other restrictive clothing, eating a healthy diet, the benefits of physical exercise, and limiting family size (through abstinence of marital relations) were also encouraged. The Popular Health Movement succeeded in reviving traditional types of healing and in promoting women as providers of medical care.

The Women's Medical Movement

The later part of the 19th century saw the emergence of the second wave of advocacy for women's health in the embodiment of the Women's Medical Movement. This era saw the creation of medical schools for women and women's hospitals in which women were able train and practice as physicians.

Female physicians faced much difficulty being accepted by male physicians as well as patients of both genders and found more opportunities for acceptance in rural and frontier environments, where physicians were scarce. The first nursing schools opened in the late 1800s, admitting both men and women. Men dominated the field of nursing in the military and in the southern part of the country, but over the course of the 20th century nursing became professionalized and evolved into a predominantly female field. Consequently, it retained less status and lower pay as compared to other male-dominated medical professions (OWH, 2002).

The Women's Medical Movement challenged prevailing medical views that women were fragile, sickly, and prone to hysteria that was controlled by their reproductive organs. Popular medical beliefs associated female hysteria to a biological disposition that was deemed inferior, even pathological, coupled with advanced education that was thought to undermine normal female development. Thus, women were advised to not pursue education, in order to restore acceptance of their femininity (Geary, 1995). Female physicians challenged this view of women by advocating education, exercise, and useful work for women as well as supporting women's right to control their fertility by limiting marital sexual intercourse. Female physicians also espoused a special rapport with female patients that made them uniquely qualified as healthcare providers of women and children (OWH, 2002; Weisman, 2000).

The Progressive Era

The Progressive Era of 1890 to 1930 advanced the roles of women and women's rights as well as women's health. Not only did women gain the right to vote in 1920 through passage of the 19th Amendment to the U.S. Constitution, this period ushered in the third wave of advocacy for women's health. Two separate and often antagonistic movements supported the creation of specific health services for women. One group of reformers consisting of white middle-class women, nurses, and female physicians from the Settlement House Movement raised public awareness regarding infant and maternal mortality at a time when national statistics were not available and prenatal care was not part of standard medical practice. These advocates influenced public policy in gaining the passage of the Sheppard–Towner Maternity and Infancy Act of 1921. This was the first federal program for the health care of women and children that established publically funded child health clinics, home visits by public health nurses, and nearly 3,000 local prenatal care clinics staffed predominantly by nurses and female physicians (Weisman, 2000).

During this time, the second group of activists advocated for the legalization of birth control. Contraceptives were not widely available to women, especially women who were poor, unmarried, and generally lacked access to private physicians. The Cornstock Law of 1873, the Act for the Suppression of Trade in, and Circulation of, Obscene Literature and Articles of Immoral Use, made it illegal to distribute information about birth control. Margaret Sanger was a nurse and social reformer who, with other advocates, challenged the Cornstock Law by disseminating birth control information and supplies. Sanger founded the first, although illegal, birth control clinic in 1916 and over a period of years established a nationwide network of family planning clinics to provide contraceptive counseling and methods to women who did not have access to private physicians. The clinics were privately funded by wealthy women and foundations, and staffed by nurses and women physicians (OWH, 2002; Weisman, 2000).

The Grassroots Movement

The fourth wave of advocacy for women's health occurred during the 1960s and 1970s when grassroots organizations led by women who were college educated challenged the authority of the nearly all-male medical profession in the delivery of health care to women, with resultant exposure of medical biases against women. Women were being excluded from making decisions about their own health care, and mainstream healthcare institutions were deemed unresponsive to women's specific needs and unwilling to engage women as partners in their healthcare decisions (Weisman, 2000). The movement advocated for reforms from a feminist perspective in areas such as unnecessary hysterectomies and cesarean sections, abortion, postpartum depression, and childbirth conditions. Women-specific alternatives were introduced, including abortion clinics, women-controlled health centers such as self-help gynecologic clinics and feminist women's clinics, and freestanding birth centers and other alternative childbirth practices (Weisman, 2000). The self-help manual *Our Bodies, Ourselves* was published in 1970 and contained validated information on issues such as heterosexuality, lesbianism, nutrition, birth control, abortion, childbearing, menopause, exercise, sexually transmitted diseases, self esteem, relationships, and the healthcare system (Geary, 1995). Written for women by women who were not medically trained, its goal was to teach women about their bodies and recognize the value of their personal experiences with the healthcare system. The book challenged women to be active in their own health care and to be critical consumers (OWH, 2002).

Women's admission to medical schools other than women's medical schools was severely restricted by quotas such that by 1960 only 7% of physicians were women. A gender discrimination suit against some medical schools in 1970 and a provision of the 1972 Civil Rights Act that prohibited gender discrimination in educational institutions paved the way for unrestricted admission of women to medical schools (OWH, 2002). Additional legal reforms gave greater rights to women, such as access to oral contraceptives, protection against employment discrimination, and equal funding for men and women in school athletic programs. Also, the Women's Health Movement had been led by white middle-class women for decades. During this period, the movement became more enriched by the inclusion of women of diverse ethnic and racial backgrounds and was joined by women's health organizations that represented African American, Latina, Asian, and Native American women. In addition, organizations that represented older women and women with disabilities joined the Women's Health Movement to advocate for their health needs.

Gains and Setbacks of the 1980s

The liberal political environment of the 1970s encouraged the Women's Health Movement to flourish and make significant gains in addressing the health needs of women. With the advent of an increasingly conservative political environment in the 1980s, setbacks in the area of reproductive rights were experienced. Anti-abortion activists attacked legalized abortion. Violence toward feminist health clinics caused many to close. In 1989 the Supreme Court handed down the Webster v. Reproductive Health Services decision, which placed increased restrictions on abortion (Nichols, 2000).

In spite of the setbacks that occurred with reproductive rights, this period saw progress with the establishment of federal task forces and agencies that were charged with the responsibility of ensuring that women's health needs were met. The Task Force on Women's Issues was formed by the U.S. Public Health Service in 1983 to ensure that women's needs were being addressed, to report on this, and to make recommendations for change. The major findings of the task force were that women were dissatisfied with current access to information and quality health care; concern that women's health was a function of the social, cultural, and economic environment; and a lack of attention by

physicians to the mental health aspects of physical disease. Major recommendations of the task force were for expansion of research to address problems unique to or prevalent in women and to increase research on contraceptive technologies for women and men (Nichols, 2000).

The National Institutes of Health (NIH) adopted a policy in 1986 that required inclusion of women in clinical research. By 1989, women leaders at the NIH found that research in women's health continued to be neglected. The Congressional Caucus for Women's Issues and Henry Waxman (D-California) requested a formal investigation of NIH research by the General Accounting Office. The investigation revealed that women were still excluded from clinical studies, and a mere 13.5% of NIH monies went toward women's health research. Furthermore, diseases that affected women disproportionately were less likely to be studied, women were more likely to be excluded from clinical trials, and women were less likely to be principal investigators conducting clinical trials. While the evidence did not suggest that women were being systematically excluded from biomedical research, the evidence did indicate that women were excluded from some studies and that the numbers of women included in studies were inadequate to detect gender differences (Nichols, 2000).

Bringing Women's Health to the National Agenda

The 1990s brought a fifth wave of advocacy for women's health, which was led by women in government, academia, medicine, and women's health advocacy and interest groups. Attention was drawn to gender inequities in society's investment in biomedical research and focused on increasing government support for women's health research and services beyond reproductive issues (Weisman, 2000). Funding for women's health research in areas such as heart disease, breast cancer, and aging processes was increased by the NIH. Policies and guidelines within the NIH were changed to include women in clinical studies. Moreover, new federal offices were created to expand the infrastructure to coordinate a women's health agenda (Weisman, 2000). The Office of Research on Women's Health (ORWH) was established in 1990 as part of the NIH in order to verify that NIH research addressed women's health needs and the inclusion of increased numbers of women, including women of racial and ethnic minorities, in clinical trials. The ORWH developed a women's health research agenda. Furthermore, the ORWH designed the Women's Health Initiative study, which was a 14-year multisite investigation of postmenopausal women that focused on the efficacy of hormone replacement therapy, diet, and exercise on coronary heart disease, breast and colon cancer, and osteoporosis (Nichols, 2000).

During this period, two other federal agencies were actively involved in women's health research. The FDA removed restrictions excluding women of childbearing potential from participating in early phases of drug testing and revised guidelines requiring sex-specific analyses of drug safety and efficacy. The U.S. Department of Health and Human Services Centers for Disease Control and Prevention (CDC) initiated screening programs for chlamydia in women and their partners, and designated Papanicolaou smears and mammography screening for underserved women (Nichols, 2000). In 1994, the CDC and the Agency for Toxic Substances and Disease Registry (ATSDR) created the Office of Women's Health to provide advocacy, guidance, leadership, and coordination of policy, programs, and activities associated with women's health both within and outside the CDC/ATSDR (U.S. Department of Health and Human Services Centers for Disease Control and Prevention [CDC], 2010).

A powerful lobby has been created by the activists in the Women's Health Movement. This lobby has alerted legislators and the public regarding the inequities that exist in women's health care. Consequently, the efforts of the lobby have been successful in making women's health an important public and political concern that commands responses from leaders in public policy, medicine, research, and government. Widespread changes from local to federal levels have been achieved (Nichols, 2000).

Women's Health and the New Millennium

The new millennium has brought many improvements to the health of the public such as findings from the Women's Health Initiative study, improvement in medications for treating HIV/AIDS, inclusion of children in clinical trials, and public health programs that target behavior-related health problems. Nevertheless, women still face many difficulties in the healthcare arena. Setbacks have occurred in advances made in the 1990s, including curtailment of funding for domestic and international reproductive health initiatives and politicizing of the women's health agenda. Millions of Americans lack health insurance or are underinsured. Women are living longer but not necessarily with a better quality of life. Unhealthy behaviors such as smoking, lack of exercise, poor diet, overeating, alcohol abuse, illicit drug use, and unsafe sex continue to threaten women's health and increase their risk of disease. Women across the United States and around the world continue to be victims of individual and societal violence.

The Role of Government in Women's Health

Federal Agencies That Promote Women's Health

The federal government plays a significant role in protecting and promoting women's health.

Through direct and indirect means, the government exercises control over many areas that influence women's health. Actions such as ensuring a safe food supply and regulating companies that provide medications to the public can impact on the maintenance of wellness in women.

During the 1990s, federal agencies and organizations devoted to women's health were established. The Office on Women's Health of the Department of Health and Human Services (DHHS) was established in 1991 and serves as the coordinating agency for all women's health initiatives throughout the agencies and offices of the U.S. DHHS, including the NIH, FDA, and CDC. The OWH also collaborates with nonprofit organizations, consumer groups, associations of healthcare professionals, tribal organizations, and state, county, and local governments. The goals of the OWH are to develop and impact national women's health policy; to develop, adapt, and replicate model programs on women's health; and to educate, influence, and collaborate with health organizations, healthcare professionals, and the public. The OWH provides leadership to promote health equity for women and girls through sex/gender-specific approaches. The OWH develops innovative programs, educates health professionals, and motivates behavior change in consumers through the dissemination of health information (OWH, 2013).

The ORWH functions as a focal point for women's health research at the NIH. The ORWH coordinates women's health research funded by the NIH and advises the NIH director and staff on matters relating to research on women's health. This office works in partnership with the NIH institutes and centers to ensure that women's health research is part of the scientific framework not only at NIH but throughout the scientific community (Office of Research on Women's Health [ORWH], 2015). The ORWH has been vital in national and international efforts to make women's health research part of the scientific and educational infrastructure. Moreover, the ORWH works with scientists, practitioners, legislators, and lay advocates to identify research priorities and set a comprehensive research agenda.

The ORWH strengthens and enhances research related to diseases, disorders, and conditions that affect women and supports research on women's health issues. The ORWH also promotes, stimulates, and supports efforts to enhance the health of women through biomedical and behavioral research on the roles of sex (the biological characteristics of being female or male) and gender (the social influences based on sex) in health and disease. Furthermore, this office ensures that research funded and supported by the NIH adequately addresses issues associated with women's health and ensures that women are appropriately represented in biomedical and behavioral research studies supported by the NIH. The ORWH develops opportunities for and supports recruitment retention, re-entry, and advancement of women in biomedical careers (ORWH, 2015).

The DHHS has implemented programs to provide for family planning, prevent sexually transmitted diseases, and reduce unintended pregnancies. The Title X Family Planning program is the only federal grant program dedicated solely to providing individuals with comprehensive family planning and related preventive health services. This program assists individuals in determining the number and spacing of their children in order to promote positive birth outcomes and healthy families. The Title X program provides access to contraceptive services, supplies, and information to women and men who want and need them. Priority for services is given, by law, to individuals from low-income families. Services are provided through a network of federally funded community-based clinics that include state and local health departments, tribal organizations, hospitals, university health centers, independent clinics, community health centers, faith-based organizations, and other public and private nonprofit agencies.

Approximately 75% of U.S. counties have at least one clinic funded by Title X that provides services as required under the Title X statute (Office of Population Affairs [OPA], 2015).

Title X provides funding for preventive services such as patient education and counseling, breast and pelvic examinations, breast and cervical cancer screening according to nationally recognized standards of care, pregnancy diagnosis and counseling, as well as sexually transmitted disease and HIV prevention, education, and counseling. Title X funding also supports training for family planning clinic personnel, data collection and family planning research aimed at improving delivery of services, as well as information dissemination and community-based education and outreach activities. Title X, by law, does not fund programs where abortion is a method of family planning (OPA, 2015).

Political Perspectives of Biomedical Research

The federal government plays an essential role in funding biomedical research. The NIH is responsible for distributing funds to private and public institutions and organizations for the purpose of conducting medical and health research. Along with the CDC and other agencies, the NIH advances basic research for the discovery of new and better methods of treatment and prevention of numerous health conditions. Funding for biomedical research is also provided by the private sector, philanthropic organizations, universities, and voluntary health agencies. Millions of dollars are invested each year by pharmaceutical companies and private corporations in order to develop new drugs, vaccines, and technologies. Such investments in biomedical research and technologies have produced advances that have increased life expectancy, improved health throughout the lifespan, and in many cases, decreased the cost of illness.

Nonetheless, discoveries of new medicines and technologies are not the only way to improve health. Approximately half of the mortality in the United States is directly or indirectly caused by unhealthy behavior choices. Research can also indicate better ways to educate people about basic measures to maintain health, such as disease prevention, eating a healthy balanced diet, exercising, maintaining a healthy weight, and avoiding tobacco and other drugs. Research on healthy behavior choices offers the potential to improve the health of millions of Americans. Promoting healthy behavior choices and the prevention of diseases are less costly, more efficacious strategies than intervention after diseases have occurred. Unfortunately, the funding for preventive programs is outdistanced by the funding of pharmaceuticals or technologies that promise the next "miracle cure" or, for the shareholder, the next source of revenue.

Research on women's health has witnessed unprecedented growth, especially in response to the inclusion of women in clinical trials. The inclusion of women in clinical trials has enabled both women and men to become the studied models for the conditions that affect them and the drugs used to treat these conditions. This trend has led to the integration of women-specific data into clinical practice and the formulation of new questions concerning women and particular diseases.

Gender-based research is research that examines the similarities and differences between women and men to learn more about the causes of disease and responses to medication. Gender-based studies identify and examine the biological and physiological differences between women and men. Females and males can manifest different symptoms of a disease, experience the course of a disease differently, or respond in dissimilar ways to pharmaceuticals. Identification and examination of gender-based differences offers a significant potential for understanding disease epidemiology and health outcomes for both women and men. Gender-based differences of various diseases and conditions will be discussed in greater detail in subsequent chapters of this book.

Basic physiological differences between men and women often influence the way they react to and metabolize drugs. Women tend to have smaller-sized organs, higher percentage of body fat, higher body water content, lower body weight, and less muscle mass. Men and women process drugs differently at the molecular level. Sex differences in the way drugs are transported within the body as well as in enzymatic action in the process of drug metabolism can affect drug reactions. Sex hormones apparently influence the effects of many drugs. In women, the menstrual cycle, pregnancy, and menopause have significant effects on how drugs react in their bodies (Society for Women's Health Research [SWHR], 2004). Differences such as age, hormonal status, race, ethnicity, and socio-economic status also affect how women metabolize drugs. The extent to which these differences prevail among the range of drugs used to prevent and treat disease is even now not fully known or understood.

FDA guidelines urge drug investigators to account for gender differences in drug metabolism throughout the development process. Also, women of childbearing age must be included in both Phase I and Phase II clinical trials.

The phases of a clinical trial are explained in **Table 1–1**. Prior to the 1990s women of childbearing age were excluded from clinical trials. However, the call for gender-specific analyses of safety and effectiveness of new drugs brought about revision of its guidelines by the FDA as well as a change of policy for the inclusion of women of childbearing age in early drug studies. Participation of women in clinical trials has resulted in representation of the population most likely to use a disease therapy and determination of any sex differences in the disease therapy. Furthermore, women's participation in clinical trials provides insight into the scientific basis for individual therapy differences and provides future directions for research (U.S. Food and Drug Administration [FDA], 2014).

Gender-based research has posed challenges as well as opportunities for pharmaceutical manufacturers. If research shows that a drug is effective for only one gender, the potential market for that drug might likely be limited and could diminish the profits of the drug company. On the other hand, targeting drugs for women or other specific populations can also allow researchers and pharmaceutical companies to create much more effective products.

Table 1–1 PHASES OF A CLINICAL TRIAL

Phase I	Involves a small-scale study designed primarily to determine safety and tolerance of a newly developed drug or therapy and optimal dose or strength of the therapy.
Phase II	Involves a larger-scale study that seeks preliminary evidence of controlled effectiveness of the drug or therapy and possible side effects. It is sometimes considered as a pilot test of the drug or therapy.
Phase III	Involves a large-scale, multiple-site randomized controlled trial that seeks evidence of the efficacy of the drug or therapy, especially in comparison to other treatments, and to monitor adverse effects.
Phase IV	Involves studies of the effectiveness of the drug or therapy in the general population. Studies focus on post-approval safety surveillance and on long-term consequences over a larger population and time scale than was possible during earlier phases.

Modified from Polit, D., & Beck, C. (2014). *Essentials of nursing research: Appraising evidence for nursing practice* (8th ed.). Philadelphia, PA: Lippincott Williams & Wilkins.

Although advances toward inclusion of women and minority groups in research studies have been made, a major barrier to the participation of women in biomedical research still remains. Many women are unable to participate in clinical trials because they lack health insurance coverage. Some insurance companies consider clinical trials experimental and, as such, are not covered under all standard health policies. Some states have passed legislation requiring health plans to pay for routine health care that a person may receive as a participant in a clinical trial.

Including women in clinical studies frequently poses challenges; however, their exclusion courts disaster through ignorance. Women, particularly those of childbearing age, present challenges to the investigation, as the researchers must consider the effects of hormonal cycling on the hypothesis being tested. Furthermore, the potential for pregnancy and possible fetal damage must be considered. These factors weigh heavily in designing and conducting any study.

Political Perspectives of Reproductive Rights

Birth control has been at the center of national attention for many years. The history and politics surrounding women's decision to control when and if to have children are long and complex. Although women today take the availability of birth control devices and information for granted, only in recent years has it been legal to use them. Over half a century ago, birth control pills were illegal in some states. Landmark legal decisions of the Supreme Court changed the status of contraception in this country. These included the 1965 decision, Griswold v. Connecticut, which struck down a statute that made the use of birth control illegal and criminalized spreading information about its use, and a 1972 decision, Eisenstadt v. Baird, that struck down a Massachusetts law that made it a felony to give contraceptives to anyone

other than married persons. The Population Research and Voluntary Family Planning Programs Law was enacted in 1970 as Title X of the Public Health Service Act. As previously discussed, Title X is a federal grant program designed to provide individuals with access to contraceptive services, supplies, and information. However, women who relied on private medical insurance to defray their medical expenses frequently were required to pay out of pocket for birth control pills since numerous insurers did not offer reimbursement for oral contraception. Recent legal victories in the reproductive rights movement increased women's access to contraception through their health insurers. In 1998, federal employees won mandated coverage for contraception via an act of Congress. Additionally, women's advocacy groups have lobbied insurers and employers to include oral contraception in covered prescription drug benefits.

Federal restrictions on contraceptive development have resulted in the likelihood of the United States lagging behind many countries in this arena. U.S. couples possibly have fewer options for contraceptive choices than couples in other developed nations. U.S. women have a responsibility to stay informed as contraceptive technology continues to evolve, and to be cognizant of the political and economic forces that might facilitate or impede the availability of contraceptive devices or agents.

For nearly a century, abortion was illegal in the United States. In 1973, the landmark Supreme Court decision Roe v. Wade legalized abortion. Nonetheless, this decision has not prevented states from imposing restrictions that limit where and when women may receive abortions. Presently, the subject of abortion rights remains at the center of major debates in the political arena of this country, most notably in the election of political representatives and the selection of Supreme Court justices. The Roe v. Wade decision did not prevent the federal government from imposing abortion restrictions in countries that receive U.S. funding. The Mexico

City Policy, or "Global Gag Rule," was first enacted between 1985 and 1993 and stipulated that nongovernmental organizations receiving U.S. assistance cannot use separately obtained non-U.S. funds to inform the public or educate their government on the need to make safe abortion available. Neither could these organizations provide legal abortion services or provide advice regarding where to get an abortion. However, exemptions were allowed in the cases of rape, incest, and pregnancy that was life-threatening to the mother, but not for a woman's physical or mental health (Change: Center for Health and Gender Equity [CCHGE], 2015).

The Global Gag Rule has had serious effects on women's health in many developing countries. Under this rule, developing countries faced the dilemma that if they agreed to the policy and accepted U.S. family planning assistance, they risked an increase in death and injuries from unsafe, illegal abortions. However, by rejecting the U.S. assistance, they would lose funding for all areas of family planning, including reduction of unplanned pregnancy, preventing HIV, and reducing maternal and infant deaths. Documentation and analysis of the impact of the Global Gag Rule has indicated that the policy restricts a basic right to speech and the right to make informed health decisions. The policy also harms the health and lives of poor women by restricting access to family planning services. Furthermore, it has been shown that the policy does not reduce incidence of abortion (CCHGE, 2015).

The Global Gag Rule was eliminated in 1993 by President Clinton but was reinstated in 2001 by President George W. Bush. President Barack Obama repealed the policy on January 23. 2009. President Obama has called for a new approach to family planning that would end the politicization of women's health on a global scale. Advocates have also been working to prevent reenactment of the policy by future presidents without approval of Congress (CCHGE, 2015).

Access to Healthcare Services, Providers, and Health Information

Advances in public health and medicine have created major improvements in the prevention, diagnosis, and treatment of diseases in women. As a result, many women are living longer and healthier lives. Over the years women have learned to seek out medical information on their own, thereby becoming informed consumers. New discoveries have lead to improved methods of disease prevention, and as such, health promotion and disease prevention have become primary goals of health care. However, health promotion and disease prevention are complicated processes. Although women have made major strides in economic, social, and political aspects of health promotion and disease prevention, women continue to encounter barriers to obtaining adequate health care. Lower socioeconomic status creates a barrier that restricts women's ability to pay for needed healthcare services and medications. It frequently prevents women from being able to pay for transportation to health facilities or engage in healthy nutrition, activities, or lifestyle choices. Many women have inadequate health insurance coverage because they are underinsured or lack health insurance altogether due to unemployment or low socioeconomic status. Cultural factors such as lack of cultural and gender sensitivity among healthcare providers causes many women to encounter discrimination because of race, ethnicity, or sexual orientation. Social factors such as language barriers or low levels of literacy increase the likelihood that women will experience difficulty in understanding medical personnel and directives or in navigating the healthcare system. Furthermore, fear of medical personnel and procedures often results in women delaying health care or avoiding it altogether.

Although many gains in women's health have been obtained, women's health activists continue to lobby for improved healthcare services and legislation that will remove barriers from access of health care. More efforts and initiatives are needed to mitigate the factors that create barriers preventing women from accessing adequate health care. These include efforts that will make health care more affordable and accessible to women of lower socioeconomic means. Efforts are needed to increase cultural sensitivity and competency among healthcare providers. Lastly, more initiatives are needed that will improve the health literacy of women.

The National Priority of Women's Health

Women's health is now recognized as a national priority, and tremendous progress has been made in expanding the scope and depth of attention to women's health and women's health research. Continued success in the women's health movement depends on several factors: political commitment; sufficient funds; educated and interested scientific and lay communities; advocacy by professionals, patients, and the public; and involvement of women, men, and communities in working for equality and recognizing gender differences. These factors have been catalysts driving the advances in women's health research and are responsible for the achievements in women's health and well-being.

Women's Health: Global Perspectives

Women's health issues have moved beyond geographical and political boundaries and have gained international visibility at the top of the worldwide health agenda. Dramatic disparities in women's health exist in resource-rich and resource-poor countries. Many factors influence women's health throughout the world. These factors encompass women's economic status, level of literacy, opportunities for employment, race and ethnicity, as well as whether women reside in urban or rural environments and the particular countries or regions of the world in which they live. Women's health is also influenced by biological, social, and cultural factors, especially gender disparities and the value society places on women (Spielberg, 2011). In particular, women and girls are frequently prevented from benefiting from quality health services. The reasons that contribute to this situation include the disproportionate burden of poverty on women, the existence of unequal power relationships between men and women, social norms that reduce education and paid employment opportunities for women, an exclusive focus on women's reproductive roles, and the potential for—or actual experience of—physical, sexual, and emotional violence (World Health Organization [WHO], 2015b).

Females comprise approximately 52% of the world's population (Spielberg, 2011). Females worldwide have an average life expectancy of 73 years as compared to 68 years for males. World population has grown to 7.2 billion people, with growth greatest in developing countries (Population Reference Bureau, 2012; U.S. Census Bureau, 2015) Life expectancy is a common indicator of the overall health and well-being of a society. Throughout the world, women tend to live longer than men (Spielberg, 2011). Moreover, notable differences exist in life expectancy between countries and regions of the world. Women of developed countries tend to have a longer life expectancy than women of developing countries (WHO, 2015c).

Childhood Mortality

When considering global childhood mortality, girls are more likely to survive infancy than boys for reasons that are unclear. Yet, some countries such as China, India, Nepal, and Pakistan have a higher mortality rate of girls relative to that of boys. Because of the dense population in China and India, the mortality rate for girls under 5 years of age for Asia as a whole (2005–2010) is higher (61 per 1,000) than for boys (56 per 1,000) (United Nations Department of Economic and Social Affairs, Population Division [UNDESA], 2010). In some societies, preferential treatment for boys in healthcare practices and nutrition, as well as the practice of female infanticide and sex-selective abortion, lead to a severe decrease in survival of baby girls. When the rate of survival of baby girls is not higher than or equivalent to the rate of survival of baby boys, this is likely a sign of specific gender-based discrimination (Spielberg, 2011).

Maternal Mortality

Women's reproductive years, mainly between the ages of 15 and 44, are years of highest risk regarding women's mortality in many parts of the world. In 2008, an estimated 358,000 women worldwide died from causes associated with pregnancy and childbirth. From a global perspective, that is 260 maternal deaths for every 100,000 live births. Although this estimate is a 34% decline from maternal deaths in 1990, developing countries account for 99% (355,000) of maternal deaths, out of which 87% of global maternal deaths are attributed to sub-Saharan Africa and South Asia. Common causes of maternal death are ascribed to direct obstetric deaths from obstetric complications that occur during pregnancy, delivery, or the post partum period. Maternal deaths are also attributed to indirect causes that result from previous existing diseases, diseases that develop during pregnancy, or diseases that were aggravated by the physiological effects of pregnancy (WHO, 2010a).

The disproportion in risk for maternal mortality between developing and developed countries and regions of the world is largely due to disparities in access to reproductive health care between resource-rich and resource-poor counties, and inequities within countries suffered by vulnerable populations and minorities. It is estimated that 99% of maternal deaths can be preventable through three types of services. These include family planning services to reduce unintended pregnancies, having a skilled attendant at deliveries, and provision of timely emergency care if obstetric complications occur (Spielberg, 2011). In developing countries, approximately 40% of births take place in a health facility and about 57% of deliveries are guided by a skilled birth attendant. Worldwide, women have a vast need for family planning services that will enable individuals and couples to decide whether or not to have children and to achieve the desired timing and spacing of children they decide to have (Spielberg, 2011).

A goal of the United Nations is to reduce maternal mortality to 213 deaths per 100,000 live births by 2015. The United Nations launched the Global Strategy for Women's and Children's Health in 2010. This strategy seeks to support the development and implementation of country-led plans to improve access to comprehensive integrated reproductive health services. The strategy also supports government initiatives to strengthen health systems to deliver high-quality healthcare services; implementation of national plans to train, retain, and deploy healthcare workers; and the development, funding, and implementation of a prioritized coordinated and innovative research agenda for women's and children's health. Presently, numerous countries are making progress toward reducing maternal mortality; however, there are still countries that have a long way to go in order to achieve this goal (WHO, 2010a).

Unsafe abortion is a procedure for terminating unintended pregnancy performed by persons who lack the necessary skills, or in an environment that is inconsistent with minimal medical standards, or both. In 2008, an estimated 21.6 million unsafe abortions took place, an increase from

19.7 million in 2003. Almost all unsafe abortions took place in developing countries. Overall, the unsafe abortion rate is approximately 14 per 1,000 women aged 15 to 44 years. Mortality attributed to unsafe abortions accounts for nearly 13% of all maternal deaths (WHO, 2011c). The World Health Organization (2011c) estimates that the number of unsafe abortions will continue to rise unless women have increased access to safe abortion and contraception, as well as stronger support to empower women with the freedom to decide whether and when to have a child. In order to reduce the number of unsafe abortions, women need access to safe and effective contraception, less restrictive abortion policies, access to sex education, and access to emergency contraception. Family planning is therefore crucial for the empowerment of women, reduction of poverty, and improvement of maternal and infant health (Spielberg, 2011).

Women's Health Issues in Adulthood

SEXUALLY TRANSMITTED INFECTIONS

Sexually transmitted infections (STIs) pose serious health risks for women worldwide. Spread person to person by sexual contact, an estimated 340 million curable new cases of STIs occur each year throughout the world in adults aged 15 to 49 years (WHO, 2013a). In developing countries the problem of STIs is prevalent to the extent that STIs and their complications are one of the top five reasons adults seek medical treatment. STIs pose serious risk for pregnant women and their unborn children. STIs can cause ectopic pregnancies, miscarriage, stillbirth, congenital infections, low birth weight, and newborn blindness. Pregnant women can transmit HIV and syphilis to their babies during pregnancy and delivery. For some women, STIs can interfere with fertility as a long-lasting complication. In some cultures, infertility can be a severe social stigma that can increase women's vulnerability to domestic abuse, divorce, and rejection by spouse, family, and community. In the presence of an untreated STI, the risk of acquiring and transmitting HIV increases tenfold. Strategies for treatment and prevention of STIs encompass education about safe sex, access to facilities for early diagnosis and treatment of disease, and actions to counteract the social prejudices and stigma surrounding STIs (Spielberg, 2011).

HIV/AIDS

Worldwide, some 33.3 million people are living with HIV infection, which is approximately 0.8% of the world's population. In 2009, an estimated 2.6 million people became newly infected with HIV (Joint United Nations Programme on HIV/AIDS [UNAIDS], 2010). Ninety five percent of new infections occur in developing countries. The hardest hit areas frequently are those where women lack economic independence, education, access to health services and information, and the ability to avoid infection (Spielberg, 2011). Africa is the most severely affected region, and sub-Saharan Africa bears an inordinate share of the global HIV burden. Seventy percent of the people infected with HIV live in sub-Saharan Africa (UNAIDS, 2010).

HIV is progressively becoming a woman's disease. More women than men live with HIV/AIDS, accounting for 52% of the total, and the disease claims the lives of over 1 million women each year. In 2009 approximately 370,000 children were infected with HIV through mother to child transmission. In recent years, the mode of transmission has shifted to where more than 80% of the HIV infections worldwide are contracted through heterosexual sex (UNAIDS, 2010). Current research geared toward preventive measures for women shows promising results. A tenofovir-based vaginal gel has shown encouraging potential as a female-initiated prevention option in reducing the acquisition of HIV infection, and may soon become viable (UNAIDS, 2010). Other strategies that have shown to be effective in HIV prevention include male circumcision, consistent use of condoms, and treatment for other sexually transmitted infections. Strategies are needed to build stronger effective prevention and treatment responses. Non-stigmatizing health services and effective referral systems across behavior and social support services for HIV, tuberculosis, and STIs are needed. Further strategies necessitate increased investment in the capacities of individuals and key communities living with HIV to organize and empower themselves, and improved communication of social and behavioral changes regarding risk and treatment (UNAIDS, 2010).

Tuberculosis

In 2009, approximately 3.3 million women contracted tuberculosis (TB) and 600,000 died from the disease (WHO, 2010b). The World Health Organization estimates that approximately 200,000 women infected with HIV died of TB in 2008. TB is acknowledged as the third leading cause of death worldwide among women between the ages of 15 and 44 years and the fifth leading cause of death among girls and women between the ages of 10 and 19 years in low-income countries (WHO, 2014a).

Once infected with TB, women in their reproductive years are more susceptible to developing active disease than men of the same age. TB can cause infertility and can contribute to numerous poor outcomes associated with reproductive health, particularly for women infected with HIV. Since the feminization of the HIV epidemic, which has produced a greater burden of HIV among women worldwide, a quarter of deaths among women with HIV are linked to TB. Moreover, factors such as poverty, malnutrition, food insecurity, living in crowded conditions, the rising use of tobacco, and increased incidence of diabetes among women can intensify the risk of TB (WHO, 2014a).

Numerous social, cultural, and economic implications occur for women who have TB. In some societies, women who are sick with TB may be stigmatized, discriminated against, and are likely to remain unmarried or become divorced. The stigma associated with TB will impact quality of life. Women with TB may be ostracized from their families and communities. A female relative sick with TB is often unable to carry out family responsibilities. As such, children of the family are frequently forced out of school or work to care for family members. Cultural and financial barriers can severely impede women with TB from seeking care. Women tend to wait almost twice as long as men to seek care for TB. Consequently care is frequently delayed until the illness is severe, leading to a poorer prognosis and greater mortality (Spielberg, 2011; WHO, 2014a). An additional concern is that TB has become more difficult and expensive to treat since multidrug-resistant forms of the disease have developed. As a result women infected with multidrug-resistant strains of TB would be required to undergo many months of complicated treatment that carries a heavy burden for them and their families (Spielberg, 2011; WHO, 2014a).

Cancer

Worldwide, cancer is a leading cause of death (WHO, 2015a). The most common sites for cancer in women are breast, lung, stomach, and colon. Breast cancer is the most widespread cancer in women, with one million new cases occurring each year. The incidence of breast cancer is highest in women from North America and northern Europe and lowest in women from Asia (Spielberg, 2011). Breast cancer is the leading cause of cancer deaths in women around the world. Approximately 521,000 deaths from breast cancer occurred in 2012 (WHO, 2015a).

Cervical cancer is the second most common type of cancer in women and is linked to genital infection with the human papillomavirus (HPV). It is estimated that 493,000 cases of cervical cancer occur each year worldwide. More than 90% of the deaths from cervical cancer occur in low-income countries where access to cervical cancer screening and treatment is scarce or nonexistent (WHO, 2013b).

The HPV infection is a common sexually transmitted infection. The risk of acquiring HPV is highest shortly after a woman begins engaging in sexual intercourse. Although most HPV infections are self-limiting and relatively harmless, persistent infection with cancer-causing strains of HPV can lead to the development of cervical cancer in women. Routine screening with Pap smears to achieve early detection of the disease is effective in decreasing the incidence of cervical cancer. Widespread screening programs that include successful treatment and follow-up of women with abnormal Pap smears have been effective in reducing cervical cancer incidence by 80%. In addition to early screening and treatment, vaccination of girls and women, age 9 years to 26 years, against HPV infection is being done to reduce the incidence of HPV-related cervical cancer (Spielberg, 2011).

Chronic Diseases

Chronic diseases are a substantial cause of disability and death among women. Cardiovascular disease and diabetes are the most common chronic diseases that women develop, with a higher incidence found among women of lower socioeconomic means. Many of the health problems that women develop as they age are associated with risk factors and unhealthy behaviors practiced in adolescence and young adulthood, such as smoking, poor diet, and sedentary lifestyle. Globally, cardiovascular diseases, such as heart attack, ischemic heart disease, and stroke, are the leading cause of death of older women (Spielberg, 2011).

Cardiovascular diseases have long been considered as problems of men, a misconception

that has led to an underestimation of the impact of cardiovascular disease in women. Women are inclined to develop heart disease later in life and are more likely to present atypical symptoms as compared to men. These dynamics likely contribute to underdiagnosis of heart disease in women. It is also important to note that nearly 10% of cardiovascular disease in women is associated with tobacco use (Spielberg, 2011).

Diabetes is another significant chronic disease that impacts on women as they age. Currently, it is estimated that 122 million women worldwide have diabetes. The incidence of diabetes is increasing most rapidly in developed countries. Many of the outcomes of diabetes affect women more severely than men (Spielberg, 2011).

Advancing Age

The population of aging women is increasing. There are approximately 336 million women aged 60 and over worldwide. The proportion of women in the population increases with age. The health of older women is influenced by genetics, environment, and a lifetime of living circumstances and experiences. Older women are more likely to live in poverty, be depressed, and lack access to health care. This is due in part to the likelihood of older women to outlive their spouses/partners, and the consequences of lost income and increased social isolation brought by the change of marital status. In many societies, older women are assuming new responsibilities of raising grandchildren because of the loss of the parents in early adulthood to disease or other causes that remove them from parenting (Spielberg, 2011).

Violence Against Women

Women are burdened not only by disease but also by violations of their human rights that directly affect their health. Violence against women is a major global public health problem. Violence against women is any act of gender-based violence occurring in public or private life that results in, or is likely to result in, physical, sexual, or mental harm or suffering to women, including threats of such acts, coercion, or arbitrary deprivation of liberty (WHO, 2014b).

Violence against women takes many forms (see **Box 1–1**) and exists in all parts of the world. The most common form is intimate partner violence. It is estimated that women between the ages of 15 and 44 are more likely to be injured or killed as a result of male-perpetrated violence than from cancer, traffic accidents, malaria, and war combined. Yearly, approximately 5,000 women worldwide are murdered by family members in the name of honor. Forced marriages and child marriages are widely practiced in many countries of Asia, the Middle East, and sub-Saharan Africa even though these practices violate the human rights of women and girls. Furthermore, as many as one in five women and one in ten men report having been sexually abused as children, making them more prone to encounter other forms of abuse later in life (WHO, 2014b). Research conducted by the World Health Organization has documented the widespread nature of gender-based violence in many countries. Among various findings that underscore the severity of the problem, a substantial number of women reported physical or sexual violence perpetrated by a husband or partner. Furthermore, a significant number of women reported that their first sexual experience was forced, and a considerable number of women reported being physically abused during pregnancy (WHO, 2005).

Numerous individual, family, and societal factors may increase the likelihood for the occurrence of violence against women. These factors comprise

Box 1–1: Forms of Gender-Based Violence

Violent acts include the following:

- Sexual, physical, or emotional abuse by an intimate partner
- Physical or sexual abuse by family members or others
- Sexual harassment and abuse by authority figures (such as teachers, police officers, employers)
- Trafficking for forced labor or sex
- Forced or child marriages
- Dowry-related violence
- Honor killings (women are murdered in the name of family honor)
- Systematic sexual abuse in conflict situations
- Female genital mutilation
- Infanticide of female infants
- Sex-selective abortion

Modified from World Health Organization. (2014b). Violence against women: Fact sheet No. 239. Retrieved from http://www.who.int/mediacentre/factsheets/fs239/en/

personal characteristics, familial characteristics, and aspects of the community and society. Potential risk factors for gender-based violence are presented in **Table 1–2**.

Common health consequences from violent acts or from the long-term effects of violence can include physical injury, death, harm to women's sexual and reproductive health, injury or death to unborn children, mental health disorders, long-term health problems, and higher rates of sexual risk-taking behaviors and substance use. The social and economic costs of gender-based violence are enormous and affect many aspects of society.

Violence against women may cause women to experience social isolation, inability to work, lost productivity and wages, and lack of participation in regular activities. Violence against women can limit women's ability to care for themselves and their children. In many situations, women do not seek help or report violence when it takes place (WHO, 2014b).

Numerous preventive strategies have been developed that are aimed at reducing risk factors. These strategies have been initiated in various communities to address the problem of gender-based violence and include increasing education

Table 1–2 POTENTIAL RISK FACTORS FOR GENDER-BASED VIOLENCE

Level of Social Category	Characteristics That Increase the Risk of Violence
Individual	Limited education Young age History of abuse and substance use
Partner	Alcohol or substance use Low education level Negative attitudes about women Witnessing domestic violence against women History of being abused as a child
Family	Marital conflicts Male dominance Economic stress Poor family functioning
Community	Gender inequality Lack of community cohesion Limited resources
Society	Traditional gender norms Cultural customs Lack of autonomy for women Restrictive laws on divorce Restrictive laws on property ownership and inheritance Social breakdown due to wars, conflicts, or disasters Military presence in a country Dislocation and displacement of populations

Modified from World Health Organization. (2014b). Violence against women: Fact sheet No. 239. Retrieved from http://www.who.int/mediacentre/factsheets/fs239/en/

and opportunities for women and girls, improving their self-esteem, and reducing gender inequities in communities. So far, these interventions have shown promising results. Additional initiatives that have shown positive outcomes consist of programs that provide support for children who have witnessed intimate partner violence, mass public education campaigns, and work with men and boys to change their attitudes toward gender inequities and acceptability of violence. Measures that reduce the consequences of violence include advocacy for victims of violence and increasing awareness of health workers regarding violence and its consequences and their awareness of available resources for abused women (WHO, 2014b).

It is essential that further evaluation of the effectiveness of preventive measures takes place. Further efforts aimed at building evidence on the scope and types of violence in different settings are essential for understanding the enormity and nature of the problem at a global level. Governments and health professionals must receive further guidance in preventing violence and in strengthening the response of the health sector to violence. Initiatives must also include dissemination of information to countries, support for national efforts to advance women's rights and prevent violence, and collaboration of international agencies and organizations to deter violence against women worldwide (WHO, 2014b).

The International Priority of Women's Health

In recent decades, extraordinary advances have been achieved in women's health, particularly in improvement in prevention and treatment of women's diseases. Great progress has been made in early screening and treatment of breast and cervical cancer, reducing maternal mortality, developing the HPV vaccine to prevent cervical cancer, and increasing the availability of family planning techniques (Spielberg, 2011). Many discoveries in women's health have led to longer lives, healthier women, and enhanced quality of life. Nevertheless, many of the basics such as regular preventative health care, family planning services, and obstetric care in sanitary conditions remain inaccessible to women around the world. Unstable political and economic situations, such as wars, poverty, political volatility, and disease pandemics continue to adversely impact women's health and quality of life. In due course, the essential aspects in solving many of the health problems of women will entail political willingness, provision of adequate resources, and women's education (Spielberg, 2011).

Research Review

Will intentionally integrating a human rights framework into women's health research advance women's freedoms, equity, and equality?

Baptiste, D., Kapungu, C., Khare, M., Lewis, Y., & Barlow-Mosha, L. (2010). Integrating women's human rights into global health research: An action framework. *Journal of Women's Health, 19*(11), 2091–2099.

The authors of this article put forth the premise that research into the etiology, diagnosis, treatment, and prevention of women's illness, and also research into women's wellness, can advance women's freedoms, equity, and human rights. The authors state that this is not an automatic process. An essential part of the process is the integration of a human rights framework into the research, which begins with recognition of the social impact of studies. The authors hypothesize that recognition of the social impact of studies can occur at two broad levels. The first level of impact is that a study can provide health benefits for women, such as a new clinical procedure or medication. While individual health outcomes may improve, the existing social templates that intensify women's vulnerability to disease conditions, such as gender inequality and discrimination, likely remain unchanged. To improve women's human rights conditions as well as health outcomes, global researchers must aim for a second level of impact. In addition to providing individualized health benefits, this deeper level decisively illuminates elements of the social and community contexts that drive women's diseases, such as cultural and social norms that disadvantage women. The authors suggest using the Scale of Change Theory as a framework to guide six strategies that target this deeper level of impact without necessarily

requiring a vast output of financial resources. The strategies include: (1) becoming fully informed of women's human rights directives to integrate them into research, (2) mainstreaming gender into research—that is, making both women's and men's concerns and experiences an integral dimension of the research so that both genders benefit equally, (3) using the expertise of local grassroots women's organizations in the setting, (4) showcasing women's equity and equality in the organizational infrastructure, (5) disseminating research findings to policy-makers to advocate for improved services, and (6) publicizing specific and global oppressions driving women's illnesses. Logistical and conceptual dilemmas in transforming a study using these principles were discussed. The authors provided a case study to illustrate how these strategies can be operationalized. A feasible approach to health researchers who desire to link women's health outcomes to social and cultural conditions through practical implementation strategies was offered.

Chapter Summary Points

- Women's health is a multifaceted, complex area of study that includes practice, education, and research, which concentrates on the physical, psychosocial, political, and economical well-being of women.
- Women's health facilitates the prevention of illness and the maintenance of wellness through screening, diagnosing, and managing conditions that are unique to women, are more common in women, are more serious in women, and have manifestations, risk factors, or interventions that are different for women.
- Women's health encompasses the entire body and brings to focus the simple recognition that men and women have some fundamentally different health needs and that women's health needs must be pursued in their own right. As such, women's health recognizes the importance of the study of gender differences.
- Women's health acknowledges the diversity of women's health needs over the life cycle and

how these needs reflect differences in race, class, ethnicity, culture, sexual preference, levels of education, and access to health care.

- The 19th and 20th centuries were periods of extraordinary developments in women's health, initiated by multiple waves of women's health movements. In order to understand the dramatic changes that have affected women's health throughout this stretch of time, it is essential to examine the social and cultural context that led up to and then underscored the resultant changes.

- The federal government plays a significant role in protecting and promoting women's health. Through direct and indirect means, the government exercises control over many areas that influence women's health.

- Research on women's health has witnessed unprecedented growth, especially in response to the inclusion of women in clinical trials, which has enabled both women and men to become the studied models for the conditions that affect them and the drugs used to treat these conditions.

- Reproductive rights have been at the center of national attention for many years. The history and politics surrounding women's decisions to control when and if to have children as well as when and if to terminate pregnancy are long and complex.

- Although women have made major strides in economic, social, and political aspects of health promotion and disease prevention, women continue to encounter barriers to obtaining adequate health care.

- Continued success in the women's health movement depends on political commitment; sufficient funds; educated and interested scientific and lay communities; advocacy by professionals, patients, and the public; and involvement of women, men, and communities in working for equality and recognizing gender differences.

- Women's health issues have moved beyond geographical and political boundaries and have gained international visibility at the top of the worldwide health agenda.

- Aspects that influence women's health throughout the world include women's economic status, level of literacy, employment opportunities, race and ethnicity, whether living in an urban or rural environment, and living in a particular country or region of the world. Women's health is also influenced by biological, social, and cultural factors, especially gender disparities and the value society places on women.

- In recent decades, extraordinary advances have been achieved in women's health, particularly in improvement in prevention and treatment of women's diseases, leading to longer lives, healthier women, and enhanced quality of life.

- Many basic healthcare services remain inaccessible to women around the world. Unstable political and economic situations, such as wars, poverty, political volatility, and disease pandemics continue to adversely impact women's health.

- The essential aspects in solving many of the global health problems of women will entail political willingness, provision of adequate resources, and women's education.

Critical Thinking Exercise

Questions for Seminar Discussion

1. What are the multiple dimensions of women's health? What does women's health encompass?
2. Discuss the diversity of women's health needs over the life cycle and how these needs reflect differences in race, class, ethnicity, culture, sexual preference, levels of education, and access to health care.
3. What is feminism? Why is a feminist model of practice essential to the health and health care of women?
4. Discuss the historical background of the women's health movements. Why is it essential to examine the social and cultural context that led up to and then underscored the resultant changes in women's health?
5. Discuss the key issues surrounding reproductive rights. Why is it imperative that women have control over their reproductive rights?
6. Why were women excluded from clinical trials in the past? What impact did this practice have on women's health care? Why is it important for women to be included in clinical trials?
7. Discuss gender-based research. What areas of health could benefit from further gender-based research?
8. Discuss the ways that government is involved in women's health.
9. Why do women continue to encounter barriers to obtaining adequate health care? What factors contribute to these barriers?
10. What are the economic, social, cultural, and political factors that can adversely influence women's health throughout the world?
11. Discuss the issues associated with worldwide childhood mortality. What are indicators of specific gender-based discrimination?
12. Discuss the disproportion in risk for maternal mortality between developing and developed countries and regions of the world. Why does this disparity exist? How can maternal deaths be prevented?
13. Discuss issues surrounding prevalent diseases of adult and older women worldwide. What economic, social, and cultural implications do these diseases and conditions have for women?
14. Discuss the forms of violence against women. What are the physical, social, and economic consequences? What factors increase women's risk for violence? Discuss measures for prevention and management of violence against women.
15. Despite extraordinary global advancements in women's health, many of the basics of health care remain inaccessible to women around the world. What factors contribute to this situation?

Internet Resources

Black Women's Health Imperative: provides information, advocacy, and resources for advancing the health and wellness of Black women. http://www.blackwomenshealth.org

Centers for Disease Control and Prevention: provides information, education and resources on disease prevention and health promotion. http://www.cdc.gov

Feminist Women's Health Center: provides comprehensive gynecological healthcare services, education, and advocacy. http://www.feministcenter.org

Global Health Council: membership alliance promoting global health through information, education, and advocacy. http://www.globalhealth.org

Kaiser Family Foundation: non-profit, private operating foundation providing non-partisan policy analysis and research of healthcare issues for policy makers and the general public. http://www.kff.org

National Organization of Women: largest organization of feminist activists in the United States providing information, education, and advocacy. http://www.now.org

Office of Research on Women's Health: provides information, education and resources on women's health research. http://orwh.od.nih.gov

Office on Women's Health: provides program coordination and oversight, information, education and resources on women's health. http://www.womenshealth.gov

Our Bodies Ourselves (Boston Woman's Health Book Collective): nonprofit public interest and consulting organization providing women's health information, education, and advocacy. http://www.ourbodiesourselves.org

Planned Parenthood Federation of America: provides reproductive healthcare services, information, education, and advocacy. http://www.plannedparenthood.org

Society for Women's Health Research: national nonprofit organization provides information, education, advocacy, and support for women's health research and research on sex differences. http://www.womenshealthresearch.org

U. S. Food and Drug Administration: information, education, and resources on safety of drugs, food, medical devices, biological products, cosmetics, radiation emitting products, veterinary drugs, and tobacco. http://www.fda.gov.

Women's Health: provides information, education, advocacy, and program coordination on women's health. http://www.cdc.gov/women/

Women's Policy, Inc.: nonpartisan, nonprofit organization ensuring informed decision making on key women's issues by policy makers at the federal, state, and local levels. http://www.womenspolicy.org

World Health Organization: information and resources on women's health around the world. http://www.who.int/en/

References

Andrist, L. (1997). A feminist model for women's health care. *Nursing Inquiry, 4*, 268–274.

Baptiste, D., Kapungu, C., Khare, M., Lewis, Y., & Barlow-Mosha, L. (2010). Integrating women's human rights into global health research: An action framework. *Journal of Women's Health, 19*(11), 2091–2099.

Change: Center for Health and Gender Equity. (2015). Global gag rule. Retrieved from http://www.genderhealth.org/the_issues/us_foreign_policy/global_gag_rule/

Donoghue, G. (Ed.). (1996). *Women's health in the curriculum: Resource guide for faculty.* Philadelphia, PA: National Academy on Women's Health Medical Education.

Geary, M. (1995). An analysis of the women's health movement and its impact on the delivery of health care in the United States. *Nurse Practitioner, 20*(11), 24–35.

Joint United Nations Programme on HIV/AIDS (2010). *Global report: UNAIDS report on the global AIDS epidemic 2010.* Geneva, Switzerland: Joint United Nations Programme on HIV/AIDS.

Nichols, F. (2000). History of the women's health movement in the 20th century. *Journal of Obstetric, Gynecologic and Neonatal Nursing, 29*(1), 56–64.

Office of Population Affairs, U.S. Department of Health and Human Services. (2011). Title X: Family planning. Retrieved from http://www.hhs.gov/opa/

Office of Research on Women's Health. (2015). About the Office of Research on Women's Health. Retrieved from http://orwh.od.nih.gov/

Office on Women's Health U.S. Department of Health and Human Services. (2002). *A century of women's health: 1900–2000.* Washington, DC.: DHHS Office on Women's Health.

Office on Women's Health U.S. Department of Health and Human Services. (2013). About the HHS Office on Women's Health. Retrieved from http://www.womenshealth.gov

Polit, D., & Beck, C. (2014). *Essentials of nursing research: Appraising evidence for nursing practice* (8th ed.). Philadelphia, PA: Lippincott Williams & Wilkins.

Population Reference Bureau. (2012). World population data sheet, 2010. Retrieved from www.prb.org/Publications/Datasheets/2012/world-population-data-sheet/fact-sheet-world-population.aspx

Society for Women's Health Research. (2004). Fact sheet: Sex differences in response to pharmaceuticals, tobacco, alcohol, and illicit drugs. Retrieved from http://swhr.org/sex-differences-in-response-to-pharmaceuticals-tobacco-alcohol-and-illicit-drugs/

Spielberg, L. (2011). Tutorial: A global perspectives on women's health. Retrieved from http://kff.org/interactive/a-global-perspective-on-womens-health-tutorial/

United Nations Department of Economic and Social Affairs, Population Division (2010). Population facts (No.2010/4). Retrieved from http://www.un.org/en/development/desa/population/publications/factsheets/index.shtml

U.S. Census Bureau. (2015). U.S. and world population clock. Retrieved from http://www.census.gov/popclock/

U. S. Food and Drug Administration. (2014). Women's health research: Women's participation in clinical trials. Retrieved from http://www.fda.gov/ScienceResearch/SpecialTopics/WomensHealthResearch/ucm131731.htm

Weisman, C. (2000). Advocating for gender-specific health care: A historical perspective. *Journal of Gender-Specific Medicine, 3*(3), 22–24.

World Health Organization. (2005). *WHO multicountry study on women's health and domestic violence against women: Initial results on prevalence, health outcomes and women's responses.* Geneva, Switzerland: World Health Organization.

World Health Organization. (2010a). *Trends in maternal mortality: 1990 to 2008. Estimates developed by WHO, UNICEF, UNFPA, and the World Bank.* Geneva, Switzerland: World Health Organization.

World Health Organization. (2010b). 2010/2011 Tuberculosis global facts. Retrieved from http://www.who.int/tb/publications/2010/factsheet_tb_2010.pdf?ua=1

World Health Organization. (2011c). *Unsafe abortion: Global and regional estimates of the incidence of unsafe abortion and associated mortality in 2008* (6th ed.). Geneva, Switzerland: World Health Organization.

World Health Organization. (2013a). Sexually transmitted infections. Retrieved from http://www.who.int/mediacentre/factsheets/fs110/en/

World Health Organization. (2013b). Women's Health: Fact sheet No. 334. Retrieved from http://www.who.int/mediacentre/factsheets/fs334/en/

World Health Organization. (2014a). Tuberculosis: Women and TB. Retrieved from http://www.who.int/tb/publications/tb_women_factsheet_251013.pdf

World Health Organization. (2014b). Violence against women. Retrieved from http://www.who.int/mediacentre/factsheets/fs239/en/

World Health Organization. (2015a). Cancer: Fact sheet No. 297. Retrieved from http://www.who.int/mediacentre/factsheets/fs297/en/

World Health Organization. (2015b). Health topics: Women's health. Retrieved from http://www.who.int/topics/womens_health/en/

World Health Organization. (2015c). World health statistics 2014. Retrieved from http://www.who.int/mediacentre/news/releases/2014/world-health-statistics-2014/en/

Chapter 2

Women's Developmental Stages and Quality of Life

Introduction

Over the past century, the life expectancy of women in the United States has increased by more than 30 years. This remarkable change is largely due to improved sanitation practices, eradication and control of communicable diseases, development of antibiotics, increasingly effective treatment of chronic diseases, and implementation of national public health policies that greatly reduced rates of death, diseases, and disability (Office on Women's Health U.S. Department of Health and Human Services [OWH], 2002). Quality of life has become a topic of great concern because realization has emerged that quality of life is as ultimately important as quantity of life.

The complex issues of women's health impact quality of life throughout the life span. Women's longer life span, unique major physiologic changes, greater tendency toward depression and mental stress, and increased risk of being victims of inter-personal violence are just a few examples of factors that can contribute to decreased quality of life in women ("Health-Related Quality of Life Among Women," 2003). Although women's life expectancy has nearly doubled, many women today can expect to live longer with the sequelae of serious injury, conditions, disorders or chronic illnesses. Certain injuries, conditions, and diseases are more prevalent among women at various points along the life cycle. These conditions can affect women's health and physical function, psychological and spiritual function, socioeconomic integrity, and family well-being, and in many cases can become life-threatening over time. Although advances have been made in many dimensions of women's health across the life cycle, the impact of women's health issues on quality of life must be acknowledged, explored, and kept in the mainstream of women's health care ("Health-Related Quality of Life Among Women," 2003; OWH, 2002). This chapter presents a starting point with perspectives on the psychological and social growth of women across the life cycle. This discussion creates a formidable setting in which to establish the conceptual model of quality of life that forms the organizing framework of this book.

A Perspective of Women's Developmental Stages Across the Life Cycle

Western culture throughout the ages has sought to partition human life into ages and stages. The need to determine order and predictability in the human life cycle has inspired a wide range of perspectives, opinions, and theories that describe predictable marker events of the life cycle. From the beginning of the 20th century up to the 1970s, major life events such as puberty, graduation, marriage, first job, first child, empty nest, retirement, widowhood, and death likely occurred for most women at predictable points in the life cycle (Sheehy, 1995). For the longest time, chronological age has stood as the criterion for normalizing the roles and responsibilities taken on by individuals throughout their lives. For example, prior to the 1970s, adulthood was considered to begin at the age of 21 and retirement to occur at age 65, thus benchmarking the lower and upper boundaries of participation in the adult world. However, since the 1970s, age norms have shifted and can no longer be considered normative. The criterion ages that have marked the movement of individuals from adolescence to young adulthood, to middle age and senescence have changed (Sheehy, 1995).

Since the post-World War II "Baby Boomer" generation came of age in the 1970s, the predictable points of life were no longer predictable. In the space of one generation, the entire shape of the life cycle became essentially altered. Social changes, economic demands, technological demands, as well as advances in health and health care have contributed to these changes. People leave childhood sooner but take longer to grow up and much longer to die. Puberty arrives earlier by several years and adolescence extends into the mid-to-late twenties. The arrival of true adulthood has been delayed until the thirties and forties. Middle age has been pushed into the fifties and the stages of life beyond the fifties have changed radically from what was experienced by pre-"Baby Boomer" generations. The gain in life expectancy in developed countries has redefined the sunset years. People entering older age are much healthier. Middle-aged and "young-old" Americans are likely to have a living parent, and this has produced unprecedented changes in family dynamics. A steady increase in the oldest old of the population has established additional life stages beyond middle age. These additional stages in the life cycle did not exist in previous generations and brought with them opportunities, discontinuities, expectations, and different social roles (Sheehy, 1995).

Passage Through Stages of Development

Adulthood proceeds by stages of development throughout the life cycle. Unlike childhood stages, which are characterized predominantly by physical and intellectual growth, stages of adult life are characterized by steps in psychological and social growth. Marker events, such as marriage, childbirth, first job, and empty nest do not define developmental stages but concrete happenings of life (Sheehy, 1995). Developmental stages of life are defined by the underlying impulses toward change that signal people from the realms of mind or spirit. Moreover, the developmental stages are influenced by the meaning individuals give to their participation in the external world, especially their perceptions and feelings about their family, social, and occupational role (Sheehy, 1995). The underlying impulses toward change signal a necessity to move on to the next stage of development. Movement from one stage to the next is actualized when a predictable crisis or turning point is encountered, which ushers in a new stage. This predictable crisis or turning point is called a passage, a crucial period of decision between progress and regression. At the point of passage, individuals are in a state of flux, feeling exposed and vulnerable, yet enjoying a heightened potential for growth. The impulse for change can be ignored or embraced. Whatever direction is chosen will result in a restructured future (Sheehy, 1995).

Although the normative benchmarks of the life cycle have shifted in the past few decades, broad, general stages of adulthood with predictable passages between them still exist, yet with a more prolonged timetable. Age norms for major life events have become highly flexible. Individuals in their twenties, thirties, and forties face drastically changed social, economic, and technologic conditions as compared to previous generations. These altered conditions generate disequilibrium

in their lives (Sheehy, 1995). Rather than a flat, linear progression through life, individuals lead cyclical lives that require starting over and over again in many domains. As a result, early and young adulthood is lived at an accelerated pace even though many of the responsibilities of full adulthood may be delayed. Middle age cannot be about coasting to retirement but must be a preparation for the sunset years. Most people who reach the sunset years (over 65) are likely to continue to work in some way or another in employment, as volunteers, or in endeavors that maintain a sense of purpose or self-worth (Sheehy, 1995).

Changes in the Life Cycle of Women

Globalization of economic competition and the progression of the women's movement have greatly contributed to the changes in the life cycle. Women have experienced a continuous expansion of opportunities, greater participation in the workforce, and assumption of multiple life roles. Social roles and developmental tasks formerly associated with one stage have been ignored or postponed. As a result, multiple life tasks accumulate in the same stage and create tremendous either/or conflicts. The shape of life stages, as well as the sequence, have been altered, and a surfeit of new choices has been made available by technological advances that diminish limitations of biology and longevity. The most radical voluntary change to the life cycle has been the reproductive revolution that has enabled women to defer childbirth by 10 to 20 years (Sheehy, 1995).

Roles of Women in Childbearing Years

Traditionally, the normative life cycle of women was perceived as bound to the reproductive aspects of their lives. The societal norms were grounded in the pre-1970s expectation that the primary and frequently preferred and exclusive roles of women orbited the private, domestic sphere of wife and mother. The normative societal roles of adult women have since shifted dramatically to include domestic and work roles that take place over the course of women's lives. Women have numerous role choices. Some women postpone marriage and children until well established in their careers, while other women may choose to marry young and simultaneously establish career identities along with roles as wives and mothers. Other women may choose to postpone their career and work lives until children have entered school or are outside the home. Still others may choose to focus on career building and economic self-sufficiency, choosing to remain child free and/or single (Shrier & Shrier, 2009). Currently the adult lives of women are all the more complex with the multiple dimensions of biology, family, and work interacting and influencing each other. The multiple dimensions influence alternatives regarding life choices and the timing of major career choices and family events (Shrier & Shrier, 2009). Consequently, the lives of women do not progress in a linear trajectory. Rather, women's lives move in a spiraling, circle-like progression in which the biologic–reproductive dimension, the family–marital dimension, and the educational–vocational dimension are bound together, interacting, overlapping, at times enhancing, and at times conflicting with one another (Seiden, 1989).

Approximately 95% of women are employed outside the home for at least part of their adult lives. The decision to work outside the home is motivated by societal expectations, financial necessity, or both. The traditional marriage in which the man is the sole breadwinner and the woman stays at home full time is found in only about 3% of American families (Shrier & Shrier, 2009). Women's labor force participation is significantly higher today as compared to the 1970s, particularly among women with children, with a large portion working full time and year round.

Moreover, women have attained progressively higher levels of education, with a tripling of the number of college degrees since the 1970s. As of 2012, approximately 70.9% of mothers with children younger than 18 years of age participated in the workforce, with greater participation more likely among women with older children (6 to 17 years of age) than mothers with younger children. Moreover, approximately 76% of unmarried mothers participate in the workforce as compared to approximately 68.5% of married mothers. The educational attainment of women in the labor force aged 25 to 64 has shown substantial increase since the 1970s. As of 2012, college degrees are held by 38% of women in the labor force as compared to 11% in 1970. The percentage of women who are high school dropouts declined from 34% in 1970 to 7% in 2012 (U.S. Bureau of Labor Statistics, 2014). These statistics underscore that the developmental phenomenon of women in their childbearing years—married or single—juggling children, career development, and educational pursuit while experiencing the maximum role demands of each has become normative. It is precisely this developmental phenomenon that makes women at this stage of their life cycle particularly vulnerable to psychosocial morbidity when faced with life-threatening diseases or conditions (Bloom & Kessler, 1994). The crucial issues of illness superimposed upon the complex role demands of women profoundly influence quality of life (Sammarco, 2001).

Roles of Women in Midlife and Beyond

From a chronological perspective, midlife is viewed as occurring from age 45 to age 65 and overlapping with old age. Old age has come to be viewed as having three periods: the young-old from ages 60 to 75; the old-old, from ages 75 to 85; and the oldest-olds, from the late 80s and beyond. Women's passage from childbearing years into midlife and beyond brings with it psychological, interpersonal, health, and economic issues that differ for each of these periods. Social class, birth cohort, ethnicity, and health contribute great inter-individual variability to women in each of these periods (Shrier & Shrier, 2009). Hence the more important indicators in determining who is young-old, old-old, or oldest-old are likely the individual differences in health and vigor rather than chronological age (Seiden, 1989).

In 1900, women were likely to live on average to about age 48 if they were white, or to age 33 if they were African-American. Moreover, many women died in childbirth or during their child-bearing years from infectious diseases (OWH, 2002). Over a century later, the 30-year increase in life expectancy signifies that greater than ever numbers of women will be reaching their 80s and beyond. The average age of menopause is 51 years. Most women can anticipate living more than 30 years post menopause if they follow guidelines for healthy diets, maintain a healthy weight, employ stress reduction measures, engage in aerobic and weight-bearing exercise, practice health-care prevention and maintenance, stay socially and intellectually engaged, and are secure financially. Many women in the postmenopausal years can enjoy lives that are physically and psychologically fulfilling and even more creative than earlier in their lives (Shrier & Shrier, 2009).

Unsurprisingly, the traditional normative roles of mid-life to older women have also shifted dramatically since the 1970s, and consequently manifest diverse issues that threaten quality of life. With the increase in life expectancy, women need to be prepared to finance an additional two decades of life. This is especially challenging since older women, especially if they are African-American or Latina, are more likely to be poor than older men (Cawthorne, 2008). Women need to acquire education, prepare career tracks, build pension and individual retirement accounts, and demand greater help from society to care for the frail elderly in their families (Sheehy, 1995).

Thus, older women are remaining in the workforce longer and postponing retirement. A vast majority of women over the age of 60 have the benefit of increased independence in lifestyle (Sheehy, 1995). Nonetheless, aging women are at risk for declining physical function and the development of chronic illnesses. Although advancing age brings with it increased emotional resilience, there is greater likelihood that older women will experience a reduction in resources of social support. The support network frequently shrinks from outliving a spouse or partner, friends, pets, or from limited social interaction associated with disability or declining health (Sammarco, 2003). Older women are more likely to transition to living on their own through late divorce or widowhood, and frequently grapple with fear and loneliness, especially after losing a spouse or partner. Older women who never had children fear having no family members alive to look after them in their old age (Sheehy, 1995).

A problem frequently cited in the literature is that the "burden of caring" is carried by women throughout the life cycle. Statistically, women care for their children and parents more so than do men. This phenomenon is likely a holdover from the time of traditional domestic arrangements of women employed in the home, when they could incorporate the care of an ill or older person into that setting (Seiden, 1989). A study of 1,666 family caregivers of cancer survivors found that 78.9% were women (Kim, Kashy, Spillers, & Evans, 2010). Most of the caregivers of older Americans are women (Cawthorne, 2008). Nonetheless, many older women face a caregiving crisis resulting from becoming the unpaid caregivers of elderly spouses, partners, parents, or even young grandchildren. Some women may have to relinquish outside employment and consequently, salary, health insurance, and pension benefits (Sheehy, 1995). Yet national surveys show that many family caregivers maintain working outside the home and few have other unpaid help to care for the ill family member (Barrett, 2004). Employed women often try to find other resources to augment their caregiving because they may not wish to—or may be unable to—forfeit their income or time to provide these services.

At the start of the second decade of the 21st century, five generations of women span the adult life cycle, with a steadily increasing aged population in the sunset years. Dramatic and evolving changes have occurred in both societal and internalized expectations of women's roles and normative life cycle since the 1970s. Today, women's adult life cycle is complex and spans multiple and varied life choices associated with family, career, and personal fulfillment. Without a doubt role strain, overload, and conflict, as well as other stresses related to efforts to combine career, family, and a personal life, may occur. For many women, multiple roles tend to be mutually enriching and result in a greater sense of well-being than experienced by women in a single role (Shrier & Shrier, 2009).

Conceptualizing Quality of Life

Quality of life is a commonly used, broad, multidimensional construct. However, the construct is often unclearly defined and poorly understood (Mandzuk & McMillan, 2005). References to quality of life have appeared in Greek philosophy, as well as in the reflections of Aristotle with respect to the universal nature of happiness and its association with "the good life" (Ferrans, 1990b, 1996). Existential quality of life has also been discussed in the writings of authors such as Kierkegaard, Satre, Maslow, Frankl, and Antonovsky (Mandzuk & McMillan, 2005).

Perceptions of quality of life emerged in America following World War II. At this time people's expectations of satisfaction, well-being, and psychological growth increased as a result of economic growth and improvements in the standard of living.

The term "quality of life" was introduced by Lyndon Johnson in his Great Society program that promoted advancing quality of life through social programs such as education and manpower, community development and housing, and health and welfare. In addition to the political arena, quality of life discussions have appeared in education, family studies, environment, and, of course, health care (Mandzuk & McMillan, 2005).

Defining Quality of Life

Extensive literature review has identified definitions of quality of life that could be grouped into five major categories: (1) normal life, (2) happiness/satisfaction, (3) achievement of personal goals, (4) social utility, and (5) natural capacity (Ferrans, 1990b). The first category of quality of life definitions focuses on one's ability to live a normal life. These definitions encompass concepts such as the ability to function at a level comparable to healthy persons or typical of the same age. Normal life definitions of quality of life can be problematic in that standards of normalcy vary widely and disagreement regarding criteria for measuring quality of life can occur (Ferrans, 1990b).

The second category of quality of life definitions focuses on an individual's happiness and satisfaction. Although not synonymous, happiness and satisfaction are closely related concepts, which have been found to behave somewhat differently across the life span in the general population. Happiness tends to decrease with advancing age whereas satisfaction tends to increase (Ferrans, 1990b). Happiness implies short-term positive feelings, while satisfaction indicates a longer-term cognitive experience, which is the outcome of a judgment of life's conditions. Accordingly, satisfaction, rather than happiness, comes closer to capturing the essence of the concept of quality of life (Campbell, Converse, & Rodgers, 1976).

The third category of definitions focuses on the achievement of personal goals. These definitions tend to be more closely aligned to the happiness/satisfaction definitions in that goal achievement results in a sense of satisfaction and failure to achieve goals results in a sense of dissatisfaction. However, the difference is that the goal achievement definitions focus specifically on the success or failure of goal achievement, rather than one's happiness/satisfaction with success or failure. The definitions of this category emphasize an individual's own goals rather than general goals that are applicable to all people (Ferrans, 1990b).

The fourth category of quality of life definitions focuses on social utility. These are definitions that characterize quality of life as the ability to lead a socially useful life, such as fulfilling socially valued roles or making contributions to the national economy through gainful employment. These definitions are frequently used in decision making concerning healthcare policy where economic matters are foremost, such as decisions pertaining to allocation of healthcare resources. Social utility definitions of quality of life can be problematic in that socially useful behavior has a wide range of meanings, and disagreement regarding measurement criteria can occur. Furthermore, discriminating prejudices can be hidden beneath the surface of apparently benign criteria. For example, if quality of life is measured in terms of earned income through gainful employment, bias against women who are homemakers or retired can result (Ferrans, 1990b).

The fifth category of quality of life definitions focuses on natural capacity. Natural capacity pertains to an individual's actual or potential physical and/or mental capabilities. These definitions are often used in decision making associated with whether to try to save a person's life or allow the person to die. These definitions are mostly used to justify decisions as to whether lifesaving measures should be continued or withdrawn in patients who are terminally ill. These definitions are clinically useful for assistance in decision making rather than guiding measurement of quality of life (Ferrans, 1990b).

The Quest for Conceptual Clarity

Quality of life has been widely addressed in the literature but, as the preceding discussion has shown, there is no consensus on the meaning of the construct. There is no consensus on how quality of life is to be conceptualized or operationalized, even within the scholarly community. Authors define quality of life in different ways and conceptualize quality of life as having differing dimensions. Consequently, achieving conceptual clarity concerning the definition of quality of life has been difficult because people often ascribe their own personal meanings without ascertaining whether their definitions are shared by others (Cella & Tulsky, 1990; Ferrans, 1990b). This lack of consensus has hindered efforts to compare findings and develop a sound theory of quality of life that can predict outcomes and inform practice.

Despite areas of conceptual disagreement surrounding quality of life, areas of conceptual agreement have been accomplished. Quality of life is nearly always conceived as multidimensional. Moreover, there is growing agreement that satisfaction with the dimensions of life seems to be the most important indicator of quality of life (Ferrans & Powers, 1985). The most frequently cited dimensions are physiological, psychological, and sociological (Donovan, Sanson-Fisher, & Redman, 1989; Fawcett, 2005; Ferrell, Wisdom, & Wenzl, 1989; Padilla, Ferrell, Grant, & Rhiner, 1990). Many scholars include a spiritual or existential domain as well (Fawcett, 2005; Padilla, Grant, & Martin, 1988). In considering the various dimensions of quality of life, it is fair to question whether all dimensions count equally in defining quality of life or if some dimensions are weighted with more importance than others. Since people differ as to how important various aspects of life are to their quality of life, especially among those of different ages and sexes, people will differ regarding which dimensions of quality of life are most important. Accordingly, it is logical to conclude that all dimensions of life do not impact equally on quality of life (Ferrans, 1990b).

Another area of conceptual agreement is that quality of life is determined not only by an evaluation of several domains of life but also by an individual's evaluation of the importance of those domains, and the construct is best studied from the perspective of the individual (Cella, 1992, 1994; Cella & Tulsky, 1990; George & Bearon, 1980; King et al., 1997; Padilla, Ferrell, Grant, & Rhiner, 1990). The individual is the only proper judge of his or her quality of life in that quality of life rests in the experience of life and the essence lies in their own evaluation of the experience. The judgment of the individual is fundamental because individuals vary in what they value in their lives (Ferrans, 1990b; Ferrans & Powers, 1985). Although the subjective perception is most essential for evaluating quality of life, objective indicators are also useful and important considerations, even though subjective and objective assessments of quality of life produce different results (Ferrans, 1990b; George & Bearon, 1980). Objective quality of life indicators include characteristics such as assets, income, education and housing, and these may supplement people's subjective quality of life evaluation (Campbell et al., 1976; Mandzuk & McMillan, 2005). Perceived quality of life involves a relationship between subjective and objective indicators of well-being. Thus it can be viewed that objective indicators influence the experience of quality of life (Campbell et al., 1976).

Health-Related Quality of Life

Health-related quality of life is a construct that has evolved over the past 30 years and includes those aspects of overall quality of life that can be clearly shown to affect health (Centers for Disease Control and Prevention [CDC], 2011). For the individual,

health-related quality of life encompasses physical and mental health and their correlates, including health risks and conditions, functional status, social support, and socioeconomic status. From the community perspective, health-related quality of life includes resources, conditions, policies, and practices that influence the health perceptions and functional status of the population (CDC, 2011). This construct excludes aspects of quality of life that are unrelated to health or do not affect health, such as cultural, political, or social attributes. For example, factors such as quality of the environment, public safety, education, standard of living, transportation, political freedom, or cultural amenities are examples of aspects that would likely be excluded from health-related quality of life (Ferrans, Zerwic, Wilbur, & Larson, 2005). However, the distinction between health-related quality of life and non-health–related quality of life cannot always be clearly determined. The argument can be made that factors such as crime, environmental pollution, lack of education, poor standard of living, lack of transportation, oppressive reproductive laws, or cultural incompetence can have very serious implications for health. In fact, in the presence of chronic illness nearly all areas of life are affected by health, and thus become "health-related." Although the construct of health-related quality of life has helped to focus attention on those aspects of overall quality of life that affect health, further work is needed to identify and clarify the critical elements of the construct and the causal relationships among them (Ferrans et al., 2005).

Quality of Life in the Context of Culture, Race, Ethnicity, Acculturation, and Humanness

Culture. Culture is defined as shared patterns of behaviors and interactions, cognitive constructs, and affective understanding that are learned through socialization. These shared patterns distinguish the members of a cultural group as well as differentiate those of another group (Center for Advanced Research on Language Acquisition, 2010). Culture is purposeful and prescribes the ways of life for a group to ensure its survival and well-being. Culture provides beliefs and values to give meaning and purpose to life (Kagawa-Singer, 2000, 2006; Spector, 2004). Culture addresses three basic and universal needs: safety and security, sense of integrity and meaning or purpose in life, and sense of belonging as an integral member of one's social network (Kagawa-Singer & Chung, 1994). Culture is fundamental to life and is an important determinant of quality of life in the context of health because it defines the purpose and prescriptions for living a meaningful life in wellness and sickness.

Culture influences perceptions of illness, of cognitive impairment, and of other physical and mental health problems. Negative perceptions and stigmatization of these conditions, in turn, influence health-related quality of life. Documentation of this relationship was shown in a cohort study of HIV-positive persons from five African countries, in which increases in HIV-related stigma over 1 year were significantly associated with decreases in life satisfaction with rates of change differing by countries (Greeff et al., 2010). Decreased life satisfaction was reflected in reduced living enjoyment, loss of control in life, decreased social interaction, and decreased perceived health status. Likewise, HIV-positive Hispanics who reported feeling stigmatized when receiving medical care had poorer physical and psychological functioning and a decreased ability to complete daily activities (Larios, Davis, Gallo, Heinrich, & Talavera, 2009).

To comprehensively operationalize the construct of culture, the measure should encompass health, ethnicity, and sociodemographic variables (Kagawa-Singer, 2006). Health characteristics include diet, physical activity, and alternative health practices such as healers and parallel or complementary health practices. Ethnic factors include parental heritage, ethnic self-identity (i.e. generation, degree of integration into mainstream society, language proficiencies, beliefs and practices, degree of personal identification and public identity, number of identity groups, and degree of overlap), interethnic social interaction choices (e.g. by circumstance or choice, by regional or community geographic residence), and religiosity and spirituality (e.g. beliefs, practices, internal/external locus of control). Sociodemographic variables consist of family structure and support system (e.g. composition and age), socioeconomic status (e.g. wealth, education, percent of money sent to home country or to support other households), generation in the United States, and reason for immigration.

Race and racism. Racial categories are based on genetic factors expressed as physical or biochemical characteristics. However, the scientific basis for making racial distinctions is weak (Hirschman, Alba, & Farley, 2000; Kagawa-Singer & Blackhall, 2001; Montagu, 1997). Many traits cross over "races," and "racial" identity can change over time. Data from the Human Genome Project and from human genome variation dispute the validity of the term "race" (Royal & Dunston, 2004). Race and other preexisting definitions of the population, such as ethnicity, religion, language, nationality, and culture, are inclined to be controversial concepts that have polarized discussions about the ethics and science of research into population-specific human genetic variation. By contrast, a wider consideration of the many historical sources of genetic variation conveys a whole-genome perspective on the ways in which existing population definitions do and do not explain how genetic variation is distributed among individuals (Foster & Sharp, 2004). Studies of health and quality of life disparities continue to use race and racial group categories to predict and understand why some people are better or worse off than others, what genetic variations exist between groups, and what behavioral, social, and environmental factors put some racial or ethnic groups at greater or lesser risk than others for poor health and health-related quality of life outcomes. Racism, the belief in the superiority of one group over another because of genetic traits, justifies the exertion of power and discriminatory action by the "superior" group over the "less superior" group. Disparities in care and reduced health and quality of life outcomes result from racially related beliefs and actions (Institute of Medicine, 2001).

Ethnicity. Ethnicity is that which holds a group together because of a common identity based on some or all of the following shared characteristics: culture, history, language, religion, genealogy, and ancestry. Ethnicity encompasses both culture and "race." Members of multicultural societies form ethnic bonds for solidarity. These bonds assure their way of life and meaning in life, particularly when the universal need for safety and security, sense of integrity and meaning or purpose in life, and sense of belonging as an integral member of one's social network are threatened (Kagawa-Singer & Chung, 1994). Ethnic mores also specify behaviors to promote or maintain health, to prevent disease or illness, and to manage seemingly random events.

Theories of culture, race, or ethnicity can contribute to strategies to promote or maintain health and well-being (Kagawa-Singer, 1995, 2006). The cultural beliefs and values that bind an ethnic group in their approach to health, and the racial identity that places an ethnic group in a position of more or less power and status in their ability to access and use the healthcare system ultimately influence health-related quality of life (Kagawa-Singer, 2001).

Acculturation. Acculturation means learning the beliefs, values, and standards of behavior of another cultural group to function comfortably in that group, typically the dominant culture, and, in the case of immigrants, the host culture. *Assimilation* means taking on the beliefs, values, and practices of the host culture and giving up those of one's own native culture. Individuals may acculturate to varying degrees without necessarily assimilating to the host culture. Acculturation can modify the significance of factors that contribute to disparities in disease incidence and mortality between ethnic groups, such as attitudes, beliefs, and behaviors regarding health or illness. Culturally influenced attitudes, beliefs, and behaviors about illness or specific diseases can, for example, delay early detection, increase consequences of late diagnosis, influence compliance with treatment plans, create mistrust or misunderstanding about the role of healthcare practitioners, and engender social stigma. Acculturation can lead to changes in the health-seeking practices of cultural groups that can narrow health disparities.

Acculturation is a multidimensional construct. A common conceptualization of acculturation encompasses the domains of preferred language, self-identity, friendship choices that determine social boundaries, standards of acceptable behavior, generation since family immigration to the host country, country of origin, and attitudes (willingness to behave in certain ways) (Suinn, Rickard-Figueroa, Lew, & Vigil, 1987). Acculturation has also been defined generically by length of residence, age at arrival in the host country, and by media influence (Marin, Sabogal, Van Oss-Marin, Otero-Sabogal, & Perez-Stable, 1987). However, these last are less important indicators of health-related quality of life. To these lists, type of neighborhood was added and language proficiency was expanded to include usage and preferences (Alarcon et al., 1999). Measures of acculturation may also be specifically determined by knowledge and practices concerning the traditions of a culture, such as knowledge and practices about the way of life of the members of the cultural group, valuation and maintenance of beliefs and non-beliefs, blood quantum, and specific cultural traditions, folklore, and language proficiency (Hishinuma et al., 2000).

Knowledge of acculturation and assimilation provides insight into health-seeking attitudes of ethnic groups, reasons for success or failure of prevention and treatment regimens, ways to best reach diverse ethnic groups with health-related messages, and strategies for opening access to health care for ethnic groups (Padilla & Perez, 1995). Acculturation is associated with health-related quality of life when demographic, medical, socioecologic, and healthcare access factors are controlled (Kim, Ashing-Giwa, Kagawa-Singer, & Tejero, 2006). However, large race or ethnic categories such as "Asian American" commonly used in research can mask the different effects of acculturation among ethnic subgroups, such as Phillipino, Korean, or Japanese. For example, Kim and colleagues found that Korean Americans reported poorer quality of life than other Asian subgroups (Kim et al., 2006). It is important for cross-cultural studies to include a measure of acculturation.

People can acculturate without assimilating into the host culture. The ability to gain sufficient knowledge about a culture to transact easily within that culture does not necessarily mean that one gives up his or her original culture. In fact, an individual can belong to several cultural groups. An understanding of the influence of culture on health-related quality of life needs to consider ethnic affiliation as well as level of acculturation and assimilation into another—usually the host—culture.

Humanness. An important philosophical question integral to the discussion of quality of life asks what it is to be human. Cultural in origin, beliefs about humanness include values about life and about quality of life compared to other desirable outcomes. Positive human criteria have been identified as minimal human intelligence, self-awareness, self-control, a sense of time, a sense of futurity, a sense of the past, the capability to relate to others, concern for others, communication, control of existence, curiosity, change and changeability, balance of rationality and feeling, idiosyncracy, and neocortical function (Fletcher, 1990). This view of humanness means that health-related quality of life assessments are made by conscious-thinking, socioemotional individuals who view their health condition or that of others in a time span encompassing past, current, and potential future health states, who view life events as not totally random but somewhat controllable, and who are unique from others.

Pertinent to this discussion is whether people from diverse cultures view humanness similarly. The indicators of humanness listed previously stem from a Judeo-Christian orientation, which is neither more nor less valid than other views. Perhaps Buddhism, Islam, or other religions or philosophies would change, add, or otherwise revise the preceding list of human criteria (Fletcher, 1990). The uniqueness of a culture is less about the array of indicators of humanness, but rather what a culture singles out and emphasizes as key components of humanness. A culture for which control of existence is the most important aspect of humanness would value health-related research differently than a culture for which balance of rationality and feeling is the key component of humanness. The first culture might emphasize cure, while the second culture might balance cure with care research. The cultural view of what it is to be human informs the relevant dimension of quality of life for that culture and the level of well-being for an individual, a group, a society, and a nation.

In a sense, health-related quality of life is not only an outcome of care, treatment, or medical decisions, but also a prescriber of behavior based on cultural beliefs, values, and norms. In the case of an infant born with severe health conditions or deformities that require extensive and prolonged medical treatment, parents and health professionals may believe that the infant has no chance for a meaningful life with even minimal quality. The parents and professionals may decide to take no action and let the infant die. This is a painful and terrifying decision fraught with ethical challenges, but a decision ultimately based on cultural norms that define a minimally acceptable health-related quality of life. These types of culturally rooted health-related quality of life decisions are made every day.

Quality of Life and Women's Health

Consideration of quality of life is essential for women's health. Quality of life is a major concern in making decisions regarding life-sustaining therapies. It figures in debates on revising treatment guidelines and practice standards. Indicators of quality of life are used in clinical practice and in clinical trials to evaluate outcomes in terms of human costs and benefits. Quality of life is significant in the healthcare system in terms of decisions

of care allocation (Ferrans, 1996). It is a prominent priority on the research agenda for health care as well as central to the national objectives for improving the health of the population of this country (CDC, 2011). Accordingly, the eminence of quality of life as an indispensable dynamic in health care confirms the significance of exploring women's health issues within the context of a quality of life framework. This process is facilitated by the selection of a definition of quality of life suitable to the purposes of this work, as well as an applicable conceptual model of quality of life relevant to women's health.

A Conceptual Model of Quality of Life for Women's Health

A conceptual model constitutes a formal explanation of a phenomenon of interest created according to the philosophical views and assumptions of the model's designer. A conceptual model allows for the efficient integration of observations and facts into an orderly scheme. The concepts of the phenomenon are assembled into a coherent structure because of their relevance to a common theme (Polit & Beck, 2012, 2014). In this context, the phenomenon of interest is quality of life, and the concepts central to quality of life and their relevance will be presented in the following discussion.

Ferrans and Powers (1992) defined quality of life as "a person's sense of well-being that stems from satisfaction or dissatisfaction with the areas of life that are important to him/her" (p. 29). The underlying ideology of this conceptualization is based on an individualistic view. Ferrans (1996) asserts that the essence of quality of life is grounded in the experience of life, and the individual is the only suitable judge of their experience. Thus, this evaluation is subjective in nature, and emphasizes the experience rather than conditions of life (Ferrans, 1996). Because individuals value different things, diverse aspects of life have varying impact on their quality of life. Hence, there is no single quality of life for all people with the same life experience. A condition that makes life intolerable for one person may be no more than a nuisance to another. Consequently, satisfaction implies an evaluation derived from comparing the desired to actual conditions of life (Ferrans, 1996).

The conceptual model (**Figure 2–1**) developed by Ferrans (1990a) describes four major domains of quality of life: health and functioning, psychological/spiritual, socioeconomic, and family. These domains are interrelated and overlapping (Ferrans, 1994). The four domains encompass 34 aspects of life, conveying the multidimensionality of the construct. The conceptual model illustrates the hierarchical relationships between the global construct of quality of life, the four major domains, and specific aspects of the domains (**Figure 2–2**) (Ferrans, 1990a). Ferrans's Conceptual Model of Quality of Life was developed based on qualitative inquiry, which determined the components of a satisfying life; extensive literature review, which revealed dimensions of life satisfaction that were assessed from representative studies; and exploratory factor analysis performed on data from study participants who completed the Ferrans & Powers Quality of Life Index. The Ferrans and Powers Quality of Life Index was designed to measure quality of life of healthy as well as ill individuals. The instrument takes into account the life domains noted by experts, the subjective evaluation of satisfaction with the domains, and the unique importance of the domains to the individual (Ferrans & Powers, 1985). The Ferrans conceptual model, which links satisfaction and quality of life, has a strong

Figure 2–1 Ferrans Conceptual Model of Quality of Life.

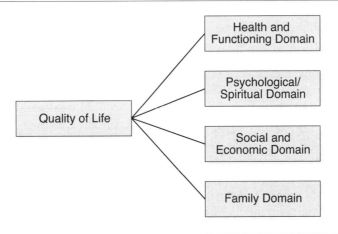

Reproduced from Ferrans, C. (1990a). Development of a quality of life index for patients with cancer. *Oncology Nursing Forum,* *77*(3, Suppl.), 15–19. Used with permission of The Oncology Nursing Society.

Figure 2–2 Hierarchical relationship between the global construct of quality and life, four major domains, and the specific aspects of the domains.

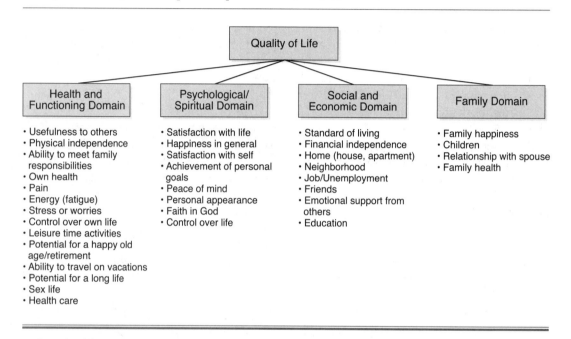

Reproduced from Ferrans, C. (1990a). Development of a quality of life index for patients with cancer. *Oncology Nursing Forum, 77*(3, Suppl.), 15–19. Used with permission of The Oncology Nursing Society.

conceptual basis, clearly distinguishes between the domains, and provides a solid example of the connection between theory and research. External validation of the conceptual model was provided by the work of Ferrell, Padilla, Grant, and their colleagues (Ferrell, Dow, Leigh, Ly, & Gulasekaram, 1995; Ferrell et al., 1992; Ferrell, Grant, & Padilla, 1991; Ferrell, Wisdom, & Wenzel, 1989, Grant et al., 1992; Padilla et al., 1990), who developed a similar conceptual model of quality of life based on qualitative analysis of data from cancer patients. Mutual validation of the two models was shown by their independent and simultaneous development on the basis of patient data from diverse samples taken from different locations in the United States (Ferrans, 1996). The Ferrans Conceptual Model of Quality of Life and the Ferrans and Powers Quality of Life Index have been used extensively, both nationally and internationally, as a basis for many research studies that have investigated the quality of life of women with a wide range of health issues. The Ferrans Conceptual Model of Quality of Life will be integrated into the analyses of women's health issues across the life cycle in subsequent chapters of this text.

Research Review

What are the predictors of quality of life in younger and older breast cancer survivors?

Sammarco, A. (2009). Quality of life of breast cancer survivors: A comparative study of age cohorts. *Cancer Nursing, 32*(5), 347–356.

The purpose of this study was to describe the differences between older and younger breast cancer survivors in perceived social support, uncertainty, quality of life, and on various demographic variables. Furthermore, this study sought to explore the role of these variables in explaining and predicting quality of life. A conceptual framework based on the Ferrans Conceptual Model of Quality of Life and the Mishel Uncertainty in Illness Theory guided this study. A descriptive research design was employed. A sample of 163 older and 129 younger breast cancer survivors was recruited from multiple sites in the New York metropolitan area and study participants completed the Northouse Social Support Questionnaire, the Mishel Uncertainty in Illness Scale Community Form, and the Ferrans and Powers Quality of Life Index-Cancer Version III. Data were analyzed using descriptive statistics, t test, chi-square, and hierarchical multiple regression.

The findings revealed that the younger cohort perceived significantly more social support than the older cohort, most notably from spouses and nurses. Both younger and older cohorts reported moderate levels of uncertainty, yet no significant difference was noted. Although both cohorts reported having acceptable overall quality of life, the older cohort reported significantly better psychological/spiritual and socioeconomic quality of life than the younger cohort. The findings also indicated that perceived social support, older age, and not having had adjuvant treatment predicted a better quality of life in breast cancer survivors, whereas uncertainty and having had a mastectomy predicted poorer quality of life. The most influential variable on the quality of life of both cohorts was uncertainty, followed by having additional illnesses, perceived social support, older age, not having had adjuvant treatment, and having had a mastectomy.

Nurses and other healthcare providers need to be mindful of the age-related differences that exist among breast cancer survivors regarding perceived social support, uncertainty, and quality of life, as well as factors that are predictive of better or poorer quality of life. This understanding will help nurses and other health practitioners to determine the resources and vulnerabilities of breast cancer survivors and better assist them in maintaining an acceptable quality of life.

Chapter Summary Points

- Over the past century, the life expectancy of women in the United States has increased by more than 30 years. With this increase in longevity, realization has emerged that quality of life is as ultimately important as quantity of life.
- Although advances have been made in many dimensions of women's health across the life cycle, the impact of women's health issues on quality of life must be acknowledged, explored, and kept in the mainstream of women's health care.
- Chronological age once stood as the criterion for normalizing the roles and responsibilities taken on by individuals throughout their lives. However, since the 1970s, age norms have shifted and can no longer be considered normative.
- Puberty arrives earlier by several years and adolescence extends into the mid- to late twenties. The arrival of true adulthood has been delayed until the thirties and forties. Middle age has been pushed into the fifties and the stages of life beyond the fifties have changed radically from what was experienced by pre-"Baby Boomer" generations.
- Women have experienced a continuous expansion of opportunities, greater participation in the workforce, and assumption of multiple life roles.
- The most radical voluntary change to the life cycle has been the reproductive revolution that has enabled women to defer childbirth by 10 to 20 years.
- Currently the lives of adult women are all the more complex with the multiple dimensions of biology, family, and work interacting and influencing each other and alternatives regarding life choices and the timing of major career choices and family events.
- The traditional normative roles of mid-life to older women have also shifted dramatically since the 1970s, and consequently manifest diverse issues that threaten quality of life.
- Quality of life is a commonly used, broad, multidimensional construct that is often unclearly defined and poorly understood.
- Authors define quality of life in different ways and conceptualize quality of life as having differing dimensions. Achieving conceptual clarity concerning the definition of quality of life has been difficult because people often ascribe their own personal meanings without ascertaining whether their definitions are shared by others.
- Multidimensionality of the construct, the importance of satisfaction with the dimensions of life, and studying the construct from the perspective of the individual are areas of conceptual agreement on quality of life.
- Health-related quality of life includes those aspects of overall quality of life that can be clearly shown to affect health.
- Culture is fundamental to life and is an important determinant of quality of life in the context of health. Culture defines the purpose and prescriptions for living a meaningful life in wellness and sickness.
- The conceptual model applied to the subsequent analysis of women's health issues across the life cycle describes four major domains of quality of life: health and functioning, psychological/spiritual, socioeconomic, and family. These domains are interrelated, overlapping, and encompass 34 aspects of life, conveying the multidimensionality of the construct.

Critical Thinking Exercise

Questions for Seminar Discussion

1. What were the traditional marker events and age criteria of the stages of the adult life cycle?
2. What global, economical, and social events in the 1970s triggered a shift in the normative roles and criterion ages of the adult life cycle?
3. In what ways did the developmental stages of the adult life cycle change since the 1970s?
4. What is entailed in the process of passage through the stages of development of the adult life cycle?
5. In view of the changes to the normative roles and stages of the adult life cycle, what challenges do adults face in passing through the stages, especially older adults?
6. How have the normative societal roles of adult women changed across the life cycle since the 1970s?
7. Describe the "burden of caring" carried by adult women throughout the life cycle. How has this tradition led to a caregiving crisis in older women?
8. What is quality of life? Why is there difficulty associated with conceptualizing the construct of quality of life?
9. Describe the categories of definitions of quality of life.
10. What limitations do some categories of quality of life definitions present in assessing quality of life?
11. What areas of conceptual agreement regarding quality of life have been achieved?
12. What is the meaning of health-related quality of life and what does it encompass?
13. What is culture and how does it influence quality of life?
14. Discuss the controversy surrounding race and racism. How is quality of life affected?
15. What is ethnicity? How do theories of culture, race, or ethnicity contribute to strategies that promote or maintain health and well-being?
16. What is the difference between acculturation and assimilation? How can acculturation influence health-related quality of life?
17. How does the cultural view of humanness shape quality of life?
18. How is consideration of quality of life essential for women's health?
19. Discuss the definition of quality of life developed by Ferrans and Powers. Explain how this definition remains consistent to the discussion of conceptual agreement.
20. Explain the Ferrans Conceptual Model of Quality of Life, the major domains, and the specific aspects of each domain.

Internet Resources

Center for Advanced Research on Language Acquisition (CARLA): provides a variety of definitions of culture. http://www.carla.umn.edu/culture/definitions.html

Center for American Progress: provides information and education about women's health and rights. http://www.americanprogress.org

Centers for Disease Control and Prevention: provides information and education about health-related quality of life. http://www.cdc.gov/hrqol/

Ferrans and Powers Quality of Life Index: provides information and education about the Ferrans and Powers Quality of Life Index for measuring quality of life. https://www.uic.edu/orgs/qli/

Healthy People 2020: Provides information about health-related quality of life and well-being. http://www.healthypeople.gov/2020/about/QoLWBabout.aspx

References

Alarcon, G., Rodriguez, J., Benavides, G., Brooks, K., Kurusz, H., & Reveille, J., with LUMINA Study Group. (1999). Systemic lupus erythmatosus in three ethnic groups. V. Acculturation, health-related attitudes and behaviors, and disease activity in Hispanic patients from the LUMINA cohort. Lupus in minority populations, nature versus nurture. *Arthritis Care and Research, 12*(4), 267–276.

Barrett, L. (2004). *Caregiving in the United States.* Washington, DC: AARP and National Alliance for Caregiving.

Bloom, J., & Kessler, L. (1994). Risk and timing of counseling and support interventions for younger women with breast cancer. *Journal of the National Cancer Institute Monographs, 16,* 199–206.

Campbell, A., Converse, C., & Rodgers, W. (1976). *The quality of American life.* New York, NY: Russell Sage Foundation.

Cawthorne, A. (2008). Center for American progress: The straight facts on women in poverty. Retrieved from https://www.americanprogress.org/issues/women/report/2008/10/08/5103/the-straight-facts-on-women-in-poverty/

Cella, D. (1992). Quality of life: The concept. *Journal of Palliative Care, 8*(3), 8–13.

Cella, D. (1994). Quality of life: Concepts and definitions. *Journal of Pain and Symptom Management, 9,* 186–192.

Cella, D., & Tulsky, D. (1990). Measuring quality of life today: Methodological aspects. *Oncology, 4*(5), 29–38.

Center for Advanced Research on Language Acquisition. (2010, January 22). What is culture: CARLA's Definition. Retrieved from http://www.carla.umn.edu/culture/definitions.html

Centers for Disease Control and Prevention. (2011). HRQOL concepts. Retrieved from http://www.cdc.gov/hrqol/concept.htm

Donovan, K., Sanson-Fisher, R., & Redman, S. (1989). Measuring quality of life in cancer patients. *Journal of Clinical Oncology, 7*(7), 959–968.

Fawcett, J. (2005). *Contemporary nursing knowledge. Analysis and evaluation of nursing models and theories* (2nd ed.). Philadelphia, PA: F. A. Davis.

Ferrans, C. (1990a). Development of a quality of life index for patients with cancer. *Oncology Nursing Forum, 77*(3, Suppl.), 15–19.

Ferrans, C. (1990b). Quality of life: Conceptual issues. *Seminars in Oncology Nursing, 6*(4), 248–254.

Ferrans, C. (1994). Quality of life through the eyes of survivors of breast cancer. *Oncology Nursing Forum, 21*(10), 1645–1661.

Ferrans, C. (1996). Development of a conceptual model of quality of life. *Scholarly Inquiry of Nursing Practice: An International Journal, 10*(3), 293–304.

Ferrans, C., & Powers, M. (1985). Quality of life index: Development and psychometric properties. *Advances in Nursing Science, 8,* 15–24.

Ferrans, C., & Powers, M. (1992). Psychometric assessment of the quality of life index. *Research in Nursing and Health, 15,* 29–38.

Ferrans, C., Zerwic, J., Wilbur, J., & Larson, J. (2005). Conceptual model of health-related quality of life. *Journal of Nursing Scholarship, 37*(4), 336–342.

Ferrell, B., Dow, K., Leigh, S., Ly, J., & Gulasekaram, P. (1995). Quality of life in long term cancer survivors. *Oncology Nursing Forum, 22*(6), 915–922.

Ferrell, B., Grant, M., & Padilla, G. (1991). Experience of pain and perceptions of quality of life: Validation of a conceptual model. *Hospice Journal, 7*(3), 9–24.

Ferrell, B., Grant, M., Schmidt, G., Rhiner, M., Whitehead, C., Fonbuena, P., & Forman, S. (1992). The meaning of quality of life for bone marrow transplant survivors. Part I: The impact of bone marrow transplant on QOL. *Cancer Nursing, 15,* 153–150.

Ferrell, B., Wisdom, C., & Wenzl, C. (1989). QOL as an outcome variable in the management of cancer pain. *Cancer, 63,* 2321–2327.

Fletcher, J. (1990). Four indicators of humanhood: The enquiry matures. In J. J. Walter & T. J. Shannon (Eds.) *Quality of life: The new medical dilemma.* Mahwah, New Jersey: Paulist Press.

Foster, M., & Sharp, R. (2004). Beyond race: Towards a whole-genome perspective on human populations and genetic variation. *Nature Reviews, Genetics, 5*(10), 790–796.

George, L., & Bearon. L. (1980). *Quality of life in older persons.* New York: Human Sciences Press.

Grant, M., Ferrell, B., Schmidt, G., Fonbuena, P., Niland, J., & Forman, S. (1992). Measurement of quality of life in bone marrow transplantation survivors. *Quality of Life Research, 1,* 375–384.

Greeff, M., Uys, L., Wantland, D., Makoae, L., Chirwa, M., Dlamini, P., … Holzemer, W. (2010). Perceived HIV stigma and life satisfaction among persons living with HIV infection in five African countries: A longitudinal study. *International Journal of Nursing Studies, 47*(4), 475–486.

Health-related quality of life among women. (2003). *Chronic Disease Notes and Reports, 16*(1), 18–22.

Hirschman, C., Alba, R., & Farley, R. (2000). The meaning and measurement of race in the U.S. census: Glimpses into the future. *Demography, 37*(3), 381–393.

Hishinuma, E., Andrade, N., Johnson, R., McArdle, J., Miyamoto, R., Nahulu, L., … Yates, A. (2000). Psychometric properties of the Hawaiian Culture Scale-Adolescent Version. *Psychological Assessment, 12*(2), 140–157.

Institute of Medicine. (2001). *Health and behavior: The interplay of biological, behavioral, and social influences.* Washington, DC: National Academy Press.

Kagawa-Singer, M. (1995). Socioeconomic and cultural influences on cancer in women. *Seminars in Oncology Nursing, 11*(2), 109–119.

Kagawa-Singer, M. (2001). From genes to social science: Impact of the simplistic interpretation of race, ethnicity, and culture on cancer outcome. *Cancer, 91*(1, Suppl.), 226–232.

Kagawa-Singer, M. (2000). Improving the validity and generalizability of studies with underserved U.S. populations expanding the research paradigm. *Annals of Epidemiology, 10*(8, Suppl.), S92–S103.

Kagawa-Singer, M. (2006). Population science is science only if you know the population. *Journal of Cancer Education, 21*(1, Suppl.), S22–S31.

Kagawa-Singer, M., & Blackhall, L. (2001). Negotiating cross-cultural issues at the end of life. *Journal of the American Medical Association, 286*(23), 2993–3001.

Kagawa-Singer, M., & Chung, R. (1994). A paradigm for culturally-based care for minority populations. *Journal of Community Psychology, 22*(2), 192–208.

Kim, J., Ashing-Giwa, K., Kagawa-Singer, M., & Tejero, J. (2006). Breast cancer among Asian Americans: Is acculturation related to quality of life? *Oncology Nursing Forum, 33*(6), E90–E99.

Kim, Y., Kashy, D., Spillers, R., & Evans, T. (2010). Needs assessment of family caregivers of cancer survivors: Three cohorts comparison. *Psycho-Oncology, 19*(6), 573–582.

King, C., Haberman, M., Berry, D., Bush, N., Hassey-Dow, K., … Underwood, S. (1997). Quality of life and the cancer experience: The state-of-the-knowledge. *Oncology Nursing Forum, 24*(1), 27–41.

Larios, S., Davis, J., Gallo, L., Heinrich, J., & Talavera, G. (2009). Concerns about stigma, social support, and quality of life in low-income HIV-positive Hispanics. *Ethnicity and Disease, 19*(1), 65–70.

Mandzuk, L., & McMillan, D. (2005). A concept analysis of quality of life. *Journal of Orthopaedic Nursing, 9,* 12–18.

Marin, G., Sabogal, F., Van Oss-Marin, B., Otero-Sabogal, R., & Perez-Stable, E. (1987). Development of a short acculturation scale for Hispanics. *Hispanic Journal of Behavioral Science, 9*, 183–199.

Montague, A. (1997). *Man's most dangerous myth: The fallacy of race* (6th ed.). Walnut Creek, CA: Alta Mira Press.

Office on Women's Health U.S. Department of Health and Human Services. (2002). *A century of women's health: 1900-2000.* Washington, DC: DHHS Office on Women's Health.

Padilla, G., Ferrell, B., Grant, M., & Rhiner, M. (1990). Defining the content domain of quality of life for cancer patients with pain. *Cancer Nursing, 13*(2), 108–115.

Padilla, G., Grant, M., & Martin, L. (1988). Rehabilitation and quality of life measurement issues. *Head & Neck Surgery, 10*(Suppl. 2), S156–S160.

Padilla, G., & Perez, E. (1995). Minorities and arthritis. *Arthritis Care and Research: The Official Journal of the Arthritis Health Professions Association, 8*(4), 251–256.

Polit, D., & Beck, C. (2014). *Essentials of nursing research: Appraising evidence for nursing practice* (8th ed). Philadelphia, PA: Lippincott Williams Wilkins.

Polit, D., & Beck, C. (2012). *Nursing research: generating and assessing evidence for nursing practice* (9th ed). Philadelphia, PA: Lippincott Williams Wilkins.

Royal, C., & Dunston, G. (2004). Changing the paradigm from 'race' to human genome variation. *Nature Genetics, 36*(11 Suppl.), S5–S7.

Sammarco, A. (2001). Psychosocial stages and quality of life of women with breast cancer. *Cancer Nursing, 24*(4), 272–277.

Sammarco, A. (2003). Quality of life among older survivors of breast cancer. *Cancer Nursing, 26*(6), 431–438.

Sammarco, A. (2009). Quality of life of breast cancer survivors: A comparative study of age cohorts. *Cancer Nursing, 32*(5), 347–356.

Seiden, A. (1989). Psychological issues affecting women throughout the life cycle. *Psychiatric Clinics of North America, 12*(1), 1.

Sheehy, G. (1995). *New passages: Mapping your life across time.* New York: Random House.

Shrier, D., & Shrier, L. (2009). Psychosocial aspects of women's lives: Work and family/personal life and life cycle issues. *Obstetrical and Gynecolological Clinics of North America, 36*, 753–769.

Spector, R. (2004). *Cultural diversity in health and illness.* Upper Saddle River, NJ: Prentice Hall.

Suinn, R., Rickard-Figueroa, K., Lew, S., & Vigil, P. (1987). The Suinn-Lew Asian Self-identity Scale: An initial report. *Educational and Psychological Measurement, 47*, 401–407.

U. S. Bureau of Labor Statistics. (2014). Women in the labor force: A databook. Retrieved from http://stats.bls.gov/cps/wlf-databook-2013.pdf

Chapter 3

Vulnerable Populations of Women

LEARNING OUTCOMES

On completion of this chapter, the learner will be able to:

1. Explain risk factors that contribute to vulnerability in women.
2. Analyze vulnerability from an individual and aggregate perspective.
3. Explain concepts that form the conceptual basis of vulnerable populations.
4. Discuss factors that contribute to health disparities in vulnerable populations.
5. Describe specific vulnerable populations of women and the significant characteristics of their health disparities.
6. Analyze how knowledge of health literacy, social justice, cultural competence, and resilience can be applied to promote well-being and positive quality of life outcomes in vulnerable populations of women.

Introduction

Over the last century, progress in public health, medicine, and technology has led to major advances in the prevention, diagnosis, and treatment of diseases in women. Consequently, countless women are enjoying longer and healthier lives, as well as improved quality of life. Despite these strides, however, significant disparity continues to exist in women's health and health care. Numerous individual and societal factors tend to place women at greater risk for health problems and increase their vulnerability to disease, injury, and psychological trauma. While women, on the whole, can be considered vulnerable, there are many subgroups of women who have greater than average risk for developing health problems and thus comprise vulnerable populations. This chapter will explore the meaning of vulnerability and what it means to be a vulnerable population. In doing so, a theoretical perspective of vulnerability in women as well as vulnerable populations of women will be provided. This chapter will also present a discussion of concepts particularly essential for the promotion of well-being and positive quality of life outcomes of vulnerable populations of women.

Vulnerability From Individual and Aggregate Perspectives

Vulnerability

In general, vulnerability means *susceptibility*. The specific implication of vulnerability in health care is *to be at risk for health problems*. People who are vulnerable are more likely to develop health problems. Certain community and corresponding individual factors are risk factors associated with the development of poor physical, psychological, or social health. Risk factors are attributes, characteristics, behaviors, or exposures that are associated with or lead to increases in the probability of occurrence of health-related outcomes (Aday, 2001).

Women can be at risk for poor physical, psychological, or social health. Some women who are not members of culturally defined populations frequently designated as being vulnerable might be vulnerable only in certain contexts. For example, emergency room nurses are vulnerable to violence. Hospital employees and visitors are vulnerable to infections. Teachers in preschool and daycare are vulnerable to a multitude of communicable diseases because of their daily contact with young children.

There is an unfortunate propensity in society to judge some vulnerable women as being at fault for their own vulnerability. For example, rape victims have often been blamed for enticing their attackers. Although people should be more cautious about personal protection in societies in which dangers exist in many contexts, this concept is quite different from blaming the victim. When a victim is blamed for his or her vulnerability, the onus of accountability is removed from the criminal and placed on the victim, which is an injustice. In the final analysis, criminals and predators need to be held accountable for criminal behavior. Victims need to be reassured that an assault is not their fault because they were simply in the wrong place at the wrong time.

Vulnerable Populations

Vulnerable populations are groups who are especially sensitive to risk factors and generally possess multiple cumulative risk factors. Vulnerable populations have a greater likelihood of developing health problems as a result of exposure to risk, or have poorer outcomes from these health problems than the rest of the population (Pacquiao, 2008). Vulnerable populations have a greater-than-average risk of developing health problems by virtue of their marginalized sociocultural status, their limited access to economic resources, or their personal characteristics such as age and gender (Aday, 2001). To illustrate this, members of ethnic minority groups have traditionally been marginalized even when they are highly educated and earning good salaries. Immigrants and the poor (including the working poor) have limited access to healthcare because of the way health insurance is obtained in the United States. Women, children, and the elderly are vulnerable to a host of healthcare problems—notably violence, but also specific health problems associated with development or aging. Developmental examples might include poor influenza outcomes for children and the elderly, psychological issues of puberty and menopause, osteoporosis and fractures, as well as Alzheimer's disease among older women.

Vulnerability is both an individual and group concept. To be a member of a vulnerable population does not necessarily mean a woman is, in fact, vulnerable. Moreover, many individuals within a vulnerable population would resist the notion that they are vulnerable, because they prefer to focus on their strengths rather than their weaknesses. These individuals might argue that *vulnerable population* is just another label that healthcare professionals use to promote a system of health care that they, the consumers of care, consider patronizing. Thus, it is important to distinguish between a state of vulnerability at any given point in time and a labeling process that further marginalizes groups of people at risk for certain health conditions. Nonetheless, the notion of a vulnerable population is a public health concept that refers to vulnerability by virtue of status, that is, some groups are at risk at any given point in time relative to other individuals or groups.

From a public health standpoint, the group concept is dominant. Consideration of aggregates helps healthcare providers increase their awareness of the health disparities and increased risk for health problems of a particular vulnerable group at any given time relative to other individuals or groups. It is critical to understand that persons who are members of a vulnerable group might not view themselves as vulnerable and may likely resent labels that imply they are not autonomous. Thus, healthcare providers should be careful to avoid labeling or stereotyping that could further marginalize the vulnerable.

Conceptual Basis of Vulnerable Populations

Numerous important concepts form the basis of vulnerable populations. These key concepts include risk, social status, social capital, human capital, access to care, cost of care, and quality of care. They influence vulnerability and are essential for understanding vulnerability as well as the nature of health care for vulnerable populations. These concepts and how they are linked to vulnerability provide a framework for describing women as a vulnerable population.

Risk

Risk is an essential underlying concept for understanding vulnerable populations. Any person can be at risk statistically by way of having the potential for certain illnesses based on genetic predisposition (Scanlon & Lee, 2007). All persons are potentially at risk for poor physical, psychological, and social health. Anyone can be vulnerable at any

particular moment as a result of circumstances in their lives or response to illness or events. People may be more or less vulnerable to poor health at different times in their lives, and there is likelihood that some individuals and groups may be more at risk than others at any given point in time (Aday, 2001).

Women who are in poor physical health, such as those having a debilitating chronic illness, may be at higher risk for poor psychological health (such as depression). Furthermore, they may be at higher risk of poor social health, such as having few supportive social contacts. Risk is cumulative. Thus persons who are in poor health and have little material (economic) and nonmaterial (psychological or social) resources to assist them in coping with illness are at greater risk for harm or neglect (Aday, 2001).

Social Status

Social status is linked with the standings that persons occupy in society that are related to age, sex, race or ethnicity, and the opportunities and rewards, such as prestige and power, they have as a result (Aday, 2001). Social status can influence vulnerability. The pervasiveness of certain diseases and the need to depend on others for help because of poor health differ throughout the life cycle. Socially defined roles that typify females at different stages of the life cycle can lead to differential exposures to health risks. For example, the dependency of infants and elderly on others, the risk-taking behaviors of adolescents, and occupation-related exposures among women in the workforce presents varying degrees of risk for illnesses or injury (Aday, 2001). Women tend to have a higher incidence of many types of illnesses as compared to men. Such disparity is frequently attributed to women's differing health needs, stress related to the complex deferential and demanding roles women play in society, and the social acceptability of women to admit their vulnerability (Aday, 2001). In addition, racial and ethnic minorities frequently have poorer health and fewer material and nonmaterial assets to meet their needs. These disparities are likely related to historical and contemporary patterns of discrimination with associated residential or occupational segregation, limited economical or educational opportunities, and disproportionate exposure to environmental risks in mainly minority neighborhoods (Aday, 2001). Consequently, women with a combination of statuses, such as being poor, elderly, and a member of a racial or ethnic minority, are in an extremely vulnerable position due to the high risk of having poor health and few material and nonmaterial resources (Aday, 2001).

Social Capital

Social capital is related to the quantity and quality of interpersonal ties among people. Members of social networks gain social capital in the form of social support and related feelings of belonging, psychological well-being, and self esteem. Social support is valuable to people in that it provides resources that enable them to achieve goals as well as helps them in coping with and minimizing the effects of negative life events or adversity on their physical and mental health. People who are members of supportive social networks experience enhanced physical, psychological, and social well-being (Aday, 2001). Communities are sources that both generate social capital and provide social capital to individuals and community members. Individuals with weak community integration or connection are most likely to have the least social capital or fewest social ties to count on. Women who likely have low social capital include those who are not married or in an otherwise committed intimate relationship, live alone, head single-parent households, have weak or nonexistent social networks of family or friends, and do not belong to any voluntary organizations such as churches or volunteer interest groups (Aday, 2001).

Human Capital

Human capital is the investment in skills and capabilities of individuals that enables them to act in a new way or improve their contributions to society. Human capital is frequently reflected by the quality of schools, housing, jobs, and income in the community. Thus, communities with poor schools, substandard housing, and high rates of unemployment likely have diminished levels of investment in the human capital or potential for productivity of the people who live there (Aday, 2001). Disparities in education and income, as well as sustained economic deprivations over the life course, are associated with wide disparities in health. Inadequate and unsafe housing can increase exposure to health risks. Consequently, women who are poorly educated, unemployed, and poorly housed are likely to lack the resources essential for coping with illness or other personal or economic adversities (Aday, 2001).

Access to Care

Access to care refers to the ability of people to find, obtain, and pay for health care. Issues associated with access to care frequently center on being able to access healthcare providers and institutions that will impart healthcare services, as well as managing financial barriers and inadequate or lack of health insurance to pay for services (Aday, 2001). Vulnerable populations are often confronted with barriers to access of care. Women, especially those who are elderly, immigrants, of lower socioeconomic means, or of racial and ethnic minorities, frequently encounter such barriers. Women in these groups commonly lack health insurance or may be challenged with language barriers, discrimination, poor health literacy, or isolation.

Cost of Care

Costs of care can be either direct or indirect. Direct costs are the dollars spent by healthcare facilities to provide care, whereas indirect costs are losses resulting from decreased patient productivity, such as absenteeism from work. Frequently, the out-of-pocket costs or cash outlays of individuals or their families are significant components of the financial burden of health care. The bulk of resources consumed in caring for vulnerable populations of women involve costs associated with treatment and loss of human productive potential (Aday, 2001).

QUALITY OF CARE

Quality of care refers to the relative inadequacy or superiority of services. Issues associated with quality of care involve characteristics of providers and institutions delivering services, treatment protocols or standards recommended or used by care providers, and the actual health consequences or outcomes of the care delivery process for patients. The effectiveness of care for many vulnerable populations of women is greatly affected by accessibility, adequacy, and acceptability. In essence, this means that outcomes of care for vulnerable populations of women are greatly influenced by what type of care they are able to get, whether the care is enough and appropriate for their needs, and whether they are willing to follow the plan recommended for treatment (Aday, 2001).

Health Disparities and Vulnerable Populations

A major characteristic of vulnerable populations is their increased risk for adverse health outcomes because of marginalization due to personal attributes, sociocultural status, or limited economic resources. Vulnerable populations commonly are affected by health disparities, which are significant differences in overall rate of disease incidence, prevalence, morbidity, mortality, or survival rates. Factors such as poverty; racial, ethnic, and gender inequalities; and access to health care contribute to health disparities.

Trends over the last five decades (the lifetime of the baby boomers) show marked changes in the demographics of the population and families, and these changes in turn have affected health disparities by way of dramatically shifting social status and social capital. A larger portion of the population is comprised of racial and ethnic minorities. The elderly population has risen from 35.5 million in 2002 to 43.1 million in 2012. It is estimated that by 2030, the elderly population will rise to 72.1 million, and 92 million by 2060 (U.S. Department of Health and Human Services, Administration for Community Living, 2015). Presently, more men and women are delaying marriage, with many choosing to live together first. Divorce rates are higher, with a concurrent increase in single-parent families. An increase in out-of-wedlock births has occurred as well as a sharp increase in maternal employment (Hofferth, 2003).

Vulnerable populations characteristically reflect health disparities associated with age, gender, race, ethnic minority, socioeconomic status and societal trends. The following discussion describes vulnerable populations of women that have been adapted from the vulnerable populations identified by Aday (2001). Significant characteristics of their health disparities are presented.

HIGH-RISK MOTHERS

This population reflects the currently high rates of teenage pregnancy and poor prenatal care, leading to birth-weight problems and infant mortality. Affected groups include very young women, African-American women, and poorly educated women, all of whom are less likely than middle-class white women to receive adequate prenatal care due to limited access to services. Although in a downward trend, the U.S. teen pregnancy and birth, sexually transmitted disease, and abortion rates are substantially higher than those of other Western industrialized countries (Centers for Disease Control and Prevention [CDC], 2011a).

Factors that increase the risk for teen pregnancy include growing up in poverty, having parents with low levels of education, growing up in a single-parent family, and having low attachment to and performance in school (CDC, 2014a).

CHRONICALLY ILL AND DISABLED WOMEN

Women who are chronically ill or disabled not only experience higher death rates as a result of heart disease, cancer, and stroke, but are also subject to prevalent chronic conditions such as hypertension, arthritis, and asthma. The debilitating effects of such chronic diseases lead to lost income resulting from limitations in activities of daily living. African-Americans are more likely to experience ill effects and to die from chronic diseases. About 27 million women in this country have disabilities and more than 50% of women over the age of 65 are living with a disability (CDC, 2014d).

WOMEN LIVING WITH HIV/AIDS

In the past decade or so, advances in tracing and treating AIDS have resulted in declines in deaths and increases in the number of people living with HIV/AIDS. This increase is also due in part to changes in transmission patterns from largely male homosexual or bisexual contact to transmission through heterosexual contact and sharing needles among intravenous drug users. Although more men than women become infected with HIV each year, it is estimated that if the current rate of new HIV infection continues worldwide, women with HIV may soon outnumber men with HIV. Women account for 23% of all people in the United States living with HIV. Women of color are disproportionately affected by HIV as compared to women of other races and ethnicities. In 2010, 64% of the total number of new HIV infections in women occurred in African-American women, 18% in white women, and 15% in Hispanic women (CDC, 2015).

MENTALLY ILL AND DISABLED WOMEN

Mental illness affects women differently than men. Some disorders occur more commonly in women as well as present with different symptoms. Numerous biological differences associated with hormones and brain structure affect mental health risks, rates of disorders, and the course of disorders. Also influential in risk and prevalence are numerous environmental and psychosocial factors, such as likelihood of women seeking treatment, likelihood of diagnosis bias, social status, and experience of abuse. Certain social and protective factors can also affect mental health, such as the effects of race, ethnicity, culture, and level of resilience (Office of the Surgeon General, 2005). Severe emotional disorders can seriously interfere with a woman's ability to function in the primary activities of daily living and interpersonal relationships, resulting in the need for prolonged mental health care.

Mental disorders that commonly affect women include anxiety disorders, attention deficit hyperactivity disorders, borderline personality disorder, postpartum depression, and schizophrenia. Women also have high incidence of unipolar and bipolar depression as well as eating disorders (CDC, 2013a; National Institute of Mental Health, 2015). Depression is twice as likely to occur in women as compared to men, and the prevalence is higher among Caucasian and Hispanic women as compared to African-American women. Early puberty is a high-risk period for specific mental disorders prevalent in adolescents, such as eating disorders.

WOMEN WHO ARE ALCOHOL AND SUBSTANCE ABUSERS

Substances that are abused include a wide array of drugs and chemicals, alcohol, and tobacco. Intoxication results in chronic disease, accidents, and, in some cases, criminal activity. Smoking has been linked to chronic diseases such as cancer, heart disease, and lung disease. Although late teen and young adult males are more likely to smoke, drink, and take drugs (CDC, 2011), the use of illicit drugs, tobacco, and alcohol, including riskier practices of binge drinking, is quite prevalent among women during their childbearing years. Substance use, abuse, and dependence among women is associated with poorer health, increased stress, psychiatric comorbidity, and increased prevalence of intimate partner violence (Simmons, Havens, Whiting, Holz, & Bada, 2009). Research findings suggest that approximately 6 out of 10 women, 18 to 44 years of age use alcohol and slightly less than one-third of women who drink in this age group binge drink (4 or more drinks within a 2-hour period) (Sidhu & Floyd, 2002). Approximately 7.6% of women who are pregnant use alcohol (CDC, 2014b). Substance use and abuse during pregnancy may result in premature birth, miscarriage, low birth weight, fetal alcohol syndrome, and places the child at risk for a variety of physical, behavioral, and cognitive problems.

WOMEN EXHIBITING SUICIDE- OR HOMICIDE-PRONE BEHAVIOR

Rates of suicide and homicide differ by age, sex, and race. Although men are four times more likely to die from suicide, women are three times more likely to report attempting suicide (CDC, 2010). Suicide rates are highest for women between the ages of 45 to 54, with poisoning as the most common method (CDC, 2012a). A substantial number of homicides in the United States are committed by intimate partners of the victims. Among women who are victims of homicide, 1 in 3 is a homicide perpetrated by an intimate partner (Paulozzi, Saltzman, Thompson, & Holmgreen, 2001).

WOMEN IN ABUSIVE FAMILIES

Children, the elderly, and spouses (overwhelmingly women) are likely targets of violence within the family. Although older children are more likely to be injured, young female children

older than 3 years of age are consistently at risk for sexual abuse. Each year, women experience approximately 4.8 million intimate partner-related physical assaults and rapes, almost twice as many as experienced by men. About 70% of deaths resulting from intimate partner violence are women and 30% are men. These numbers underestimate the problem, since many acts of intimate partner violence are unreported (CDC, 2012b).

HOMELESS WOMEN

It was estimated that on any given night in 2014, 578,000 persons were homeless and nearly 70% were living in emergency shelters or transitional housing, while 31% were living unsheltered. Homelessness has a severe impact on the lives of people. People who are homeless suffer disproportionately high rates of other chronic diseases and communicable infections, have poorer mental health than average, are more likely to engage in substance abuse, and are frequently the victims of violence. The mortality rate of homeless people is 4 to 9 times higher than that of people who are not homeless (CDC, 2014c).

Women who are homeless are likely victims of domestic violence. In addition to the previously discussed health problems of the homeless, many homeless women have experienced severe physical or sexual assault perpetrated by an intimate partner. Domestic violence increases the likelihood for women to become homeless because victims of domestic violence often lack support networks and financial resources due to isolation by their abusers. Furthermore, homeless women who are victims of domestic violence frequently suffer from anxiety, panic disorder, major depression, and substance abuse (National Alliance to End Homelessness [NAEH], 2015).

IMMIGRANT AND REFUGEE WOMEN

Following the 1965 Immigration Act and its emphasis on family unification, women have immigrated to the United States in large numbers. Of the overall 41.3 million foreign-born immigrants in this country, 51%, or 21.2 million, immigrants are female. Globally, 48% of the immigrant population is female, making the United States the world's top destination for female immigrants (Ruiz, Zong, & Batalova, 2015).

In the United States, immigrant women are more likely to be older, and widowed, divorced, or separated than immigrant men. Immigrant women are more likely to be unemployed and live in poverty than native born women. Moreover, immigrant women are less likely to have health insurance than immigrant men and native born women (Ruiz et al., 2015). Immigrant women are among the most vulnerable and exploited people in American society. They are largely voiceless, isolated, and afraid. Frequently immigrant women do not know their rights, and are vulnerable to abuse, exploitation, sexual harassment, and sexual violence (Southern Poverty Law Center, 2011).

Health care for women who are immigrants, refugees, and temporary residents is complicated by diversity of languages, health practices, food choices, culturally based definitions of health, and previous experiences with American bureaucracies. Some immigrants may have infectious diseases of personal or public health significance; others often have untreated chronic conditions such as vitamin deficiencies, diabetes, or hypertension. Many immigrants and refugees arrive with both infectious and chronic conditions. Healthcare providers are often unfamiliar with screening recommendations and diseases endemic to the immigrants' countries of origin and are unprepared to deal with language, social, and cultural barriers encountered in caring for the new arrivals. Furthermore, immigrants and refugees frequently experience demands imposed by their new environment that compete with their perception of need for health care, and subsequently create additional health challenges (CDC, 2013b).

Lesbian, Bisexual, and Transgender Women

Although a widely diverse community, lesbian, bisexual, and transgender (LBT) women are a vulnerable and historically underserved population who frequently lack access to needed health care and social services. They frequently experience barriers to care and services such as lack of health insurance coverage, low income, lack of access to culturally competent health and social service providers, and cultural beliefs about health care and health providers that decrease utilization of available services (Berberet, 2005).

LBT women are at higher risk for diseases and conditions such as heart disease, cancer, depression, and HIV infection and tend to have higher incidence of smoking, obesity, and stress. LBT women are less likely than heterosexual women to seek medical care and routine health screenings such as mammography and Pap tests due to fear of discrimination or previous negative experiences with healthcare professionals. LBT women are apt to have a higher tendency toward alcohol and drug abuse than heterosexual women. Moreover, many healthcare providers may be uninformed regarding specific health issues of LBT women, and often will not inquire about sexual orientation when taking personal health histories. Many LBT women fear sexual orientation bias among healthcare providers and this fear serves as a significant barrier to care, even among women who have adequate financial resources or health insurance coverage (Berberet, 2005; Cochran, 2012; Dutton, Koenig, & Fennie, 2008).

Incarcerated Women

More than one million women are under criminal justice supervision. Over 200,000 women are incarcerated in prisons and jails in the United States, a number that has grown 800% over the last three decades. Approximately two-thirds of incarcerated women are there for non-violent crimes, many for drug-related crimes. African-American women represent 32.6% of incarcerated women and Hispanic women 16%. Nearly two-thirds of incarcerated women are mothers, with close to 77% having been the primary caregivers for their children prior to incarceration (Women's Prison Association, 2009).

Incarcerated women are more likely to be of low socioeconomic status and have low levels of education. A substantial number of incarcerated women have history of alcohol and substance abuse and have been victims of physical and sexual abuse. Incarcerated women are more likely to suffer mental illness and have HIV infection (Sentencing Project, 2007). They also are more likely to suffer from poor nutrition, and have elevated risk of reproductive health problems, including high-risk pregnancies and sexually transmitted diseases. In addition to experiencing numerous health disparities, incarcerated women are often underserved in receiving adequate health care (Clark, et al., 2006).

Key Factors That Influence the Care of Vulnerable Women

The care of vulnerable women can be influenced by any number of factors that can increase or diminish access to care, quality of care, and cost of care, as well as affect individual and social resources for coping with vulnerability. The following discussion explores selected factors associated with health vulnerability that are fundamental to establishing a theoretical perspective of care for vulnerable women. Health literacy, social justice, cultural competence, and resilience are highlighted as essential areas in which intervention can promote well-being and positive quality of life outcomes in vulnerable women.

LITERACY AND HEALTH LITERACY

Literacy. Literacy has been defined as the use of printed information to maneuver in society, meet one's goals, and develop one's knowledge and abilities (Kirsch, Jungeblut, Jenkins, & Kolstad, 2002). This definition has been expanded to include comprehension and retention of verbal and gestural information (Doak, Doak, & Root, 2001). The National Adult Literacy Survey (NALS) was conducted in 1992, and again in 2003. The NALS remains the largest study on adult literacy carried out in this country.

The original NALS data suggested that one-fourth to one-third of American adults are functionally illiterate and approximately an equal number have marginal literacy skills that disallow full functioning in society. Essentially, half of the adult population in the United States has poor to nonexistent skills in reading, listening, and computation. Minor proportions of the participants of the NALS survey were learning disabled (5%) and spoke English as a second language, if at all (15%). However, most of the participants were white and born in America. Although education correlated with literacy, adults with a tenth-grade education tended to read at the seventh- to eighth-grade level. Participants receiving Medicaid had an average of a fifth-grade reading level. One-third of the NALS sample demonstrated basic functionality in understanding and using written information. Only 20% of the sample demonstrated a level of proficiency in handling information to perform complex reading and computational tasks (National Center for Education Statistics, 2015).

The NALS was re-administered in 2003 and the results showed a slightly worsening trend. In fact, the NALS data suggested that certain groups fared much worse in their literacy skills than the general population. These groups included the poor, elderly, immigrants, people who did not finish high school (disproportionately represented by Hispanic, African-American, and Asian-Pacific participants), people with physical, mental, or health conditions that disallowed participation in work or school settings, and people with mental health problems (National Center for Education Statistics, 2015).

Participants in the lowest literacy level had difficulty with performing usual tasks of daily living based on printed information and in performing complex tasks that required following directions and computation. Interestingly, members of the group considered having no or minimal functional literacy did not acknowledge themselves as vulnerable, related to their illiteracy.

A meta-analysis of U.S. studies on literacy reviewed literature spanning 1963 through 2004 and, based on a pool of 85 articles, essentially validated the same prevalence rates mentioned earlier. The findings concluded that limited literacy is highly prevalent, negatively affects health, and is consistently associated with education, ethnicity, and age (Paasche-Orlow, Parker, Gazmararian, Neilsen-Bohlman, & Rudd, 2005).

Literacy has been discussed as currency in the United States because those with less literacy are much less likely to meet the needs of daily living and to pursue life goals (Kirsch et al., 2002). From this perspective, illiteracy has the potential to create health risks and exacerbate existing health conditions. Although all humans are vulnerable, certain segments of the community are much more vulnerable to ill health in terms of initial susceptibility and in their responses (Aday, 2001). Illiteracy is related to social status and access to health care. Persons with poor reading skills who are unable to perform basic literacy functions, such as reading a bus schedule or following directions in completing a task generally have low social status outside of their immediate social ties. Low social status is often associated with low-paying jobs that offer no or minimal healthcare insurance. Low status also can affect a provider's perception of the abilities of a patient. Care may be "edited," and based, at times, on misperceptions (Aday, 2001).

Social status has been associated with poor health in that persons with low social status are more likely to use disproportionately more healthcare services, receive substandard care and less information about their illness, and be presented with fewer options (Duncan, Daly, McDonough, & Williams, 2002). Persons with low literacy have much greater difficulty in accessing human capital, that is, jobs, schools, income, and housing than persons with functional literacy skills (Kirsch et al., 2002). Furthermore, persons who are illiterate tend to lack social capital in that they are more likely to be single or divorced, live in single-parent homes, and be loosely connected to their own communities.

Access to care can be seriously challenged when people have low literacy skills. Accessing care in the United States most often requires complex language skills that are involved with identifying and evaluating possible providers of care, negotiating appropriate entry points into the healthcare system, contacting and communicating needs to obtain an appointment, successfully traveling to and finding the actual site of care, interpreting written materials, and relating to clock and calendar skills. People with low literacy skills are frequently denied access to health care by virtue of their inability to successfully negotiate these tasks.

Illiteracy affects cost of care and the quality of care. It is a significant component of patient adherence to care regimens and hospitalizations in numerous circumstances, such as pregnancy, diabetes, AIDS, asthma, advanced age, sexually transmitted diseases, cardiac surgery, rheumatoid arthritis, psychiatric conditions, women's health, rural residents, immigrants, mental health, older adults, and payer status (Agency for Health care Research & Quality [AHRQ], 2004; Baker et al., 2002; Institute of Medicine [IOM], 2003). Without exception, populations within the context of these circumstances have high prevalence of illiteracy in proportions that mirror the findings from the NALS data. People with literacy problems commonly do not understand instructions and demonstrate less comprehension of their illness or condition.

Consequences of illiteracy include both poorer health outcomes and increased healthcare costs.

In fact, costs of health care may be as much as four times greater for those who read at or below a second grade level than for the general populace (U.S. Department of Health and Human Services, 2000). It is estimated that low literacy increases annual healthcare expenditures by $73 billion in 1998 dollars (National Academy on an Aging Society, 2015). Research has shown that people with documented low literacy have a 52% higher risk of hospital admission as compared to those with functional literacy, even after controlling for age, social and economic factors, and self-reported health (Baker et al., 2002). Low literacy is also associated with higher use of expensive emergency services (AHRQ, 2004). Furthermore, client illiteracy was reported as the highest predictor of poor asthma knowledge and ineffective use of metered-dose inhalers (Williams, Baker, Honig, Lee, & Nowlan, 1998).

Acknowledging the pervasive influence of illiteracy on the quality of care in the United States, the IOM (2003) has identified literacy as one of the top three areas that cut across all other priorities for improvement in the nation's health. Literacy is required for self-management and collaborative care, the other two priority cross-cutting areas.

Health literacy. Since the mid-1990s, the term *health literacy* has been used in medical literature to address the literacy problem. Health literacy is defined as the ability of an individual to obtain, process, and understand basic health information and services needed to make appropriate health decisions. Health literacy encompasses the ability to read and comprehend instructions on prescription bottles, appointment slips, and other essential health-related materials required to successfully function as a patient. It includes the ability to understand basic health information, the ability to effectively handle the healthcare system, and the ability to understand consent forms. Health literacy necessitates reading, listening, analytical, decision making, computation, and application skills as well as the ability to apply these skills to

health situations (American Medical Association, 1999; Glassman, 2014).

Illiteracy specifically increases health risks in women. Women with no or low literacy cannot read or interpret informational pamphlets, directions on prescribed or over-the-counter medications, or diet instructions. A mismatch of vocabulary and skill is problematic and inability to comprehend graphics and pictures pose additional, and for many patients, insurmountable challenges (Doak et al., 2001). Literacy is a complex skill that necessitates much more than simply reading words. It includes many components, such as decoding, comprehension, and retention of information. The development of literacy involves a series of stages. It is not a "free-standing skill" yet requires integration of related life skills to navigate the healthcare system, effectively perform self-care, and make healthcare decisions.

Health and health care add unique aspects to the concern for women's literacy. Health and health care can have a temporary or long-term effect on literacy skills. Situations such as anesthesia due to surgery, blood loss, or acute pain may temporarily impair one's decoding, comprehension, and recall skills. Sustained medical conditions can interfere with mentation, cognition, and attention on a longer-term basis. Delayed mental development, neurological conditions such as Alzheimer's disease and stroke, and psychological disorders such as depression or anxiety may impair literacy skills and the ability of the patient to interact effectively with providers. Sensory impairments can adversely affect literacy. Visual difficulties were in fact associated with a substantial number of NALS participants that tested in the lowest level of literacy (Kirsch et al., 2002).

Healthcare providers have contributed to the health literacy dilemma. In the past, providers, in their listening, speaking, and written interactions with patients have had a tendency to ignore the literacy variable in care, and as such, increased the literacy challenge for their patients

(Doak et al., 2001). The readability level of written healthcare instructions, booklets, and informed consent forms is often substantially higher than the reading skills of patients in the general care population (Cutilli, 2007; Doak et al., 2001; Fobis & Aligne, 2002). Providers tend to seriously underestimate the literacy problem in patients, tend not to be knowledgeable about illiteracy, are frequently inattentive to the literacy needs of patients, and interact differently with patients who admit to literacy problems (Doak et al., 2001; Schillinger et al., 2003). Patients with low literacy are likely to experience difficult interactions with healthcare providers and tend to avoid seeking care because of stigma and shame (Arthur, Geiser, Arriola, & Kripalani, 2009; Katz, Jacobson, & Kripalani, 2007).

Functional illiteracy directly creates health vulnerability in women. Illiteracy is pervasive in patient populations, and healthcare providers cannot rely on self-disclosure or education level to identify all patients with health literacy needs. Women with the greatest health needs are also the same individuals who do not have the tools to navigate the complex U.S. healthcare system. Currently there is a major mismatch between patient literacy skills and provider communication styles and health materials. Solutions addressing this intersection of healthcare needs and illiteracy include interventions that will identify those with literacy deficits as well as close the gap between health information and low-literacy individuals. Efforts at this level involve improved literacy screening measures, using multiple education strategies, addressing the needs of patients with limited English proficiency, and incorporating technology to address the learning needs of low-literacy patients. Although these strategies may well lessen the gap between the provider's style of oral and written communication and the patient's level of literacy skill, they may essentially be skirting the core issue related to vulnerability.

As discussed earlier, literacy problems create health risks. By using methods that ignore or accommodate the literacy deficit, providers essentially propagate the illiteracy problem by perpetuating the predominant tertiary care focus in the current system of health care. Literacy affects women's lives in foundational ways through the creation of social stigma and prejudicial attitudes, and diminishing the ability to navigate within complex systems throughout society that include health care and beyond to housing and money management. Literacy is a core driver of vulnerability in this country and needs to be addressed as an integral aspect of health care. Providers need to improve their own sensitivity and skills in working with low-literacy patients. They can improve the health of their patients by increasing patient literacy. Strategies that involve partnering with communities and community-wide agencies, such as schools, community centers, and libraries, can help to develop patient literacy skills, and thereby decrease their health risk.

SOCIAL JUSTICE

The ethical principle of justice is often defined in the forms of social, distributive, and market justice. A common definition of social justice is a concern for the equitable distribution of societal benefits and burdens (Redman & Clark, 2002). Social justice is also, albeit less often, defined as changing social relationships and institutions to promote equitable relationships (Drevdahl, Kneipp, Canales, & Dorcy, 2001). Social justice is also considered as doing what is best for an individual or group according to their needs and the fundamental principle that human beings have inalienable rights (Pacquiao, 2008). Distributive justice is fair, equitable, and appropriate distribution of resources according to justified norms that structure the terms of social cooperation (Beauchamp & Childress, 2001). Market justice posits that people are entitled only to goods and services that they acquire according to guidelines of entitlement (Young, 1990).

Upon closer examination, certain distinctions become apparent between these forms of justice. Social justice is concerned with making equitable—that is, fair and just—the balance between societal benefits and burdens. It posits that social rights exist, but that collateral responsibilities come with those rights (Lebacqz, 1986). Social beings are meant to both give and receive, using equity (being just, fair, and impartial) as a framework for relating to one another. Equity implies that persons must conduct themselves with reasonableness and moderation when exercising their rights. Distributive justice involves equality more than equity; this concept is used more often to discuss the allocation or distribution of services and goods in society (Young, 1990). Equality focuses on giving the same access and resources to different groups (Sellers and Haag, 1992). Social justice advocates explore social relationships including how those relationships form the basis for the allocation of goods and services (Young, 1990). Social justice focuses on equity, because many theories of social justice assert that "equal" does not mean "just" (Lebacqz, 1986). Thus, the concepts of social and distributive justice are somewhat parallel, yet have different primary foci of study (Drevdahl et al., 2001).

Market justice is based on honoring the rights of people who have earned entitlement to privileges. Market justice allows inequality as long as those inequalities result from a fair market system. In other words, only those who earn rights can receive their entitled privileges in a market system. Individuals who earn no rights do not have secured privileges. Rather than being a parallel model to social justice, market justice is an opposing model. These two viewpoints diametrically oppose each other yet exist simultaneously.

Although somewhat distinct, all forms of justice may coexist to varying degrees. For example, some healthcare services in the United States are given as needed, such as care to children who are orphaned. In other cases, minimal health care is given, such as the medical and dental benefits associated with Medicaid. Persons who can afford more treatment or faster treatment may get those services as well if they can pay a particular price, such as to health clinics that offer expanded services to clients who can pay access fees.

Social injustice is created by oppressive situations. Social injustice is often conceptualized as a personal act with social justice as the individual response to that act (Liaschenko, 1999; Olsen, 1993), or in a wider, more complex perspective in which unequal distribution of resources and access influences healthcare delivery, health status, and health actualization or achievement of optimal health (Austin, 2001). Social justice is fundamental to advocating for elimination of health disparities by ensuring the basic human right to access to quality health care (Pacquiao, 2008). To be effective in promoting justice, injustice must be dealt with on many fronts, specifically antecedents of injustice, the processes of injustice, and the results of injustice in society (Holland & Henriot, 1983). This concentration on the creation and recreation of injustice will help to focus attention on points of intervention. Social justice can then be addressed in terms of social justice awareness, amelioration, or transformation (Holland & Henriot, 1983).

Social justice awareness. Social justice awareness involves exploring how one perceives others as vulnerable or privileged. Awareness requires asking critical questions about how systems of domination and oppression promote categorizations such as *vulnerability* and *privilege*. Social justice awareness is temporal; an ongoing process that requires viewing from different angles, contexts, and frames of reference. Social justice awareness of an issue of major health and social concern to women may involve conducting a self-interview as well as client interviews on how the issue affects women's health. The healthcare professional would explore how health is related to the health or social issue and record her/his own thoughts prior to interviewing clients affected or not affected by the issue.

The next step would be to interview women who are and those who are not affected by the health or social issue. These women would be asked how the issue may or may not influence their health, and their thoughts would be recorded. A literature review would then be conducted on aspects of the issue and health. The initial thoughts should be compared to the knowledge gained in the interview and review of relevant literature. It is likely that awareness of the relationship between the issue and health will increase.

Social justice amelioration. Social justice amelioration entails addressing the immediate results or antecedents to unjust conditions. In the short term, social justice amelioration remedies urgent or semi-urgent concerns, but it does not change the conditions that continue to create the injustice. Amelioration requires a direct attempt to address the situation of the clients who are affected by the health or social issue. However, the situation is often addressed by treating the most immediate concerns of a person affected by the issue. The conditions that created the issue remain.

Social justice transformation. Social justice transformation involves redressing unjust conditions by changing the structures that cultivate those unjust situations. Transformation directs individual actions toward long-range, methodical solutions to unjust situations. Social justice transformation also necessitates critically deliberating about the conditions that produced the injustice. A critical exploration into the conditions that created the injustice and the relationship of the injustice to health services allocation, current health status, or future health attainment are necessary as part of any attempt to change or develop just health and social policies that would restructure the system.

A social justice agenda recognizes that vulnerable populations of women are not treated equally in society. Social justice gives moral privilege to the needs of the most vulnerable group in an effort to promote justice within society at large. As vulnerability among women is minimized or eliminated, the moral agency of those privileged can be simultaneously elevated. Social justice is an essential concept in promoting just health and social relationships for vulnerable women in society.

CULTURAL DIVERSITY AND CULTURAL COMPETENCE

Cultural diversity has become a priority in health care owing to the changing demographics and economics of the growing multicultural world and the long-standing disparities in the health status of people from culturally diverse backgrounds (Campinha-Bacote, 2003). Women from culturally diverse backgrounds are often at risk for marginalization, in which they experience discrimination, poor access to health care, and resultant illnesses and traumas from environmental dangers or violence that make them vulnerable to a wide range of health problems (Hall, 1999; Hall, Stevens, & Meleis, 1994).

Cultural competence is important and particularly useful for healthcare providers in caring for women who are vulnerable. It necessitates being sensitive to the differences in culture of one's constituents and behaving in a way that is respectful of a person's values and traditions while performing those activities or procedures necessary for the person's well-being. Cultural competence is based on an insightful understanding of culture and its substantial influence in the lives of people. This depth of understanding advances respect for, and minimizes negative consequences of, cultural differences (Pacquiao, 2008).

In the United States, care that is culturally competent is acknowledged as a pathway to remove barriers to access to health care and reduce health disparities. Promotion of cultural competence is entrenched in a commitment to preserve and protect fundamental human rights. Advocacy for social justice is intrinsic in culturally competent care of vulnerable populations. (Pacquiao, 2008).

Although the literature presents many methods and ideas for developing cultural competence, there is general agreement that cultural competence occurs on affective, cognitive, and behavioral levels, and self-awareness is a key indicator of success. A variety of methods are available for developing cultural competence in healthcare professionals. Immersion programs provide an exceptional way to induce cultural competence, although they are costly and time consuming. Immersion programs are powerful learning experiences at all levels because they enable participants to experience different cultures out of their usual safe context. Simulation is another method for developing cultural competence, and these activities provide a setting in which participants can practice communication and problem solving as well as develop self-awareness (Meltzoff & Lenssen, 2000). Cross-cultural communication exercises can help in the development of skills needed to overcome barriers in this regard (Shapiro, Hollingshead, & Morrison, 2002). Preparation of didactic materials for developing knowledge about groups is a useful point of reference for healthcare providers who provide care to diverse patients. Didactic materials frequently provide information regarding diverse cultural groups such as perceptions of illness, patterns of kinship and decision making, and comfort with touch. Multicultural training courses are also available, and are easier and less costly to operate than immersion programs.

Resilience

Resilience is the ability of individuals to adapt in the face of adversity, trauma, or tragedy. It is a characteristic that allows people to adapt to significant sources of stress that can result from family and relationship problems, or workplace and financial stressors (Newman, 2003). Resilience is also viewed as the capability to bounce back in spite of considerable stress or adversity (Place, Reynolds, Cousins, & O'Neill, 2002), and as the

ability to cope successfully despite adverse circumstances (Rutter, 1985). It is an ability to adjust easily to or recover quickly from illness, change, depression or misfortune (*American Heritage Dictionary*, 2006; *Merriam-Webster*, 2011). Resilience is viewed as both a personality trait and as a dynamic process (Luthar, Cicchetti, & Becker, 2000). This dynamic process is highly influenced by protective factors and enables people to recover from adversity and go on with their lives (Dyer & McGuinness, 1996).

Concept analyses of resilience identified antecedents and consequences of the concept. *Antecedents* are events or incidents that occur before the occurrence of the concept and *consequences* are circumstances that result from the concept (Walker & Avant, 2005). Findings indicate that the main antecedent of resilience is adversity (Earvolino-Ramirez, 2007). In addition to adversity, three other antecedents were identified. These were interpretation of the event as either physically or psychologically traumatic, the cognitive ability to interpret adversity, and a realistic worldview as opposed to false optimism or depressive attitude (Gillespie, Chaboyer, & Wallis, 2007). Consequences of resilience were found to be integration, control, adjustment, growth (Gillespie et al., 2007), effective coping, mastery, and positive adaptation (Earvolino-Ramirez, 2007). Concept analyses also revealed defining attributes, which are clusters of characteristics most frequently associated with the concept and most frequently present when the concept occurs (Walker & Avant, 2005). Defining attributes of resilience were found to be rebounding/reintegration, high expectancy/self-determination, positive relationships/social support, self-esteem/self-efficacy, flexibility, sense of humor, hope, and coping (Earvolino-Ramirez, 2007; Gillespie et al., 2007). The importance of conducting concept analyses lies in the acquisition of knowledge about the concept of resilience that contributes to the construction of theoretical models that will test the concept. Research then progresses to examine the effectiveness of strategies and interventions that enhance resilience in vulnerable populations.

Resilience has been studied in various situations of vulnerable women. For example, in an investigation of body image dissatisfaction and resilience in college women, findings suggested that women who had a positive relationship with their parents were more resilient and therefore demonstrated less body image dissatisfaction (McGrath, Wiggin, and Caron, 2010). In a phenomenological study of Asian immigrant women in the United States who survived child sexual abuse, resilience strategies reported by these women included the use of silence, sense of hope, South Asian social support, social advocacy, and intentional self-care. The findings suggested that these strategies allowed the women to heal and move on with their lives (Singh, Hays, Chung, & Watson, 2010).

Elderly women often face adversity in their older years, as evidenced by decreasing functional status, declining health, increased stress, poorer living conditions, and experiencing negative life events (Hildon, Montgomery, Blane, Wiggins, & Netuveli, 2010). Factors that are salient to resilience in older women have been identified. Having social connectedness with family, friends, and community provided a support mechanism as well as allowed older women to extend themselves to help others. Spiritual grounding was also important to older women in providing a higher power to lean on, which provided meaning and purpose to their lives. Resilient older women were found to take a "head-on" approach to adversity to move forward through life challenges (Kinsel, 2005). Terminally ill older adults facing death exhibit resilient behaviors by redefining self, embracing religion and spirituality in times of uncertainty, maintaining social relationships, and defending their independence as the end of life approaches (Nelson-Becker, 2006).

Additional research needs to be conducted on resilience and resilient attributes to enhance the resilience process in vulnerable populations of women. Obtaining increased understanding of how some women remain resilient despite facing adversity will likely lead to successful implementation of strategies and interventions for others.

Research Review

What are the ethical challenges of conducting research with vulnerable populations of women?

Mkandawire-Valhmu, L., Rice, E., & Bathum, M. (2009). Promoting an egalitarian approach to research with vulnerable populations of women. *Journal of Advanced Nursing, 65*(8), 1725–1734.

A history of human rights abuses that have occurred worldwide in human subject research has brought recognition of the need for further development of standard ethical guidelines for conducting research with human subjects. Although ethical standards have been instituted globally, and advances have been made to help protect the rights of research participants, research activities have also expanded and become more complex, especially regarding research with vulnerable populations. The need to include women, ethnic minorities, and members of other vulnerable groups, who historically have been underrepresented in research, is substantial. Scholars are thus confronted with the question of how to conduct this research in an ethical and respectful manner.

The authors used feminist qualitative research perspective in their discussion of issues surrounding conducting research with diverse populations of vulnerable women. Feminist research is a method of engaging with women during the research process and in writing about women's lives, that prevents further marginalization and contributes to their liberation.

Recognizing the need for increased understanding of low income women with limited education and limited access to health care, the authors conducted three separate but similar research studies using focus groups and individual interviews with low income women from Malawi, women diagnosed with schizophrenia in the United States, and rural indigenous Aymara women of the highlands of Peru. An important issue that came to light in the conduct of these three studies was how power disparities between researchers and participants influenced women's decisions to participate in the studies and give informed consent. The authors strongly perceived that women might have based their decisions to participate in the research studies on the unequal power between themselves and the researcher or the healthcare provider/agency worker facilitating recruitment. The authors posited that participation in research by women of lower socioeconomic strata may be done out of obligation to the researcher who is perceived as possessing greater power and privilege than themselves. Moreover, many women might be fearful of displeasing their healthcare providers, and this fear might lead them to participate in research as an effort to please their providers. Low literacy levels of women who participated in the studies were acknowledged as an influential factor associated with power differentials between the researchers and participants that affected the informed consent process.

In addition to concerns regarding women's true motivations for participating in research, the authors described dilemmas related to compensation of participants for taking part in a study. Compensation of too high a value could be perceived by participants as coercive due to their financial need, and compensation of too low a value could be perceived by participants as devaluation of their input into the research.

The authors recognized that nursing researchers need to develop and implement studies with vulnerable populations, and be cognizant that power dynamics have implications for recruitment and informed consent procedures. The authors recommend that research be guided by feminist principles, which will mandate researchers to ensure that research activities contribute to the development of policy that will positively benefit participants and their communities. Furthermore, inclusion of members of vulnerable populations in current debates that stem from ethical dilemmas in research with vulnerable populations will assist in informing policy that guides how research is conducted.

Chapter Summary Points

- Vulnerability means susceptibility. The specific implication of vulnerability in health care is to be at risk for health problems.
- Vulnerable populations have a greater-than-average risk of developing health problems by virtue of their marginalized sociocultural status, their limited access to economic resources, or their personal characteristics such as age and gender.
- On the whole women are a vulnerable population.
- Significant concepts form the conceptual basis of vulnerable populations, such as risk, social status, social capital, human capital, access to care, cost of care, and quality of care.
- These concepts influence vulnerability and are essential for understanding vulnerability as well as the nature of health care for vulnerable populations.
- Vulnerable populations commonly are affected by health disparities, which are significant differences in overall rate of disease incidence, prevalence, morbidity, mortality, or survival rates.
- Factors such as poverty; racial, ethnic, and gender inequalities; and access to health care contribute to health disparities.
- Vulnerable populations of women include high-risk mothers, the chronically ill and disabled, women with HIV/AIDS, the mentally ill and disabled, alcohol and substance abusers, women who exhibit suicidal or homicidal behavior, abused women, homeless women, immigrants and refugees, lesbian, bisexual, and transgender women, and incarcerated women.
- The care of vulnerable women can be influenced by any number of factors that can increase or diminish access to care, quality of care, and cost of care, as well as affect individual and social resources for coping with vulnerability.
- Health literacy, social justice, cultural competence, and resilience are essential areas in which intervention can promote well-being and positive quality of life outcomes in vulnerable populations of women.

Critical Thinking Exercise

Questions for Seminar Discussion

1. Discuss the meaning of vulnerability with respect to individuals and groups.
2. How can identifying a group as a vulnerable population cause further marginalization and patronization?
3. What are vulnerable populations and why are they at risk for health problems?
4. What factors marginalize women and increase their vulnerability?
5. Discuss the concepts of risk, social status, social capital, and human capital. How are these concepts linked to women as a vulnerable population?
6. Discuss access to care, cost of care, and quality of care. How are these concepts linked to women as a vulnerable population?

7. How have the changes in the demographics of populations and families over the past 5 decades influenced health disparities in women?
8. What are the specific populations of vulnerable women? What factors specifically increase their vulnerability and health disparities?
9. How do lack of literacy and health literacy influence vulnerable populations of women?
10. Discuss how social justice awareness, amelioration, and transformation might be applied to injustices experienced by vulnerable populations of women.
11. How can cultural competence remove barriers to access of care and decrease health disparities among vulnerable populations of women?
12. Discuss antecedents, consequences, and defining characteristics of resilience. How can nurses and other healthcare providers enhance the resilience of vulnerable populations of women?

Internet Resources

Administration on Aging/Administration for Community Living: information and education about home and community-based services to assist the elderly. http://www.aoa.gov

Agency for Health Research and Quality: information and education to improve the quality, safety, efficiency, and effectiveness of health care for Americans. http://www.ahrq.gov/

Centers for Disease Control and Prevention: information and education about health conditions of vulnerable women. http://www.cdc.gov/

National Academy on an Aging Society: information and education about the aging population in America. http://www.agingsociety.org/

National Alliance to End Homelessness: information and education about homelessness in the United States. http://www.endhomelessness.org/

National Center for Education Statistics: information about education and literacy in the United States. http://nces.ed.gov/

Office of Minority Health and Health Disparities: information and education about health disparities of vulnerable populations. http://www.cdc.gov/omhd/default.htm

Office of Women's Health: information and education about women's health. http://www.womenshealth.gov/

The San Diego LGBT Community Center: information and education about the lesbian, gay, bisexual, transgender, and HIV community. http://www.thecentersd.org/

U.S. Department of Health and Human Services Health Resources and Service Administration: information and education about health literacy. http://www.hrsa.gov/publichealth/healthliteracy/index.html

Women's Prison Association: information and education about women and criminal justice. http://www.wpaonline.org

References

Aday, L. (2001). *At risk in America*. San Francisco, CA: Jossey-Bass.

Agency for Health care Research and Quality. (2004). Literacy and health outcomes (Evidence Report/Technology Assessment No. 87). Retrieved from www.ahrq.gov

American Medical Association. (1999). Health literacy report of the Council on Scientific Affairs Ad Hoc Committee on Health Literacy. *Journal of the American Medical Association, 10*(6), 552–557.

Arthur, S., Geiser, H., Arriola, K., & Kripalani, S. (2009). Health literacy and control in the medical encounter. A mixed-method analysis. *Journal of the National Medical Association, 101*(7), 677–683.

Austin, W. (2001). Nursing ethics in an era of globalization. *Advances in Nursing Science, 24*, 1–18.

Baker, D., Gazmararian, J., Williams, M., Scott, T., Parker, R., Green, D., ... Peel, J. (2002). Functional health literacy and the risk of hospital admission among Medicare managed care enrollees. *American Journal of Public Health, 92*(8), 1278–1283.

Beauchamp, T., & Childress, J. (2001). *Principles of biomedical ethics* (5th ed.). New York: Oxford University Press.

Berberet, H. (2005). The San Diego LGBT Community Center lesbian bisexual and transgender needs assessment 2005. Retrieved from http://www.thecentersd.org/programs/womens-resource-center/wrc-needs-assessment.pdf

Campinha-Bacote, J. (2003). Many faces: Addressing diversity in health care. *The Online Journal of Issues in Nursing, 18*(1), Manuscript 2. Retrieved from www.nursingworld.org/MainMenuCategories/ANAMarketplace/ANAPeriodicals/OJIN/TableofContents/Volume8 2003/No1Jan2003/AddressingDiversityinHealthCare.aspx

Centers for Disease Control and Prevention. (2010). Understanding suicide. Fact sheet 2010. Retrieved from http://www.cdc.gov/ViolencePrevention/pdf/suicide-FactSheet-a.pdf

Centers for Disease Control and Prevention. (2011). Health, United States, 2010: With special feature on death and dying. Retrieved from http://www.cdc.gov/nchs/data/hus/hus10.pdf

Centers for Disease Control and Prevention. (2012a). Suicide: Facts at a glance. Retrieved from http://www.cdc.gov/violenceprevention/pdf/Suicide-DataSheet-a.pdf

Centers for Disease Control and Prevention. (2012b). Understanding intimate partner violence. Fact sheet 2012. Retrieved from http://www.cdc.gov/violenceprevention/pdf/IPV_factsheet-a.pdf

Centers for Disease Control and Prevention. (2013a). Burden of mental illness. Retrieved from http://www.cdc.gov/mentalhealth/basics/burden.htm

Centers for Disease Control and Prevention. (2013b). Health considerations for newly arrived immigrants and refugees. Retrieved from http://wwwnc.cdc.gov/travel/yellowbook/2014/chapter-9-health-considerations-for-newly-arrived/before-arrival-in-the-united-states

Centers for Disease Control and Prevention. (2014a). About teen pregnancy. Retrieved from http://www.cdc.gov/teenpregnancy/AboutTeenPreg.htm

Centers for Disease Control and Prevention. (2014b). Excessive alcohol use and risks to women's health. Retrieved from http://www.cdc.gov//alcohol/fact-sheets/womens-health.htm

Centers for Disease Control and Prevention. (2014c). National Homeless Person's Memorial Day. Retrieved from http://www.cdc.gov/Features/Homelessness/index.html

Centers for Disease Control and Prevention. (2014d). Women with disability. Retrieved from http://www.cdc.gov/ncbddd/disabilityandhealth/women.html

Centers for Disease Control and Prevention. (2015). HIV among women. Retrieved from http://www.cdc.gov/hiv/risk/gender/women/index.html

Clark, J., Herbert, M., Rosengard, C., Rose, J., DaSilva, K., & Stein, M. (2006). Reproductive health care and family planning needs among incarcerated women. *American Journal of Public Health, 96*(5), 834-838.

Cochran, S. (2012). Lesbian and bisexual health fact sheet. Retrieved from http://www.womenshealth.gov/publications/our-publications/fact-sheet/lesbian-bisexual-health.cfm

Cutilli, C. (2007). Health literacy in geriatric patients: An integrative review of literature. *Orthopaedic Nursing, 26*(1), 43–48.

Doak, C., Doak, L., & Root, J. (2001). *Teaching patients with low literacy skills* (2nd ed.). Philadelphia: Lippincott, Williams, & Wilkins.

Drevdahl, D., Kneipp, S., Canales, M., & Dorcy, K. (2001). Reinvesting in social justice: A capital idea for public health nursing. *Advances in Nursing Science, 24*, 19–31.

Duncan, G., Daly, M., McDonough, P., & Williams, D. (2002). Optimal indicators of socioeconomic status for health research. *American Journal of Public Health, 92*(7), 1151–1158.

Dutton, L., Koenig, K., & Fennie, K. (2008). Gynecologic care of the female to male transgender man. *Journal of Midwifery and Women's Health, 53*, 331–337.

Dyer, J., & McGuinness, T. (1996). Resilience: An analysis of the concept. *Archives of Psychiatric Nursing, 10*(5), 276–282.

Earvolino-Ramirez, M. (2007). Resilience: A concept analysis. *Nursing Forum, 42*(2), 73–82.

Fobis S., & Aligne, C. (2002). Poor readability of asthma management plans found in national guidelines. *Pediatrics, 109,* e52.

Glassman, P. (2014). Health literacy. Retrieved from http://nnlm.gov/outreach/consumer/hlthlit.html

Gillespie, B., Chaboyer, W., & Wallis, M. (2007). Development of a theoretically derived model of resilience through concept analysis. *Contemporary Nurse, 25*(1), 124–135.

Hall, J. (1999). Marginalization revisited: Critical, post-modern, and liberation perspectives. *Advances in Nursing Science, 22*(1), 88–102.

Hall, J., Stevens, P., & Meleis, A. (1994). Marginalization: A guiding concept for valuing diversity in nursing knowledge development. *Advances in Nursing Science, 16*(4), 23–41.

Hildon, Z., Montgomery, S., Blane, D., Wiggins, R., & Netuveli, G. (2010). Examining resilience of quality of life in the face of health-related and psychosocial adversity of older ages: What is "right" about the way we age? *Gerontologist, 50*(1), 36–47.

Hofferth, S. (2003). The American family: Changes and challenges for the 21st century. In H. Wallace, G. Green, & K. Jaros (Eds.), *Health and welfare for families in the 21st century.* (pp. 71–79). Sudbury, MA: Jones & Bartlett.

Holland, J., & Henriot, P. (1983). *Social analysis: Linking faith and justice.* Maryknoll, NY: Orbis Books.

Institute of Medicine (IOM). (2003). *Priority areas for national action: Transforming health care quality.* Washington, DC: National Academies Press.

Katz, M., Jacobson, E., & Kripalani, S. (2007). Patient literacy and question-asking behavior during the medical encounter: A mixed-methods analysis. *Journal of General Internal Medicine, 22*(6), 782–786.

Kinsel, B. (2005). Resilience as adaptation in older women. *Journal of Women & Aging, 17*(3), 23–39.

Kirsch, I., Jungeblut, A., Jenkins, L., & Kolstad, A. (2002). Adult literacy in America: A first look at the findings of the National Adult literacy Survey (3rd ed.). Retrieved from http://nces.ed.gov/pubs93/93275.pdf

Lebacqz, K. (1986). *Six theories of justice.* Minneapolis, MN: Augsburg.

Liaschenko, J. (1999). Can justice coexist with the supremacy of personal values in nursing practice? *Western Journal of Nursing Research, 21*(1), 35–50.

Luthar, S., Cicchetti, D., & Becker, B. (2000). The construct of resilience: A critical evaluation and guidelines for future work. *Child Development, 71*(3), 543–562.

McGrath, R., Wiggin, J., & Caron, R. (2010). The relationship between resilience and body image in college women. *Internet Journal of Health, 10*(2), 21p, 2010588933.

Meltzoff, N., & Lenssen, J. (2000). Enhancing cultural competence through simulation activities. *Multicultural Perspectives, 2*(1), 29–35.

Mkandawire-Valhmu, L., Rice, E., & Bathum, M. (2009). Promoting an egalitarian approach to research with vulnerable populations of women. *Journal of Advanced Nursing, 65*(8), 1725–1734.

National Academy on an Aging Society. (2015). Fact sheet: Low health literacy skills increase annual health care expenditures by $73 billion. Retrieved from http://www.agingsociety.org/agingsociety/publications/fact/fact_low.html

National Alliance to End Homelessness. (2015). Domestic violence. Retrieved from http://www.endhomelessness.org/pages/domestic_violence

National Center for Education Statistics. (2015). National assessment of adult literacy. Retrieved from http://nces.ed.gov/NAAL/index.asp?file=AssessmentOf/Health/HealthLiteracyResults.asp&PageID=158

National Institute of Mental Health. (2015). Women and mental health. Retrieved from http://www.nimh.nih.gov/health/topics/women-and-mental-health/index.shtml

Nelson-Becker, H. (2006). Voices of resilience: Older adults in hospice care. *Journal of Social Work in End-of-Life & Palliative Care, 2*(3), 87–106.

Newman, R. (2003). Providing direction on the road to resilience. *Behavioral Health Management, 23*(4), 42–43.

Office of the Surgeon General. (2005). Surgeon general's workshop on women's mental health. Retrieved from http://www.surgeongeneral.gov/topics/womensmentalhealth/#01

Olsen, D. (1993). Populations vulnerable to the ethics of caring. *Journal of Advanced Nursing, 18,* 1696–1700.

Pacquiao, D. (2008). Nursing care of vulnerable populations using a framework of cultural competence, social justice, and human rights. *Contemporary Nurse, 28,* 189–197.

Paasche-Orlow, M., Parker, R., Gazmararian, J., Neilsen-Bohlman, L., & Rudd, R. (2005). The prevalence of limited health literacy. *Journal of General Internal Medicine, 20,* 175–184.

Paulozzi, L., Saltzman, L., Thompson, M., & Holmgreen, P. (2001). Surveillance for homicide among intimate partners–United States, 1981–1998. *MMWR, 50*(S S 03), 1–6. Retrieved from http://www.cdc.gov/mmwr/preview/mmwrhtml/ss5003a1.htm

Place, M., Reynolds, J., Cousins, A., & O'Neill, S. (2002). Developing a resilience package for vulnerable children. *Child and Adolescent Mental Health, 7*(4), 162–167.

Redman, R., & Clark, L. (2002). Service-learning as a model for integrating social justice in the nursing curriculum. *Journal of Nursing Education, 41*, 446–449.

Resilience. (2006). The American heritage dictionary of the English language (4th ed.). Retrieved from http://dictionary.reference.com/browse/resilience

Resilience. (2011). Merriam-Webster online dictionary. Retrieved from http://www.merriam-webster.com/dictionary/resilience

Ruiz, A., Zong, J., & Batalova, J. (2015). Immigrant women in the United States. Retrieved from http://www.migrationpolicy.org/article/immigrant-women-united-states#Age and Marital Status

Rutter, M. (1985). Resilience in the face of adversity: protective factors and resistance to psychiatric disorders. *British Journal of Psychiatry, 147*, 598–611.

Scanlon, A., & Lee, G. (2007). The use of the term vulnerability in acute care: Why does it differ and what does it mean? *Australian Journal of Advanced Nursing, 24*(3), 54–59.

Schillinger, D., Piette, J., Grumbach, K., Wang, F., Willson, C., Daher, C., … Bindman, A. (2003). Physician communication with diabetic patients who have low literacy. *Archives of Internal Medicine, 163*(1), 83–90.

Sellers, S., & Haag, B. (1992). Achieving equity in nursing education. *Nursing and Health Care, 13*(3), 134–137.

Sentencing Project. (2007). Women in the criminal justice system. Retrieved from http://www.sentencingproject.org/doc/publications/womenincj_total.pdf

Sidhu, J., & Floyd, R. (2002). Alcohol use among women of childbearing age, 1991–1999. *MMWR Weekly, 51*(13), 273–276. Retrieved from http://www.cdc.gov/mmwr/preview/mmwrhtml/mm5113a2.htm

Shapiro, J., Hollingshead, J., & Morrison, E. (2002). Primary care resident, faculty, and patient views of barriers to cultural competence and skills needed to overcome them. *Medical Education, 36*, 749–759.

Simmons, L., Havens, J., Whiting, J., Holz, J., & Bada H. (2009). Illicit drug use among women with children in the United States: 2002–2003. *Annals of Epidemiology, 19*(3), 187–193.

Singh, A., Hays, D., Chung, Y., & Watson, L. (2010). South Asian immigrant women who have survived child sexual abuse: resilience and healing. *Violence against Women, 16*(4), 444–458.

Southern Poverty Law Center (2011). Immigrant women. Retrieved from http://www.splcenter.org/what-we-do/immigrant-justice/in-this-section/immigrant-women

U.S. Department of Health and Human Services. (2000). *Healthy People 2010: Understanding and improving health.* Washington, DC: National Academies Press.

U.S. Department of Health and Human Services, Administration for Community Living. (2015). Administration on Aging (AoA): Future growth. Retrieved from http://www.aoa.acl.gov/Aging_Statistics/Profile/2013/4.aspx

Walker, L., & Avant K. (2005). *Strategies for theory construction in nursing* (4th ed.). Upper Saddle River, NJ: Pearson Prentice Hall.

Williams, M., Baker, D., Honig, E., Lee, T., & Nowlan, A. (1998). Inadequate literacy as a barrier to asthma knowledge and self-care. *Chest, 114*, 1008–1015.

Womens Prison Association. (2009). Quick facts: Women & criminal justice-2009. Retrieved from http://www.wpaonline.org/wpaassets/Quick_Facts_Women_and_CJ_2009_rebrand.pdf

Young, I. (1990). *Justice and the politics of difference.* Princeton, NJ: Princeton University Press.

Chapter 4

Enhancing Women's Health, Wellness, and Quality of Life

LEARNING OUTCOMES

On completion of this chapter, the learner will be able to:

1. Explain factors that contribute to stress in women.
2. Describe measures for stress relief and enhancement of well-being in women.
3. Analyze the effects of obesity and overweight on health, wellness, and quality of life.
4. Explain the importance of nutrition and healthful diet for disease prevention and enhancement of well-being and quality of life.
5. Distinguish the importance of physical activity for disease prevention, health promotion, and enhancement of quality of life.
6. Describe complementary and alternative therapeutic modalities that may reduce risk of disease, promote well-being, and enhance quality of life.

Introduction

Women's lifestyles have changed dramatically over the past several decades. The accelerated and hectic pace of women's lives exposes them to frequent and intense stress. Some common intense stressors that women face daily include managing multiple role demands, experiencing conflicting domestic and employment related responsibilities, dealing with rapid and abrupt cultural and technological changes, and navigating an uncertain economy. An estimated 43% of all adults suffer adverse health effects associated with stress, and 75% to 90% of all visits to primary care physicians are for complaints or disorders related to stress (American Psychological Association, 2007). Stress has been linked to the six leading causes of death: heart disease, cancer, lung ailments, accidents, liver cirrhosis, and suicide. Stress has also been declared a workplace hazard by the Occupational Safety and Health Administration (American Psychological Association, 2007).

Within the American population, an indicative sign of stress is the ever-expanding waistline. Alarmingly, obesity has reached epidemic proportions. Average Americans consume more food and exercise considerably less than Americans in previous generations. Despite evidence documenting the fact that healthful eating and regular exercise help people live longer, healthier, happier lives, many women continue to follow unhealthful eating patterns and lead sedentary lives. Along with these dramatic changes in women's lifestyles, various indices of health have spiraled even further downward: cancer, diabetes, heart disease, and scores of stress-related illnesses. Without a doubt, stress, obesity, and physical inactivity can substantially impact women's health, well-being, and quality of life.

This chapter explores stress, weight maintenance, and physical activity and the overall role these factors play in influencing women's health, well-being, and quality of life. The role of stress reduction, healthful diet, and regular exercise in the maintenance of health and well-being are highlighted. Selected complementary and alternative therapeutic modalities that women commonly use to promote health, prevent disease, and enhance well-being and quality of life are also explored.

Stress

Stress is the experience of a perceived, real, or imagined threat to one's mental, physical, emotional, or spiritual well-being, which results in a series of physiological responses and adaptations known as the stress response. The stress response is comprised of several physiological mechanisms which, when activated, prepare the body to defend itself against, or escape from, a perceived threat (fight-or-flight response). The fight-or-flight response consists of four stages:

Stage 1: The brain receives stimuli from one or more of the five senses—for example, a scream, the smell of smoke, or the sight of an oncoming car veering out of control.

Stage 2: The brain interprets the stimulus as either a threat or non-threat. If the stimulus is interpreted as a non-threat, the response ends. If the stimulus is deciphered as an actual threat, the brain then activates the nervous and endocrine system to quickly prepare for defense and/or escape.

Stage 3: The body remains in a state of arousal until the threat is resolved.

Stage 4: The body returns to homeostasis, which is a state of physiological calmness, once the threat is gone.

Adrenaline and cortisol, released during the stress response, produce a variety of physical responses for the preparation of movement and energy production. A summary of these physiological responses is presented in **Box 4–1**.

Box 4–1: Physiological Responses to Stress

- Elevation in heart rate to pump oxygenated blood to working muscles
- Elevation in blood pressure to deliver blood to working muscles
- Increase in respiratory rate to supply working muscles with oxygen for energy metabolism
- Peripheral vasodilatation of arteries in areas of greatest muscle mass (arms and legs)
- Elevation of serum glucose for metabolic processes during muscle contractions
- Mobilization of free fatty acids as an energy source for prolonged activity (such as running)
- Increase in blood coagulation and decrease in clotting times in the event of bleeding

- Increase in muscular strength
- Decrease in gastric movement and abdominal blood flow to increase perfusion to vital organs and working muscles
- Increase in perspiration to cool body core temperature

Types of Stress

Stress can be perceived as a positive motivating or inspiring factor—a factor that is neither positive nor negative with no consequential effect—or a negative factor, termed *distress*. Distress is often abbreviated as simply stress, and can be acute or chronic. Acute stress is the type that surfaces, is quite intense, and disappears quickly. Acute stress can be helpful for energizing or motivating a person. Chronic stress does not appear so intense, yet lingers for prolonged periods of time. Chronic stress can overload a person and cause emotional symptoms such as edginess and distorted thinking. Chronic stress is believed to be the type of stress associated with disease because the body experiences prolonged exposure to the physiological effects of the stress response. It is believed that as much as 70% to 85% of all diseases and illnesses are stress related.

Stress is experienced when an individual is exposed to any type of stressor. A stressor is a situation that causes or promotes stress. Any situation that is perceived as a threat is a stressor, and this can vary considerably from person to person. Stressors can range from daily annoyances to life altering events, and how individuals experience and react to them depends on how the stressor is perceived. Acute stress is frequently caused by rapid-onset stressors that may occur unexpectedly. The stress response is usually set in motion before a full analysis of the situation is made, but ultimately the body will return to a calm state. Chronic stressors may give some advance warning yet manage to cause physical arousal nevertheless. Chronic stressors frequently merit more attention because their prolonged physical impact is likely more significant. Some of the most common stressful life events in women's lives are presented in **Box 4–2**.

Box 4–2: Common Stressful Life Events

Common stressful life events in women's lives include:

- Death of a spouse
- Death of a close family member
- Divorce
- Losing a job
- Major personal illness or injury
- Marital separation

(continues)

The Wellness Perspective

Wellness is the balance, integration, and harmony of the physical, intellectual, emotional, and spiritual aspects of the human condition. As such, the four components of total well-being, physical, mental, emotional, and spiritual, are closely linked and interwoven into one interconnected living system. While for the purposes of academic study these parts are often approached separately, in reality the whole is greater than the sum of the parts and all parts must be considered as one system. When applied to maintenance of health, this holistic wellness perspective indicates that all aspects of an individual must be treated equally and each considered part of the whole. Stress profoundly affects all components of wellness in the following ways.

Stress and Physical Well-Being

Physical well-being is described as the optimal functioning of the major physiological systems. As previously noted, the effects of prolonged stress can be harmful due to repeated or extended exposure of the body to the physiological effects of the stress response. During the stress response, adrenaline and cortisol increase blood pressure, heart rate, and blood sugar levels. As a result, chronic stress can contribute to the development of a variety of health problems. These include mental health disorders (such as depression and anxiety), obesity,

heart disease, high blood pressure, cardiac arrhythmias, menstrual problems, and acne and other skin problems (Office on Women's Health [OWH], 2010).

Although the body can adapt to the physiological effects of chronic stress, pathological repercussions can occur, ultimately causing disease. Selye (1978) studied the physiological effects of chronic stress and identified the General Adaptation Syndrome as adaptations that occur in the body as a result of repeated exposure to stress. These stress-induced changes are presented in **Box 4–3**. Many of these physiological changes are subtle and often go unnoticed until permanent damage has occurred. In the General Adaptation Syndrome, the body tries to accommodate stress by adjusting to it. Selye (1978) described the following three stages of the general adaptation syndrome.

Stage of alarm reaction. In the stage of alarm reaction, the first stage of the stress response is activated and the classic fight-or-flight response occurs. Several body systems are activated. Initially, the nervous system and endocrine system respond, followed by the cardiovascular, pulmonary, and musculoskeletal systems.

Stage of resistance. In the stage of resistance, the body endeavors to revert to a state of homeostasis. However, because the perception of threat continues, complete homeostasis is not obtained. The body remains activated or aroused, usually at a

Box 4–3: Physiological Adaptations Resulting From Repeated Exposures to Stress

- Enlargement of the adrenal cortex
- Constant release of stress hormones; corticosteroids released from the adrenal cortex
- Atrophy or shrinkage of lymphatic glands (thymus gland, spleen, and lymph nodes)
- Significant decrease in white blood cell count
- Bleeding ulcerations of the stomach and colon
- Death of the organism

lesser intensity than experienced during the alarm stage, but enough to cause a higher metabolic rate in some organ tissues. One or more organs may, in effect, remain activated, and as a result, enter the third and final stage.

Stage of exhaustion. During this stage, one or more of the body's organs targeted by specific metabolic processes can no longer meet the demands placed upon it. The organ or organs fail to function properly. This can result in failure or death of the organ. Depending upon which organ fails or dies (such as the heart), this can result in the death of the organism as a whole.

Stress and Mental Well-Being

Mental or intellectual well-being is considered as the ability to gather, process, recall, and exchange or communicate information. Exposure to stress can impair cognitive function and decrease the processing and recall abilities needed to make sound decisions, as well as the ability to communicate them. Stress can impair one's ability to focus, concentrate, and remember. Evidence suggests that cognitive dysfunction is likely attributed to the effects of the stress hormones cortisol and noradrenalin on the prefrontal cortex of the brain, which controls working

memory and is where new information is processed and stored (Institute of HeartMath, 2014).

Stress and Emotional Well-Being

Emotional well-being is the ability to feel and express the entire range of human emotions and control them without being controlled by them. The range of human emotions spans a continuum from anger to love and every emotion in between. From a holistic perspective, the expression of all emotions is considered healthy, since denying the ability to feel and express any emotion suggests an emotional imbalance. Expression of emotions allows a release of feelings, known as a catharsis.

Positive emotions such as joy, bliss, and love are considered by many people as healthy emotions, whereas anger and fear are thought of as unhealthy. Actually, anger and fear are also healthy emotions when used specifically for their intended purpose, to get out of harm's way. Both anger and fear are survival emotions, intended to last long enough to get out of physical danger. Healthy emotions can quickly become unhealthy when they remain longer than the intended purpose for which they serve. Left unresolved, unhealthy emotions can cause serious problems in the mind-body-spirit dynamics of optimal health.

Ideally, anger, fear, and the various ways these emotions manifest are protective. When danger is sensed, these emotions summon an alarm to move rapidly into a state of physical survival. Both anger and fear are intended to last long enough to remove an individual from physical danger, be it seconds or minutes, not much longer. When feelings of anger or fear linger beyond the amount of time needed to reach a place of safety, emotions are not controlled, rather emotions become controlling. This can compromise emotional well-being. Retaining feelings of anger or fear instead of letting these feelings go can make individuals feel emotionally drained, which signifies that the healthy emotion has become unhealthy. Prolonged anger, fear, grief, and depression are classic and common examples of the unhealthy emotions that are widespread among women in today's society.

Anger and fear are key stress emotions. Anger is the fight response and fear is the flight response. Anger is manifested in various ways, such as guilt, envy, impatience, indignation, intimidation, intolerance, frustration, rage, prejudice, and hostility. Fear is also manifested in numerous ways, such as doubt, embarrassment, anxiety, apprehension, insecurity, and paranoia. Anger and fear are widespread throughout society and are a part of the human landscape.

Often anger is suppressed, which can result in the development of various physical problems, such as migraine headaches, ulcers, liver problems, hypertension, and rheumatoid arthritis. Women more than men tend to suppress anger. Some people feel guilty about feeling angry and substitute feelings of anger for obsessive behaviors, such as excessive eating, excessive drinking, excessive shopping, and sex. People who self-mutilate are thought to be punishing themselves for their anger, substituting cutting behaviors for anger. Some people mismanage anger through explosive or aggressive behavior. Using intimidation as a main outlet of anger, individuals may engage in road rage, foul language, bullying, or hostility in response to a perceived threat. Explosive behavior is more common in men but can be exhibited in women as well. Some mismanage anger through passive-aggressive behavior. Sarcasm is a common manifestation of this type of mismanaged anger. In each of these types of mismanaged anger, prolongerd anger results in individuals being controlled by their anger rather than being able to control it.

Fear is a response to physical danger, yet it is rare that individuals encounter actual physical danger that would require a person to run and hide. Nevertheless, the emotion is there in the event circumstances require it. In today's society, self-promoted feelings of fear and worry are prevalent. The reasons are associated more with a perceived sense of failure, rejection, and the unknown than to any actual physical danger. Some common pervasive chronic stressors associated with fear and anxiety include credit card debt, struggling relationships, loss of a job, and terminal illness. Whereas anger is an energizing emotion, fear is energy-depleting. Nonetheless, like unresolved anger, over time, chronic fear and the stress hormones associated with it can be toxic to the body.

It is important to reiterate that not all stress is bad. Good stress is an essential part of life, as are all emotions associated with it. Joy, compassion, love, and happiness are indispensable to optimal health. These emotions generate an entire pharmacopeia of beneficial neuropeptides that enhance the immune system. Emotional well-being is actually a balance of emotional experiences. If a balance of the full emotional spectrum with frequent exposure to the emotions associated with good stress is not sought, then all aspects of one's personal wellness paradigm are affected. Thus, combining peak experiences, joyful moments, and comic relief with an array of coping skills and relaxation techniques is fundamental for maintaining emotional well-being.

Stress and Spiritual Well-Being

Spiritual well-being is regarded as the maturation of higher consciousness through the development of a strong personal value system, a meaningful purpose in life, and having strong, insightful, nurturing relationships with both one's self and others. Stress can produce a series of obstacles on the path to spiritual development, making the path to one's higher self more difficult if not entirely inaccessible. These obstacles, which can be specific or abstract human characteristics and/or related behaviors, undermine the maturation process of human spirituality to the detriment of spiritual health and total well-being. Obstacles to spiritual maturation may include laziness, greed, despair, anger, fear, low self-esteem, unresolved loss, substance addictions, and co-dependency. These obstacles perpetuate the stress response. One of the most significant obstacles to spiritual evolution is the stress emotion fear. While obstacles may impede the progress of one's spiritual maturation, distractions can derail spiritual maturation, sometimes indefinitely. Distractions are behaviors and/or material possessions that divert individuals from making progress on their spiritual path.

Whereas behavioral changes such as smoking cessation and eating a balanced diet can enhance physical well-being, intervention techniques can be employed to enhance the development of inner resources and behaviors associated with spiritual health. A common intervention is meditation, which includes many styles of increasing self-awareness. Meditation, along with other techniques that reduce stress and enhance physical, mental, emotional, and spiritual well-being will be discussed later in this chapter.

Similarities and Differences in Gender Response to Stress

Women in contemporary society face special stressors. Many women, including those with young children, are members of the paid workforce. Yet women are still more likely than men to assume the majority of domestic responsibilities in caring for dependent family members and in doing household chores. Juggling domestic responsibilities with employment responsibilities can sap women of their energy and cause stress that affects both their home life and their work life.

The fight-or-flight response is considered the prototypic human response to stress. Although fight-or-flight may characterize the primary physiological responses to stress for both men and women, it has been posited that behaviorally, responses to stress by women are more marked by a pattern of "tend and befriend" (Taylor et al., 2000). *Tending* involves nurturing activities that are designed to protect the self and offspring and that promote safety and reduce distress. *Befriending* refers to the creation and maintenance of social networks that may aid in this process (Taylor et al., 2000). As such, while both men and women have a built-in dynamic for survival of physical danger, women also have an inherent nurturing response for their offspring and a means to befriend others. As a result, women are more prone to create a strong social support system, which is an invaluable coping technique.

It is believed that the female response to stress is tied into their DNA and manifested through a combination of brain chemistry and hormones—in particular, oxytocin. Evidence suggests that oxytocin is associated with calming, relaxation, and increased sociability, which is believed to enhance nurturing and befriending tendencies in women. Oxytocin is released in women and, to a lesser degree, in men, in response to stress. The effects of oxytocin are enhanced by estrogen in the female brain and are inhibited by androgens in the male brain. Male response to stress, on the other hand, is associated with sympathetic arousal enhanced by testosterone, which is associated with increased aggression that augments the fight response to stress (Taylor et al., 2000). Thus, while male response to stress is prone to sympathetic arousal and to a fight-or-flight pattern that is, at least in part, organized and activated via androgens, female stress responses do not show these androgen links. Instead, female stress responses may be tied, at least in part, to the release of oxytocin and its biobehavioral associations to caregiving behavior. Oxytocin is posited to trigger attachment processes between mothers and offspring, and it may also be implicated in other close social bonds (Taylor et al., 2000).

Not only do women and men differ in their stress physiology, they frequently perceive, appraise, and respond to stress differently. Women tend to internalize their stress, which can lead to feelings of failure and self-blame. Women are more likely to experience physical symptoms of stress than men. In response to stress, women tend to take care of those closest to them and draw support from family and friends. Men are more likely to have the fight-or-flight response, whereby they cope by "escaping" into a relaxing activity or distraction (OWH, 2010). Men might respond positively with physical activity, or negatively with aggression and substance abuse.

There also seem to be gender-specific behaviors associated with discussing and solving problems. Men tend to think their way through by looking for solutions to problems, whereas women tend to prefer talking about their problems. Women bond quickly by sharing confidences. However, the downside of talking about stressors is that merely talking about them tends to perpetuate rather than solve one's stressors. While talking may strengthen female friendships, it might also increase anxiety and depression if solutions are not introduced quickly.

Coping With Stress

When a situation or event is perceived as a stressor, an individual will likely feel vulnerable and threatened. In order to survive the threat, whether minimal or substantial, a coping strategy is employed to manage the stress. Each stressor will require its own coping strategy. For most people, some coping strategies are second nature when a minimal

stressor is encountered. A course of action is taken with little or no conscious thought given. However, when numerous stressors of increasing intensity are encountered with manifestation of a great deal of tension, routine coping strategies may be ineffective. This may result in feelings of mental fatigue, immobilization, and mental paralysis until a more effective coping strategy or combination of strategies is engaged.

Coping is the process of managing demands that are judged as taxing or exceeding an individual's resources (Lazarus & Folkman, 1984). Coping is comprised of both cognitive and behavioral efforts in order to manage the stressor. The managing process involves some or all of the following: an increased awareness process of oneself, the situation, and the environment; palliative coping, which is an emotional regulation process; and instrumental coping, which is a series of behavioral changes (Lazarus & Folkman, 1984). Coping does not just involve using one or several techniques. It also involves possessing and implementing a frame of mind of self-efficacy, which is the belief that one can successfully accomplish a specific task. Self-efficacy allows access to inner resources including self-confidence, faith, willpower, and self-reliance. The possession and implementation of self-efficacy tends to divide those who choose effective coping strategies from those who choose non-effective coping strategies. One's dominant coping style may be a function of one's personality.

Each stressor undergoes primary appraisal to determine the extent of damage. Then the stressor undergoes a secondary appraisal, and a series of coping responses are aligned with the stressor to see which would be the best course of action. These coping responses may be action oriented (time management or assertive behavior) or intrapsychic (acceptance). The responses used to cope with stress may result from internal resources or external resources. Inner resources may include characteristics such as willpower, sense of humor, creativity, sense of reason, self-efficacy, faith, and optimism. External resources may include time, money, and social support from friends and family (Lazarus & Folkman, 1984).

Coping skills can enable an individual to reduce harmful environmental conditions and/or tolerate or adjust to negative events or realities. Coping skills enable an individual to maintain a positive self-image and to maintain emotional equilibrium and satisfying relationships with others. Coping responses can bring about three outcomes: to regain emotional status quo, to resume normal activities interrupted by the stressor, or to feel psychologically overwhelmed (Lazarus & Folkman, 1984).

Coping strategies that are successful in dealing with the cause of perceived stressors necessitate four basic components. The first component is an increased awareness of the stressor, which requires a clear focus and full perspective of the situation at hand. Stressors tend to encourage a myopic view that distorts both focus and perspective. An effective coping strategy will clarify the true nature of the problem and open one's view to a host of possibilities. The second component involves some aspect of information processing. The dynamics of information processing involve adding, subtracting, changing, and manipulating sensory input to deactivate the perception of the stressor before physical damage occurs. This necessitates a secondary appraisal. Information processing also encompasses assessing all available resources that can be employed in peaceful confrontation. The third component involves the results of information processing, which will likely include a new series of actions or modified behaviors. These actions, combined with the new cognitive approach, engage the stressor from all sides. The fourth component, and perhaps the most important, is peaceful resolution.

An effective coping strategy must work toward a satisfactory resolution. Without successful resolution of the stressor, the coping technique will be less effective. Even though some coping strategies may appear appropriate for a specific situation, they may not achieve a peaceful resolution, in which case a new strategy should be selected.

Coping strategies may be positive or negative. Positive coping strategies are effective in dealing with stress through accomplishing a peaceful resolution. The goal of an effective strategy is not merely to survive but thrive in the face of adversity. On the other hand, negative coping strategies provide no enlightened resolution. They perpetuate perceptions of stress and further ineffective responses in a vicious circle. Negative coping strategies include avoidance of the problem or inhibition of action, victimization, emotional immobility (worrying), hostile aggression, and self-destructive addictive behaviors, such as drinking, drugs, and food binging.

Certain personality types are associated with certain coping strategies. People who exhibit Type A behaviors, codependent behaviors, and helpless–hopeless behaviors are likely to make use of a negative coping style and feel victimized by their stressors. On the other hand, people who exhibit components of a hardy personality, self-actualization or sensation seeking (Type R), are more likely to confront rather than avoid problems, take calculated risks, and see their stressors through to peaceful resolution.

Hundreds of coping strategies exist. Each may be used alone, or several may be used together for a stronger defense against the effects of perceived stress. There are numerous positive coping strategies from which to choose. The strategies that particularly emphasize increased awareness and information processing include journaling, art therapy, cognitive restructuring, humor therapy, dream therapy, and creative problem solving. Coping skills that emphasize behavior change or implementing a course of action include time management, assertiveness training, social orchestration, and communication skills. It is important to note that coping techniques are skills, and as such, their effectiveness increases with practice. No coping strategy will work as a defense against all perceived stress. It is important to have as wide an assortment of strategies as possible from which to choose in order to facilitate resolution of stressors.

Overweight and Obesity

Maintaining a healthy weight requires attaining balance between the amount of calories consumed and the amount of calories burned by physical activities. Body weight can be evaluated by calculating a weight-for-height ratio, or body mass index (BMI). The BMI is calculated by dividing the body weight in pounds by height in inches squared, multiplied by 703. This measurement is closely correlated with total body fat, but does not measure body fat. A person who has a large body frame, a lot of muscle mass, and little fat may have a BMI above the healthy range but may still be healthy. Women who have an abundance of fat and little muscle mass may have a BMI in the healthy range but may not be at their healthy weight. BMI results and their designations are presented in **Table 4–1**. Estimations of body fat and body fat distribution may also be done with measurements of skinfold thickness and waist circumference, calculation of waist-to-hip circumference ratios, and techniques such as ultrasound, computed tomography, and magnetic resonance imaging (MRI) (Centers for Disease Control and Prevention [CDC], 2012a).

In addition to total weight, weight distribution is a significant concern. A person with body fat distribution that favors the upper body is referred to as "apple" shaped. A person with body fat distribution that favors the hips and thighs is referred to as "pear" shaped, and this is generally subcutaneous fat. Women with apple-shaped body fat distribution tend to develop considerable visceral fat and are at higher risk for developing type 2 diabetes, coronary artery disease, hypertension, gallbladder disease, and polycystic ovarian syndrome (Savard &

Svec, 2005). Waist measurement is also a loose indicator for risk of developing heart disease, cancer, and other chronic diseases. Women with a waist size greater than 35 inches and men with a waist size greater than 40 inches likely have higher risk for developing such diseases.

Causes of Weight Gain

The causes of weight gain are multifaceted. Body weight is influenced by genetic, behavioral, environmental, cultural, and socioeconomic factors. Some individuals may have a genetic predisposition toward weight gain or a genetic propensity to eat more than they need for energy. Others may have a genetic tendency toward diminished capacity to use dietary fats as fuel, or an increased tendency to store body fat (CDC, 2013). Genes can be a direct cause of obesity in disorders such as Bardet–Biedl syndrome and Prader–Willi syndrome (CDC, 2012b). For the vast majority of people, becoming overweight and obese results from excess calorie consumption and/or inadequate physical activity. Thus, when a woman consumes more calories than are expended in physical activity, she will gain weight. The amount of calories consumed can be offset by calories burned through physical activities, and can help a person maintain or lose weight.

Weight gain is normally viewed from an individual perspective. Individuals who are overweight or obese are frequently held responsible for overindulging or overeating, whereas those who maintain a healthy weight or lose weight are praised for their discipline. Although this perspective contains elements of truth, viewing the issue from a population-based perspective can generate insight into the problems of overweight, obesity, and difficulty in

Table 4–1 Body Mass Index Ranges

	Underweight	Healthy	Overweight	Obese
BMI	Below 18.50	18.50–24.99	25.00–29.99	30.00 and above

maintaining healthy weight. Factors that can influence the decision of whether to exercise can include availability of free time to exercise, access to safe and satisfying places to walk, run, or play sports, monetary costs involved with exercise such as cost of gym memberships, and conflicts with employment. Similar factors can influence a woman's ability to maintain a healthy diet. A woman may live in an area where healthful foods are unavailable, inconvenient, or considerably more expensive than foods high in fat and sugars. The processed food industry employs a variety of strategies to sell its often unhealthy products. For example, increasing portion sizes is a tactic that markets the idea that customers are getting a better deal for their money. These tactics make a handsome profit for the fast food and carbonated beverage industry at the cost of consumers taking in excess, unneeded calories without adding nutrients to their diet.

The Incidence and Prevalence of Obesity

Obesity is a complex, multifactorial chronic illness. The incidence and prevalence of overweight and obesity have increased dramatically in both men and women among all population groups. Currently 34.9%, or 78.6 million, American adults and 17%, or 12.7 million children and adolescents, are obese (CDC, 2014). In the United States, as of 2005, 28% of men, 34% of women, and nearly 50% of non-Hispanic African-American women were obese (Olshansky et al., 2005). Across racial groups, the rate of obesity is highest in non-Hispanic African-Americans at 47.8%, followed by 42.5% for Hispanics, 32.6% for non-Hispanic whites, and 10.8% for non-Hispanic Asians. The rate of obesity is higher among middle-aged adults 40 to 59 years of age (39.5%) than among younger adults 20 to 29 years of age or adults over the age of 60 (35.4%) (Ogden, Carroll, Kit, & Flegal, 2014).

Between 1988–1994 and 2005–2008 the prevalence of obesity increased in adults at all levels of income and education (Ogden, Lamb, Carroll, & Flegal, 2010). Evidence suggests that among women, and specifically non-Hispanic white women, obesity prevalence increases as income decreases. Generally, 42% of women with income below 130% of the poverty level are noted to be obese, and 29% of women with income at or above 350% of the poverty level are obese. For non-Hispanic white, non-Hispanic African-American, and Mexican-American women, prevalence is comparable, yet trends are only significant for non-Hispanic white women. In this case, 39.2% of those with income below 130% of the poverty level are noted to be obese, whereas 27.5% of non-Hispanic white women with income at or above 350% of the poverty level are obese (Ogden et al., 2010).

Among women with a college degree, the prevalence of obesity is lower than among those with some college education. College-educated women are less likely to be obese than women who have less than a high school diploma. Evidence suggests that 23.4% of women with a college degree are obese, whereas 42.1% of women with less than a high school education are obese. Non-Hispanic white and Mexican-American women with college degrees are significantly less likely to be obese compared with those with less than a high school education. Among non-Hispanic white, non-Hispanic African-American, and Mexican-American women, the prevalence of obesity among those with a college degree is significantly lower than among women with some college (Ogden et al., 2010).

Health Consequences of Obesity

Evidence suggests that as weight increases to the levels of overweight and obesity, the subsequent risks for developing health problems also increases. Health consequences that can result from overweight and obesity are listed in **Box 4–4** and summarized below. The health problems associated with overweight and obesity in adults are complex and often interrelated. It is not unusual for overweight and obese individuals to manifest multiple health problems.

Box 4–4: Health Consequences of Overweight and Obesity

- Coronary heart disease
- Type 2 diabetes
- Cancers (endometrial, breast, gallbladder, and colon)
- Hypertension
- Dyslipidemia (for example, high total cholesterol or high levels of triglycerides)
- Stroke
- Metabolic syndrome
- Liver disease
- Gallbladder disease
- Sleep apnea and respiratory problems
- Obesity hypoventilation syndrome
- Osteoarthritis
- Gynecological problems (abnormal menses, infertility, polycystic ovarian syndrome)

Modified from National Heart, Lung, and Blood Institute. (2012). What are the health risks of overweight and obesity? Retrieved from http://www.nhlbi.nih.gov/health/health-topics/topics/obe/risks#

CORONARY HEART DISEASE

A rise in the risk of coronary heart disease is associated with increased BMI. Being overweight or obese can lead to increased plaque buildup along the lining of the coronary arteries, also known as atherosclerosis. Plaque buildup in the arteries can narrow or block the coronary arteries and consequently reduce blood flow to the heart muscle, which can lead to angina or myocardial infarction. Overweight and obesity can also lead to heart failure (National Heart, Lung, and Blood Institute [NHLBI], 2012).

HYPERTENSION

Being overweight or obese can increase the risk of developing high blood pressure (NHLBI, 2012).

Numerous factors contribute to hypertension in the overweight or obese individual, such as atherosclerotic narrowing of the arteries and increased oxygen demand caused by excessive body mass.

STROKE

Being overweight or obese enhances atherosclerotic plaque buildup in the arteries. Plaques can rupture causing a blood clot to form. A blood clot in the brain can disrupt blood flow to brain tissue and cause a stroke. The risk of stroke increases as BMI increases.

TYPE 2 DIABETES

Risk for developing type 2 diabetes is high in overweight and obese individuals (NHLBI, 2012).

In overweight individuals, the cells in the body become less sensitive to the insulin that is released from the pancreas. Evidence suggests that fat cells are more resistant to insulin than muscle cells. Thus, in overweight and obese individuals, insulin will likely become less effective overall due to overabundance of fat cells. As such, glucose levels increase in the blood due to insulin-resistant tissue instead of being taken into the cells to be used as energy. Diabetes is a leading cause of early death, coronary heart disease, stroke, kidney disease, and blindness (NHLBI, 2012).

ABNORMAL BLOOD LIPIDS

Being overweight or obese increases the risk for developing abnormal blood lipids. This includes having high levels of triglycerides and LDL cholesterol, and low levels of HDL cholesterol. Having abnormal levels of these blood lipids increases the risk of coronary heart disease.

METABOLIC SYNDROME

Metabolic syndrome identifies a group of risk factors that increase the risk for heart disease and other health problems, including diabetes and stroke. Although it is possible to develop one of these risk factors singularly, the risk factors tend to occur together. Metabolic syndrome will be diagnosed if at least three of the following risk factors are exhibited (NHLBI, 2012):

- Abdominal obesity (having extra fat in the waist area: an "apple shape")
- Elevated (higher than normal) triglyceride level or being on medication to treat high triglycerides
- Lower than normal HDL cholesterol level or being on medication to treat low HDL levels
- Hypertension or being on medication to treat high blood pressure
- Elevated fasting blood glucose or being on medication to treat diabetes

CANCER

Being overweight or obese increases the risk of developing cancer of the breast, endometrium, colon, and gallbladder (NHLBI, 2012).

OSTEOARTHRITIS

Individuals who are overweight or obese are at higher risk for developing osteoarthritis because the extra weight can cause more pressure and wear on body joints such as knees, hips, and lower back. Osteoarthritis occurs if the tissue that protects the joints is worn away (NHLBI, 2012).

SLEEP APNEA

Individuals who are overweight or obese have increased risk for sleep apnea. Sleep apnea is a common disorder in which pauses in breathing or shallow breathing occur during sleep. Obese or overweight individuals may develop sleep apnea due to having increased fat stored around the neck. This leads to narrowing of the airways which makes it more difficult to breathe.

OBESITY HYPOVENTILATION SYNDROME (OHS)

Individuals who are obese or overweight have increased risk for developing OHS. In OHS, obese individuals have difficulty breathing deeply. They will hypoventilate, which results in increased carbon dioxide levels and decreased oxygen levels in the blood. OHS can lead to serious complications and even death (NHLBI, 2012).

REPRODUCTIVE PROBLEMS

Obesity can increase the risk of developing reproductive problems such as irregular menstrual cycle, amenorrhea, infertility, and polycystic ovarian syndrome (NHLBI, 2012).

GALLBLADDER DISEASE

Being overweight or obese increases the risk of developing gallbladder disease—in particular, developing gallstones. Being overweight also may increase the risk of developing an enlarged gallbladder, which can become dysfunctional (NHLBI, 2012).

Obese and overweight children and adolescents have increased health risks as well, especially for type 2 diabetes. Type 2 diabetes was once a rare occurrence in American children, but it is now becoming increasingly present in overweight and obese children. Children who are overweight are also more likely to become overweight or obese adults with the same risks for disease (NHLBI, 2012).

Obesity and Mortality

Evidence suggests that overweight and obesity, particularly during midlife, is associated with an increased risk of death (Adams et al., 2006). It has been predicted that unless effective population-level interventions are developed, obesity may cause a decline in life expectancy during the 21st century. Furthermore, the youth of today may, on average, live less healthy and possibly shorter lives than their parents. The health and life expectancy of minority populations is predicted to suffer the greatest impact from obesity because these subgroups tend to have limited access to health care, and childhood and adult obesity has increased the most rapidly in these groups (Olshansky et al., 2005).

Economic Burden of Obesity and Overweight

Obesity imposes a substantial economic burden on the healthcare system. It is estimated that the annual medical burden of obesity has risen to almost 10% of all medical spending and could amount to more than $147 billion per year (in 2008 dollars) (Finkelstein, Trogdon, Cohen, & Dietz, 2009). Across all payers (both private and public sectors), per capita medical spending for an obese person is $1,429 higher per year, or roughly 42% higher, than for someone of normal weight. Moreover, as a result of the Part D prescription drug benefit, the obesity-attributable prescription drug costs to Medicare are $7 billion for the noninstitutionalized population. Even though pharmaceutical, medical, and surgical treatment options for obesity are available, costs attributable to obesity almost totally result from treating the diseases and conditions that obesity produces (Finkelstein et al., 2009).

What these figures do not reflect are the indirect costs that are measured in terms of lost productivity, premature disability, and early death. Healthcare costs and the possibility of complications from surgery for obese and overweight individuals are higher than those for people of healthy weight. Added costs may exist at the individual or household level. Overweight or obese individuals may need to purchase specially designed chairs or beds to support them, specialty clothing, and higher than average numbers of medications. This can present a significant cost burden to families. In addition, people who are overweight or obese are subject to discrimination and social stigmatization. Consequently, they may be vulnerable to low self-esteem and depression, which may further decrease productivity.

Another area of significant expenditure is the billions of dollars spent by overweight and obese people in addressing weight concerns. These expenditures include health club memberships, home exercise equipment, diet books, weight loss aids, and participation in weight loss programs. It is estimated that 45 million people attempt to lose weight each year and spend $33 billion on weight loss products (Boston Medical Center, 2014).

Healthy Weight Loss

In order to achieve weight loss, an individual needs to burn more calories than he or she ingests. This is more difficult to achieve than it sounds. Millions of Americans have limited opportunities to exercise. Many cities and suburbs have been designed with cars, not pedestrians, in mind so walking can be unpleasant or dangerous. Some neighborhoods are unsafe, and being outside is a safety risk. Advertisements and commercials for weight loss constantly promote ways that their products and methods can help people lose weight, yet their claims are often biased, inaccurate, or exaggerated. Consequently, achieving healthy weight loss can be challenging.

The means to successful weight loss lies with increasing the basal metabolic rate (BMR) by exercise, not by cutting calories. When a woman endeavors to lose weight by cutting calories her body responds as it would to starvation, by burning fewer calories, thus lowering the BMR. Moreover, much of the weight lost on a low-calorie diet results from lost muscle tissue and lost water weight. Less muscle tissue results in a lower BMR. As a result, the more weight that is lost by dieting, the more the BMR will decrease, and there is greater likelihood that the weight will be regained. Although calorie reduction does have a role in weight loss, exercise helps solve the metabolic problem. Exercising regularly is necessary for any weight control program. Exercise increases the metabolic rate by building muscle and preventing muscles from shrinking as a result of weight loss. Adding exercise to a diet program helps keep the BMR steady and facilitates keeping the weight off. A benefit of exercise is that it will burn calories. In addition, the metabolism remains higher for several hours after exercise, so calories are burned at a higher rate even during inactivity. Along with promoting weight loss, exercise seems to affect the body in a more complex, integrated way. Exercise brings appetite and energy expenditure into balance and trims the physical profile even without weight loss. Exercise helps to improve overall health by decreasing the blood pressure, improving cholesterol levels, strengthening the cardiovascular system, reducing risk of type 2 diabetes, and decreasing stress.

A food diary can help some women facilitate their weight loss by allowing them to identify their eating and exercising patterns. All meals, snacks and drinks should be recorded in the diary. Review of the dietary notes recorded over a few days enables a woman to objectively examine her eating habits and set realistic goals for weight loss based on a healthful diet. Progress is monitored through the food diary as well as weekly (not daily) checks with the scale. Upon achieving reasonable weight loss, women can then focus on weight maintenance through healthful eating and exercise.

Unhealthy Weight Loss

American women relentlessly worry, think, and obsess over weight loss. Huge profits are made by promoters of diet books, programs, and plans that prey on women's insecurities about their weight and offer easy solutions in the form of their new products. When women fail to lose weight, or gain back weight they have lost, they frequently blame themselves, even though the diets may be flawed, ineffective, or unrealistic.

Dieting without exercise is an ineffective weight loss modality. A chronic pattern of dieting, known as "yo-yo dieting" or weight cycling, entails losing weight and regaining it repeatedly. Weight cycling takes place when restraint in food consumption is replaced by disinhibition. The more difficult it is for a person to attain a healthy weight, the more likely it is that rebound weight gain will occur (Outland, Madanat, & Rust, 2013). Weight cycling can put the health of the individual at risk. It can decrease insulin sensitivity, which increases the risk of developing type 2 diabetes (Outland et al., 2013). Evidence suggests that there are strong and consistent associations between body weight variability and negative health outcomes—in particular, mortality from coronary heart disease. Evidence also suggests that weight cycling may have negative psychological and behavioral consequences with increased risk for psychopathology, life dissatisfaction, and binge eating (Brownell & Rodin, 1994). People who engage in weight cycling may also store more fat in the abdominal area with each failed diet, which, as discussed earlier, can have serious health risks.

Another unhealthy diet modality is diet supplements. Weight loss supplements commonly contain stimulants, which can produce elevated heart rate, heart attacks, nervousness, insomnia, headaches, seizures, or death. Diet supplements are not subjected to the same testing standards as substances regulated by the Food and Drug Administration. Thus, supplements may have a higher rate of contaminations or contraindications not stated on warning labels.

Alcohol should be omitted from weight loss efforts because it provides empty calories that contribute to weight gain without any nutritional benefit. Alcohol also affects the BMR by slowing the rate that the body burns fat, and thus encourages the storage of body fat.

Popular Weight Loss Modalities

Some popular diet plans promote specific eating regimens to achieve maximum weight loss. Some of these include high carbohydrate/very low fat regimens or high protein/high fat/low carbohydrate regimens. Often people are not able to lose weight with these diet regimens because of the mistaken belief that they could eat unlimited amounts of certain foods. The truth is that excessive calories, regardless of food source, will cause weight gain.

Some diet programs are based on providing a nutritionally balanced dietary plan, support, and dietary education. These include Weight Watchers, Nutrisystem, and Jenny Craig. Depending on the program, subscribers purchase dietary plans and have access to counseling or regular membership meetings. These programs provide prepared meals and snacks, and support the dieter with counseling, coaching, and/or education. They advocate weight loss and maintenance approaches that emphasize healthful eating habits, following a nutritionally balanced diet, portion control, and physical activity.

Severely overweight and obese individuals may turn to gastrointestinal surgery (bariatric surgery), to achieve weight loss. Bariatric surgery, which alters the digestive process, promotes weight loss by closing off parts of the stomach to make it smaller. Such procedures that reduce the size of the stomach are known as "restrictive operations" since they restrict the amount of food that the stomach can hold. Other bariatric surgeries are known as malabsorptive operations. These combine stomach restriction with a partial bypass of the small intestine. The goal of a malabsorptive operation is to create a direct connection from the stomach to the lower portion of the small intestine, which then bypasses segments of the digestive tract that absorbs calories and nutrients. People who have had these surgeries often find eating and swallowing extremely painful, and each meal becomes an ordeal. Although weight is lost, patients may experience problems in the postoperative period, such as the "dumping" syndrome, whereby rapid ejection of stomach contents into the small intestines after eating produces uncomfortable and distressing physical symptoms. Bariatric surgical procedures are appropriate only for severely obese people who have not been able to control their weight with diet, exercise, and appropriate pharmaceutical modalities, and who exhibit adverse health conditions related to their obesity.

Physical Activity

Women who are physically active derive health benefits throughout the life cycle. Physical activity is an activity that brings health benefits and signifies movement of a moderate intensity lasting a few minutes or more. Thus, many common activities can constitute physical activities. Exercise is a purposeful session of physical activity performed in order to improve health. Physical activity can be done in the form of intense exercise sessions or in the form of more moderate-intensity activities, such as walking or yoga. Physical fitness is the ability to meet routine physical demands while sustaining a reserve to meet sudden physical demands. Fitness is a relative state that has different meaning to different individuals. For example, the state of physical fitness of a firefighter will likely differ from the state of physical fitness of a ballet dancer. Each may differ in muscle strength, flexibility, and workout goals.

One's state of fitness may change over time. However, it is apparent that fitness provides significant short- and long-term health benefits. Evidence suggests that women who exercise just one hour per week or more are 33% less likely to die from cancer, 50% less likely to die from cardiovascular disease, and 66% less likely to die early as compared to women who do not exercise (Hu et al., 2004).

The Benefits of Physical Activity

Regular physical activity is essential for individuals of all ages to achieve and maintain a healthy body weight, prevent chronic disease, and promote psychological well-being. Physical activity also helps to improve cognitive functioning and prevent falls in older adults (U.S. Department of Health and Human Services, 2008). The physical and psychological benefits of regular physical activity can improve the quantity and quality of life. Adults and children of all age groups and body types, including those with disabilities, can reap substantial benefits from regular physical activity. The physical and psychological benefits of regular physical activity are summarized in **Box 4–5**.

Of particular significance is the fact that regular exercise decreases risk of death and injury from

---

Box 4–5: Physical and Psychological Benefits of Regular Physical Activity

- Decreased risk of early death
- Decreased risk of developing coronary heart disease, stroke, and cancers of the breast, lung, and colon
- Decreased risk of developing osteoporosis, type 2 diabetes, and depression
- Lowered blood pressure and serum cholesterol
- Improvement of aerobic capacity, muscle strength, and muscle endurance
- Increased cognitive functioning and decreased symptoms of depression
- Improvement in ability of older adults to complete day-to-day tasks
- Improvement in cognitive function of older adults and reduction in the risk of falls
- Maintenance of healthy muscles, joints, and bones
- Weight control, muscle building, and fat reduction
- Reduction of symptoms and severity of diabetes and arthritis

Modified from U.S. Department of Health and Human Services. (2008). 2008 Physical activity guidelines for Americans. Retrieved from http://www.health.gov/paguidelines/guidelines/

heart disease, which is the leading cause of death in the United States. Physical activity improves overall cardiovascular function and affects other risk factors for heart disease. Regular physical activity can reduce stress, lower blood pressure, build lean body weight, reduce body fat, and improve serum cholesterol levels. Exercise can reduce the risk of developing chronic diseases such as colon cancer, type 2 diabetes, osteoporosis, and obesity. Physical activity is essential for maintaining the health of muscles, bones, and joints. It is essential for ensuring normal skeletal development and increasing bone mass and density. Physical activity also slows the rate of bone loss in women as they age, which is significant for reducing the risk of osteoporosis. Regular physical activity is instrumental in improving balance and coordination, which decreases the risk of fall-related fractures in older women.

Exercise burns calories and increases lean body weight. This is a significant benefit for preventing obesity and its risk for numerous chronic diseases, as well as for improving individuals' overall sense of well-being. Many individuals who exercise regularly report that they feel better when they engage in exercise. Evidence suggests that aerobic exercise is potentially valuable, along with medication if necessary, as a complementary therapy for depression (Brosse, Sheets, Lett, & Blumenthal, 2002). Evidence also suggests that regular exercise may decrease anxiety and depression that may appear during pregnancy (Da Costa, Rippen, Drista, & Ring, 2003). Research also suggests that people who regularly exercise report feeling happier and better about themselves, and generally experience a better quality of life than people who do not (Elevsky et al., 2005; U.S. Department of Health and Human Services, 2008). Other research findings confirm that exercise is associated with various psychological benefits such as decreased stress, increased sense of well-being, and improvements in cognitive function and mood (U.S. Department of Health and Human Services, 2008). Appropriate exercise during pregnancy

promotes numerous physical and psychological benefits, such as improved psychological well-being, potentially shorter labor, and speedier recovery after childbirth.

For significant health benefits, adults should engage in at least 2.5 hours per week of moderate intensity (e.g. brisk walking or gardening) or 1.25 hours per week of vigorous-intensity aerobic physical activity (e.g. jogging or kick-boxing), or an equivalent combination of both vigorous and moderate intensity activity. In addition, muscle strengthening activities should be performed on at least 2 days per week. Additional health benefits would be acquired by engaging in physical activity beyond this amount (U.S. Department of Health and Human Services, 2008). However, even small amounts of physical activity are better than none at all.

Physical inactivity is a serious national problem. It is estimated that more than half of the adults in this country do not get enough physical activity to provide important health benefits. Evidence suggests that women are less likely than men to be physically active. Results from the 2007–2009 National Health Interview Survey indicated that 14.7% of women met the recommendations for adequate physical activity, compared to 21.1% of men (U.S. Department of Health and Human Services, 2011). In every age group, women were less likely than men to meet the recommendations for adequate physical activity. The percentage of both men and women reporting adequate physical activity generally decreased as age increased (U.S. Department of Health and Human Services, 2011). Adequate physical activity was noted to differ by poverty status and race and ethnicity. Generally, women with household incomes of 200% or more of poverty (18.8%) were more than twice as likely to report adequate physical activity as compared to those with incomes below 200% of poverty (8.6%). This difference in income was consistent within each racial and ethnic group (U.S. Department of Health and Human Services, 2011). Overall, non-Hispanic

White (16.9%), non-Hispanic women of multiple races (16.0%), and non-Hispanic American Indian/Alaska Native women (14.9%) reported the highest levels of adequate physical activity. Fewer non-Hispanic African-American (9.4%), Hispanic (9.5%), and non-Hispanic Asian women (10.3%) reported engaging in adequate physical activity. These racial and ethnic differences were consistent within both income groups (U.S. Department of Health and Human Services, 2011).

Elements of Physical Fitness

American women in general are not active enough in their daily activities to be naturally fit. Women in today's society who desire to become physically fit will need to make a commitment of time and energy to exercise. Physical fitness is comprised of four major areas.

CARDIOVASCULAR ENDURANCE

Cardiovascular endurance is the ability to sustain vigorous physical activity for an extended period of time. Cardiovascular endurance is considered the most crucial component of fitness. It is a reflection of the ability of the heart to pump blood efficiently through the body. Increasing cardiovascular endurance augments the capability of the heart, blood vessels, and blood to deliver oxygen to the cells of the body and then remove waste products. Even though muscles can draw on quick sources of energy for short-term exertion, sustained exercise beyond a minute or two requires that muscles receive oxygen from the blood. This type of physical activity is called aerobic exercise. With repeated physical exercise the heart is better able to deliver oxygenated blood to the muscles with greater efficiency and muscles have improved capacity to utilize oxygen. This coupled capability is known as the training effect. The heart rate at rest and the heart rate at exertion decreases as a result of this regular exercise. In addition, the heart is able to recover from the stress of exercise more quickly.

MUSCULAR STRENGTH

Muscular strength is the total force that groups of muscles produce in one effort, such as jump, lift, or heave. The most effective way to increase muscle strength is by working out with weights, either free weights or weight machines. Gains in muscle strength are produced most quickly from heavy resistance and few repetitions.

MUSCULAR ENDURANCE

Muscular endurance is the ability to execute repeated muscular contractions over a span of time without tiring. Muscle endurance requires strength and increases by repetition, working at a moderate level of intensity, and building up to a specified goal. Endurance building exercises include push-ups, situps, and pullups.

FLEXIBILITY

Flexibility is the ability to move joints through their full range of motion. Flexibility is effectively improved by static stretching exercises that apply steady pressure without excessive bouncing. Flexibility varies from person to person as well as from joint to joint. Men tend to be less flexible than women due to skeletal, muscle mass, and body composition differences. Good flexibility is protective against muscle pulls and tears since muscles that are short and tight are more likely to be overstretched. Care should be taken in selecting exercises that increase flexibility, as some movements may cause injury to the lower back and knees. Stretching certain muscle groups can help prevent or relieve pain. For example, stretching hamstrings and lower back muscles may relieve lower back pain, and stretching calf muscles may help avert leg cramps.

Regular exercise can affect the ratio of lean muscle to fat weight by reducing excess body weight through energy expenditure and by increasing the overall metabolic rate of the body. The body burns calories during the period of physical exercise as well as for a few hours afterward, which is known as *afterburn*. Exercise performed for a longer period at a more intense level will keep the BMR elevated for a longer period of time. Regular exercise improves overall muscle tone and contributes to a trimmer appearance. In addition, exercise can improve balance, coordination, and agility.

Conditioning Programs

Conditioning programs or training regimens are comprised of physical activities that improve fitness. Such programs may consist of either aerobic training or strength training. Aerobic training will increase the ability of the body to use oxygen and improve cardiovascular endurance. Strength training will augment the size and strength of specific muscles and body areas. The most effective fitness programs combine aerobic exercise with strength training. Jointly, aerobic exercise and strength training exercise impart better benefits than either form of exercise alone. Joined with a healthy diet, this combination program may likely be the most efficient strategy for weight loss. Calorie consumption while working out, as well as the resultant muscle mass from strength training will boost the basal metabolic rate further because muscle will consume more energy than will fat.

WARM-UP

Before beginning an aerobic or strength training session, a warm-up is important. A warm-up primes the body for exercise by slowly increasing the heart rate and blood flow, increasing temperature of the muscles, and enhancing the function of muscles. The risk of sports related injury is decreased by adequate warming up. Sudden exercise without adequate warm-up may cause changes in blood pressure as well as abnormal heart rate and blood flow. This could be dangerous, especially for older individuals. Jogging in place or stationary cycling can be done for a full body warm-up 5 to 10 minutes to raise body temperature.

STRENGTH TRAINING

Like aerobic exercise, strength training can help prevent or delay many of the negative consequences associated with aging or inactivity. The amount of muscle that a strength training program provides depends on three factors: intensity (the amount of weight lifted or pulled), repetitions (the number of times the weight is lifted or pulled), and frequency (the number of sessions in a given period). Experts generally concur that an individual should use enough weight in order to just barely perform 8 to 12 repetitions in a row. A good frequency is considered to be two to three sessions per week.

Strength training often necessitates working out against moderate resistance to tone muscles and build muscle endurance. Resistance can be provided by free weights, dumbbells, barbells, or weight machines. Resistance can also be provided by one's body weight such as in performing push-ups or pull-ups. The benefits of strength training are summarized in **Box 4–6**.

Men tend to have more muscle mass than women, particularly in the upper body. Gender differences in size, hormones, and normal activity levels likely explain this discrepancy. Women who engage in strength training however gain strength at the same rate as men. Many women do not engage in strength training out of concerns about becoming unflatteringly muscular. A moderate program will not create noticeable muscle bulk in men or women but will produce a firmer, trimmer physique.

AEROBIC EXERCISE

Aerobic exercise imparts benefits that are different than those gained from strength training. Along with significantly raising the heart rate, aerobic exercise appears to lower serum cholesterol levels and blood pressure. Improvements in cardiovascular fitness as well as the ability of the heart and lungs to deliver oxygenated blood to the muscles

Box 4–6: The Benefits of Strength Training

- Well-toned muscles help maintain good posture, and may help prevent injuries.

- Muscle strength produces benefits in daily living by increasing stamina and self-confidence.

- Strength training increases bone density, thereby helping to delay or minimize osteoporosis and vulnerability to fractures.

- Injury prevention, especially for musculoskeletal injuries induced by exercise, such as runner's knee or shin splints, which are injuries caused by muscle weaknesses, imbalances, and joint instability.

- Maintaining a strong back through strength training protects it from injury. Lower back pain frequently results from weakness of back and abdominal muscles, both of which help support the back.

- Strength training helps improve poor posture, which is a source of many back problems.

are additional benefits that strength training does not generally provide. Running, bicycling, and swimming are examples of aerobic exercise.

Aerobic exercise has three significant components. These components include intensity, duration, and frequency. These components influence the amount of health benefits provided by any exercise program. Each of these components is equally important. Exercise intensity is determined by work per unit of time. The target heart rate is a heart rate obtained during aerobic exercise. It signifies the minimum level of exertion at which cardiovascular fitness can increase for an individual in a specific age group. The target heart rate is an informative indicator by which exercise intensity may be monitored. Exercise duration is the length of time of a single exercise session. To derive benefits to the heart, aerobic exercise must be intense enough to elevate the heart rate and must continue for a specified length of time, depending on the intensity of the workout. To derive the most benefits from aerobic exercise, the aerobic activity should last for 30 minutes or more (U.S. Department of Health and Human Services, 2008).

Cool-Down

After intensive exercise, a cool-down is important. A cool-down consists of gradually slowing down from exercise by exercising at a slow but steady rate for 5 to 10 minutes. This less intensive exercise helps to prevent muscle stiffness and potentially dangerous sudden drops in blood pressure that occur when vigorous exercise is abruptly stopped. After exercise, stretching is important to protect against injury.

Gender Similarities and Differences in Physical Fitness

Numerous psychological, social, cultural, and historical issues influence how women think about fitness and exercise. In the past, women were stereotyped as the weaker sex and were not encouraged to become as physically fit as men. Sociocultural prejudices have customarily limited women's access to and their full participation in sports. Significant developmental tasks of childhood include growth of self-esteem and self-confidence with physical activity. Thus, due to lack of encouragement, young girls often lacked the self-esteem and confidence necessary for participation in sports as they grew older. Title IX legislation was passed in 1978, which mandated that public schools provide equal funding for girls' sports. Nonetheless, since the passage of Title IX, opportunities, resources, and perhaps most importantly, encouragement for physical fitness has not been equally distributed to children, regardless of gender. A new generation of women's sports groups and sports stars has revised the societal rule that says only male athletes can be admired.

Men have traditionally surpassed women in physical competition. Men are able to run longer and faster, jump higher and farther, lift more and longer. A common belief has been that men are inherently gifted physically whereas women are not. However, in recent years, women have become more competitive in all athletic arenas. These advances naturally generate several questions that seek to better define gender similarities and differences in sports and exercise. It is difficult to resolve these issues since young boys and girls have not been raised with equivalent levels of emphasis, encouragement, and training in physical fitness.

Men and women differ biologically and the effect of these differences on athletic performance is not entirely understood. Although no apparent differences exist between male and female musculature, the fact that men are stronger than women reflects the larger absolute quantity of their muscle mass. Women seem to be half as strong as men in the upper body regions of the shoulders, arms, and backs, and two-thirds as strong in the legs and lower body, primarily attributed to men having larger muscle fiber areas and greater lean body weight (total weight minus body fat). Commonly, 25% of a woman's body weight is composed of fat as compared to 15% of the body weight of a man. Having extra body fat may be a hindrance in sports such as running whereas it may be an advantage in sports such as swimming. In addition, women also tend to have lower blood volume, about 5% less hemoglobin, smaller hearts, and less lung capacity than men.

Women's performance in endurance sports has improved dramatically in recent years. Women have gained increasing recognition as proficient athletes, either in competition with each other or in mixed sports. The gender gap in such sports is gradually narrowing. Similar levels of absolute performance may or may not reach the same levels in male and female professional athletes. As such, it is essential that women do not allow prejudice or feelings of inferiority to prevent them from attaining their own most favorable fitness levels. Achieving the levels of fitness that best reflect an individual's personal inclination and goals is the responsibility of an adult of either gender.

Exercise and Older Women

As women age, exercise becomes more important. Many problems that are commonly associated with aging include increased body fat, decreased muscle mass, decreased muscle strength and flexibility, decreased bone mass, decreased metabolism, and slower reaction time. Such problems are frequently signs of inactivity that can be reduced or prevented by exercise. Physical disability in the elderly is mainly caused by decreased muscle strength. Critical components of maintaining the ability to walk and remaining independent are retaining muscle strength and flexibility. Falls are responsible for 80% of the injuries requiring a hospital visit in people over the age of 65 years. Exercise can significantly improve balance, coordination, and bone strength when combined with calcium and vitamin D supplements. This combination can greatly decrease the likelihood and severity of falls (Kannus, Sievanen, Palvenen, Jarvinen, & Parkkari, 2005).

In addition to improving physical fitness, exercise can decrease the risk of developing type 2 diabetes and osteoporosis, as well as reduce the symptoms associated with these diseases. The pairing of muscle strengthening and aerobic exercises may likely be the best method for prevention of these chronic debilitating illnesses. Exercise can engender a sense of well-being as well as ease symptoms of depression, which can commonly occur among elderly women.

Complementary and Alternative Therapeutic Modalities

Complementary and alternative therapeutic modalities are an array of healthcare approaches with a history of use or origins outside of mainstream medicine. Nearly 40 % of Americans use alternative or complementary healthcare approaches for specific conditions or to maintain overall well-being. In addition, more women than men use complementary or alternative health practices (National Center for Health Statistics, 2010). Complementary therapeutic modality generally refers to the use of a non-mainstream approach together with conventional medicine. An alternative modality refers to the use of a non-mainstream approach in place of conventional medicine. Most people use non-mainstream approaches along with conventional medicine. The boundaries between complementary practices and conventional medicine may overlap and change with time (National Center for Complementary and Integrative Health [NCCIH], 2014b).

This selection of non-mainstream healthcare approaches may also be considered as part of integrative medicine or integrative health care. Integrative health care is the assimilation of various non-mainstream health practices into treatment and health promotion. Consumers of complementary and alternative medicine (CAM) commonly perceive benefits to health or well-being. Moreover emerging evidence suggests that some of the perceived benefits of complementary and alternative therapeutic practices are real or meaningful, yet overall, the scientific evidence about many of the modalities is limited. In several instances, a lack of reliable data makes it difficult for people to make informed decisions about using integrative health care (NCCIH, 2014b).

Alternative and complementary healthcare approaches generally fall into one of two subgroups: natural products and mind and body practices. Natural products include a variety of substances that include herbs (also known as botanicals), vitamins and minerals, and probiotics. Natural products are widely marketed as dietary supplements and readily available to consumers. Some natural products have been studied in large, placebo-controlled trials. Research findings have indicated that numerous natural products have failed to show anticipated effects. Research is ongoing on other natural products to determine whether they are effective and safe. Although some findings indicate that various natural products may be helpful, more needs to be learned about the effects of these products in the human body, as well as their safety and potential interactions with medicines and with other natural products (NCCIH, 2014b).

Mind and body practices consist of a large and diverse group of procedures or techniques administered or taught by a trained practitioner or teacher. Mind and body practices generally include acupuncture, massage therapy, meditation, movement therapies, relaxation techniques, spinal manipulation, tai chi, qigong, yoga, hypnotherapy, and healing touch. Of these practices, deep breathing, meditation, chiropractic and osteopathic manipulation, massage, yoga, progressive relaxation, and guided imagery are most commonly used by adults. Depending on the practice, the amount of research on mind and body approaches differs widely. Research in acupuncture, yoga, spinal manipulation, and meditation has been plentiful, and evidence suggests that some of these practices seem to hold promise in pain management. Other practices have had little research to date (NCCIH, 2014b).

In addition to natural products and mind and body practices, there are other complementary and alternative health approaches that may not neatly fit into either natural products or mind and body practices. Ayurvedic medicine from India and traditional Chinese medicine are ancient systems of healing that are associated with particular cultures. Each incorporates specific universal principles into a system of living and medicine. Alternatively, homeopathy and naturopathy are therapeutic disciplines that are not associated with specific cultures, yet they focus on natural health promotion and healing (NCCIH, 2014b). Commonly used natural products, mind and body practices, and other complementary and alternative health approaches will be further discussed in the remainder of this chapter.

Natural Products

In the United States, natural products are used by more than 38 million people. Herbal supplements are one form of natural product commonly used by women. An herb is a plant or plant part (such as leaves, flowers, or seeds) utilized for its scent, flavor, and/or possible health-related properties. An herbal supplement may contain a single herb or mixtures of herbs. The law requires that all of the herbs contained in a supplement must be listed on the product label (NCCIH, 2014d). The herbal medical tradition, also known as herbalism, has a long history of use outside of conventional medicine, yet, with improvements in analysis and quality control, the use of herbal supplements has become more mainstream. Moreover, advances in clinical research have shown the value of herbal medicine in the treatment and prevention of disease (University of Maryland Medical Center [UMMC], 2013i).

HISTORY OF HERBAL MEDICINE

The use of herbs for medicinal purposes extends back prior to recorded history. The first recorded evidence of herbal use appeared as early as 3,000 BC in ancient Chinese and Egyptian papyrus writings that described medicinal uses for plants. Herbs have long been used by indigenous cultures (such as African and Native American) in their healing rituals. Other cultures developed traditional medical systems, such as Ayurveda and traditional Chinese medicine, in which herbal therapies became an integral part (UMMC, 2013i). During medieval times, the use of herbal medicine developed and spread throughout Europe. Originally in medieval Europe, herbal medicine was practiced as a woman's art, however toward the 13th century the traditional female village herbalist became displaced by Christian monks, graduates of male-only medical colleges, and members of barber-surgeon guilds (EBSCO, 2012a). When chemical analysis first became accessible in the early 19th century, scientists began to extract and modify the active ingredients from plants. The name for the extracted chemical, "drugs" was derived from the old French word for herb, which was "drogue" (EBSCO, 2012a). Later, chemists began manufacturing their own version of plant compounds and, as time went on, the use of herbal medicines decreased in favor of drugs. Nearly 25% of pharmaceutical drugs are derived from botanicals (UMCC, 2013i).

THE PROBLEM OF REPRODUCIBILITY

Several factors have contributed to the predominance of chemical drugs over herbs. Currently, a crucial issue with herbs is the problem of reproducibility. Scientists, for the most part, are uncertain as to what specific ingredient in a particular herb works to treat a condition or illness. The beneficial effect of an herb may be due to the many ingredients it contains that work together. A number of factors affect the chemical makeup of an herb and establish how effective an herb will be. These include the type of environment (climate, insects, soil quality) in which a plant grew, where it was grown, plants that grew nearby, as well as how and when it was harvested and processed (EBSCO, 2012a; UMMC, 2013i). Such variability poses a significant problem for people who want to use herbs medicinally as opposed to using herbs for taste and fragrance.

Because a great deal of variation is possible, it is difficult to ascertain whether one batch of an herb is equivalent in effectiveness to another. The desire to solve this problem has been a motivating factor for discovering the active ingredients of herbs and purifying them into single-chemical drugs. The majority of common herbs that possess an identifiable active ingredient have already been processed into drugs. Popular herbs that are currently used do not contain any known, single active ingredients. As such, no simple way to determine the effectiveness of a given herbal batch exists (EBSCO, 2012a; UMMC, 2013i).

Herbal standardization is a method that can partially overcome this problem. In this process, an extract of the entire herb is made and the liquid is boiled off until the concentration of some ingredient reaches a certain percentage. This ingredient is not usually the active ingredient; it is a "tag" or "handle" used for standardization purposes. The extract is then manufactured into tablets or capsules or bottled as a liquid, with the concentration of the tag ingredient identified on the label. Partial standardization is not perfect because two products that have the same concentration of tag ingredients may still vary widely in other unlisted or even unidentified active ingredients. Even so, this method of partial standardization is better than nothing, and it permits a particular amount of reproducibility. Thus, whenever possible, consumers are encouraged to use standardized herbal extracts and the actual products that were tested in double-blind studies (EBSCO, 2012a).

The World Health Organization has recently estimated that 80% of people around the world rely on botanicals for a portion of their primary health care. In the United States, interest in returning to natural or organic remedies, combined with public dissatisfaction with the cost of prescription medications, has resulted in a significant increase in use of herbal supplements over the past 30 years (UMMC, 2013i). The U.S. Dietary Supplement Health and Education Act (DSHEA) of 1994 classified herbal supplements as dietary supplements. Unlike prescription drugs, herbal supplements can be sold without having been tested for safety and effectiveness. Consequently, herbal supplements must be produced according to quality manufacturing practices (UMMC, 2013i).

HERBAL SUPPLEMENTS AND SAFETY

It is commonly believed that herbs are naturally safer and gentler than drugs. However no rational justification for this belief exists. Even though herbal supplements are natural products, being natural does not guarantee that the products are safe. Herbs are plants that contain one or more drugs and, as such, may produce side effects, especially if consumed in dosages high enough to produce substantial benefits (EBSCO, 2012a). Herbal supplements may contain a variety of compounds and all of its ingredients may not be known. Some herbal supplements may damage the liver, interact with medications, or pose risks if an individual has medical problems or is going to have surgery. Many herbal supplements have not been tested on pregnant or lactating women or on children. Numerous herbal supplements are under investigation in an effort to identify active ingredients and to understand their effects in the body. In addition, the label of an herbal supplement may not accurately distinguish what is actually contained in the supplement. Analysis of the substance may occasionally find differences between labeled and actual ingredients. The herbal supplement may not contain the correct plant species or the amount of ingredients may be lower or higher than stated on the label. The possibility also exists that the herbal supplement may be contaminated with other herbs, pesticides, metals; or may be adulterated with unlabeled, illegal ingredients (NCCIH, 2014d).

Although there is a lack of scientific evidence that supports the effectiveness of herbal supplements, women over the centuries have used herbal remedies safely and effectively. Women who wish to take herbal supplements should do so according to the following safety guidelines (NCCIH, 2014d):

1. Herbal supplements should be taken under the guidance of a healthcare provider who has been properly trained in herbal medicine.
2. Women should refrain from taking herbal supplements on a daily basis over an extended period of time.
3. Women should refrain from taking large quantities of any one herbal supplement.
4. Women should use only standardized and tested herbal supplements that are labeled with ingredients and quantities on the package.
5. Women should check expiration dates and lot numbers of the products they purchase.
6. Women who are pregnant, attempting to become pregnant, or who are lactating should avoid taking herbal supplements.
7. Women with certain medical conditions, who plan to have surgery or who are taking prescription medications should avoid taking herbal supplements.
8. Herbal supplements should not be given to babies or young children.

HERBAL REMEDIES COMMONLY USED BY WOMEN

Women commonly use herbs for regulation of hormones, reduction of water retention, mood elevation, and relief of menstrual and menopausal problems. When used wisely and cautiously, the most popular medicinal herbs are at least reasonably safe. Some herbal supplements generally used by women are discussed here.

BLACK COHOSH (ACTAEA RACEMOSA, CIMICIFUGA RACEMOSA)   The black cohosh plant belongs to the buttercup family and is native to North America. Black cohosh was used in Native American medicine

and was a home remedy in 19th century America. It has been used for rheumatism (arthritis and muscle pain), and more recently as a folk or traditional remedy for menopausal symptoms such as hot flashes, night sweats, and vaginal dryness. Other uses of black cohosh include relief of menstrual irregularities, relief of premenstrual syndrome, and to induce labor. Fresh or dried underground stems and roots of black cohosh are used to make strong teas (infusions), capsules, solid extracts used in pills, or liquid extracts (tinctures) (NCCIH, 2012a).

Research findings are mixed on the effectiveness of black cohosh in relieving menstrual symptoms. Evidence suggests that black cohosh, whether used alone or in combination with other herbal supplements, failed to relieve hot flashes and night sweats in perimenopausal or postmenopausal women. Most current research studies on black cohosh have been less than 6 months long, thus safety of long-term use has not been determined. Further research is being conducted to investigate the potential effects of black cohosh on hot flashes and other menopausal symptoms. At the present time not enough reliable data exists to ascertain the effectiveness of black cohosh in treating rheumatism and other conditions (NCCIH, 2012a).

There are some safety concerns of black cohosh. It is unknown if black cohosh causes liver problems, as evidence is not definitive; however, women who have a liver disorder or develop symptoms of liver problems while taking black cohosh should consult their healthcare provider. Side effects of black cohosh include stomach discomfort, headache, and rash. Overall, results of clinical trials of black cohosh for menopausal symptoms have not found serious side effects. Black cohosh should not be mistaken for blue cohosh (*Caulophyllum thalictroides*). Blue cohosh has different characteristics, treatment uses, and side effects. Black cohosh is sometimes given with blue cohosh to stimulate labor; however, this treatment has caused adverse outcomes in newborns, which seem to be associated with blue cohosh (NCCIH, 2012a).

CALENDULA (*CALENDULA OFFICINALIS*) Calendula, or pot marigold, is a plant whose yellow flower petals have been used for medicinal purposes since the 12th century. Calendula belongs to the same family as daisy, chrysanthemum, and ragweed. It is native to southwestern Asia, Western Europe, Macronesia, and the Mediterranean area, and is now grown as an ornamental plant throughout the world. Calendula is not the same as the annual marigold plant that is frequently grown in gardens. Calendula contains high levels of flavonoids, which are plant-based antioxidants that protect body cells from damage caused by unstable free radical molecules. In addition, calendula may protect against inflammation, viruses, and bacteria (UMMC, 2013a).

The traditional use of calendula has been as a treatment for stomach upset and ulcers, and to relieve menstrual cramps; however, no scientific evidence exists to support that calendula works for these conditions. Currently, calendula is not commonly taken by mouth except when used in very small amounts in homeopathic preparations. Calendula is frequently used as a topical remedy that has been shown in animal studies to help wounds heal faster, likely by increasing blood flow and oxygen to the affected area, which helps to stimulate growth of new tissue. Improvement in skin hydration and firmness has also been noted with calendula use (UMMC, 2013a). In addition, the dried flower petals of the calendula plant are used in ointments, tinctures, and washes for treatment of burns, bruises, cuts, and the minor infections they cause (UMMC, 2013a). Evidence suggests that calendula is helpful in preventing dermatitis or skin inflammation in patients receiving radiation therapy for breast cancer, and is a safe and effective remedy for diaper rash. Calendula is also used for the treatment of hemorrhoids, nosebleeds, varicose veins, proctitis, and conjunctivitis.

The use of calendula ointments to heal first-degree burns and sunburns is frequently recommended by professional homeopaths. In children, calendula is sometimes used to treat ear infections, and a few scientific studies have found no side effects. However, there is not enough evidence to support whether calendula is actually effective in treating ear infections (UMMC, 2013a).

Although calendula is generally considered safe for topical use, it should not be applied to an open wound without a doctor's supervision. Women with allergies to plants in the daisy or aster family, including chrysanthemums and ragweed, may develop an allergic reaction to calendula, usually in the form of a skin rash. Calendula should not be used by pregnant and breastfeeding women. There is a possibility that calendula could interfere with conception, so couples trying to get pregnant should not use calendula. There is no evidence to indicate there are any interactions between calendula and conventional or herbal medications. In theory, taking calendula orally may interact with sedatives, high blood pressure medications, and medications to treat diabetes. Therefore, women should consult with their physicians before combining these drugs with calendula (UMMC, 2013a). Calendula may cause sleepiness and drowsiness. Taking it with other herbs and supplements that have this same effect might cause too much sleepiness. Some of these include 5-HTP, calamus, California poppy, catnip, hops, Jamaican dogwood, kava, St. John's wort, skullcap, valerian, yerba mansa, and others (Natural Medicines Comprehensive Database, 2014).

CHASTEBERRY (*VITEX AGNUS CASTUS*) Chasteberry is the fruit of the chaste tree, a small, shrub-like tree that grows in the Mediterranean region and in central Asia. Monks in the Middle Ages believed that the plant promoted chastity, and used chasteberry to decrease sexual desire. Women have used chasteberry for thousands of years to relieve menstrual problems and stimulate lactation. Presently, chasteberry is considered a folklore, or traditional, remedy for menstrual problems and is used by women to relieve premenstrual syndrome, menopausal symptoms, some types of infertility, and acne. Liquid or solid extracts are prepared from the dried, ripe chasteberry. The extracts are then made into tablets or capsules (NCCIH, 2012b).

Evidence suggests that chasteberry is likely beneficial for premenstrual syndrome. However, because the studies were not well designed, firm conclusions cannot be drawn. Some study findings suggest that chasteberry may help relieve breast pain and some types of infertility; however, once again, reliable scientific evidence is lacking as to whether chasteberry has any effect on these conditions. Studies investigating how chasteberry works in the body as well as how it may affect premenstrual syndrome are currently being conducted (NCCIH, 2012b).

Although chasteberry has not been associated with serious side effects, women need to be aware that chasteberry can cause gastrointestinal problems, acne-like rashes, and dizziness. Chasteberry may also affect the levels of certain hormones such as prolactin and luteinizing hormone, and it indirectly increases the ratio of progesterone to estrogen. Women who are pregnant, taking oral contraceptives, or have hormone-sensitive conditions such as breast cancer, should avoid using chasteberry. Chasteberry may also affect the dopamine system in the brain. Therefore, women who take dopamine-related drugs for Parkinson's disease, or certain antipsychotic medications, should not use chasteberry (NCCIH, 2012b).

DONG QUAI (ANGELICA SINENSIS)   Dong quai is a fragrant perennial plant that grows at high altitudes in the cold damp mountains of China, Korea, and Japan. A member of the celery family, the plant has smooth purplish stems and umbrella-shaped clusters of white flowers and produces winged fruits in July and August. The yellow-brown thick-branched roots are used for medicinal purposes. The plant matures in 3 years and the root is harvested and then processed into tablets, powders, and other forms of medicine (UMMC, 2013b).

Dong quai has been used for centuries as a tonic, medicine, and spice in China, Korea, and Japan. It is frequently used in traditional Chinese medicine in combination with other herbs. Dong quai is used for treatment of women's reproductive problems such as dysmenorrhea, and to improve blood flow. Occasionally referred to as the "female ginseng," dong quai is sometimes suggested for relief of cramps, irregular menstrual cycles, amenorrhea, infrequent periods, premenstrual syndrome, and menopausal symptoms, such as hot flashes (UMMC, 2013b). Although very few research studies have been conducted on the use of dong quai in humans, some lab tests suggest that dong quai contains compounds that may help reduce pain, open blood vessels, and stimulate and relax the muscles of the uterus. Some researchers are uncertain whether dong quai acts like estrogen or blocks estrogen in the body. Because research findings have been inconclusive, more studies are needed to see whether dong quai is safe and effective (UMMC, 2013b).

The essential oil of dong quai should not be ingested because it contains a small amount of cancer-causing substances. Women who have chronic diarrhea or abdominal bloating should avoid using dong quai. Dong quai at high doses may make women more sensitive to sunlight and cause skin inflammation and rashes. Therefore women using dong quai should avoid direct exposure to sunlight or use sunscreen when outdoors. It is uncertain if dong quai acts like estrogen, thus women who are at risk of hormone-related cancers, including breast, ovarian, and uterine cancers, should not use dong quai. Women who are pregnant should avoid using dong quai since it may cause the uterus to contract and increase the risk of miscarriage. Lactating women should not use dong quai since it is unknown if the herb is safe to use when breastfeeding. Dong quai should not be given to children (UMMC, 2013b).

Women who take anticoagulants such as warfarin (Coumadin) or antiplatelet drugs such as clopidogrel (Plavix) should avoid dong quai because it may increase the risk of bleeding. Dong quai may also increase the risk of bleeding when used with many other herbs and supplements that act as blood thinners, such as feverfew, fish oil and other omega-3 fatty acids, garlic, ginger, ginkgo, ginseng, licorice, Chinese skullcap, and turmeric. Research is lacking on interactions between dong quai and hormone medications such as estrogens, progesterones, oral contraceptives, tamoxifen, or raloxifene. Dong quai should be avoided by women who are taking hormonal medications without the supervision of a physician. Both dong quai and St. John's wort increase photosensitivity. Therefore women should consult their physicians before taking these herbs together.

ECHINACEA (*ECHINACEA PURPUREA, ECHINACEA ANGUSTIFOLIA, ECHINACEA PALLIDA*)   Echinacea, currently one of the most popular herbs in this country, is a perennial herb native to southern Canada and the midwestern region of North America. Echinacea has tall stems and bears single pink or purple flowers. The plant has a large central seed cone that is usually purple or brown in color (UMMC, 2013c).

Echinacea has been used for more than 400 years by Native Americans as a general "cure-all," and to treat infections and wounds. Throughout history, echinacea has been used to treat malaria, scarlet fever, syphilis, diphtheria, and blood poisoning. Its use was prevalent during the 18th and 19th centuries. However, after antibiotics were introduced, the use of echinacea declined in this country. Interest in echinacea picked up throughout the 20th century, and its use became especially popular in Germany, where most of the scientific research on this herb has been conducted. Currently, echinacea is used to boost the immune system and help the body to fight infections, shorten the duration of common colds and flu, and reduce symptoms such as sore throat, cough, and fever (UMMC, 2013c).

Three species of echinacea are commonly used for medicinal purposes, *Echinacea purpurea*, *Echinacea angustifolia*, and *Echinacea pallida*. Several chemicals play a role in the therapeutic effects of echinacea: polysaccharides, glycoproteins, alkamides, volatile oils, and flavonoids. The chemicals found in the roots of the plant differ from those found in the upper parts. The roots are noted to have high concentrations of volatile oils (odorous compounds) and the above-ground parts of the plant have higher concentrations of polysaccharides, which are known to trigger immune system activity. These active substances combine to produce the beneficial effects of echinacea. Evidence suggests that the above-ground portion of *Echinacea purpurea* is the most effective. In Germany, echinacea is government-regulated and the above-ground parts of the plant are approved for treatment of colds, upper respiratory tract infections, urinary tract infections, and slow-healing wounds. The root portion of *Echinacea pallida* is approved for treating flu-like infections (UMMC, 2013c).

The results of several laboratory and animal studies indicate that the active substances contained in echinacea enhance the function of the immune system, relieve pain, decrease inflammation, and have hormonal, antiviral, and antioxidant effects. Hence, professional herbalists suggest echinacea for treatment of urinary tract infections, vaginal yeast infections, ear infections, athlete's foot, sinusitis, hay fever, and slow-healing wounds. Emerging evidence suggests that echinacea extract may have antiviral effects on the development of cold sores triggered by the herpes simplex (HSVI) when taken prior to infection. The ability of echinacea to treat or prevent the common cold is under debate. Evidence is conflicting as to whether the herb is effective in preventing or reducing the severity of the common cold. Echinacea preparations tested in clinical trials differ widely. Different products use different parts of the plant, which explains the varied effectiveness among diverse echinacea products. Thus it is important that women choose high-quality preparations and consult their healthcare providers for recommendations (UMMC, 2013c).

Echinacea products may contain one, two, or all three species of the herb, and are available in extracts, tinctures, tablets, capsules, or ointments. Echinacea is often combined with other immune-boosting herbs, vitamins, and minerals. It is important that women desiring to use echinacea buy products with guaranteed potency or standardized extracts made by reputable established companies that distribute their product through trustworthy and knowledgeable establishments (UMMC, 2013c).

Women should avoid using echinachea if they have tuberculosis, HIV/AIDS, diabetes, connective-tissue disorders, multiple sclerosis, autoimmune disorders, and possibly liver disorders. Echinachea may decrease the effectiveness of immunosuppressive therapy. Therefore women who are organ transplant recipients and who must take immunosuppressant medications should not use echinacea.

Although rare, allergic reactions to echinacea may develop, ranging from mild rash to anaphylaxis. The risk for allergic reactions to echinacea may be increased in women with asthma and other allergies. Women with allergies to plants in the daisy family, such as ragweed, chrysanthemums, marigolds, and daisies, should avoid taking echinacea. Oral ingestion of echinacea may cause temporary numbing and tingling on the tongue, as well as gastrointestinal upset. Because evidence regarding the safety of echinacea in pregnant and lactating women is sparse, women who are pregnant or breastfeeding should consult their healthcare provider (UMMC, 2013c).

Evening Primrose Oil (*Oenothera Biennis*)
Native throughout the United States, this wildflower grows as a circle of leaves around evening primrose stems after the first year it is planted. During the second year of growth, flowers bloom after sunset, June through September, or on overcast days. The leaves grow at alternating levels on both sides of the stem (UMMC, 2013d).

Originally the seeds were used for food by Native Americans, who also made poultices from the entire plant to heal bruises. The root of evening primrose was taken back to England and Germany by European settlers, where it was used for food (UMMC, 2013d). The oil found in the seeds of evening primrose is high in the essential fatty acids linolenic acid and gamma-linolenic acid. Both linolenic acid and gamma-linolenic acid are omega-6 fatty acids. The body uses essential fatty acids as building blocks for a variety of molecules. Another essential fatty acid is omega-3, which is found in fish oil. A balance of omega-6 and omega-3 fatty acids in the body is necessary for good health (UMMC, 2013d). Although many North Americans tend to consume too much omega-6 oil in their diets, there are different types of omega-6 fatty acids. Some omega-6 fatty acids are healthier, such as that found in evening primrose oil. Gamma-linolenic acid is also found in spirulina (a blue-green algae), borage, hemp, and black currant oil (UMMC, 2013d).

Evening primrose oil is used to relieve symptoms of premenstrual syndrome, rheumatoid arthritis, Raynaud's phenomenon, diabetic peripheral neuropathy, mastalgia, and menopausal symptoms; however, scientific evidence regarding effectiveness of treatment for these conditions is limited. More research is needed. Research findings indicate that evening primrose oil is useful for relieving the itchiness, crusting, edema, and redness from eczema and dermatitis. Evening primrose oil can be used by both adults and children for the treatment of skin conditions (UMMC, 2013d).

Evening primrose oil is considered safe to use when women adhere to recommended dosages. Adverse effects are rare and mild if they occur, and may include nausea, stomach pain, and headache. The presence of stomach pain and loose stools may indicate that the dose is too high. Omega-6 supplements, including gamma-linolenic acid and evening primrose oil, should not be used by women who have epilepsy or other seizure disorders, bleeding problems, or a blood disorder. It is uncertain if evening primrose oil is safe in pregnant or lactating women. Thus, women should consult their physicians prior to use (UMMC, 2013d). Because of the risk of drug interactions, women who are using the following medications should consult their physicians before using evening primrose oil: anticoagulants and blood thinners such as aspirin, wafarin, and clopidogrel; antihypertensive drugs; phenothizines; anti-seizure drugs; and antidepressants, such as citalpram, escitalopram, fluoxetine, paroxetine, and sertraline (UMMC, 2013d).

GARLIC (*ALLIUM SATIVUM*) Garlic is an edible bulb from a plant in the lily family and has been used medicinally for 5,000 years. Garlic originally was native to central Asia but is now grown throughout the world. The plant grows to the height of 24 inches or more, and the compound bulb of the plant is used medicinally. Each bulb contains between 4 and 20 cloves and each clove weighs about 1 gram (UMMC, 2013e).

Garlic's long history of use as food as well as medicine dates back to the time the Egyptian pyramids were built and it has been used as a treatment for a wide variety of ailments. Gravediggers in 18th-century France drank wine mixed with crushed garlic with the belief it would protect them from the plague. In World Wars I and II, garlic was given to soldiers to prevent gangrene (UMMC, 2013e). Garlic has been used as an antiseptic to prevent wound infections. Nowadays, garlic is used to prevent atherosclerosis, hypertension, elevated cholesterol, and to boost the immune system. A regular dietary intake of garlic may also help protect against cancer. As people age, free radicals can build up in the body and can contribute to the development of heart disease, Alzheimer's disease, and cancer. The rich antioxidants in garlic may be effective in fighting off free radicals and may reduce or help prevent damage that free radicals can cause to body tissue over time (UMMC, 2013e).

Medicinally, garlic is most frequently considered as an herb used for heart disease and atherosclerosis; however, evidence has been inconsistent. Some study findings suggest that garlic may help prevent heart disease, slow down atherosclerosis, and lower blood pressure between 5% and 8% (UMMC, 2013e). Garlic appears to have blood thinning properties, which can be helpful in preventing heart attacks and strokes. The effectiveness of garlic in lowering elevated blood cholesterol levels has not been supported by current research findings. Research findings suggest that garlic may be helpful in preventing colds and shortening the duration of cold symptoms in people who did have colds (UMMC, 2013e). Garlic might strengthen the immune system and help the body fight diseases such as cancer. Population studies suggest that people who eat more garlic, raw or cooked, may be less likely to get cancer of the colon, stomach, or esophagus (UMMC, 2013e).

Garlic supplements may be made from fresh, dried, freeze-dried, aged, or garlic oil extracts. Supplements made from each of these sources may have different effects on the body since not all garlic contains the same amount of active ingredients. Thus, the label should be read carefully and standardized garlic products used to get the most benefits (UMMC, 2013e). It is also important to follow the directions of a healthcare provider who is experienced in herbal medicine. The U.S. Food and Drug Administration has listed garlic as Generally Recognized as Safe; however, garlic has side effects, which include upset stomach, bloating, bad breath, and body odor. A stinging sensation on the skin from may be caused by handling too much fresh or dried garlic, or it may cause skin lesions. Although less common, garlic may cause headache, fatigue, loss of appetite, muscle aches, dizziness, and allergic reactions. People with thyroid problems and ulcers should seek medical advice before taking garlic as a supplement (UMMC, 2013e).

Because garlic has blood thinning properties, too much garlic may increase the risk for bleeding during or after surgery. Garlic may also interact with anticoagulants and blood thinning medications, such as warfarin, clopidogrel, or aspirin. In addition, garlic may interact with non-steroidal anti-inflammatory agents such as ibuprofen, naproxen, and some prescription medications to increase the risk of bleeding (UMMC, 2013e). Garlic may interfere with the actions of isoniazid, oral contraceptives, and cyclosporine, making these drugs less effective. Garlic may also interfere with blood levels of protease inhibitors used for treatment of HIV/AIDS, making them ineffective. These drugs include amprenavir, fosamprenavir, indinavir, nelfinavir, ritonavir, and saquinavir (UMMC, 2013e).

GINGER (*ZINGIBER OFFICINALE*)   Ginger is a root, or rhizome, native to Asia, that has been used as a spice and herbal medicine for thousands of years. The rhizome is a knotted, thick, beige underground stem. The above-ground stem of the plant is about 12 inches tall with long, narrow, ribbed, green leaves, and white or yellowish-green flowers. The active components of the ginger root are believed to be volatile oils and pungent phenol compounds, such as gingerols and shogaols. Ginger is available in tinctures, extracts, capsules, and oils. It may be purchased fresh and made into a tea, and is found in a wide variety of food and drinks such as ginger bread, ginger snaps, ginger sticks, and ginger ale (UMMC, 2013f).

Ginger has a long history of medicinal use in Asian, Indian, and Arabic herbal traditions. It has been used in China as an herbal treatment for indigestion, stomach upset, diarrhea, and nausea for more than 2,000 years. Ginger has also been used to treat arthritis, colic, heart conditions, headache, common cold, flu-like symptoms, and painful menstrual periods (UMMC, 2013f). Currently, healthcare professionals may recommend ginger to help prevent or treat nausea and vomiting from motion sickness, pregnancy, and cancer chemotherapy. Ginger is also used to treat mild stomach upset, reduce pain of osteoarthritis, and may even be used in heart disease (UMMC, 2013f).

Research evidence suggests that ginger might be helpful in reducing some symptoms of motion sickness with fewer side effects than caused by conventional prescription or over-the-counter medications used for nausea (UMMC, 2013f). However, some studies have found that ginger may not work as well as scopolamine for motion sickness. Evidence also suggests that ginger is helpful in reducing nausea and vomiting associated with pregnancy (UMMC, 2013f). Research findings indicate that ginger may also be helpful in reducing the severity and duration of nausea related to chemotherapy. However, more research is needed to reach a definitive conclusion. Conflicting results have been obtained as to whether ginger is helpful in reducing nausea and vomiting after surgery. Some studies found that ginger did reduce nausea following surgery; however, some study findings indicate that ginger did not help reduce postoperative nausea, but might have in fact increased it. More research in this area is needed (UMMC, 2013f).

Ginger has been used in traditional medicine for hundreds of years to reduce inflammation. While some evidence suggests that ginger may be helpful in relieving pain from osteoarthritis, some findings indicate that ginger is no more effective in reducing symptoms of osteoarthritis than ibuprofen or placebo. Furthermore, ginger may take several weeks to work. Preliminary study findings also suggest that ginger may be helpful in lowering cholesterol as well as preventing blood from clotting, which can be useful in treating heart disease. However, more research is needed in this area (UMMC, 2013f).

Ginger rarely produces side effects; however, in high doses ginger may cause mild heartburn, diarrhea, belching, mouth irritation, or stomach upset. Some of these side effects may be avoided when ginger supplements are taken with meals or in capsule form (UMMC, 2013f). Individuals with gallstones should consult their physician before taking ginger. Women who are pregnant or breastfeeding, who have heart conditions, or who have diabetes should be equally cautious and also consult their physician before taking ginger (UMMC, 2013f). Ginger may increase the risk of bleeding and should not be taken with antico-agulants or blood thinning medications such as warfarin, clopidogrel, or aspirin. Individuals with bleeding disorders should not take ginger. Ginger may lower blood sugar and should not be taken with diabetes medications. Ginger may also lower blood pressure and should not be taken with high blood pressure medications (UMMC, 2013f).

GINKGO (*GINKGO BILOBA*)   The ginkgo is the oldest surviving species of tree and dates back 300 million years. The ginkgo died out in Europe during the Ice Age; however, the tree survived in China, Japan, and other parts of East Asia. Some trees can live as long as 1,000 years, and the trees have been cultivated widely for medicinal and cer-emonial purposes (EBSCO, 2013). The ginkgo is a tough, hearty tree that can grow to a height of 120 feet. It has short branches with fan-shaped leaves and inedible fruits that are malodorous. The inner seed of the fruit may be poisonous. In autumn, the leaves turn brilliant colors. In the United States, the ginkgo is sometimes planted along urban streets (EBSCO, 2013).

In traditional Chinese medicine, ginkgo seeds and leaves were utilized for treatment of numer-ous health problems, especially asthma and other respiratory illnesses. However, in the 1950s, the medical possibilities of ginkgo leaf extracts rather than seed-based remedies were investigated by German researchers (EBSCO, 2013). Thus, mod-ern research findings are based on standardized ginkgo biloba extract made from the dried green leaves, which differs from the traditional Chinese herb. Comparisons drawn between the two types are not correct. The standardized extract is highly concentrated and appears to be more effective in treating health problems than the non-standard-ized leaf alone (UMMC, 2013g).

Although more than 40 components have been discovered in ginkgo, only two are thought to have medicinal properties: flavonoids and terpenoids. Evidence has shown that flavonoids, which are plant-based antioxidants, protect nerves, blood vessels, the heart muscle, and the retina from dam-age. Terpenoids, such as ginkgolides, have been shown to improve blood flow by dilating blood vessels and decreasing the stickiness of platelets (UMMC, 2013g).

In Europe, ginkgo is used widely for treating Alzheimer's disease. At first it was thought that ginkgo improved blood flow to the brain. However, current evidence suggests that ginkgo protects nerve cells damaged in Alzheimer's disease. Evidence also suggests that ginkgo is just as effective as standard drugs for treating Alzheimer's disease and vascular dementia as well as other severe forms of memory and mental function decline. Evidence suggests that ginkgo may help people with Alzheimer's disease improve cognitive functions of thinking, learning, and memory, have an easier time performing daily activities, improve social behavior, and reduce feel-ings of depression. While the findings of several stud-ies indicate that ginkgo might work as well as some prescription Alzheimer's medications to delay the symptoms of dementia, ginkgo has not been tested against all of the drugs prescribed to treat Alzheimer's disease. Even though ginkgo is sometimes recom-mended to prevent Alzheimer's disease and demen-tia, and some study findings have suggested it might help, other study findings have not supported this claim (EBSCO, 2013; UMMC, 2013g).

Evidence suggests that ginkgo may be helpful in treating intermittent claudication, which is pain resulting from decreased blood flow to the legs. People with intermittent claudication experience difficulty walking due to extreme pain. Some stud-ies have shown that ginkgo may work as well as prescription medication in improving pain-free walking distance, although other studies have not supported this claim (EBSCO, 2013).

Evidence indicates that ginkgo may be effec-tive in relieving symptoms of premenstrual syn-drome, most notably breast pain and emotional disturbance. Research findings suggest that ginkgo may also be helpful in relieving anxiety, relieving vertigo, enhancing memory and thinking, preserving vision in people with age-related macular degeneration disease and glaucoma, and reducing symptoms associated with Raynaud's phenomenon. However, more research is needed in these areas (EBSCO, 2013; UMMC, 2013g).

Ginkgo is relatively safe to use; however, since safety for use in pregnant women has not been established, pregnant and lactating women should avoid using ginkgo. Side effects include stomach upset, headaches, skin reactions, and dizziness (UMMC, 2013g). The *Ginkgo biloba* fruit or seed should not be eaten. Some people who have taken ginkgo have reported internal bleeding; however, it was unclear whether the bleeding was associated with ginkgo or occurred for some other reasons, such as a combination of ginkgo and blood-thinning drugs. Thus, individuals who take anticoagulants such as warfarin, blood-thinning medications such as clopidogrel, or nonsteroidal anti-inflammatory drugs such as ibuprofen, should consult with their physicians before taking ginkgo (UMMC, 2013g). Individuals who are scheduled for surgery or dental procedures should stop taking ginkgo at least 36 hours prior to the procedure due to the risk of bleeding, and should inform their physicians that they take ginkgo. Due to the risk of seizures, ginkgo should not be taken by individuals who have epilepsy, since ginkgo may decrease effectiveness of anticonvulsant medication such as carbamazepine and valproic acid (EBSCO, 2013; UMMC, 2013g). Individuals with diabetes should consult their physicians before taking ginkgo, as ginkgo may elevate or lower insulin and blood sugar levels. Ginkgo should be avoided by anyone taking selective serotonin reuptake inhibitor antidepressant drugs such as citalopram, escitalopram, fluoxetine, fluvoxamine, and paroxetine. Individuals who take alprazolam for anxiety should avoid ginkgo, as it may decrease the effectiveness of alprazolam (EBSCO, 2013; UMMC, 2013g). Ginkgo

may lower blood pressure. Thus, those taking high blood pressure drugs, especially calcium channel blockers, should avoid taking ginkgo. Individuals who take antibiotics in the aminoglycoside family should avoid ginkgo since it may increase risk of damage to the auditory nerve, and consequently, hearing loss (EBSCO, 2013; UMMC, 2013g).

Ginseng (*Panax Quinquefolius, Panax Ginseng*)   For thousands of years, the ginseng plant has been used in traditional Chinese medicine. Asian or Korean ginsengs (*Panax ginseng)* are the same plants but grown in different regions, and American ginseng (*Panax quinquefolius)* is a relative in the same species, and is native to North America. Both Asian/Korean ginseng and American ginseng contain the same active ingredients, which researchers believe are ginsenosides. These plants should not be confused with Siberian ginseng or Eleuthero (*Eleutherococcus senticosus),* which is a completely different plant and does not have the same active ingredients (UMMC, 2013h).

The leaves of the ginseng plant grow in a circle around a straight stem. The umbrella-shaped flowers are yellowish-green, grow in the center of the plant, and produce red berries. The taproot of the ginseng plant is gnarled in appearance and resembles a small human body with stringy shoots that look like "arms" and "legs." Wrinkles around the neck of the root indicate the age of the plant. Ginseng can be used for medicinal purposes after it has grown for about 6 years (UMMC, 2013h). Asian ginseng supplements are produced from the ginseng root and the long, thin offshoots called root hairs. Both Asian or Korean and American ginseng contain ginsenosides and saponins, which are ginseng's active ingredients. Asian ginseng also contains glycans (panaxans), polysaccharide fraction DPG-3-2, peptides, maltol, B vitamins, flavonoids, and volatile oil (UMMC, 2013h).

Ginseng is one of the most popular herbs used in the United States and it has been researched for a number of conditions. Some studies of Asian or

Korean ginseng have used a combination of herbs, thus it is not always possible to definitively identify the effectiveness of ginseng in the results (UMMC, 2013h). It is believed that Asian ginseng boosts the immune system and likely helps the body resist infection and disease. Evidence suggests that ginseng may increase the number of immune cells in the blood and improve the response of the immune system to a flu vaccine. In addition, research findings indicate that ginseng may reduce the risk of getting a cold as well as shorten the duration and intensity of a cold (UMMC. 2013h).

Asian ginseng appears to have antioxidant properties. Antioxidants are helpful in ridding the body of free radicals, which can damage DNA and contribute to a number of conditions such as heart disease and diabetes. Preliminary evidence suggests that Asian ginseng may improve the symptoms of heart disease in people, and likely decrease "bad" LDL cholesterol levels as well as raise "good" HDL cholesterol (UMMC, 2013h). Some studies found that Asian ginseng may lower blood pressure, while other studies found that it increased blood pressure (UMMC, 2013h). While it has been found in some studies that both American and Asian ginseng may lower blood sugar levels in people with type 2 diabetes, other studies have found that Asian or Korean ginseng raises blood sugar levels. It is believed that the ginsengosides in American ginseng may lower blood sugar levels, whereas different ginsengosides in Asian ginseng might elevate blood sugar levels (UMMC, 2013h).

Some studies have found that Asian ginseng may be helpful in improving thinking or learning, especially when used in combination with Gingko biloba. While some evidence suggests that Asian ginseng may be helpful in improving physical strength and endurance, some studies found no effect at all. Even so, athletes frequently take Asian ginseng to increase endurance and strength (UMMC, 2013h).

Asian ginseng is sometimes referred to as an "adoptogen," which is believed to be a substance that helps the body better cope with mental or physical stress. Some research findings have suggested that Asian ginseng may reduce the risk of some types of cancer; however, more research is needed before any definitive conclusions can be drawn (UMMC, 2013h).

The use of red Korean (Asian) ginseng has been investigated for its effect on menopausal symptoms and it was found that it may relieve some of the symptoms of menopause such as improving mood, particularly feelings of depression, and giving a sense of well-being. The ginseng was used in combination with a vitamin and mineral supplement. However, another study found no effect (UMMC, 2013h).

Women who use Asian ginseng may experience nervousness or sleeplessness, especially if taken at high doses or combined with caffeine. Although rare, other side effects may include high blood pressure, insomnia, restlessness, anxiety, euphoria, diarrhea, vomiting, headache, nosebleed, breast pain, and vaginal bleeding (UMMC, 2013h). Asian ginseng should be taken with food to avoid low blood sugar, even in individuals without diabetes. Individuals with diabetes should consult with their physicians before taking ginseng. People with high blood pressure should avoid taking Asian ginseng without consulting their physicians. People with low blood pressure and those who are sick should be cautious, and consult their physicians (UMMC, 2013h). Individuals with bipolar disorder should avoid taking ginseng, as it may increase the risk of developing mania. People with autoimmune diseases such as rheumatoid arthritis, lupus, or Crohn's disease should consult with their physicians before taking Asian ginseng, since theoretically Asian ginseng may increase the activity of an already overactive immune system (UMMC, 2013h). Women who are pregnant or breastfeeding should avoid using Asian ginseng. In addition, women who have a history of breast cancer should avoid using Asian ginseng. Since Asian ginseng may have blood-thinning properties, it should not be taken at least 7 days before surgery to decrease the risk of bleeding during or after a surgical procedure (UMMC, 2013h).

Women who take certain medications should not use Asian ginseng without first consulting with their physicians. Asian ginseng may interact with angiotensin-converting enzyme (ACE) inhibitors used to treat high blood pressure. These medications include captopril, benazepril, enalapril, lisinopril, fosinopril, ramipril, perindopril, quinapril, moexipril, and trandolapril (UMMC, 2013h). Asian ginseng may make certain heart medications, such as calcium channel blockers, work differently than intended. These medications include amlodipine, diltiazem, and nifedipine (UMMC, 2013h). Asian ginseng may increase the risk of bleeding, especially for women taking anticoagulants and blood-thinners such as warfarin, aspirin, or clopidogrel. Ginseng may increase the effects of caffeine, possibly causing nervousness, sweating, insomnia, or irregular heartbeat. Ginseng may interact with diabetes medications and insulin, causing lower blood sugar levels, and increasing the risk of hypoglycemia (UMMC, 2013h). Asian ginseng may boost the immune system and interact with drugs taken to treat an autoimmune disease or drugs taken after organ transplant. Ginseng may increase the stimulant effect and side effects of stimulants taken for attention deficit hyperactivity disorder, including amphetamine, dextroamphetamine, and methylphenidate (UMMC, 2013h). Ginseng may interact with monoamine oxidase inhibitor (MAOI) antidepressants, causing headaches, tremors, and mania. MAOI antidepressants include phenelzine, isocarboxazid, tranylcypromine (UMMC, 2013h). Asian ginseng may impede the painkilling effects of morphine and interfere with the effectiveness of furosemide. Because Asian ginseng may interact with medications that are metabolized by the liver, those taking any medications should consult with their physicians before taking Asian ginseng (UMMC, 2013h).

GREEN TEA (*CAMELLIA SINENSIS*)   For hundreds of years tea has been grown in China and India and is the most widely consumed beverage in the world, second only to water. Tea is consumed by millions of people worldwide. It is only in the last couple of decades that health benefits have been assigned to this common ancient beverage (University of Maryland Shore Regional Health [UMSRH], 2014a). Green tea has been used in traditional Chinese and Indian medicine as a stimulant, diuretic, astringent, and to improve heart health. Green tea has also been used for treating gas, regulating body temperature and blood sugar, promoting digestion, and for improving mental processes (UMSRH, 2014a).

The main varieties of tea derived from the leaves of the *Camellia sinensis* plant are green, black, and oolong. Tea was originally cultivated in East Asia, and the plant grows as large as a shrub or tree. Tea now grows throughout Asia and parts of the Middle East and Africa. People who live in Asian countries commonly drink green and oolong tea, while Americans more commonly drink black tea. Green tea is produced from unfermented tea leaves, oolong tea from partially fermented tea leaves, and black tea from fully fermented tea leaves. The less-processed green tea reportedly contains the highest concentration of polyphenols (UMSRH, 2014a). These substances are known to possess strong antioxidant properties and may be important in preventing cancer. The antioxidant effects of polyphenols appear to be stronger than vitamin C. The antioxidants are protective against the damage caused by free radicals to body tissues. Free radicals can contribute to the aging process as well as the development of a number of health problems such as cancer and heart disease. Antioxidants in green tea can neutralize free radicals and may reduce or prevent the damage they cause. The polyphenols in green tea give it a somewhat bitter flavor (UMSRH, 2014a).

The polyphenols are classified as catechins. There are six primary catechin compounds in green tea: catechin, gallaocatechin, epicatechin, epigallocatechin, epicatechin gallate, and apigallocatechin gallate, also known as EGCG. EGCG is the most active and most extensively studied. Other components of green tea include caffeine, theobromine, and theophylline, which produce stimulant effects. The amino acid compound L-theanine has a calming effect on the nervous system (UMSRH, 2014a).

Evidence suggests that green tea may be helpful in reducing the risk of atherosclerosis and coronary heart disease. Researchers are uncertain as to why green tea lowers cholesterol and triglyceride levels but have noted that polyphenols might block cholesterol from being absorbed in the intestines. Evidence also suggests that green tea may help reduce harmful LDL cholesterol in the blood (UMSRH, 2014a).

Findings of several population-based studies suggest that both green and black teas may help protect the body against cancer. Scientists have determined from findings in early clinical studies that the polyphenols in tea, especially green tea, may play an important role in preventing cancer, killing cancer cells, and stopping cancer cells from growing. Both laboratory and human subject studies have been conducted that focused on bladder, breast, ovarian, colorectal, esophageal, lung, pancreatic, prostate, skin, and stomach cancers, but results have been mixed. More research is needed in this area (UMSRH, 2014a).

Green tea may help reduce inflammation associated with Crohn's disease and ulcerative colitis, and may help protect the liver from toxic substances as well as help treat viral hepatitis. It may be helpful in controlling blood sugar levels, lowering hemoglobin A1c levels in borderline diabetics, and may help prevent the development and progression of type 1 diabetes (UMSRH, 2014a). Research findings also suggest that green tea extract may help boost metabolism and burn fat, which may improve weight loss and maintenance in overweight and moderately obese people. Green tea may help prevent dental cavities, reduce the inflammation and cartilage breakdown associated with arthritis, treat genital warts, and prevent symptoms of cold and flu (UMSRH, 2014a).

Green tea should not be taken by those with high blood pressure, kidney problems, liver problems, stomach ulcers, or psychological disorders,

especially anxiety. Women who are pregnant or breastfeeding should also avoid green tea. Women with diabetes, glaucoma, or osteoporosis should consult with their physicians before taking green tea or green tea extract (UMSRH, 2014a). Individuals who drink large amounts of green tea over long periods of time may experience irritability insomnia, heart palpitations, and dizziness. Signs of caffeine overdose include nausea, vomiting, diarrhea, headaches, and loss of appetite. Women with signs of caffeine overdose should decrease caffeine intake and consult with their physicians (UMSRH, 2014a).

Green tea may interact with a variety of medications. Individuals who take adenosine should avoid taking green tea. The caffeine in green tea may reduce the sedative effects of benzodiazepines such as diazepam and lorazepam. Individuals taking beta-blocker blood pressure medications such as propranolol and metropolol may experience blood pressure elevation from the caffeine in green tea (UMSRH, 2014a). Individuals who take warfarin should avoid taking green tea, as the vitamin K in green tea can render warfarin ineffective. In addition, green tea should not be taken with aspirin since this combination may increase the risk of bleeding (UMSRH, 2014a). Women who are taking chemotherapeutic medications such as doxorubicin and tamoxifen should consult with their physicians before drinking green or black tea or taking tea extracts while undergoing chemotherapy (UMSRH, 2014a).

Individuals who take ephedrine should avoid taking green tea, as the combination may cause agitation, tremors, insomnia and weight loss. Individuals who take lithium should avoid green tea, as green tea has been shown to reduce serum lithium levels, thereby decreasing its effectiveness (UMSRH, 2014a). Green tea may also reduce the absorption of folic acid into the blood. Those who take MAOI antidepressants such as isocarboxazid, moclobemide, phenelzine, and tranylcypromine should not take green tea, as green tea combined with these medications can precipitate a hypertensive crisis (a severe elevation in blood pressure)

(UMSRH, 2014a). Individuals who take quinolone antibiotics should consult with their physicians before taking green tea. While evidence suggests that green tea may increase the effectiveness of quinolone antibiotics, the risk of side effects is also increased. Green tea, especially caffeinated green tea, may also interact with acetaminophen, carbamazepine, dipyridamole, estrogen, fluvoxamine, methotrexate, mexiletine, phenobarbital, theophylline, and verapamil. Individuals who take these medications should consult with their healthcare provider before using green tea (UMSRH, 2014a).

St. John's Wort (*Hypericum Perforatum*)

The medicinal use of St. John's wort dates back to ancient Greece, when the herb was used to treat various illnesses, including "nervous disorders." Throughout the ages the use of St. John's wort continued as a treatment of nervous disorders, and as such, was classified as a nervine (a treatment for nervous disorders) in the 1800s (EBSCO, 2012b).

St. John's wort is a shrub-like plant with yellow flowers that grow in clusters. The flowers have oval, elongated petals. The plant is believed to be native to Europe, parts of Asia and Africa, and the western United States. Both the flowers and leaves are medicinal (UMMC, 2013j).

St. John's wort has anti-inflammatory, antibacterial, and antiviral properties and has been used as a topical remedy to help heal wounds and burns. In the United States, St. John's wort is one of the most frequently purchased herbal products. The active components of St. John's wort that have been studied include hypericin and pseudohypericin, which are found in both the leaves and flowers. However, researchers have begun to consider that other compounds may be responsible for the healing properties of this herb and are now investigating its essential oils and flavonoids. Research is ongoing (UMMC, 2013j).

An extensively studied area of St. John's wort action has been in treatment for depression. An impressive body of evidence suggests that St. John's wort may help treat mild to moderate (not severe) depression with fewer side effects than most prescription antidepressants. St. John's wort has been shown to work just as effectively as selective serotonin reuptake inhibitors (SSRIs) such as fluoxetine, citalopram, and sertraline. St. John's wort does not cause loss of sex drive, which is one of the most common side effects of antidepressants (UMMC, 2013j). However, St. John's wort interacts with various medications. Women who take St. John's wort must do so only under the guidance of a healthcare provider. Those with severe depression, who are unable to function day to day or have thoughts about harming themselves or others, should not try to treat themselves with herbs. They should consult with their physicians for appropriate treatment (UMMC, 2013j).

St. John's wort has been investigated for use with other conditions. Evidence suggests that it may be helpful in relieving symptoms of premenstrual syndrome, such as cramps, irritability, food cravings, and breast tenderness. St. John's wort, used in combination with black cohosh, may help improve mood and anxiety during menopause (UMMC, 2013j). There is also some evidence suggesting that St. John's wort, used alone, may help improve the mood of people with seasonal affective disorder (SAD). SAD is a depressive type of mood disorder that occurs during winter months due to lack of sunlight. SAD is commonly treated with light therapy. Evidence suggests that light therapy used in combination with St. John's wort is more effective (UMMC, 2013j). The antibacterial properties of St. John's wort may also help to fight inflammation. Topical application of St. John's wort may help relieve symptoms associated with minor wounds and skin irritations such as eczema, minor burns, and hemorrhoids (UMMC, 2013j).

Women who use St. John's wort may experience some mild side effects such as stomach upset, hives or other skin rashes, fatigue, restlessness, headache, dry mouth, and feelings of dizziness or mental confusion. Photosensitivity may also be experienced. Light-skinned women who take St. John's wort should wear protective clothing when out in the sun and use sunscreen with at least SPF 15 or higher. Sunlamps, tanning booths, or tanning beds should be avoided (UMMC, 2013j).

St. John's wort should not be taken by individuals who have severe depression, bipolar disorder, schizophrenia, attention deficit disorder, attention deficit hyperactivity disorder, or Alzheimer's disease. St. John's wort should not be stopped abruptly. Dosage should be gradually lowered before discontinuing use. St. John's wort may interfere with fertility and becoming pregnant. It should not be taken by women who are pregnant or breastfeeding. Since St. John's wort can interact with medications used during surgery, individuals who are to undergo surgery should discontinue St. John's wort at least 5 days or more before the surgical procedure (UMMC, 2013j).

Since St. John's wort can interact with many medications, women should consult with their physicians prior to use. St. John's wort can render certain drugs ineffective and potentiate the effects of others. St. John's wort can increase the side effects of tricyclic antidepressants, selective serotonin reuptake inhibitors, and monoamine oxidase inhibitors, leading to a dangerous condition called serotonin syndrome. Women who take these antidepressants should not use St. John's wort (UMMC, 2013j). St. John's wort may decrease effectiveness of antihistamines such as loratadine, cetirizine, and fexofenadine. Individuals who take the over-the-counter cough medication dextromethorphan should avoid St. John's wort, as it can increase the risk of side effects, including serotonin syndrome (UMMC, 2013j). St. John's wort should not be used with medications used for treating migraines such as naratriptan, rizatriptan, sumatriptan, and zolmitriptan, as it can increase the risk of side effects, including serotonin syndrome. Women who take clopidogrel should avoid St. John's wort because it may increase the risk of bleeding. St. John's wort can also potentiate the sedative effects of anticonvulsants, such as phenytoin and valproic

acid; barbiturates; alcohol; benzodiazepines, such as diazepam; and drugs to treat insomnia, such as zolpidem, zaleplon, eszopiclone, and ramelteon. Women who take these medications should not take St. John's wort (UMMC, 2013j). Women who use aminolevulinic acid, a drug that increases photosensitivity of the skin, should not use St. John's wort to avoid dangerously increasing the sensitivity of their skin to the sun (UMMC, 2013j).

Women who take digoxin should avoid St. John's wort since it can decrease the effectiveness of digoxin. St. John's wort may decrease the effectiveness of oral contraceptives, and may increase the risk of unplanned pregnancy. St. John's wort can also decrease the effectiveness of immunosuppressive drugs taken for treatment of autoimmune disorders or organ transplant, such as adalimumab, azathioprine, cyclosporine, etancrcept, methotrexate, mycophenolate mofetil, and tacrolimus, and should thus be avoided (UMMC, 2013j). St. John's wort should not be taken by women who use any kind of antiretroviral medications for the treatment of HIV and AIDS. Women who take theophylline or Xanax should avoid St. John's wort due to risk of decreased effectiveness (UMMC, 2013j). Women who take warfarin should avoid St. John's wort since it may reduce the effectiveness of the anticoagulation action of this drug. Since St. John's wort is metabolized by certain liver enzymes, it may interact with other medications that are metabolized by the same enzymes. Therefore women should avoid St. John's wort if they take antifungal drugs such as ketoconazole, itraconazole, and fluconazole; statins such as astorvastatin, lovastatin, and simvastatin; imatinib, irinotecan; some calcium channel blockers, and any medication metabolized by the liver (UMMC, 2013j).

Mind and Body Practices

Mind and body practices use the power of thoughts and emotions to influence physical health. Most ancient healing practices that have produced many of the mind and body practices used today emphasize the link between body and mind, and essentially tap the healing forces within the human body to attain wellness. Mind and body practices condition the mind to focus on the body without distraction (UMSRH, 2014c). This state of focused concentration is believed to help a person to improve their health. Research conducted on various mind and body practices has shown solid evidence that many of these practices actually fight disease and promote health. Today mind and body practices are no longer viewed with suspicion and are taught at many prestigious medical schools in the United States and around the world (UMSRH, 2014c).

When the body is physically or emotionally stressed, the release of stress hormones affects all organs and systems. The body's natural capacity to heal may be diminished. Mind and body practices promote relaxation of body and mind, which reduces the level of stress hormones in the blood and enhances function of the immune system (UMSRH, 2014c).

Mind and body practices encourage relaxation, improve coping skills, reduce tension and pain, and lessen the need for medication. As such, these practices can help people with many health problems (UMSRH, 2014c). Numerous mind and body practices are used in combination with medication to treat pain. They are often effective in the treatment of anxiety and depression and may be helpful in treating many diseases, such as cancer, high blood pressure, asthma, heart disease, obesity, insomnia, diabetes, chemotherapy-related pain, nausea, and vomiting, fibromyalgia, stomach and intestinal problems, and menopausal symptoms (UMSRH, 2014c).

Mind and body practices are generally very safe and work well when combined with conventional medical care. Each technique may have its own risks and side effects. Women who have concerns should consult with their healthcare providers (UMHRSC, 2014c).

A variety of mind and body practices commonly used by women include the following.

Acupuncture

Acupuncture dates back thousands of years. It has been practiced in China as a key component of traditional Chinese medicine. It is also practiced in other parts of Asia. Acupuncture refers to a group of procedures that use a variety of techniques to stimulate specific points on the body, known as the meridian system. The meridian system is a network of hundreds of interconnected points throughout the body which allows for the passage of energy, or *chi*, between the physical and subtle bodies of the energy field. Each meridian connects one or more vital organs. When energy is congested or blocked in any meridian, the health of the associated organ will suffer. Acupuncture is considered the primary means to ensure the free flow of energy through the meridians by placing tiny bulb-like needles at various gates (acupuncture points) along the meridian pathways to unblock energy congestion. Although Western medicine does not quite acknowledge the concept of chi or meridians, it does recognize many remarkable outcomes of acupuncture in the treatment of chronic illnesses in which Western medicine has proven less than effective.

Extensive studies on acupuncture have focused in particular on back and neck pain, osteoarthritis and knee pain, and headache. Evidence suggests that acupuncture may help ease types of pain that are often chronic in nature, such as low back pain, neck pain, and osteoarthritis/knee pain. Acupuncture may also help reduce the frequency of tension headaches and prevent migraine headaches (NCCIH, 2014a). However, evidence about the value of acupuncture for other health issues is uncertain, and research is ongoing. Areas of investigation include the effectiveness of acupuncture in relieving symptoms of menopause, reducing pain and discomfort associated with chemotherapy, and the effectiveness of acupuncture versus simulated acupuncture and usual care in relief of pain (NCCIH, 2014a). Scientists are only now beginning to understand the effects of acupuncture on the brain and body and how best to measure these effects. Research findings indicate that many factors such as expectation and belief, which are unrelated to acupuncture needling, may play important roles in the effectiveness of acupuncture on pain (NCCIH, 2014a).

Acupuncture is a safe procedure when performed correctly by experienced, well-trained practitioners using sterile needles. Acupuncture that is not performed properly can cause serious side effects. Complications may result from improper delivery of treatments or from use of unsterile needles. When delivered improperly, acupuncture can cause serious adverse effects such as infections, punctured organs, collapsed lungs, and injury to the central nervous system (NCCIH, 2014a).

Women should not use acupuncture to postpone consulting a healthcare provider about a health problem. When an acupuncturist is used, his or her credentials should be checked. Most states require that acupuncturists hold a license, certification, or registration to practice acupuncture. Although the quality of care is not ensured by a license, it does indicate that the practitioner has met certain standards associated with knowledge and practice of acupuncture (NCCIH, 2014a). Some conventional medical practitioners may also practice acupuncture. Women should ask about their training and experience before selecting a practitioner for treatment. Women should also inquire about the estimated number of treatments needed and the cost of each treatment. Some insurance companies may cover the cost, but some do not (NCCIH, 2014a).

CHIROPRACTIC

Chiropractic is a healthcare profession that provides a complementary health approach that is widely used in this country. The term chiropractic is derived from the Greek words *cheir*, which means hand, and *praxis*, which means practice, and refers to a treatment done by hand. Chiropractic focuses mainly on the relationship between the structure of the body, chiefly the spine, and its functioning, as coordinated by the nervous system. It is believed that the relationship between the spine and functioning of the nervous system affects health (NCCIH, 2012c).

Although spinal adjustment/manipulation is a central part of treatment in chiropractic care, it is not synonymous with chiropractic. Spinal manipulations, manipulations of other parts of the body, and a variety of other treatments are commonly used to correct alignment problems, achieve pain relief, improve function, and encourage the natural ability of the body to heal itself (NCCIH, 2012c). Other healthcare providers such as physical therapists or osteopathic physicians also may use spinal manipulation in order to achieve healthcare goals for patients (NCCIH, 2012c).

Chiropractic care is mainly sought for relief of low back pain but is also commonly sought for other kinds of musculoskeletal pain such as neck and shoulder pain, headaches, and problems of the hands and feet (NCCIH, 2012c). Evidence suggests that spinal manipulation seems to benefit some people with low back pain, headaches, neck pain, upper and lower extremity joint problems, and whiplash-associated injuries (NCCIH, 2012c). Research findings have not shown effectiveness of chiropractic care in treating asthma, hypertension, and menstrual pain. Evidence is inconclusive regarding effectiveness of chiropractic care in treating fibromyalgia, mid-back pain, premenstrual syndrome, sciatica, and temporalmandibular joint disorders (NCCIH, 2012c).

Chiropractors commonly take a detailed health history during the initial visit and conduct a physical examination with special focus on the spine. Other diagnostic tests or examinations, such as x-rays, may also be performed. If chiropractic care is deemed suitable, a treatment plan will be formulated (NCCIH, 2012c). In subsequent visits, a chiropractor may perform one or more of various adjustments and other manual therapies available in chiropractic care. Directed mainly to the spine, chiropractic manipulation entails using the hands or a device to apply controlled rapid force to a joint. The aim is to increase range and quality of motion in the area being treated, and to help restore health (NCCIH, 2012c). Another type of manual therapy that may be applied is joint mobilization. Spinal adjustments and other manual therapies may be combined with several other treatment approaches such as heat and ice, electrical stimulation, relaxation techniques, rehabilitative and general exercise, dietary supplements, and counseling about weight loss, diet, and other life style factors (NCCIH, 2012c).

Women who use chiropractic care may experience side effects that include temporary headaches, tiredness, and discomfort in the areas of the body that received treatment. Rare serious complications such as stroke, cauda equine syndrome (pinched nerves in the lower spinal canal), and deterioration of herniated discs have been reported but it is unclear whether spinal manipulation actually caused such complications. Nevertheless, an important focus of ongoing research of chiropractic care is safety (NCCIH, 2012c).

Chiropractic practitioners graduate from 4-year chiropractic colleges accredited by the Council on Chiropractic Education. Chiropractic training programs include academic work as well as clinical training in caring for patients. Coursework commonly includes study in biomedical sciences, public health, and research methods. Some chiropractors wishing to specialize in certain fields may pursue 2 to 3 years of postgraduate residency for training (NCCIH, 2012c). To become licensed to practice, graduates need to pass a national certification examination. Chiropractic is regulated individually by each state and most states require chiropractors to earn continuing education credits annually to maintain licensure. The scope of practice varies from state to state in such areas as dispensing and selling dietary supplements and the use of other complementary healthcare approaches such as acupuncture or homeopathy (NCCIH, 2012c).

Women who desire chiropractic care should ask the practitioner about his or her education and licensure. Women should mention any health conditions they may have and inquire if the chiropractor has any specialized training or experience in the condition for which care is being sought. Women should ask about cost of treatment, insurance coverage, and any out-of-pocket costs. Chiropractic care is covered by many insurance plans, health maintenance organizations, Medicare, and state workman's compensation systems (NCCIH, 2012c). Women should also tell the chiropractor about prescription, over-the-counter medications, and dietary supplements they take. If any dietary supplements are suggested by the chiropractor, women should inquire about possible interactions. Women should inform their healthcare providers regarding any complementary health approaches they use in order to maintain safe and coordinated health care (NCCIH, 2012c).

Massage Therapy

Massage has been used as a healing modality for over 4,000 years. Massage has been and continues to be an important component of traditional Chinese medicine. For centuries, massage has been practiced as a healing technique worldwide in nearly every culture (UMSRH, 2014b). During the mid 19th-century, a contemporary form of massage, Swedish massage, was introduced to this country. By the end of the 19th century, Swedish massage had taken firm hold among physicians as a respected therapeutic practice. In the early 20th century, massage became overshadowed by new technologies and drug therapies, and thus became dormant. During the 1970s interest in massage therapy was rekindled and grew steadily over the years. Today there are over 125,000 massage therapists in practice in the United States, with ever-increasing numbers to meet the demands of over 80 million massage appointments annually (UMSRH, 2014b).

Massage is a treatment during which a therapist manipulates muscles and other soft tissues to improve health and well-being. Massage may range from gentle stroking and kneading of muscles and other soft tissues to deeper manual procedures. Massage is effective in relieving muscle tension, decreasing stress, and inducing feelings of calmness. Massage not only affects the body as a whole, it especially affects the activity of the musculoskeletal, lymphatic, circulatory, and nervous systems (UMSRH, 2014b).

Human touch can achieve both physical and emotional healing. Certain massage techniques may either stimulate or calm the muscles and tissues of the body to achieve a desired goal. The massage of soft tissue transmits electrical signals both locally and throughout the body. These signals, along with healing properties of touch, help heal damaged muscle, improve circulation, clear waste products via the lymphatic system, increase the activity of the immune system, relieve pain and tension, and cause a calming effect. Massage may also improve well-being by stimulating the release of endorphins and decreasing the levels of certain stress hormones (UMSRH, 2014b).

Nearly 100 different massage and body work techniques are practiced, each designed to achieve a specific goal. In the United States, the massage techniques that are most commonly practiced include the following.

AROMATHERAPY MASSAGE   This technique involves massaging essential oils from plants into the skin to enhance the healing and relaxation effects of the massage. The essential oils are thought to stimulate two structures deep in the brain that store emotions and memory, evoking a powerful effect on mood (UMSRH, 2014b).

CRANIOSACRAL MASSAGE   Gentle massage is applied to the head and spine in order to correct imbalances and restore the flow of cerebrospinal fluid to these areas (UMSRH, 2014b).

LYMPHATIC MASSAGE   The flow of lymph is enhanced by light rhythmic strokes throughout the body. Manual lymphatic drainage is the most popular form of lymphatic massage and aims to drain excess lymph (UMSRH, 2014b).

MYOFASCIAL RELEASE   Trained physical therapists or massage therapists use gentle pressure and body positioning to relax and stretch muscles, fascia, and associated structures (UMSRH, 2014b).

POLARITY THERAPY   The flow of energy within the body is stimulated and balanced to enhance well-being and healing (UMSRH, 2014b).

REFLEXOLOGY   Reflexologists believe that hands and feet contain reflex points, or direct connections to specific organs and structures throughout the body. Special thumb and finger massage techniques are applied to the reflex points to provide reciprocal healing to the corresponding organ (UMSRH, 2014b).

ROLFING   This technique consists of application of deep pressure to fascia in order to stretch, lengthen, and achieve more flexibility of the fascia. The aim of rolfing is to realign the body's ideal skeletal structure to achieve energy conservation, tension release, and better function (UMSRH, 2014b).

SHIATSU   A widely used technique in traditional Chinese medicine, shiatsu is the application of gentle finger and hand pressure to specific areas of the body to enhance the flow of energy (chi) through the energy pathways of the body (meridians) (UMSRH, 2014b).

SWEDISH MASSAGE   This technique incorporates a variety of strokes and pressures designed to improve the flow of blood to the heart, remove waste products from tissues, stretch ligaments and tendons, and relieve physical and emotional tension (UMSRH, 2014b).

TRIGGER POINT MASSAGE   This technique incorporates application of pressure to tender areas where muscles have been damaged (trigger points) to relieve pain and muscle spasm (UMSRH, 2014b).

Integrative Touch   This gentle type of massage incorporates mild, noncirculatory techniques to meet the needs of hospitalized patients or patients in hospice care (UMSRH, 2014b).

Compassionate Touch   This technique enhances quality of life for ill, elderly, or dying patients through the combination of focused one-on-one attention, intentional touch, and sensitive massage with communication (UMSRH, 2014b).

Massage is thought to enhance healing, increase energy, decrease recovery time from injury, relieve pain, and improve relaxation, mood, and well-being. It is helpful for relieving a variety of musculoskeletal problems such as low back pain, osteoarthritis, fibromyalgia, sprains and strains (UMSRH, 2014b). Massage may also relieve depression in people with chronic fatigue syndrome, chronic constipation (when performed in the abdominal area), reduce swelling, relieve sleep disorders, and enhance self-image. Evidence suggests that massage may reduce stress and improve mental alertness in the workplace (UMSRH, 2014b). Some research findings indicate that deep tissue massage lowers blood pressure levels; other findings suggest that massage may have immediate beneficial effects on pain and mood in people with advanced cancer (UMSRH, 2014b).

Research findings indicate that massage is likely an effective therapy with mothers and newborns. Mothers who are trained to massage their babies frequently feel less depression and have a better emotional bond with their infants (UMSRH, 2014b). Newborns massaged by their mothers tend to cry less and are more alert, sociable, and active. Evidence also suggests that babies who receive regular massage therapy likely gain weight faster, sleep better, have less gas or colic, and have better body awareness and better digestion (UMSRH, 2014b).

Massage is generally considered safe. An extremely vigorous massage technique may cause pain or other rare adverse side effects. Women who are pregnant should be very cautious and find a therapist trained specifically to perform massages on pregnant women (UMSRH, 2014b). Although massage may help diabetics regulate blood sugar over time, women who are diabetics should closely monitor their blood sugar, as massage may lower blood sugar. Diabetics who receive massages on a regular basis should monitor blood sugar levels often to assess fluctuations over time (UMSRH, 2014b). People who have heart failure, kidney failure, phlebitis, cellulitis, blood clots in the legs, bleeding disorders, or contagious skin conditions should avoid massage. People with mental impairment, osteoporosis, high fever, low platelets or white blood cell counts should avoid massage (UMSRH, 2014b). People with rheumatoid arthritis, goiter, eczema, and other skin lesions should avoid massage during periods of exacerbation and consult with their physicians. People who have cancer should consult with their physicians before considering massage, as skin may be fragile or damaged from chemotherapy or radiation therapy (UMSRH, 2014b). People on medications should discuss their medications with the massage therapist, as massage may influence absorption or activity of oral and topical medications (UMSRH, 2014b).

Continued research is needed to further determine effectiveness of massage therapy as a treatment modality for other health problems and conditions, as well as cost effectiveness of massage therapy in comparison to other treatments (UMSRH, 2014b).

Qigong and Tai Chi

Qigong   Qigong is an ancient Chinese healthcare system that dates back to about 4,000 years. Qigong incorporates physical postures, breathing techniques, and focused intention. The term qigong is composed of two Chinese words: qi (pronounced chee), which refers to the life-force or vital energy that flows through all things in the universe, and gong (pronounced gung), which refers to accomplishment or skill cultivated through steady practice. The term qigong means cultivating energy. Qigong is a system practiced for maintenance of health, healing, and increasing vitality (National Qigong Association [NQA], 2015).

The practices of qigong, whether for martial, medical, or spiritual purposes, involve a posture (either moving or stationary), breathing techniques, and mental focus. It is believed that some practices increase qi, some practices circulate qi, and some practices use qi to cleanse and heal the body, store qi, or release qi to help heal others. Practices of qigong vary from soft, simple internal styles such as tai chi, to vigorous, challenging external styles such as kung fu. Most forms of qigong consist of slow, gentle movements that can be easily modified for the physically challenged and for all age groups (NQA, 2015).

The practice of qigong as a healthcare system is not a cure-all, but it is believed to be highly effective. Qigong is a widely practiced form of alternative complementary health care throughout the world. It creates an awareness of and influences dimensions of the body and mind that are addressed in traditional exercise programs. The integration of the meridian system of qi, mind intent, and breathing techniques is believed to increase the benefits of exercise exponentially (NQA, 2015). The practice of the gentle rhythmic movements of qigong may help reduce stress, build stamina, increase vitality, and enhance functioning of the immune system. Qigong may also enhance cardiovascular, respiratory, circulatory, lymphatic, and digestive functions; however, not enough rigorous scientific research exists to confirm if qigong is actually effective in these claims. Research evidence does suggest, however, that qigong reduces high blood pressure and the incidence of falling among the elderly population (NQA, 2015). Also considered important is that qigong reestablishes the connection between mind, body, and soul. The integration of these

three aspects of being is believed to encourage a positive outlook on life and helps eliminate harmful behaviors and attitudes. Qigong helps to create a balanced life style, and enhances harmony, stability, and enjoyment (NQA, 2015).

TAI CHI   Tai chi is closely related to qigong in that both forms are energy-based exercises practiced to improve health and well-being. Both forms involve gentle movement, focused awareness, and breathing techniques (NCCIH, 2010b). Tai chi originated in ancient China as a martial art and a means of self defense. As time passed, tai chi was practiced for health purposes as well. The philosophical underpinnings of tai chi incorporate yin and yang, which are opposing forces in the body, and qi, the vital energy, or life force, in the body. It is believed that practicing tai chi will maintain a healthy balance of yin and yang, which will enhance the flow of qi (NCCIH, 2010b).

Tai chi is practiced by individuals alone or in groups. Among Chinese people, tai chi is commonly practiced in neighborhood parks in the early morning, before going to work (NCCIH, 2010b). Although numerous forms of tai chi are practiced, all involve slow, relaxed, graceful movements, each movement flowing into the next. The body moves continuously, and correct posture is essential. People practicing tai chi must also focus and put aside distracting thoughts, and breathe in a deep and relaxed, focused manner (NCCIH, 2010b).

Tai chi is practiced for a variety of health-related reasons. It may be practiced for benefits associated with low-impact, weight-bearing, aerobic exercise. It helps improve physical conditioning, muscle strength, coordination, and flexibility, and it helps to improve balance and reduce the risk of falls, especially in the elderly. Tai chi may also help to reduce pain and stiffness from osteoarthritis, improve sleep, and enhance overall well-being (NCCIH, 2010b).

Research is ongoing on tai chi to learn more about how it works and the possible effects it may have on health and chronic diseases and conditions. Several studies have focused on the elderly and the effectiveness of tai chi in preventing falls, improving cardiovascular fitness, improving immune system functioning, enhancing functional capacity in breast cancer patients, improving quality of life of persons with HIV infection, and improving overall well-being (NCCIH, 2010b). Research findings of studies that examined both tai chi and qigong practices indicate that the strongest and most consistent evidence of health benefits of tai chi or qigong is in bone health, cardiopulmonary fitness and factors associated with preventing falls, improving quality of life, and in improving self-efficacy (NCCIH, 2010a). Evidence also suggests that tai chi may be effective in reducing blood pressure (NCCIH, 2010b). Additional research is warranted to definitively determine the benefits of tai chi as a treatment modality (NCCIH, 2010b).

Tai chi is considered a relatively safe practice, although it should not be used as a replacement for conventional care or to delay seeing a physician for a medical problem. As with any exercise regimen, overdoing it may result in soreness or sprains. Pregnant women, women with joint problems, osteoporosis, back pain, fractures, hernia, or other medical conditions should consult with their physicians before beginning a tai chi program of exercise (NCCIH, 2010b). Tai chi should not be practiced immediately following a meal, when very tired, or if one has an active infection. Individuals who have not exercised in a while should consult with their physicians before starting tai chi practice (NCCIH, 2010b).

Licensing of tai chi instructors is not required and practice is not regulated by state or federal government. Traditionally, a student learns from a master instructor. There is no standard training of instructors. Students who are experienced may become instructors by gaining a master instructor's approval. Those who wish to practice tai chi with an instructor should inquire about the instructor's training and experience (NCCIH, 2010b).

RELAXATION TECHNIQUES

The stresses and demands of modern society can cause people to push themselves, physically and mentally, to the limits of well-being. Stress-related disorders account for the majority of visits to healthcare providers. Excessive stress is detrimental to health and the immune system. Relaxation techniques are procedures that help to facilitate coping with stress and promote long-term health by slowing down the body and quieting the mind. Relaxation techniques commonly involve refocusing attention (purposely noticing areas of tension), increasing body awareness, and exercises (such as meditation) to connect the body and mind. When implemented daily, relaxation techniques can promote a healthier perspective on stressful conditions. A large body of research evidence underscores the beneficial effects of relaxation on health and well-being. Relaxation techniques can be categorized into four major types, which are described here.

AUTOGENIC TRAINING Autogenic training involves the use of visual imagery and body awareness to create a deep state of relaxation. A person imagines a peaceful place and then concentrates on different physical sensations, moving from feet to head. For example, the person might concentrate on warmth and heaviness in the arms and legs, easy, natural breathing, or a calm heartbeat.

BREATHING With breathing techniques, a person places one hand on the chest, the other hand on the abdomen. The person inhales slowly and deeply, with the abdomen pushing against the hand. Each breath is held, and then slowly exhaled.

PROGRESSIVE MUSCLE RELAXATION Progressive muscle relaxation consists of slowly tensing and then relaxing each muscle group individually. A person begins tensing and relaxing muscle groups in the toes, and ends with those in the head.

MEDITATION   Meditation involves inducing a mode of consciousness that quiets the mind from external and internal noise to gain clarity. Many types of meditation are practiced but the most popular forms in this country are transcendental meditation, in which the person repeats a *mantra*—a single word or phrase, and mindfulness meditation, in which the person focuses attention on their thoughts and sensations. Regardless of the type of meditation, most have four elements in common: a quiet location with as few distractions as possible; a focus of concentration, such as a specially chosen word or set of words; a comfortable posture, such as sitting, lying down, or walking; and an open attitude that allows distractions to come and go naturally without judging them (NCCIH, 2014c).

When the body enters a state of deep relaxation, a set of physiological changes occur in response. The relaxation response entails a decrease in heart rate, blood pressure, muscle tension, and rate of breathing. The physiological changes of the relaxation response are opposite the fight-or-flight response to stress, which is increased heart rate, increased blood pressure, and increased respiratory rate (UMSRH, 2014d). A positive effect of learning the relaxation response is that it helps to offset ill effects of the fight-or-flight response. Learning the relaxation response will, over time, allow the development of a greater state of alertness. Techniques such as meditation and progressive muscle relaxation help to develop the relaxation response. Relaxation techniques are now a recommended form of treatment for many stress-related disorders (UMSRH, 2014d).

Relaxation techniques are associated with numerous positive health outcomes. Evidence suggests that meditation can help reduce stress hormone levels and improve a person's quality of life. Evidence also suggests that relaxation techniques likely reduce the perception of pain as well as enhance the immune response. Meditation may be helpful in the treatment of post-traumatic stress

disorder and may break substance abuse patterns in drug and alcohol abusers (UMSRH, 2014d). It has been shown that relaxation techniques can enhance coping skills in migraine sufferers, reduce stress, and improve mood in cancer patients. Overall, research findings indicate that with consistent practice, relaxation techniques may potentially reduce symptoms or improve outcomes in a variety of health conditions, including premenstrual syndrome, pain, irritable bowel syndrome, anxiety, infertility, high blood pressure, high cholesterol, diabetes, panic disorders, chronic tension headaches, fibromyalgia, insomnia, psoriasis, arthritis, and attention deficit hyperactivity disorder. It is essential that usual medical care and advice are followed for these conditions as well. Relaxation techniques should complement usual medical care, not replace it (UMSRH, 2014d).

Relaxation techniques are very safe; however, rare side effects have been associated with their use, such as increased anxiety because of a heightened awareness of body sensations, pain, heart palpitations, muscle twitching, and crying spells. This may be related to the process of relaxing and reflecting inward such that strong emotions are allowed to come to the surface (UMSRH, 2014d). Individuals with schizophrenia and other forms of psychosis should avoid relaxation techniques. Although many relaxation techniques may be self-taught, anyone with a specific medical or psychological disorder or concern should consult a healthcare professional or therapist who teaches relaxation techniques as part of their therapeutic practice (UMSRH, 2014d).

YOGA

The practice of yoga dates back thousands of years to ancient India. As a mind-body therapy, yoga connects the body, breath, and mind to energize and balance the whole person. Yoga has various styles that typically combine physical postures, breathing techniques, meditation, and a distinct philosophy to improve overall well-being. Yoga is practiced in this country by millions of people of all ages and fitness levels. While yoga is also a spiritual practice for many, most people in western culture practice yoga for exercise or to reduce stress. Hatha yoga is the most common form of yoga practiced in the United States and Europe. Hatha yoga emphasizes physical postures known as asanas, with the aim of balancing the opposites in one's life. During the asanas, flexing is followed by extension, a rounded back is followed by an arched back, and physical exercises are followed by meditation (UMSRH, 2014e).

The more popular styles of Hatha yoga include Ashtanga, Bikram, Iyengar, Integral, Kundalini, and Viniyoga, among others. Ashtanga yoga is a vigorous workout that requires constant movement from one posture to another. Bikram, one form of hot yoga, is a series of 26 asanas done in a room that is heated to 95 to 100 degrees. Bikram yoga warms and stretches the muscles, ligaments, and tendons, and purifies the body through perspiration. Integral yoga is a gentle form of yoga that includes meditation, breathing techniques, and chanting. Iyengar yoga requires great attention to detail, exact alignment of the body, and maintaining postures for long periods of time. Kundalini yoga accentuates the effects of breath on the asanas in order to free energy in the lower body to move upward. Viniyoga modifies asanas to each person's needs or abilities with synchronization of breaths and postures. The body is led into a posture by breath (UMSRH, 2014e).

Scientists are not quite certain how yoga brings about good health. Some think that, similar to other mind-body practices, yoga reduces stress. Others believe that yoga causes release of endorphins from the brain. Evidence suggests that yoga can decrease heart rate, promote muscle relaxation, and increase breathing capacity (UMSRH, 2014e). The breathing techniques, known as pranayama, increase blood flow and decrease oxygen consumption. This brings more oxygen to the brain and enhances the way oxygen is used in the body. Breathing techniques increase the amount of air drawn into the lungs, which helps a person feel more alert and focused. Asanas offer a gentle to intense workout that increases strength, flexibility, and balance. Meditation calms the mind and provides both physical and emotional relaxation, which assists in reducing blood pressure, chronic pain, anxiety, and cholesterol levels (UMSRH, 2014e).

The benefits of yoga include improved fitness, increased relaxation and self-confidence, and decreased stress and anxiety. People who practice yoga tend to have good posture, flexibility, coordination, sleep habits, and digestion. Although yoga does not cure any disease, it is a highly effective complementary therapy that helps treat a wide range of health problems (UMSRH, 2014e). Evidence suggests that yoga may be helpful in treating anxiety and stress, rheumatoid arthritis and osteoarthritis, chronic back pain, depression, diabetes, epilepsy, hypertension, hormonal problems, irritable bowel syndrome, lung diseases, and migraine (UMSRH, 2014e). Yoga may also be helpful as an additional therapy in reducing stress and strengthening the immune system in cancer patients. When combined with a healthy diet, yoga may also be helpful in treating people with heart disease by lowering blood pressure, decreasing stress, and reducing frequency and severity of episodes of chest pain. In people with carpal tunnel syndrome, yoga postures that stretch and strengthen joints in the upper body may increase grip strength and decrease pain (UMSRH, 2014e).

Yoga is low impact and generally safe for healthy people. However, done incorrectly it can cause injury. Thus it is essential that yoga is practiced with a trained instructor. Individuals may experience stiffness as their bodies become accustomed to different asanas (UMSRH, 2014e). Although the risk for injury is very low, certain types of stroke and pain from nerve damage are rare possible side effects. Pregnant women should be cautious and avoid certain postures. Special classes designed for pregnant women are available. People who have specific medical conditions such as sciatica, glaucoma, and hypertension should consult with their physicians and modify or avoid certain postures that may be unsafe. In such cases a gentler form of yoga may be more suitable (NCCIH, 2013c).

Ancient Healing Systems

An ancient healing system is a system of health care that has been practiced for thousands of years and is associated with a particular culture. Ancient healing systems are rooted in a philosophical or spiritual tradition of each particular culture. Two ancient healing systems, Ayurveda and traditional Chinese medicine, are discussed here.

AYURVEDA

Ayurveda originated in India over 3,000 years ago and is one of the oldest medical systems in the world. Ayurveda remains a traditional healthcare system in India and promotes the use of herbal compounds, special diets, and other unique health practices. The term *Ayurveda* is derived from the Sanskrit words *ayur,* which means life, and *veda,* which means science or knowledge (NCCIH, 2013a). Many Ayurvedic practices were handed down by word of mouth before written records existed. The fundamental concepts of Ayurvedic medicine encompass universal interconnectedness among people, their health, and the universe; the constitution of the body (prakriti); and life forces (dosha). Based on these principles, Ayurvedic physicians prescribe individualized treatments encompassing herbal compounds, diet, exercise, and life style recommendations. Ayurvedic medicine is used by the majority of the population of India, either exclusively or in combination with conventional Western medicine. It is also practiced in a variety of forms in Southeast Asia (NCCIH, 2013a).

Although some studies have investigated the use of Ayurvedic medicine for specific conditions, not enough well-controlled clinical trials and systematic research reviews have been conducted to provide evidence of effectiveness. The clinical trials that have been conducted have been small, had research design problems, or lacked appropriate control groups. Therefore, results have been inconclusive (NCCIH, 2013a).

Various products and practices are used in Ayurvedic medicine. Ayurvedic products in the United States are regulated as dietary supplements and thus are not required to meet the same safety and effectiveness standards as conventional medications. Ayurvedic products may contain herbs only or herbs combined with metals, minerals, or other materials. If some of these products are used improperly or without the direction of a trained practitioner, they may be harmful. Various products may cause side effects or interact with conventional medications (NCCIH, 2013a). There is also the potential for Ayurvedic products to be toxic, as some may contain levels of lead, mercury, and/or arsenic that exceed the standards for acceptable daily intake. In addition, certain Ayurvedic practices such as massage, special diets, and cleansing techniques may have side effects. Women who are pregnant or breastfeeding should use caution and consult their physicians if considering using Ayurvedic medicine. It is essential that women inform their healthcare providers about any Ayurvedic products or practices they use in order to ensure safe and coordinated care (NCCIH, 2013a).

TRADITIONAL CHINESE MEDICINE

Chinese medicine dates back 2,500 years and is rooted in the ancient philosophy of Taoism. This ancient healing system encompasses a variety of practices including acupuncture, Chinese herbal medicine, diet therapy, moxibustion, tai chi, and qigong. In this country, Americans use traditional Chinese medicine chiefly as a complementary health approach.

The fundamental concepts of traditional Chinese medicine are based on the following beliefs:

1. The human body is a miniature version of the larger surrounding universe.
2. Harmony between yin and yang, two opposite yet complementary forces, supports health. Imbalance between these forces results in disease.
3. The five elements of fire, earth, wood, metal, and water symbolize all phenomena including the stages of human life. These elements also explain the functioning of the body and how it changes during disease.
4. Qi is the vital energy that flows through the body and executes multiple tasks in maintaining health (NCCIH, 2013b).

Although traditional Chinese medicine is widely used throughout China, and has limited use in the West, as rigorous scientific evidence of its effectiveness is sparse. It is difficult for researchers to investigate traditional Chinese medicine because the treatments are frequently complex and are rooted in ideas that are very different from those of conventional Western medicine (NCCIH, 2013b). The majority of studies conducted on traditional Chinese medicine have focused on specific techniques and practices—chiefly acupuncture and Chinese herbal therapies. Numerous systematic reviews have been conducted of studies of traditional Chinese medicine approaches for various medical conditions. Research findings have been largely inconclusive as to whether traditional Chinese medicine is effective in treating these conditions (NCCIH, 2013b).

The safety of the various practices in traditional Chinese medicine varies. Tai chi and qigong are considered safe for most people but may cause soreness or sprains if overdone or until the individual gets accustomed to the exercise. Acupuncture is considered safe when performed by an experienced practitioner using single-use sterile needles (NCCIH, 2013b). Moxibustion involves burning an herb above the skin to apply heat to acupuncture points. Complications may include allergic reactions, burns, and infection. Both moxibustion and cupping, which involves applying a heated cup to the skin to create a slight suction, may temporarily mark the skin. Information on other practices in traditional Chinese medicine is scarce (NCCIH, 2013b).

The herbal products used in traditional Chinese medicine are commonly marketed in this country as dietary supplements. The regulations for dietary supplements are less stringent than the regulations for prescription and over-the-counter medications. Chinese herbal products may not contain the ingredients listed on the packaging, or may be contaminated with toxins, drugs, or heavy metals. Moreover, some herbs may have serious side effects, may interact with drugs, or may be unsafe for people with certain medical conditions (NCCIH, 2013b).

Traditional Chinese medicine should not be used as a replacement for conventional medical care or as a reason to postpone or delay consulting with a healthcare provider regarding a medical problem. Individuals should not self-treat with herbal remedies. The use of herbal remedies should be supervised by a healthcare provider or professional with expertise in herbal medicine (NCCIH, 2013b). Individuals should inquire regarding the training and expertise of the traditional Chinese medicine practitioner they are considering, and women who are pregnant or breastfeeding should consult with their healthcare provider if considering using traditional Chinese medicine. It is essential that women inform their healthcare providers about any complementary health approaches they use in order to ensure safe and coordinated care (NCCIH, 2013b).

Research Review

What are the reasons older Americans use CAM?

Tait, E., Laditka, J., Laditka, S., Nies, M., Racine, E., & Tsulukidze, M. (2013). Reasons why older Americans use complementary and alternative medicine: Costly or ineffective conventional medicine and recommendations from health care providers, family, and friends. *Educational Gerontology, 39*, 684–700.

Few studies have examined the reasons older Americans use CAM. The authors of this study addressed this shortcoming by examining four specific reasons why older adults use CAM. Two of the reasons were related to conventional medicine, in that CAM was used because conventional medicine did not help or because conventional medicine was too expensive. The other two reasons were associated with common sources of recommendations to use CAM, that is, recommendations from healthcare providers and recommendations from family, friends, or coworkers. Of particular interest to the authors were differences in the influence of the four reasons by gender, age, chronic conditions, income, and insurance status. The authors hypothesized that women were more likely than men to use CAM, African-Americans and Hispanics were more likely than whites to use CAM, the younger old were more likely to use CAM than the oldest old, and those with chronic conditions were more likely to use CAM than those without them. In addition, the authors hypothesized that those with less income and those who were uninsured were more likely to use CAM due to the cost of conventional medicine.

Data were obtained from the 2007 U.S. National Health Interview Survey and its Complementary and Alternative Medicine supplement. A sample of 10,096 respondents above the age of 50 represented 89.5 million adults. Logistic analyses adjusted for the sampling design and were weighted for national representation. The findings indicated that a sample representing 25 million older adults reported using CAM because it was recommended by a healthcare provider. Other reasons for use of CAM were recommendations by family, friends, or coworkers (20.2 million), ineffective conventional medicine (5.2 million), and expense of conventional medicine (4.0 million). Adjusted results indicated that women were more likely than men to use CAM for all four reasons. African-Americans and Hispanics were less likely to use CAM than whites for most of the reasons. The uninsured were much more likely to use CAM because conventional medicine was too expensive, and those with higher incomes were less likely to use CAM. In addition, older adults with chronic conditions, particularly musculoskeletal conditions or depression were more likely to use CAM for most of the reasons.

These findings suggest that healthcare providers are likely to recommend CAM to older patients for chronic conditions. These recommendations may be reinforced by limited effectiveness of conventional medical treatment for these conditions, as well as its cost. These findings may be useful in helping healthcare providers identify patients most likely to use CAM, especially those using CAM for chronic illnesses, and those who may be at higher risk for adverse interactions between CAM and conventional medical therapies.

Chapter Summary Points

- The accelerated and hectic pace of women's lives exposes them to frequent and intense stress.
- Common intense stressors women face daily include managing multiple role demands, experiencing conflicting domestic and employment-related responsibilities, dealing with rapid and abrupt cultural and technological changes, and navigating an uncertain economy.
- Chronic stress is believed to be associated with disease because the body experiences prolonged exposure to the physiological effects of the stress response. The majority of diseases and illnesses are likely stress related.
- Although fight-or-flight may characterize the primary physiological responses to stress for both men and women, it has been posited that behaviorally, responses to stress by women are more marked by a pattern of "tend and befriend."
- Coping is the process of using both cognitive and behavioral processes to manage demands that are judged as taxing or exceeding an individual's resources.
- Maintaining a healthy weight requires attaining balance between the amount of calories consumed and the amount of calories burned by physical activities.
- As weight increases to the levels of overweight and obesity, the subsequent risks for developing health problems also increases.
- The means to successful weight loss lies with increasing the BMR by exercise, not by cutting calories.
- Ineffective weight loss efforts include starvation or hunger, dieting without exercise, weight cycling, and using diet supplements.
- Severely overweight and obese individuals may turn to bariatric surgery to achieve weight loss.
- Physically active women derive health benefits throughout the life cycle.
- Physical activity is activity that brings health benefits and signifies movement of a moderate intensity lasting a few minutes or more.
- More than half of the adults in this country do not get enough physical activity to provide important health benefits. Women are less likely than men to be physically active.
- The four major areas of physical fitness include cardiovascular endurance, muscular strength, muscular endurance, and flexibility.
- Complementary therapeutic modality is the use of a non-mainstream approach together with conventional medicine, whereas alternative therapeutic modality is the use of a non-mainstream approach in place of conventional medicine.
- Alternative and complementary healthcare approaches generally fall into one of two subgroups: natural products and mind and body practices.
- Mind and body practices consist of a large and diverse group of procedures or techniques administered or taught by a trained practitioner or teacher.
- Herbal supplements are natural products, and there is no guarantee that these products are safe. Some herbal supplements may damage the liver, interact with medications, or pose risks if an individual has medical problems or undergoes surgery.

- Mind and body practices emphasize the link between body and mind, and tap the healing forces within the human body to attain wellness. Mind and body practices condition the mind to focus on the body without distraction.
- Mind and body practices are generally safe and work well when combined with conventional medical care.
- Ayurveda and traditional Chinese medicine are two ancient healing systems that prescribe individualized treatments encompassing herbal compounds, diet, exercise, and life style recommendations.

Critical Thinking Exercise

Questions for Seminar Discussion

1. What factors contribute to stress in women?
2. How does stress affect women's well-being and quality of life?
3. How do women differ from men in their response to stress?
4. What are the basic components of successful coping strategies?
5. What positive coping strategies are available to help women cope with stress?
6. What factors influence weight gain in women?
7. How does overweight and obesity affect health, well-being, and quality of life?
8. How do healthy weight loss strategies compare and contrast with unhealthy weight loss strategies?
9. Why is physical inactivity a national problem?
10. What are the four major elements of physical fitness?
11. How do women differ from men in physical fitness?
12. How can exercise improve health, well-being, and quality of life of women of all ages?
13. Why are complementary and alternative therapeutic modalities popular among women?
14. What is the problem of reproducibility in herbal supplements?
15. What safety measures should women take when using herbal remedies?
16. What herbal remedies are commonly used by women? What is the state of research evidence regarding these herbal remedies?
17. What safety measures should women take when using mind and body practices?
18. What is the state of research evidence regarding mind and body practices?
19. How can mind and body practices improve health, well-being, and quality of life?
20. What are ancient healing systems? What safety issues should be considered by women who use Ayurvedic or traditional Chinese medicine?

Internet Resources

The Academy of Integrative Health and Medicine: provides information and resources for women, families, and professionals. http://aihm.org/

American Chiropractic Association: provides information and resources for women, families, and professionals. http://www.acatoday.org/

American Holistic Health Association: provides information and resources for women, families, and professionals. http://ahha.org/

The American Institute of Stress: Provides information, education, and resources regarding management of stress for women, families, and professionals. http://www.stress.org/

Ayurvedic-Medicines.org: provides information and resources about Ayurvedic medicine. http://www.ayurvedic-medicines.org/

The Center for Mind-Body Medicine: provides information and resources for women, families, and professionals about mind-body medicine. http://cmbm.org/

Centers for Disease Control and Prevention: Division of Nutrition, Physical Activity, and Obesity (NPAO): provides information and resources for women, families, and professionals about nutrition, physical activity, and obesity. http://www.cdc.gov/nccdphp/dnpao/index.html

National Center for Complementary and Integrative Health: the lead agency of the federal government for scientific research on complementary and integrative health approaches. https://nccih.nih.gov/

Traditional Chinese Medicine World Foundation: provides information and resources for women, families, and professionals about traditional Chinese medicine. http://www.tcmworld.org/

References

Adams, K., Schatzkin, A., Harris, T., Kipnis, V., Mouw, T., Ballard-Barbash, R., ... Leitzman, M. (2006). Overweight, obesity, and mortality in a large prospective cohort of persons 50 to 71 years old. *New England Journal of Medicine*, *355*(8), 763–778.

American Psychological Association. (2007). How Does Stress Affect Us? *PsychCentral*. Retrieved from http://psychcentral.com/lib/how-does-stress-affect-us/0001130

Boston Medical Center. (2014). Nutrition & weight management. Retrieved from http://www.bmc.org/nutritionweight/services/weightmanagement.htm

Brosse, A., Sheets, E., Lett, H., & Blumenthal, J. (2002). Exercise and the treatment of clinical depression in adults: recent findings and future directions. *Sports Medicine*, *32*(12), 741–760.

Brownell, K., & Rodin, J. (1994). Medical, metabolic, and psychological effects of weight cycling. *Archives of Internal Medicine*, *154*(12), 1325–1330.

Centers for Disease Control and Prevention. (2012a). Defining adult overweight and obesity. Retrieved from http://www.cdc.gov/obesity/adult/defining.html

Centers for Disease Control and Prevention. (2012b). Adult obesity causes & consequences. Retrieved from http://www.cdc.gov/obesity/adult/causes/index.html

Centers for Disease Control and Prevention. (2013). Genomics and health. Retrieved from http://www.cdc.gov/genomics/resources/diseases/obesity/index.htm

Centers for Disease Control and Prevention. (2014). Adult obesity facts. Retrieved from http://www.cdc.gov/obesity/data/adult.html

Da Costa, D., Rippen, N., Drista, M., & Ring, A. (2003). Self-reported leisure time physical activity during pregnancy and relationship to psychological well-being. *Journal of Psychosomatic Obstetrics and Gynaecology*, *24*(2), 111–119.

EBSCO. (2012a). Herbal medicine. Retrieved from http://therapy.epnet.com/nat/GetContent.asp?siteid=EBSCO&chunkiid=37432

EBSCO. (2012b). St. John's wort. Retrieved from http://therapy.epnet.com/nat/GetContent.asp?siteid=EBSCO&chunkiid=31050

EBSCO. (2013). Ginkgo. Retrieved from http://therapy.epnet.com/nat/GetContent.asp?siteid=EBSCO&chunkiid=21740

Elavsky, S., McAuley, Motl, R., Konopack, J., Marquez, D., Hu, L., … Diener, E. (2005). Physical activity enhances long-term quality of life in older adults: efficacy, esteem, and affective influences. *Annals of Behavioral Medicine*, *30*(2), 138–145.

Finkelstein, E., Trogdon, J., Cohen, J., & Dietz, W. (2009). Annual medical spending attributable to obesity: Payer and service-specific estimates. *Health Affairs*, *28*(5), w822–w831.

Hu, F., Willet, W., Li, T., Stampfer, M., Colditz, G., & Manson, J. (2004). Adiposity as compared with physical activity in predicting mortality among women. *New England Journal of Medicine*, *351*(26), 2694–2703.

Institute of HeartMath. (2014). Stress and cognitive decline. Retrieved from http://www.heartmath.org/free-services/articles-of-the-heart/stress-and-cognitive-decline.html

Kannus, P., Sievanen, H., Palvenen, M., Jarvinen, T., & Parkkari, J. (2005). Prevention of falls and injuries in elderly people. *Lancet*, *366*(9500), 1885–1893.

Lazarus, R., & Folkman, S. (1984). *Stress, appraisal, and coping*. New York: Springer.

National Center for Complementary and Integrative Health. (2010a). Tai chi and qi gong show some beneficial health effects. Retrieved from https://nccih.nih.gov/research/results/spotlight/071910.htm

National Center for Complementary and Integrative Health. (2010b). Tai chi and qui gong. Retrieved from https://nccih.nih.gov/health/taichi/introduction.htm

National Center for Complementary and Integrative Health. (2012a). Black cohosh. Retrieved from https://nccih.nih.gov/health/blackcohosh/ataglance.htm

National Center for Complementary and Integrative Health. (2012b). Chasteberry. Retrieved from https://nccih.nih.gov/health/chasteberry

National Center for Complementary and Integrative Health. (2012c). Chiropractic: An introduction. Retrieved from https://nccih.nih.gov/health/chiropractic/introduction.htm

National Center for Complementary and Integrative Health. (2013a). Ayurvedic medicine: An introduction. Retrieved from https://nccih.nih.gov/health/ayurveda/introduction.htm

National Center for Complementary and Integrative Health. (2013b). Traditional Chinese medicine. Retrieved from https://nccih.nih.gov/health/whatiscam/chinesemed.htm

National Center for Complementary and Integrative Health. (2013c). Yoga for health. Retrieved from https://nccih.nih.gov/health/yoga/introduction.htm

National Center for Complementary and Integrative Health. (2014a). Acupuncture: What you need to know. Retrieved from https://nccih.nih.gov/health/acupuncture/introduction

National Center for Complementary and Integrative Health. (2014b). Complementary, alternative, or integrative health: What's in a name? Retrieved from https://nccih.nih.gov/health/whatiscam

National Center for Complementary and Integrative Health. (2014c). Meditation: What you need to know. Retrieved from https://nccih.nih.gov/health/meditation/overview.htm

National Center for Complementary and Integrative Health. (2014d). Using dietary supplements wisely. Retrieved from https://nccih.nih.gov/health/supplements/wiseuse.htm

National Center for Health Statistics. (2010). National health interview survey. Retrieved from http://www.cdc.gov/nchs/data/nhis/brochure2010January.pdf

National Heart, Lung, and Blood Institute. (2012). What are the health risks of overweight and obesity? Retrieved from http://www.nhlbi.nih.gov/health/health-topics/topics/obe/risks#

National Qigong Association. (2015). What is qigong? Retrieved from http://nqa.org/resources/what-is-qigong/

Natural Medicines Comprehensive Database. (2014). Calendula. Retrieved from http://www.nlm.nih.gov/medlineplus/druginfo/natural/235.html

Office on Women's Health. (2010). Stress and your health. Retrieved from http://www.womenshealth.gov/publications/our-publications/fact-sheet/stress-your-health.pdf

Ogden, C., Carroll, M., Kit, B., & Flegal, K. (2014). Prevalence of childhood and adult obesity in the United States,

2011–2012. *Journal of the American Medical Association*, *311*(8), 806–814.

Ogden, C., Lamb, M., Carroll, M., Flegal, K. (2010). *Obesity and socioeconomic status in adults: United States 1988–1994 and 2005–2008. NCHS data brief no 50.* Hyattsville, MD: National Center for Health Statistics.

Olshansky, S., Passaro, D., Hershow, R., Layden, J., Carnes, B., Brody, J., … Ludwig, D. (2005). A potential decline in life expectancy in the United States in the 21st century. *New England Journal of Medicine*, *352*(11), 1138–1145.

Outland, L., Madanet, H., & Rust, F. (2013). Intuitive eating for a healthy weight. *Primary Health Care, 23*(9), 22–28.

Savard, M., & Svec, C. (2005). *The body shape solution to weight loss and wellness.* New York: Atria Publishers.

Selye, H. (1978). *The stress of life.* New York: McGraw Hill.

Tait, E., Laditka, J., Laditka, S., Nies, M., Racine, E., & Tsulukidze, M. (2013). Reasons why older Americans use complementary and alternative medicine: Costly or ineffective conventional medicine and recommendations from health care providers, family, and friends. *Educational Gerontology, 39*, 684–700.

Taylor, S., Klein, L., Lewis, B., Gruenwald, T., Gurung, R., & Updegraff, J. (2000). Biobehavioral responses to stress in females: Tend-and-befriend, not fight-or-flight. *Psychological Review, 107*(3), 411–429.

University of Maryland Medical Center. (2013a). Calendula. Retrieved from http://umm.edu/health/medical/altmed/herb/calendula

University of Maryland Medical Center. (2013b). Dong quai. Retrieved from http://umm.edu/health/medical-reference-guide/complementary-and-alternative-medicine-guide/herb/dong-quai

University of Maryland Medical Center. (2013c). Echinacea. Retrieved from http://umm.edu/health/medical-reference-guide/complementary-and-alternative-medicine-guide/herb/echinacea

University of Maryland Medical Center. (2013d). Evening primrose oil. Retrieved from https://nccih.nih.gov/health/eveningprimrose

University of Maryland Medical Center. (2013e). Garlic. Retrieved from http://umm.edu/health/medical-reference-guide/complementary-and-alternative-medicine-guide/herb/garlic

University of Maryland Medical Center. (2013f). Ginger. Retrieved from http://umm.edu/health/medical-reference-guide/complementary-and-alternative-medicine-guide/herb/ginger

University of Maryland Medical Center. (2013g). Gingko biloba. Retrieved from http://umm.edu/health/medical-reference-guide/complementary-and-alternative-medicine-guide/herb/ginkgo-biloba

University of Maryland Medical Center. (2013h). Ginseng. Retrieved from http://umm.edu/health/medical-reference-guide/complementary-and-alternative-medicine-guide/herb/asian-ginseng

University of Maryland Medical Center. (2013i). Herbal medicine. Retrieved from http://umm.edu/health/medical/altmed/treatment/herbal-medicine

University of Maryland Medical Center. (2013j). St. John's wort. Retrieved from http://umm.edu/health/medical-reference-guide/complementary-and-alternative-medicine-guide/herb/st-johns-wort

University of Maryland Shore Regional Health. (2014a). Green tea. Retrieved from http://umshoreregional.org/health/medical/altmed/herb/green-tea

University of Maryland Shore Regional Health. (2014b). Massage. Retrieved from http://umm.edu/system-hospital-sites/shore-health/health/medical/altmed/treatment/massage

University of Maryland Shore Regional Health. (2014c). Mind-body medicine. Retrieved from http://umm.edu/system-hospital-sites/shore-health/health/medical/altmed/treatment/mindbody-medicine

University of Maryland Shore Regional Health. (2014d). Relaxation techniques. Retrieved from http://umm.edu/system-hospital-sites/shore-health/health/medical/altmed/treatment/relaxation-techniques

University of Maryland Shore Regional Health. (2014e). Yoga. Retrieved from http://umm.edu/system-hospital-sites/shore-health/health/medical/altmed/treatment/yoga

U.S. Department of Health and Human Services. (2008). 2008 Physical activity guidelines for Americans. Retrieved from http://www.health.gov/paguidelines/guidelines/

U.S. Department of Health and Human Services, Health Resources and Services Administration, Maternal and Child Health Bureau. (2011). *Women's Health USA 2011.* Rockville, MD: U.S. Department of Health and Human Services.

Chapter 5

Eating Disorders

LEARNING OUTCOMES

On completion of this chapter, the learner will be able to:

1. Explain the incidence, etiology, and genetic links of eating disorders in adolescent and young women.
2. Describe risk factors and risk reduction for adolescent and young women with eating disorders.
3. Discuss how gender disparities influence awareness, diagnosis, and treatment of eating disorders.
4. Analyze current screening, diagnostic, and treatment practices associated with eating disorders.
5. Discuss threats to quality of life of adolescent and young women created by eating disorders.
6. Explore implications for enhancing quality of life outcomes in adolescent and young women with eating disorders.

Introduction

Eating disorders are devastating and complex mental illnesses that commonly occur in adolescent girls and young women. Eating disorders frequently exist together with other mental disorders such as depression, anxiety, or substance abuse. A combination of biological, psychological, and sociocultural dynamics contribute to the development of eating disorders, and each disorder has distinctive symptoms and adverse physical sequelae. Eating disorders that are untreated are frequently accompanied by life-threatening medical and psychiatric complications. This chapter explores the issues of eating disorders that develop in adolescent and young women. The significant impact of eating disorders on the quality of life of adolescent and young women is also discussed.

Incidence

In the United States, the prevalence of eating disorders is widespread. It is estimated that as many as 20 million females and 10 million males suffer from eating disorders such as anorexia nervosa or bulimia nervosa (National Eating Disorders Association [NEDA], 2015b). In addition, millions of individuals are afflicted with binge eating disorder. There are likely many more cases of eating disorders that are not reported because of the secretiveness and shame associated with these conditions (NEDA, 2015b).

Eating disorders commonly develop in women and girls. The female-to-male ratio of incidence of anorexia nervosa and bulimia nervosa ranges from 6:1 to 10:1 (Franco, 2012). The lifetime prevalence among women of anorexia nervosa is 0.9%, and 1.5% for bulimia nervosa, as compared to the lifetime prevalence among males of 0.3% for anorexia and 0.5% for bulimia (Hudson, Hiripi, Pope, & Kessler, 2007). Women tend to develop eating disorders between the ages of 12 to 35. The average age of onset for eating disorders is 19 years old for anorexia nervosa, 20 years old for bulimia nervosa, and 25 years old for binge eating disorder (Hudson et al., 2007).

Eating disorders are prevalent in industrialized societies that have an abundance of food, and thinness among women is considered attractive. Countries in which eating disorders are most common include the United States, Canada, Europe, Australia, and South Africa (Franco, 2012). Nonetheless, the rates of eating disorders have risen in Asia, particularly in Japan and China, where women have been influenced by culture change and modernization. In the United States, eating disorders have become common among young Hispanic, Native American, and African-American women, but at rates that are lower than among white women (Franco, 2012). When considering the prevalence of eating disorders in diverse groups of women, the lifetime prevalence of anorexia nervosa is 0.14% in African-American women, 0.12% in Hispanic women, 0.12% in Asian women, and 1.5% in white women. The lifetime prevalence of bulimia nervosa is 1.9% in African-American women, 1.91% in Hispanic women, 1.42% in Asian women, and 2.3% in white women. The lifetime prevalence of binge eating disorder is 2.36% in African-American women, 2.31% in Hispanic women, 2.67% in Asian women, and 2.7% in white women (Brown, Cachelin, & Dohm, 2009).

Eating disorders have the highest mortality rate of any mental illness. In fact, the mortality rate associated with anorexia nervosa is 6 to 12 times higher in females as compared to the general population, adjusting for age (Academy for Eating Disorders [AED], 2011). For females 15–24 years old, the mortality rate associated with anorexia nervosa is 12 times higher than the mortality rate associated with all causes of death. Furthermore, about 20% of individuals suffering from anorexia nervosa will die prematurely from complications associated with their eating disorder, including heart problems, organ failure, malnutrition, and suicide (National Association of Anorexia Nervosa and Associated Disorders [ANAD], 2015). Mortality rates for specific eating disorders are estimated to be 4% for anorexia nervosa and 3.9% for bulimia nervosa (Crow et al., 2009).

Despite having the highest mortality rate of any mental disorder, the mortality rates of individuals with eating disorders vary significantly between studies and sources. The large variance in mortality rate is likely related to reported deaths being attributed to specific medical complications rather than the diagnosis of an eating disorder that compromised a person's health.

Ethnic Considerations

A common misconception about eating disorders is that they are diseases of middle class or upper class white females who are pathologically engrossed with trying to achieve a stereotyped unrealistic ideal of thinness and beauty. This misconception continues despite empirical evidence that suggests ethnic minority women are not immune to developing eating disorders. In fact, evidence suggests that eating disorders are likely significant problems for African-American, Hispanic, Asian and other diverse ethnic groups of women (Brown et al., 2009). Information about eating disorders among ethnic minority women is sparse because little research on eating disorders has been conducted using participants from racial and ethnic minority groups. Nonetheless, reports of eating disorders among ethnic minority women are increasing. This may be due to increased *reporting* of the eating disorders and not an actual rise in incidence. Factors that probably influence the rate of reporting eating disorders among ethnic minority women include under-reporting of problems by individuals, and under- or misdiagnosing by treatment providers, which may be attributed to the mistaken belief that women from racial and ethnic minorities are immune to developing eating disorders (NEDA, 2015a).

The prevalence of eating disorders among ethnic minority women varies depending on the eating disorder syndrome or symptom under consideration and the population in question. It is likely that cultural factors influence the etiology of eating disorders in ethnic minority women. As such, recognition and treatment of eating disorders and associated problems in ethnic minority women cannot be implemented effectively on a large scale until a greater understanding of culture as well as contextual variables is gained (Brown, et al., 2009).

Etiology and Risk Factors

Eating disorders are serious mental illnesses that are manifested by a variety of unhealthy eating and weight control habits that become obsessive, compulsive, and/or impulsive in nature. Eating disorders almost always begin as diets but these disorders are much more complicated than unhealthy eating habits or desire to lose weight. Individuals who have eating disorders are also likely to suffer from low self-esteem/self-worth and have mental illnesses such as depression, anxiety disorders, and substance abuse problems. Numerous biological, social, cultural, and environmental factors are believed to contribute to the development of eating disorders, and these

factors are inextricably linked (Striegel-Moore & Bulik, 2007). The presence of these risk factors can increase an individual's vulnerability to eating disorders, and, when combined with triggering life events, they may increase the likelihood of developing a disorder.

Sociocultural Factors

The female beauty ideal of extreme thinness that is prevalent in Western culture as well as objectification of the female body have been acknowledged as significant factors that influence the development of eating disorders in young women. Women are exposed to the thin ideal, internalize this ideal, and experience a discrepancy between themselves and the ideal. This discrepancy, in turn, can lead to body dissatisfaction, dietary restraint, and restriction (Striegel-Moore & Bulik, 2007). For some women, restraint and/or restriction may lead to overeating, which amplifies concerns of body image and can initiate additional restraint and/or purging. Objectification of the female body increases the risk of developing eating disorders by placing the value of women primarily on their appearance, and this emphasis reinforces the need to pursue attractiveness (Streigel-Moore & Bulik, 2007).

Psychological Factors

Feminist theorists have suggested that two elements of feminine identity, as defined by Western culture, contribute to women's enhanced risk for eating disorders. Women are socially conditioned to place high importance on interpersonal relationships and have a tendency to define themselves in terms of their relationships with others. Thus, the relational point of reference increases women's vulnerability to the judgment of others, especially during adolescence. The ability to successfully engage in interpersonal relationships often becomes linked to self-worth. Physical attractiveness is a powerful determinant of interpersonal success. Failed relationships may be experienced as fundamental insults on individual identity and may engender feelings of self-doubt and low self-esteem. In a society where beauty and femininity are inextricably linked, women are likely to place a high priority on achieving the culturally defined beauty ideal because of increased motivation to attain social approval and meaningful interpersonal relationships. Hence there is emphasis on the importance of beauty for interpersonal attraction (Sargent, Stein, & Rosen, 2009).

Although a compelling sociocultural influence, not all girls or women develop eating disorders in this cultural climate. Other factors exist that may amplify or diminish the risk that arises from the thin beauty ideal. Social pressure to be thin, for example, frequently takes the form of media images, peer teasing, or admonishments to lose weight. In higher social classes of society, more attention is presumably paid to and more resources are available for attaining the beauty ideal. Personality traits such as perfectionism can increase one's desire to comply with social norms. Having increased social anxiety may amplify an individual's susceptibility to social feedback. Being heavy or obese moves one's body further away from the ideal. High impulsivity may make restrictive eating challenging and increase

the risk for binge eating. Individual differences in biological responses to starvation and the reward value of starvation or eating can also be influential (Streigel-Moore & Bulik, 2007).

Identity impairments have been thought to contribute to the development of eating disorders. Women who lack a clear and consistent sense of self due to impaired identity formation may be more vulnerable to cultural pressures for achieving the unrealistic stereotypic cultural ideal body image (Sargent et al., 2009). Positive self-schemas serve to motivate and direct patterns of daily behavior; lack of positive identity can lead to self-confusion, dissatisfaction, and high reliance on body weight as a source of self-definition and esteem (Sargent et al., 2009).

Crucial phases of adolescent and adult life with related life stressors also are associated with the development of eating disorders. Critical life events may precipitate the onset of an eating disorder in vulnerable individuals (Sargent et al., 2009). Significant stress, when coupled with inadequate coping resources, can combine with other risk factors to increase a person's vulnerability to developing an eating disorder. Potential triggers for developing eating disorders are presented in **Box 5–1**.

Box 5–1: Potential Triggers for Eating Disorders

Eating disorders may be triggered in vulnerable girls and women by:

- Environmental changes (changes in school, moving to a new home or city)
- Family changes (parental divorce, birth of a child, increased familial stress)
- Loss of a loved one (through death or breakup of a relationship)
- Trauma
- Uncomfortable feelings about adult sexuality or unwanted sexual advances
- Maturity fears
- Increased familial responsibility or caretaking

- Dieting to promote weight loss (often for an upcoming special event)
- Industry pressure to maintain a certain physical appearance
- Teasing or being bullied
- Rejection
- Threats to physical safety or security
- Academic difficulties
- Peer pressure (including pressure from team sports)
- Chronic illness, especially one that may affect weight or appearance
- Other significant loss or disappointment

Occupational Factors, Athletics, and Other Activities

Several sports, occupations, and disciplines that place undue emphasis on body weight and appearance tend to contribute to a higher incidence of eating disorders among participants. Ballet dancers, models, and entertainment personalities frequently experience social and occupational pressure to be thin. The more a person is involved in these types of activities, especially at advanced levels, the more likely they are to experience pressure about body shape and weight. Athletes involved in sports that emphasize appearance, weight requirements, or endurance, such as gymnastics, figure skating, track and field, swimming, jockeying, wrestling, rowing, and bodybuilding, often face weight restrictions that may lead to unhealthy attempts at weight control. Parents and coaches may exert undue pressure on participants to maintain sometimes unrealistic weight goals to enhance performance in the discipline (Sargent et al., 2009). The misconception that a lower body weight improves performance, pressures and weight restrictions on athletes training for a sport since childhood or on elite athletes, and the presence of psychological factors can also contribute to an athlete developing an eating disorder.

The female athlete triad refers to three interrelated problems of female athletes: disordered eating, amenorrhea, and osteoporosis. This is a dangerous condition because the lack of nutrition resulting from disordered eating can cause a reduction in estrogen levels, cessation of menstrual periods, and loss of calcium and bone density. Separately, disordered eating, cessation of menstruation, and osteoporosis are all serious conditions. Together they create acute health risks that may become irreversible and possibly life threatening. Adolescent girls are at particular risk for the female athlete triad because of the active biological changes and growth spurts they experience at this time, the insecurities that accompany adolescence (including peer and social pressures), and the increased focus on thinness for females.

Biological Factors

Perinatal factors such as having been born prematurely, being small for one's age, and having suffered birth trauma such as cephalohematoma can increase the risk for developing anorexia nervosa. Girls who have experienced an early puberty tend to have increased risk for developing eating disorders. Puberty brings with it biological changes in body weight, shape, and size with increased deposition of body fat. Girls and young women who suffer from chronic illnesses such as diabetes mellitus also have increased risk for developing eating disorders (Katzman & Golden, 2008).

Evidence suggests that genetic or inherited components play a significant role in the development of eating disorders. Research findings indicate a higher incidence of diagnosed eating disorders in first-degree female relatives and monozygotic twin offspring of patients with anorexia nervosa and bulimia nervosa. Moreover, children of patients with anorexia nervosa have a tenfold greater lifetime risk of developing anorexia nervosa than the general population (Franco, 2012; Striegel-Moore & Bulik, 2007).

Serotonin is involved in the regulation of eating as in the mechanisms of feeding, fasting, and satiety, and is thought to be associated with eating disorders. Serotonin also plays a role in body image and perception abnormalities, and other characteristics related to eating disorders such as seasonality of symptoms, prevalence in females, onset after stressful life events, and associated psychiatric traits such as depression, anxiety, impulsivity, and addiction. Serotonin dysregulation may lead to the disruption of complex control mechanisms that may eventually manifest as eating disorders ("Genetic factors have a role in the development and treatment of eating disorders," 2005). Research findings suggest that dysfunction of the serotonin system affects feeding behaviors—in particular, the satiety response. Molecular genetics research regarding anorexia nervosa and bulimia nervosa risk has explored mood and appetite, with particular focus in the serotonergic system (serotonin receptor and transporter genes) and the dopaminergic system (dopamine receptor and transporter genes), as well as other genes believed to be central to the etiology of eating disorders. Associations between mutations in the gene encoding the serotonin transporter, SLC6A4, and increased risk of anorexia nervosa have been obtained but its role

in other eating disorders is as yet unclear. Investigations are ongoing ("Genetic factors," 2005; Striegel-Moore & Bulik, 2007).

Degree of Risk of Eating Disorders

Risk factors increase the probability of developing a harmful outcome, while protective factors identify individuals at lower risk for developing a disorder or a higher probability of favorable outcomes. Presently, the understanding of risk and pathology of eating disorders far exceeds that of protective factors and resilience (Steiner et al., 2003). The degree of risk for developing eating disorders varies according to the presence of risk and protective factors, which generally operate in a probabilistic manner. As such, females who grow up in Western culture have greater probability for developing an eating disorder but do not necessarily develop an eating disorder later in life. The majority of females brought up in Western cultures do not have eating disorders (Steiner et al., 2003).

It is likely that particular developmental periods exist in which exposure to risk factors have greater influence on the later development of eating disorders. These critical periods are markedly significant in that the disturbances within them likely lead to qualitative changes and a future inability to draw level with the normal course of development (Steiner et al., 2003). Puberty, for example, is acknowledged as a critical period for eating disorder development in young adolescent girls. Before puberty, the presence of body image disturbance and weight preoccupation is rare. The occurrence of puberty influences normal body fat development, and girls face the outlook of the restricted societal view of an ideal woman's body. They may quickly develop a negative body image if their own bodies are not congruent with the societal ideal. This negative body image develops at a time when other psychosocial changes are taking place. Girls advance from elementary to middle school. Peer influence increases and parental influence decreases, and subsequently there is a growing sense of self-consciousness in relation to one's peers. During this crucial window, developing a negative body image may considerably increase vulnerability to developing an eating disorder in a way that it might not during a different developmental period (Steiner et al., 2003). The mechanism of how risk factors lead to the development of eating disorders is complex, and it is unlikely that a single risk factor is the cause of any eating disorder. A convergence of multiple risk factors, which interact with protective factors and have an effect over time eventually determines why one individual may develop an eating disorder and another will not (Steiner et al., 2003).

Risk Reduction

Prevention efforts are becoming increasingly effective in reducing risk factors for developing eating disorders. Beneficial prevention measures include targeting those most at risk, addressing cultural support for eating disorders, and increasing protective factors against eating disorders. Formal prevention programs geared toward reducing the risk of developing eating disorders and presented in schools to both genders, or through organizations such as the Girl Scouts, have been successful (Franco, 2012).

Prevention efforts may fail or inadvertently encourage disordered eating if the sole purpose of the efforts is to warn the public about signs, symptoms, and dangers of disordered eating. In order to be effective, prevention programs must also address the cultural obsession with slenderness as a physical, psychological, and moral issue. In addition, the objectification of women must be addressed by examining the roles of men and women in society (Levine & Smolak, 2005). The most effective efforts at prevention are those that try to reach children early, include parents, and encourage community involvement. Interactive

and participatory prevention efforts are best whenever possible, as strictly didactic presentations may be counterproductive, especially for those in high-risk populations. It is essential for prevention efforts to support the enhancement of protective factors that may reduce the risk of developing eating disorders. Protective factors include high self-esteem, high self-efficacy, optimism, creativity, spirituality, a supportive family network, positive role models, participation in extracurricular activities, problem-solving skills, and participation in non-elite sports (Levine & Smolak, 2005).

Programs that teach media literacy have become increasingly popular in recent years and have produced promising results. These efforts encourage critical viewing of media images to reduce the impact of unhealthy messages pertaining to weight and body image. Effective media literacy programs emphasize awareness of media use, analysis of media content, activism involving letters of praise or protest sent to advertisers, advocacy for healthy alternative media messages, and increased understanding of who has access to mass media in order to participate in media in positive ways (Levine & Smolak, 2005).

Gender Similarities and Differences

Males and females with eating disorders tend to be similar regarding physiologic and psychological characteristics, age of onset and premorbid characteristics, psychiatric comorbidity, and susceptibility to parental and media influences (Weltzin, 2012). Females with eating disorders are inclined to outnumber males by a sizeable margin. Lifetime prevalence is approximately 1.75 to 3 times as high among females as males for anorexia nervosa, bulimia nervosa, and binge eating disorder. However, gender disparity is reversed for subthreshold binge eating disorder. The lifetime prevalence of subthreshold binge eating disorder is 1.9% in males as compared to 0.6% in females. The 12-month prevalence of binge eating disorder is also consistently disparate, with 0.8% in males and 0.4% in females (Hudson et al., 2007). The extent of gender differences in symptomatology depends on the particular eating disorder. There is greater likelihood that girls and women will manifest weight dissatisfaction, dieting for weight control, and use of purging than boys or men. On the other hand, males tend to adopt fewer oral control and dietary restraint behaviors, are less preoccupied with body shape, and show less desire for thinness than women (Gadalla, 2009). There is also a greater tendency for boys and men to manifest binge eating and excessive exercise for weight control (Striegel-Moore et al., 2009).

Although commonly seen in females with eating disorders, body dissatisfaction and distorted sense of body image may also appear in males. Males with eating disorders frequently experience muscle dysmorphia, which is an extreme concern with becoming more muscular. Hence, unlike the female desire to achieve thinness, males with muscle dysmorphia see themselves as smaller than they actually are and want to gain weight and bulk up. To that end, males are more likely to use steroids or other harmful drugs to increase muscle mass (NEDA, 2015c). A history of obesity along with a history of weight-based victimization tends to be more common among males with eating disorders than females. Involvement in sports likely presents a slightly greater risk factor in males than in females. Evidence suggests that males participate more frequently than females in an occupation or athletic team in which control of weight is important for good performance. Alcoholism and physical abuse are other factors that may increase the risk of eating disorders in males (Weltzin, 2012).

There appears to be a greater tendency for males with anorexia nervosa or bulimia nervosa to declare a homosexual or bisexual orientation as compared with females (Weltzin, 2012). Moreover, the higher risk of homosexual males for developing eating disorders as compared to heterosexual males may be attributed to an amplified emphasis on physical appearance relative to gay culture (Striegel-Moore & Bulik, 2007).

Males with eating disorders are inclined to be underdiagnosed and undertreated. Males likely do not consider themselves at risk for eating disorders and tend to experience fewer severe symptoms (Gadella, 2009). Males, especially adolescent males with eating disorders, may experience a sense of stigmatization in having developed what is perceived as a "female" disease (Weltzin, 2012). These adverse feelings may prevent them from coming forward to care providers. Cultural biases and lack of treatment facilities dedicated for males with eating disorders can also act as barriers to seeking treatment (Gadella, 2009). Consequently, males with eating disorders have a tendency to experience a significant lag between onset and treatment. Healthcare providers may have a decreased index of suspicion for eating disorders in males as compared to females, which may delay diagnosis until the disorder is well established or has reached dangerous proportions. Eating disorders in males are likely to be diagnosed in the presence of substantial psychiatric comorbidity or accompanied by severe medical complications (Weltzin, 2012).

Diagnosing Eating Disorders

Eating disorders are configurations of behaviors, thoughts, and feelings that are cultivated over a period of time. Diagnosis of an eating disorder is made when the person's symptoms meet the diagnostic criteria given in the *Diagnostic and Statistical Manual of Mental Disorders, 5th Edition* [DSM-V] (American Psychiatric Association [APA], 2013). The DSM-V provides descriptions of signs, symptoms, research findings, and guidelines that enable healthcare providers to classify mental illnesses and determine the best descriptive category for an individual's condition or problem. These criteria are evidence-based and reflect the state of current knowledge. The DSM-V has established diagnostic criteria for the diagnosis of anorexia nervosa, bulimia nervosa, and binge eating disorder.

Anorexia Nervosa

Anorexia nervosa is a devastating, life-threatening eating disorder that occurs in both males and females. However, it predominantly affects adolescent girls and young women. It is a biopsychological syndrome in which physiological and psychological manifestations are entangled. Anorexia nervosa is characterized by self-starvation and excessive weight loss. Women may exhibit an extreme fear of weight gain, an obsession with their weight, and persistent behavior to prevent weight gain (APA, 2013).

Anorexia nervosa has been categorized into two subtypes: Binge-Eating/Purging and Restricting Type. Individuals with Binge-Eating/Purging Type exhibit binge eating and also purging behaviors. Purging may involve self-induced vomiting or misuse of laxatives, enemas, or diuretics. Some individuals with this subtype may not binge eat but regularly purge after eating small amounts of food. Individuals with Restricting Type do not exhibit binge eating or purging. Weight loss is accomplished by dieting, fasting, and/or excessive exercise (APA, 2013).

Physical symptoms of anorexia nervosa include significant loss of weight, refusal to eat, amenorrhea, and denial of unusual eating behaviors or weight change. As the metabolism of an anorexic person slows down to adjust to the lack of nourishment, other symptoms occur, such as muscle weakness, constipation, brittle hair and nails, lethargy, and lowered body temperature, which produces constant feelings of coldness and slowness. Psychological symptoms of anorexia nervosa include distorted body image, confusion of self-image, sense of being incompetent, depression, and withdrawal from others. Individuals also become socially withdrawn as the disorder progresses, and believe that weight, shape, or being thin is the predominant

reference for establishing personal value or self-worth. Other identifiable psychological features include frustration over becoming overweight, fear of losing control over eating, loss of judgment relative to the requirement of food as a basic need for the body, and an unrealistic sense of body image.

Women with anorexia nervosa frequently exhibit obsessive-compulsive behaviors, such as obsessing about becoming fat. Thus they will compulsively exercise or practice odd eating rituals to avoid becoming fat. Other compulsive behaviors may consist of frequent weighing, looking in the mirror, and taking body measurements. Women with anorexia are also obsessed with food and eating, and will often cook, prepare, and shop for food for others. They will eat in secret and reject food in public.

Anorexia nervosa usually develops in early to late adolescence. A general characteristic of the anorectic personality is a feeling of overall ineffectiveness as a person. The typical anorexic woman is highly self-critical, has poor self-esteem, and believes that she is inadequate in most areas of personal and social functioning. The woman with anorexia nervosa frequently feels powerless and unable to control many areas of her life, and thus establishes power over her food intake and weight. Because of her perfectionist tendencies, the woman with anorexia nervosa believes that the ultimate sign of control is a "perfect" body. Symptoms of depression, with large mood swings, are commonly seen in women with anorexia nervosa.

Bulimia Nervosa

Bulimia nervosa is a serious, potentially life-threatening eating disorder characterized by cyclic binge eating followed by purging. An individual purges in order to undo or counteract the effects of binge eating. Bulimia usually begins with extreme hunger as a result of long periods of food deprivation from fasting or dieting. The hunger is followed by attempts at eating while still trying to control weight. Women with bulimia often maintain normal body weight but are extremely dissatisfied with their bodies. Some bulimics have reported that in their pre-adolescent years, they gained feelings of self-control and power through this self-denial. The situation progresses to out-of-control binges and purges because the artificial elimination methods have relieved the feeling of being "stuffed," and the bulimic believes this is a good way to lose weight.

Binges frequently occur when bulimics believe that they have passed a self-imposed limit on acceptable food intake. Thus, they feel defeated and usually gorge themselves until they are interrupted or the food runs out. During such binges, the caloric intake may range from 2,000 to 3,000 calories and commonly lasts for less than 2 hours but has been reported to last as long as 8 hours. The binge foods of choice are usually high-calorie, easily ingested "junk" food that requires little preparation and can be obtained while keeping the binge secret from others. Bulimics use several modes of purging, including vomiting, diuretics, laxatives, fasts, enemas, diet pills, and excessive exercise (APA, 2013). The number of different methods of purging is a stronger index of the severity of the woman's condition than the frequency of use of any one type.

The binge–purge cycle may occur anywhere from one to three times weekly to an average of 14 or more episodes per week. The cycle often begins in response to a strong negative emotion. Other triggers may include interpersonal stressors, boredom, dietary restraint, and negative feelings regarding body weight, body shape, and food (APA, 2013). After the binge, some women initially feel relaxed and soothed, but then these feelings turn to shame, guilt, and self-hatred. The bulimic woman then feels the need to purge to relieve the fear of weight gain and to regain a sense of control and purity. After the purge, bulimics may feel relieved that they have controlled their weight, but guilty and negative about

succumbing to the cycle again. These feelings of guilt invariably lead the bulimic to perpetuate the behavior.

Women afflicted with bulimia often appear to be independent high achievers and are of normal weight. Bulimia nervosa has traditionally affected adolescents and young adult females from middle-class backgrounds, but it affects other groups of women as well. Bulimics are often perfectionists, obsessive-compulsive, depressed, intense, insecure, sensitive to rejection, anxious to please, and dependent on others. They may be socially isolated as a result of their all-consuming preoccupation with food and weight and their struggle to hide their eating behavior. The majority of women who suffer from bulimia nervosa are aware that their eating habits are abnormal but may believe that they have the ultimate weight control secret that allows them to be able to eat yet not gain weight. Other factors thought to contribute to the development of bulimia nervosa include family problems, maladaptive behavior, self-identity conflicts, history of sexual abuse, and cultural overemphasis on physical appearance. In addition to the psychological problems, bulimia nervosa can cause a variety of physical problems, such as hypoglycemia, slowed metabolism, spontaneous regurgitation, erosion of tooth enamel, tooth loss, mineral deficiencies, and bleeding or sores in the mouth and esophagus.

The bulimic woman will likely exhibit evidence of binge eating. This may include the disappearance of large quantities of food in short periods of time, or the discovery of wrappers and containers indicating that large amounts of food have been consumed. The individual may also exhibit signs of purging behaviors, including frequent trips to the bathroom after meals, presence of wrappers or packages of laxatives or diuretics, and signs of having vomited. The bulimic will often follow a rigidly excessive exercise program despite weather, fatigue, illness, or injury. The bulimic may also demonstrate unusual swelling of the cheeks or jaw, discoloration or staining of the teeth, and calluses on the back of the hands or knuckles from self-induced vomiting (APA, 2013).

Binge Eating Disorder

Binge eating disorder is characterized by compulsive overeating without attempting to purge. Women with binge eating disorder frequently experience episodes of consuming very large quantities of food but do not engage in behaviors that prevent weight gain, such as self-induced vomiting. Women with binge eating disorder frequently feel out of control during the binge eating episode. Signs that binge eating is out of control include eating more rapidly than normal, eating when not hungry, eating to the point of discomfort, eating alone due to shame about the behavior, and feeling self-disgust, depressed, or guilty afterward (APA, 2013).

Binge eating disorder is different from non-purging bulimia nervosa in that individuals with non-purging bulimia binge after periods of fasting and use excessive exercise as a way to compensate for their binges. Binge eating episodes may be triggered by negative emotion, boredom, interpersonal stressors, and negative feelings about body weight, body shape, and food (APA, 2013). Some women may develop binge eating disorder after a period of weight loss diets and restrictive eating. Others may use binging as a calming mechanism unrelated to previous dieting or restrictive behaviors. Most are obese and have a long history of weight fluctuation. However, women of normal weight also can be affected. Those with binge eating disorder are at high risk for medical problems associated with obesity in addition to depression and anxiety due to guilt and feelings of self-disgust. These include high blood pressure, high cholesterol levels, heart disease, diabetes mellitus, gallbladder disease, and musculoskeletal problems. Many individuals affected with binge eating disorder have reported histories of major family dysfunction and childhood abuse.

Other Specified Feeding or Eating Disorder (OSFED)

OSFED is a condition with numerous variations of disordered eating that do not meet the full criteria for anorexia nervosa or bulimia nervosa. These include atypical anorexia with normal weight, bulimia nervosa with less frequent behaviors, binge eating disorder with lesser occurrences, purging disorder without binge eating, and night eating syndrome (excessive nighttime food consumption) (APA, 2013).

Women with OSFED have physical and behavioral symptoms that are of shorter duration or less severe than full-blown anorexia or bulimia nervosa. Moreover, those who develop an eating disorder in the OSFED category exhibit the same medical complications and degree of psychological distress as seen in those who meet the full diagnostic criteria of anorexia nervosa or bulimia nervosa.

Unspecified Feeding or Eating Disorder

Unspecified feeding or eating disorders are conditions which present with symptoms characteristic of a feeding or eating disorder that cause clinically significant distress in social, occupational, or other important functioning areas. However, these symptoms do not meet the full criteria for any of the disorders in the feeding and eating disorders diagnostic class. This category is used in situations in which the clinician elects not to specify the reason that the criteria are not met for a specific feeding and eating disorder and also includes conditions in which there is insufficient information to determine a more specific diagnosis (APA, 2013).

The spectrum of signs and symptoms of eating disorders is presented in **Table 5–1**. The signs and symptoms are grouped into different behavior categories for the sake of clarity. Girls and women with an eating disorder may exhibit some or all of these symptoms. Many of the signs and symptoms listed can also be caused by other illnesses. Thus, it is important that a thorough professional assessment and medical exam be done by the healthcare provider in order to rule out other physical conditions or illnesses and obtain a proper diagnosis of an eating disorder.

Table 5–1 SUMMARY OF SIGNS AND SYMPTOMS OF EATING DISORDERS

Food Behaviors	Appearance and Body Image	Exercise Behaviors	Thoughts, Beliefs, Feelings	Physical Complaints	Other Behaviors
Denies hunger	Significant weight loss	Exercises even when injured or overly tired	Suicidal thoughts	Low blood pressure and heart rate	Self-mutilating behaviors
Only eats a few "safe" foods	Refuses to maintain minimum normal weight	Exercises compulsively	Difficulty expressing feelings unrelated to food or weight	Decreased coordination	Denial of symptoms
Avoids eating with others	Shows intense fear of gaining weight		Depression (may include feelings of anger, shame, or guilt)	Headaches	Substance use or abuse
Cooks for others but does not eat what is prepared	Spends time inspecting self in mirror		Self-critical and/or a perfectionist	Dental problems, swollen glands, discolored teeth	Suicidal gestures
Is ritualistic about food	Entertains magical thinking about weight		Overly concerned with opinions of others	Hair loss (on head and sometimes eyelashes)	Frequent use of laxatives or diuretics
Has rules about eating	Seeks to emulate thin people		Extremes in thinking ("all or nothing" thinking)	Dry skin, bruises	
Restricts eating or maintains severe dieting	Wears baggy clothes to hide weight loss		Low self-esteem, feelings of worthlessness	Bloodshot eyes	
Purges (self-induced vomiting)	Weighs self frequently		Mood fluctuations, irritability	Insomnia, poor sleeping habits	
Makes frequent trips to bathroom after eating	Has negative body image		Difficulty concentrating	Constipation, gastrointestinal problems	

Table 5–1 Summary of Signs and Symptoms of Eating Disorders (*continued*)

Food Behaviors	Appearance and Body Image	Exercise Behaviors	Thoughts, Beliefs, Feelings	Physical Complaints	Other Behaviors
Hoards food	Abuses diet pills or prescription medications		Isolated, withdrawn	Frequent complaints about feeling cold	
Vague or secretive eating patterns	Weight fluctuates		Impaired relationships	Fatigue or hyperactivity	
Overuses caffeine	Appears pale and frail			Complaints of nausea	
Skips meals	Fears fat in food and on body			Dizziness or fainting	
Chews food and spits it out before swallowing				Growth of fine, downy body hair (lanugo)	
Preoccupied with food content and ingredients				Abdominal cramps, bloating	
Makes excuses for not eating, plays with food on plate, moves it around instead of eating				Marks on the backs of hands from self-induced vomiting	
Suffers intense guilt after eating					
Food is continuously missing in the house					
Eats large quantities when upset, constantly eating, or feels unable to stop					
Fears running out of food					

Treatment

Women and girls with eating disorders tend to be intensely secretive about the disorder. However, friends and family members of individuals affected by these disorders often suspect the problem due to the nature of restrictive eating, binging, purging, or excessive exercise behaviors. Many friends and family members try to ignore their suspicions for the sake of protecting the individual's privacy or a wish to refrain from interfering. Women with bulimia nervosa or binge eating disorder are often able to identify themselves. Conversely, women with anorexia nervosa are often in denial about their condition and usually are brought to treatment by concerned family members. Many women enter therapy to treat an eating disorder only after being persuaded to do so by the people in their lives. It thus becomes extremely important for friends and family members to confront the women in their lives when they suspect disordered eating, and to provide them with support in finding the appropriate help. As with all health interventions, sensitivity and care should be taken when discussing eating disorders with individuals, and one needs to understand the very central and painful role the disorder plays in the woman's life.

Adequate nutrition, reducing excessive exercise, and eliminating purging behaviors are the foundations of treatment for eating disorders. A treatment plan must be individualized to the patient's needs and can include an interdisciplinary approach comprised of individual, group, or family psychotherapy, medical care and monitoring, nutritional counseling, and medications (NIMH, 2011). Severity of the disorder and need for hospitalization is determined by the patient's weight and cardiac and metabolic status. Patients may receive outpatient treatment, inpatient treatment, partial hospitalization, or treatment in a residential setting as per individual need. Patients with life-threatening complications or extreme psychological problems require inpatient hospitalization to treat problems caused by malnutrition or to ensure they eat enough if they are severely underweight.

Anorexia Nervosa

The goals of treatment for anorexia nervosa in female patients encompass restoration to a healthy weight associated with the return of menses and normal ovulation in female patients, and normal physical and sexual growth and development in adolescents. Treatment goals also include management of physical complications, enhancement of patients' motivation to cooperate in the restoration of healthy eating patterns and to participate in treatment, and provision of education regarding healthy nutrition and eating patterns. The goal of treatment is to help patients reassess and change core dysfunctional cognitions, attitudes, motives, conflicts, and feelings related to the eating disorder, and to treat associated psychiatric conditions, including deficits in mood and impulse regulation and self-esteem and behavioral problems. In addition, treatment seeks to enlist family support and provide family counseling and therapy where appropriate and to prevent relapse (APA, 2010).

An interdisciplinary team approach involving a physician, a nutritionist, and a therapist is recommended. Inpatient nutritional rehabilitation is recommended for severely underweight patients to restore weight and reverse acute medical complications. Most medical complications are reversible with nutritional rehabilitation. Complications that may not be reversible include osteopenia, growth retardation, and structural brain changes (Katzman & Golden, 2009).

Nutritional rehabilitation focuses on restoring weight, normalizing eating patterns, achieving normal perceptions of hunger and satiety, and correcting biological and psychological sequelae of malnutrition. Expected rates of controlled weight gain are 2 to 3 lbs per week in the inpatient setting and 0.5 to 1.0 lbs per week in the outpatient setting (APA, 2010). Oral, enteral, and parenteral methods of refeeding may be employed. Close medical monitoring is essential to avoid the development of refeeding syndrome, a potentially fatal complication involving severe electrolyte and fluid shifts associated with refeeding a malnourished patient (AED, 2011). In addition to refeeding, nutritional rehabilitation encompasses weight maintenance interventions.

Psychological therapy is an essential component of treatment and is implemented during hospitalization and continued after discharge. Psychosocial interventions focus on helping patients to understand and cooperate with their nutritional and physical rehabilitation. In addition, psychosocial interventions aim to help patients understand and change the behaviors and dysfunctional attitudes related to their eating disorder, as well as improve their interpersonal and social functioning. Psychosocial interventions also address comorbid psychopathology and psychological conflicts that reinforce or maintain eating disorder behaviors (APA, 2010).

Psychotherapeutic modalities can be individual, group, and family based. Some modalities for individual therapy used with patients with anorexia nervosa include dynamic expressive–supportive therapy and cognitive behavioral therapy (Franco, 2012). Individual therapy may be more suitable for adult women, while family therapy may be more suitable for adolescents.

Evidence supports the usefulness of family therapy in treating adolescents with anorexia nervosa. A family therapy modality frequently used with adolescents is the Maudsley Approach. In this conjoint family therapy format, parents of adolescents are directed to take complete control over their anorexic child's eating and weight, and are coached to find effective means for doing so. Once the adolescent is compliant with parental authority, external control is gradually decreased. In later stages of therapy,

resolution of the eating disorder is explicitly linked to the adolescent's right to age-appropriate autonomy (Wilson, Grilo, & Vitousek, 2007).

Pharmacological therapy tends to be less effective in patients with anorexia nervosa than in patients with bulimia nervosa. Medications may be used in treating anorexia nervosa following weight restoration. Medications help patients maintain weight, sustain normal eating behavior, and can also be helpful in managing associated psychiatric symptoms. Anorexia nervosa patients who have depression or obsessive-compulsive behaviors that persist in spite of or in the absence of weight gain may be given selective serotonin reuptake inhibitors (SSRIs) such as fluoxetine (Franco, 2012). SSRIs are frequently used in combination with psychotherapy. Adverse reactions from drugs such as tricyclic antidepressants and monoamine oxidase inhibitors are more pronounced in malnourished individuals, and as such, use of these drugs should be avoided in anorexia nervosa patients. The U.S. Food and Drug Administration (FDA) has issued a black box warning that antidepressants may worsen depression and increase the risk of suicidal thinking and behavior in adolescents and young adults. The FDA has also issued a black box warning against use of bupropion in patients with eating disorders because of the likelihood that the drug may increase the risk of seizures in these patients. Low-dose antipsychotics may be given to decrease agitation and psychotic thinking. These drugs may increase appetite significantly, which could be distressful to the patient, especially if the patient is not psychotic. Anti-anxiety drugs such as benzodiazepines may be given to treat extreme anticipatory anxiety regarding eating (Franco, 2012).

Weight gain through nutritional rehabilitation—sufficient intake of dietary protein, carbohydrates, and fats—is recommended to treat physiological complications of malnutrition from semistarvation, including osteopenia and osteoporosis. Although no specific hormonal therapy or vitamin supplements have been shown to be efficacious in increasing bone mineral density, supplemental calcium and vitamin D are often recommended especially when calcium intake is inadequate for growth and maintenance and a patient lacks daily exposure to sunlight (Yager et al., 2012). Evidence suggests that zinc supplements may foster weight gain in some patients, and thus patients may benefit from daily multivitamin tablets that contain zinc (APA, 2010).

Bulimia Nervosa

The profound emaciation associated with anorexia nervosa patients is usually not seen in patients with bulimia nervosa. The weight of most patients with bulimia tends to be within normal body weight parameters. However, medical complications from frequent binging/purging behaviors are likely and need to be corrected.

The goals of treatment for patients with bulimia nervosa include reduction and, where possible, elimination of binge eating and purging, treatment of physical complications, enhancement of patients' motivation to cooperate in the restoration of healthy eating patterns and participation in treatment, and provision of education regarding healthy nutrition and eating patterns. Treatment also aims to help patients reassess and change core dysfunctional thoughts, attitudes, motives, conflicts, and feelings related to the eating disorder. Treatment goals also include management of associated psychiatric conditions, including deficits in mood and impulse regulation, self-esteem, and behavior; enlistment of family support and provision of family counseling and therapy where appropriate; and prevention of relapse (APA, 2010).

Nutritional interventions focus on reducing and eliminating binge eating and purging behaviors, encouraging healthy eating behaviors, eliminating foods that trigger binging, and following a structured dietary plan of eating three normal meals a day. Sufficient nutritional intake can avert craving and encourage satiety. Assessment of nutritional intake is essential for all patients, even those with a normal body weight (or normal BMI), because normal weight does not guarantee appropriate nutritional intake or normal body composition. Patients of normal weight should receive nutritional counseling in order to help decrease food restriction, augment the variety of foods eaten, and encourage healthy but not compulsive exercise patterns (APA, 2010).

Cognitive behavioral therapy is considered an effective psychological intervention for patients with bulimia nervosa. In this modality, cognitive and behavioral procedures are designed to enhance motivation for change, replace dysfunctional dieting with a regular and flexible pattern of eating, reduce undue concern over body shape and weight, and avoid relapse. Treatment usually encompasses 16 to 20 sessions of individual therapy over a period of 4 to 5 months. Cognitive behavioral therapy has also been successfully applied as group therapy (Wilson et al., 2007). Some patients who do not respond initially to cognitive behavioral therapy may have better success with interpersonal therapy or therapy with the SSRI fluoxetine (APA, 2010).

Antidepressants are useful in decreasing the frequency of disordered eating in bulimia nervosa patients, as well as treating comorbid depression, anxiety, obsessions, and specific impulse-disorder syndromes. Fluoxetine is the only SSRI approved by the FDA for treating bulimia nervosa and appears to be effective in reducing binge eating and purging behaviors, decreasing relapse, and improving eating attitudes (NIMH, 2011). Sertraline has also shown efficacy in treatment of bulimia in randomized controlled trials. Evidence suggests that fluoxetine is helpful in treating adolescent patients (APA, 2010). SSRIs such as sertraline, paroxetine, citalopram; tricyclic antidepressants such as imipramine, nortryptyline, and desipramine;

and the monoamine oxidase inhibitor, tranylcypromine, have demonstrated efficacy in several studies (Franco, 2012). However, these drugs are not recommended as initial treatment (APA, 2010). Combining medication with cognitive behavioral therapy has been shown to be superior to either therapy alone (Shapiro et al., 2007). Careful attention to the black box warnings associated with antidepressants is essential. Potential benefits and risks of antidepressant treatment must be discussed with patients and families if such medications are to be prescribed (APA, 2010).

Other Specified Feeding or Eating Disorders

Except for binge eating disorder, evidence to guide the treatment of the various eating disorders included under the category of Other Specified Feeding or Eating Disorders (OSFED) is scarce. Current practice guidelines recommend that patients with subsyndromal anorexia nervosa or subsyndromal bulimia nervosa receive treatment similar to that of patients who fulfill all criteria for these diagnoses (APA, 2010).

Binge Eating Disorder

Weight loss and reduction of symptoms of binge eating may be achieved through engaging patients in behavioral weight control programs that incorporate low- or very-low-calorie diets. It is essential that patients be counseled that weight loss is often not maintained and binge eating may recur when weight is gained. Patients with binge eating disorder may benefit from a range of approaches including various combinations of diets, behavior therapies, interpersonal therapies, psychodynamic psychotherapies, non-weight-directed psychosocial treatments, and even some "non-diet/health at every size" psychotherapy modalities for binge eating and weight loss or stabilization. Programs that focus on decreasing binge eating rather than on weight loss may be more efficacious for patients with a history of repeated weight loss followed by weight gain ("yo-yo" dieting) or patients with an early onset of binge eating (APA, 2010).

Individual or group cognitive behavioral therapy is considered effective for managing the behavioral and psychological symptoms of binge eating disorder. Interpersonal therapy and dialectical behavior therapy may also be effective for behavioral and psychological symptoms and can be regarded as alternatives. The efficacy of self-help and guided self-help cognitive behavioral therapy programs and their use as an initial step in a sequenced treatment program has been supported by considerable evidence (APA, 2010). Other modalities that use a "non-diet" approach that focuses on self-acceptance, improved body image, better nutrition and health, and increased physical movement have been tried, as have addiction-based 12-step approaches, self-help organizations, and treatment programs based on the Alcoholics Anonymous model. However, no systematic outcome studies of these programs are available (APA, 2010).

Treatment with SSRI antidepressants may be effective in achieving at least a short-term reduction in binge eating behavior but not with substantial weight loss. Dosages tend to be at the high end of the recommended range. Topiramate, an anticonvulsant medication, is effective for binge reduction and weight loss; however, adverse effects may limit its clinical usefulness for some individuals. Zonisamide, an antiseizure medication, may be helpful in achieving weight loss; however, it may also cause adverse side effects. For most binge eating disorder patients, combining antidepressant medication with their behavioral weight control and/or cognitive behavioral therapy regimen does not enhance binge suppression when compared with medication alone (APA, 2010). Nevertheless, some medications may generate additional weight reduction and have associated psychological benefits. Orlistat, a weight loss medication, when added to a guided self-help cognitive behavioral therapy program, may yield additional weight reduction. While fluoxetine combined with group behavioral treatment may not aid in binge cessation or weight loss, it may reduce depressive symptoms (APA, 2010).

Quality of Life Issues Associated With Eating Disorders

Eating disorders have enormous impact on the totality of the lives of girls and young women, the population most vulnerable to these conditions. Widespread impact is felt on the physical, psychological, and social aspects of life. Eating disorders are distinguished by the significant propensity to evolve, become chronic, or follow patterns of relapses and recurrences, and to have a high mortality rate (Pradierna, Quintana, Arostegui, Gonzalez, & Horcajo, 2000). Quality of life issues and concerns associated with eating disorders are commonly multidimensional and encompass health and physical functioning, psychological and spiritual well-being, socioeconomic integrity, and family well-being. Disabling physical symptoms of eating disorders, such as weight loss and cardiac dysfunction, often demand urgent attention of healthcare professionals, and may override other issues. However, from the perspective of women with eating disorders, physical symptoms may be of less concern than the impact of the disorder on other areas of life (Jones, Evans, Bamford, & Ford, 2008). Thus, it is important for healthcare providers not to lose sight of quality of life issues beyond the physical ramifications and to carefully weigh appraisals of quality of life from patients with eating disorders.

Issues Affecting Health and Physical Functioning

Health and physical functioning issues for women with eating disorders are varied. Some issues are caused by starvation or malnutrition and some may be caused by purging methods such as vomiting and laxative use, excessive exercise, or extreme weight gain from binging. A summary of complications that affect health and physical functioning in patients with eating disorders is presented in **Table 5–2**. Many complications are serious; some are life threatening. Death may result from a variety of medical complications of eating disorders such as heart failure, liver failure, kidney failure, stroke, seizure, gastric rupture, pancreatitis, and suicide. Women who develop serious or life-threatening complications must be monitored closely and referred for appropriate treatment. Most complications can be reversed with nutritional rehabilitation and recovery. Specific treatment guidelines for anorexia nervosa, bulimia nervosa, and binge eating disorder have been previously discussed.

Treatment for eating disorders is available through a variety of professionals, levels of care, treatment modalities, and treatment programs. The length of time a woman has been ill, the severity of the eating disorder, and the presence of medical or other complications determine the level of care, how many healthcare professionals are involved, and whether going to a treatment program is an appropriate choice.

Treatment in a structured setting, such as a day treatment program or residential facility, is often recommended when symptoms are out of control and /or could become dangerous. If medical or psychiatric symptoms are already at a dangerous level and the medical risks are significant, then a hospital or other appropriate 24-hour care setting may be required. Indicators that help to determine the need for an inpatient care setting are presented in **Box 5–2**.

Table 5–2 COMPLICATIONS AFFECTING HEALTH AND PHYSICAL FUNCTIONING OF PATIENTS WITH EATING DISORDERS

Body System	Complications
Cardiovascular	Bradycardia, orthostatic hypotension, cardiac dysrhythmias, heart failure, mitral valve prolapse, heart murmurs, cardiomyopathy, pericardial effusion
Fluid and Electrolytes	Dehydration, hypokalemia, metabolic alkalosis, hyponatremia, kidney infection and failure
Gastrointestinal	Obstipation, constipation, delayed gastric emptying, malabsorption syndrome, liver dysfunction or failure, esophageal rupture, bowel perforations, ulcers, gastritis, pancreatitis, Barrett's esophagus
Skeletal	Osteopenia, osteoporosis, fractures, arrested skeletal development
Neuromuscular	Organic brain syndrome, seizures, brain damage, shrinkage of gray and white matter, peripheral neuropathies, generalized muscle weakness
Hematologic	Anemia, leukopenia, thrombocytopenia
Oropharyngeal	Dental decay, gum damage, pharyngeal erythema, swollen salivary glands
Reproductive	Arrested maturation, infertility, amenorrhea, polycystic ovarian syndrome, complications with pregnancy
Endocrine/Metabolic	Euthyroid sick syndrome, hypercortisolism, partial diabetes insipidus, elevated cholesterol levels, hypothermia, hypoglycemia, hyperglycemia
Integumentary	Lanugo growth, hypercarotenemia, skin bruising, alopecia

Box 5–2: Indicators for Inpatient or Residential Care for Eating Disorders

Indicators that help determine the need for inpatient medical or psychiatric treatment setting

- Cardiovascular dysfunction
- Dehydration
- Electrolyte abnormalities
- Rapid weight loss of 15% to 25% of ideal body weight (weight loss less than this usually requires hospitalization rather than residential)
- Continued weight loss (1 to 2 pounds per week) in spite of competent psychotherapy
- Multiple episodes of binge/purge behaviors with little or no reduction
- Outpatient treatment failure: no improvement or getting worse
- Suicidal thoughts or gestures (such as self-cutting)

(continues)

> ## Box 5–2: Indicators for Inpatient or Residential Care for Eating Disorders (*continued*)
>
> - No support system, abusive family situation, or support system that sabotages treatment
> - Inability to perform activities of daily living
> - Increase in impulsive behaviors such as drugs, shoplifting, risky sexual behaviors, etc.
> - Co-occurring psychiatric disorder that requires hospitalization

Women who are not medically unstable or actively suicidal yet still require or desire 24-hour care may benefit from residential programs that provide a smaller, more personal environment than is offered in a hospital setting. In a residential treatment facility, a patient lives at the facility that offers extended care (usually no longer than 6 months), including group and individual psychotherapy, medical and nutritional monitoring, patient education, and alternative therapies. Residential treatment facilities are intended to be home-like settings where patients can practice coping skills learned in therapy sessions within a structured, supervised program. Residential treatment is not intended for patients who have acute medical or psychiatric symptoms. Length of stay and costs vary.

Day treatment and partial hospitalization programs offer alternatives to help women transition from 24-hour care and provide a step-down level of care that is more than outpatient care yet allows women to live at home. In these programs, women spend about 7 to 12 hours per day, 5 days per week at a program site and receive at least two supervised meals and one snack, and a majority of their time is spent in group therapies and individual counseling. Nutritional and medical needs are closely monitored. At the end of each day's program, patients return to their homes (Tantillo, MacDowell, Anson, Tallie, & Cole, 2009). This method provides greater structure and patient accountability. Day treatment and partial hospitalization programs are becoming more prevalent, in part due to the fact that they are less costly

than 24-hour programs. Insurance companies often require them as a first step before they will authorize 24-hour care.

Transitional or supported housing offers another alternative that allows individuals with eating disorders to move away from 24-hour care while still providing guidance and structure in a home with other recovering patients, where residents can practice relationship and daily living skills. The overall goal of transitional housing is to help integrate individuals with eating disorders into the community and allow them to lead fulfilling and satisfying lives outside a hospital or institutional setting. The setting provides a safe living environment in which women may receive individual counseling or case management in order to improve problem-solving and daily living skills. Residents may participate in support groups, be given meals, and receive transportation to appointments and events in the community (Tantillo et al., 2009). Transitional living houses are not meant to be used instead of residential care because they do not provide enough supervision and structure.

For some women who participate in partial hospitalization programs, returning to the home in the evening following 7 hours of intensive therapeutic programming is stressful. This stress can hinder recovery, and may increase recidivism due to an unsupported or harmful living environment (Tantillo et al., 2009). Evidence suggests that combining partial hospitalization with transitional or supportive housing may be more effective in enhancing recovery, lowering the risk of relapse, and improving health-related quality of life than attending partial hospitalization alone. Returning to a transitional home following an intensive day in partial hospitalization provides residents with additional support during high-risk times in the evening and on weekends. This support can fortify residents in preparation for their ongoing recovery by specifically targeting health-related quality of life issues and generalization of treatment skills to community living (Tantillo et al., 2009).

Another level of care that can either be used as an initial step up, providing more than outpatient therapy alone, or a step down from more structured care, is intensive outpatient programs. This option allows for more structure, support, education, and monitoring than traditional outpatient care. Additional therapeutic activities and some meals are provided. These programs meet a few days per week, for a few hours, either in the daytime or evening. In traditional outpatient care, a patient meets with one or more treatment providers one to three times per week in an office setting. Sessions may typically last 45 minutes to an hour. Outpatient care is generally provided by collaboration between a physician, psychotherapist, and registered dietician.

Issues Affecting Psychological and Spiritual Functioning

PSYCHOLOGICAL ISSUES

In addition to physical symptoms, eating disorders are often accompanied by a substantial psychological burden on quality of life. Women with eating disorders commonly experience irritability, worry, social withdrawal, social anxiety, insomnia, poor self-esteem, distorted body image, unusual eating attitudes and behaviors, and a relentless pursuit of thinness. Women with eating disorders frequently exhibit personality problems such as impulse control, affect regulation, perfectionism, obsessionality, and rejection sensitivity.

Certain psychiatric conditions frequently coexist with eating disorders. Depression occurs in as many as 40% to 70% of those with eating disorders. Other psychiatric disorders including anxiety, social phobia, obsessive-compulsive disorder, body dysmorphic disorder, attention deficit hyperactivity disorder, and post-traumatic stress disorder may also be exhibited. Personality disorders as well as disorders arising from substance use and abuse may also coexist with eating disorders.

Psychotherapy is a cornerstone of comprehensive treatment for women with eating disorders. The four main psychotherapeutic approaches to treatment that are generally accepted as useful with eating disorders are psychodynamic therapy, cognitive behavioral therapy, interpersonal therapy, and dialectical behavioral therapy.

PSYCHODYNAMIC THERAPY Psychodynamic therapy focuses on dealing with a person's past experiences and underlying psychological issues. Determining the root cause of maladaptive behaviors and resolving those underlying issues removes the necessity for continuing the maladaptive behaviors. However, it is now generally accepted that in addition to resolving underlying issues, patients also need to resolve current issues involving food, weight, and relationships in order to break serious behavioral patterns associated with eating disorder symptoms.

COGNITIVE BEHAVIORAL THERAPY Cognitive behavioral therapy is based on the belief that affect and behavior are largely determined by the way a person structures the world through cognitions (thoughts and beliefs), based on attitudes and assumptions developed from previous experiences. It is a combination of behavioral techniques and aspects of cognitive therapy designed to identify, reality-test, and correct distorted cognitions. This form of therapy tends to be more successful with bulimia nervosa and binge eating disorder patients than with anorexia nervosa patients.

Cognitive behavioral therapy targets symptom behaviors such as binge eating, purging, and restricting behaviors. Dysfunctional thoughts about body shape and weight are managed with the goal of developing alternative thought patterns and behaviors. Monitoring food patterns, challenging faulty cognitions, and identifying triggers to eating disorder behaviors are all important aspects of this approach.

Interpersonal Therapy Interpersonal therapy focuses on difficulties in relationships. It is a short-term focal psychotherapy designed to help patients identify and modify interpersonal problems rather than focusing on specific food- and weight-related behaviors. Patients are helped to understand the role of interpersonal relationships in the development and maintenance of eating disorder symptoms.

Dialectical Behavioral Therapy Dialectical behavioral therapy is a combination of cognitive behavioral therapy, interpersonal therapy, and mindfulness training. Mindfulness helps a person to develop greater inner awareness. This form of therapy was originally developed to treat people who had problems with impulse control, self-destructive behaviors, volatile moods, and problems in relationships, all of which are commonly found in individuals with bulimia. Dialectical behavioral therapy works on dealing directly with the behavioral symptoms, and addresses interpersonal relationships. It focuses on helping patients build skills in a variety of areas to cope with emotions and handle problems without resorting to self-destructive or self-defeating behaviors. The mindfulness aspect of therapy helps patients to become more conscious of their inner and outer world.

As discussed earlier, treatment of an eating disorder involves comprehensive care that has been individualized according to the needs of the patient. This comprehensive, team-based approach is most effective, and incorporating a variety of therapies enhances treatment effectiveness and yields the best treatment outcomes.

Spiritual Issues

A critical aspect of the recovery process is the commitment of the individual. Early treatment dropout adversely affects the prognosis for recovery. Ending treatment prematurely can lead to a relapse of symptoms. Discouragements, doubts, fears, and lapses in motivation can hinder progress and dissuade patients from continuing with treatment. Women with eating disorders need to understand that recovery is an often difficult process that involves changes over time. Recovery also takes place in a process of growth and change, in which self-discovery leads to a greater sense of completeness, empowerment, and well-being.

Eating disorders can erode women's spirituality when the condition becomes the sole focus of their lives. The disorder replaces God or a higher power, family, and friends as a source of support, comfort, and love in their lives (Berrett, Hardman, O'Grady, & Richards, 2007). Eating disorders also generate spiritual disconnection of self from the body, nature, and society, whereby individuals can lose touch with spirituality and meaning in their lives (Berrett et al., 2007; Matusek & Knudson, 2009). Women with eating disorders tend to believe that the eating disorder will provide the solution to their emotional, relationship, and spiritual problems (Berrett et al., 2007).

In some cases, eating disorders may have dimensions of religious justification and asceticism. Some women may link their disordered eating behavior to spiritual beliefs and practices, such as self-sacrifice in reparation for imagined wrongdoing, or self-denial and fasting sanctioned by the church. In extreme cases, self-sacrifice can approach a death wish, where death from starvation is perceived as the ultimate punishment or redemption and escape from sinning and greed (Marsden, Karagianni, & Morgan, 2007).

Overcoming an eating disorder requires attention to the whole human being in all its mental, physical, emotional, social, and spiritual richness. Recovery often requires an all-encompassing change in lifestyle so as to develop a greater, different, or revised sense of self, to foster new relationships, and to find different ways of relating to others, with the ultimate purpose of promoting a sense of purpose and direction in life (Matusek & Knudson, 2009). A reconnection to the spiritual, sacred, and soulful aspects of life frequently diminishes the need in patients for disordered eating behaviors. Incorporation of spiritual perspectives and interventions into the care of women with eating disorders is an important consideration that can assist in treatment and recovery (Marsden et al., 2007). Attending to the spiritual growth and well-being during inpatient treatment may help reduce depression and anxiety, relationship distress, social role conflict, and eating disorder symptoms (Richards, Berrett, Hardman, & Eggett, 2006).

Issues Affecting Socioeconomic Integrity

Women with eating disorders experience numerous social and economic burdens that can greatly impact quality of life. They are often high consumers of medical and social care due to the chronic nature of the disorders and the numerous associated complications and co-morbidities (Simon, Schmidt, & Pilling, 2005). In a study that examined the overall costs of treatment for a cohort of adolescent patients with anorexia nervosa, average cost of treatment in one year ranged from $33,105 to $83,736. This included all inpatient care at baseline and during treatment as well as outpatient care. The majority (72%) of costs were attributed to medical hospitalization, with an additional 9% of outpatient costs for medical monitoring, and 19% for psychiatric care (Lock, Couturier, & Agras, 2008). The costs for adults with anorexia nervosa are likely higher than adolescent costs due to the fact that adults with eating disorders are more resistant to treatment, do not stay in treatment, and tend not to respond to treatment (Lock et al., 2008).

Limited access to care based on insurance benefit restrictions has historically posed a barrier to the recovery process. However, passage of the Mental Health Parity and Addiction Equity Act (MHPAEA) in October 2008 has mandated insurance companies to cover major mental illnesses on a par with physical illnesses. The Patient Protection and Affordable Care Act (Affordable Care Act) has made MHPAEA applicable to the individual health insurance market and qualified health plans in the same manner and to the same extent as MHPAEA applies to health insurance issuers and group health plans (United States Department of Labor, 2014).

This parity, or equivalence, in insurance coverage has made it easier to obtain treatment for a wide range of mental illnesses, including eating disorders. However, each state can decide what diagnoses are included as coverable mental illnesses. Thus, some states include eating disorders as coverable mental illnesses and some do not.

In states that require parity for eating disorders, coverage varies. Not all health insurance plans provide coverage for eating disorders. Some may cover treatment only if the eating disorder is so severe as to require medical stabilization in a hospital setting. Benefits may be denied if individuals are not sick enough to warrant the level of care required. Also, insurance companies routinely limit the number of days of treatment for eating disorders that are reimbursed. Treatment for eating disorders is commonly extensive and long-term. Unfortunately, physicians may have to discharge patients too early if adequate coverage or resources to continue treatment are lacking. Early discharge from treatment is associated with relapse or, in extreme cases, death (Eating Disorders Coalition for Research, Policy, & Action, 2008).

Women commonly develop eating disorders during adolescence and young adulthood, although older patients are being seen in increasing numbers. Eating disorders impose significant indirect and intangible costs on patients, families, communities, employers, society, and the healthcare system. Issues such as premature death, higher healthcare claims, worries about affordability of health care, lost productivity, absenteeism, lost wages, workplace accommodation, and increased use of human resource services are encountered and impact substantially on quality of life (Simon et al., 2005).

Eating disorders also influence social functioning. The majority of eating disorders develop during adolescent and young adult years when women are in secondary school, higher education, or at the beginning of their working careers, times that place women at crucial stages of psychosocial and educational development. Consequently, impairment in education and occupation is likely (Simon et al., 2005). Social isolation is common among those with eating disorders, which may further restrict social networks and access to social support. (Simon et al., 2005).

Issues Affecting Family Well-Being

Eating disorders have considerable impact on family well-being and quality of life. While each patient with an eating disorder faces her own unique challenges, illness severity, and timeline for recovery, the burden of care on family members can be considerable regardless of these factors. The burden of care comprises objective and subjective domains. Objective burden of care encompasses time spent caring for the affected family member, assistance with activities of daily living, and financial support. Subjective burden of care encompasses distress, strain, and level of satisfaction (de la Rie, van Furth, de Koning, Noordenbos, & Donker, 2005; Hillege, Beale, & McMaster, 2006). Family caregivers not only manage the burdens associated with the eating disorder but also face additional challenges related to comorbid conditions such as depression, anxiety, self-injury, or substance abuse. Family caregivers often face substantial unmet needs of their own and consequently frequently experience poor quality of life (de la Rie et al., 2005).

Family caregivers experience a range of emotional responses including distress, anger, frustration, despair, fear, and guilt (Highet, Thompson, & King, 2005; Hillege et al., 2006). An eating disorder may sometimes bring a family together and unify family members; however, it can just as frequently fracture families and disintegrate family ties. Social interactions within the family are affected, which can cause marital strain, substantial stress on sibling relationships, and rifts among family members. The emotional pressures can undermine the ability of the family to cope with the impact of caring for a family member with an eating disorder, and coping mechanisms can be negatively affected and depleted (Hillege et al., 2006).

Eating disorders can encroach upon every part of family life and become all-consuming, with unrelenting demands on the family caregiver and other family members. Financial concerns become worrisome. Caregivers often experience substantial financial drain due to health insurance, hospitalization, and therapists. They also may experience anxiety and uncertainty about how to continue paying for treatment when benefits run out. The trajectory of eating disorders commonly contains hidden costs such as transportation costs, frequent hospitalizations, food fads, additional family care costs, and time missed at work, which add to the distress of financial concerns (Hillege et al., 2006).

Families of patients with eating disorders often experience social isolation. This may be by choice of family caregivers in an effort to manage a situation they feel outsiders do not understand. The stigma of a mental illness such as an eating disorder can engender discriminatory attitudes and negative feelings in others, including uninformed health professionals (Björkman, Angelman, & Jönsson, 2008; Stewart, Schiavo, Herzog, &

Franko, 2008). Families may feel shame, humiliation, and exclusion from their social networks, which can intensify feelings of being alone and unsupported (Highet et al, 2005). Seclusion from social networks deprives the family of sharing the burden of care with others, which further depletes their limited coping resources (Hillege et al., 2006). Lack of understanding and compassion on the part of healthcare professionals can cause family caregivers to feel excluded from the treatment process, which can further fuel feelings of anxiety or frustration (Highet et al., 2005). Negative attitudes of healthcare professionals may be perceived by family caregivers and patients, creating barriers to obtaining effective care and services (McMaster, Beale, Hillege, & Nagy, 2004).

Family quality of life can be improved through measures aimed at lessening the destructive impact of eating disorders on family functioning and relational harmony within the family structure. Families should be acknowledged as integral to the recovery of their loved ones with eating disorders and included in the treatment process (Hillege et al., 2006). Addressing the needs of patients through symptom treatment helps to alleviate the burden of care experienced by family caregivers. Nonetheless, the specific needs of family caregivers and other family members must also be taken into account. The treatment team should provide individual and family teaching, counseling, and education as well as comprehensive social support for the complex emotional, relational, and life changes that families experience (Highet et al., 2005).

Implications for Healthcare Providers

Strategies to improve the quality of life of adolescent girls and women with eating disorders need to begin with early diagnosis and subsequent early initiation of treatment to maximize recovery. However, the secretive nature of individuals with eating disorders makes early diagnosis and treatment initiation particularly challenging for healthcare providers, as eating disorders are often revealed only when the patient reaches emaciation and/or experiences severe health problems (Walker & Lloyd, 2011). Thus it is essential to increase public awareness that eating disorders are a significant public health problem and prevention efforts are warranted. Prevention efforts that target adolescent girls and young women who are at high risk, such as those who exhibit early warning signs, appear to be more effective than universal programs that are directed at, for example, an entire grade in a high school.

Eating disorders encompass a complex combination of biological, psychological, and social factors. These patients can be challenging. They frequently deny the presence of a problem and are often resistant to treatment. It is not unusual for healthcare providers who are untrained in the subtleties of eating disorder pathology to feel frustration, anger, and negative attitudes toward eating disorder patients, especially when patients become irrational, non-compliant, and highly resistant to treatment. Healthcare providers who lack specialized training may become ineffective in the recovery process of their patients. Thus it is essential that healthcare providers who treat individuals with eating disorders obtain disorder-specific training in the course and outcomes of the disorders as well as in treatment models with the strongest evidence base (Walker & Lloyd, 2011).

A comprehensive, team-based approach provides the most effective treatment for eating disorders and yields the best treatment outcomes. It is essential that team members agree on criteria for the different levels of care that may be required during the treatment process so that patients experience a competent, complementary, and unified treatment team. To avoid panic and confusion, members of the healthcare team should establish criteria for, and goals of, any day treatment or inpatient treatment ahead of time in case the need for these levels of treatment arises. These criteria and goals should also be discussed with the patient, family caregivers and significant others and, when possible, agreed upon before any admission. It is important to establish guidelines for what constitutes higher levels of care early in eating disorder treatment, and such planning may reduce the need for involuntary hospitalization. Unless a patient is an adolescent, involuntary hospitalizations are difficult to enforce, and, for adults, should be considered only when absolutely necessary.

Healthcare providers should be cognizant of the spiritual dimension of eating disorders in their patients. Spiritual issues may pose an impediment to treatment, or they may be employed to improve motivation and treatment adherence. Spirituality should be considered an integral part of holistic care and should be addressed repeatedly throughout treatment. Clinical teams who may feel ill-equipped or uncomfortable in addressing spiritual issues should liaise with multi-faith chaplaincies or spiritual resources as appropriate (Marsden et al., 2007).

The inclusion of family caregivers in the treatment process is of primary importance in the maintenance of quality of life. Collaboration is especially important for communication and improved outcomes. Healthcare providers should be mindful of providing families with appropriate access to treatment information, especially practical advice and guidance on how to interact with their loved ones with eating disorders (McMaster et al., 2004). Healthcare providers also need to be mindful of the vital role of social support in the treatment plan, especially with respect to family caregivers. Social support is a significant moderator of family caregiver distress, an important predictor of care burden, a predictor of changes in burden and depression, and a buffer against the negative impact of caregiving (Winn, Perkins, Murray, Murphy, & Schmidt, 2004). Improving access to information concerning the eating disorder, along with providing social support to patients and family caregivers could greatly enhance quality of life.

Special Concerns of Age and Ethnicity

Although women commonly develop eating disorders during adolescence and young adulthood, eating disorders may also appear in older women, both with and without a history of an eating disorder. Healthcare providers may be less likely to suspect an eating disorder in an older woman, especially if the individual has been functional for most of her adult life. Symptoms of an eating disorder may be dismissed in older women, so persistence in finding help and treatment with a qualified eating disorder professional is vital for this cohort. Thorough medical assessments are essential. Physical illnesses, such as cancer, diabetes, Parkinson's disease, cardiovascular illness, and certain infections can result in weight loss, so obtaining an accurate diagnosis is important. Healthcare providers should consider and rule out loss of appetite related to other mental illnesses, such as depression and dementia. Such illnesses can coexist with eating disorders. Complications of eating disorders are similar in younger and older women, but older patients may be more vulnerable to these complications.

Treatment approaches tend to differ between younger and older patients. Family therapy tends to be more effective in adolescent patients, while individual therapy tends to work better with adult patients, although some treatment programs combine both approaches with positive results. The issues and concerns of adolescent girls, such as puberty, peer pressure, or first dating experiences naturally differ from those of adult women, so the treatment approach for an older woman with an eating disorder should be carefully selected and appropriate to address the issues pertinent to the psychosocial life stage of the individual. Inclusion of family in the treatment process of either younger or older women is, without a doubt, essential for recovery.

Risk factors for and pathways to disordered eating among ethnic minority women are as diverse and unique as the cultural contexts in which they exist. Information about the multifaceted nature of eating disorders in ethnic minority women is scarce. Despite suffering levels of distress similar to white women, women of ethnic minority groups have been shown to be more reluctant to seek treatment. Consequently, eating disorders have largely gone underdetected and undertreated in ethnic minority women (Brown et al., 2009).

Various factors have been considered as to why ethnic minority women tend not to seek treatment. Barriers to seeking treatment, from the perspective of minority women, can include feelings of shame or stigma, cultural perceptions of psychological disturbances that might minimize or interpret differently the seriousness of the problem, turning to alternate forms of therapy, belief that seeking therapy is a sign of character weakness, preference for family or informal support systems in times of need, distrust of counselors or fear that they will be hostile or cold, and difficulty in navigating the mental health system (Cachelin, Rebeck, Veisel, & Striegel-Moore, 2001). System barriers to treatment include language barriers, financial constraints, lack of health insurance, inaccessible healthcare facilities, time conflicts, long waits, lack of transportation, lack of child care, and lack of ethnically representative professional staff. Minority women who are less acculturated to American society are less likely to seek treatment for eating disorders (Cachelin et al., 2001). Healthcare providers need to recognize that women from ethnic minority groups do develop eating disorders and need adequate treatment. Further research is needed to define the extent and depth of the problems associated with underdetection and undertreatment of minority women with eating disorders.

Research Review

Will quality of life be impacted as a person moves along the trajectory towards an eating disorder?

Sanftner, J. (2011). Quality of life in relation to psychosocial risk variables for eating disorders in women and men. *Eating Behaviors, 12*, 136–142.

The purpose of this study was to investigate whether quality of life is impacted in women and men who develop the thoughts, feelings, and/or behaviors (i.e., the psychosocial risk factors) that increase the likelihood of developing an eating disorder. A cross-sectional, correlational design was used. A mid-sized Midwestern university was used as the setting for this study, from which a representative sample of 266 women and 114 men was drawn from the student population. Study participants completed questionnaires that measured both generic and eating disorder-specific quality of life, body dissatisfaction, objectified body consciousness, internalization of sociocultural ideals, and restrained eating. The mean age of female participants was 19.88, with a range between 18 and 46 years. For male participants, mean age was 20.65 with a range between 18 and 53 years. Mean body mass index (BMI) for the females was 25.25 with a range of 17.68 to 43.26. Mean BMI for the males was 26.25 with a range of 19.18 to 39.72. Self-identified ethnicity of the female participants was comprised of 87.2% European American, 4.1% African-American, 0.4% Latina/Hispanic, 0.8% Asian, 0.4% Native American, 0.4% Pacific Islander, 1.9% multiethnic, and 0.8% other ethnicity. Self-identified ethnicity of the male participants was comprised of 86.0% European American,

5.3% African-American, 1.8% Latino/Hispanic, 0% Asian, 0% Native American, 0% Pacific Islander, 4.4% multiethnic, and 1.8% other ethnicity. Data were analyzed with descriptive statistics, comparative statistics, correlational statistics, and multivariate analyses.

Findings revealed that women reported significantly higher levels of psychosocial risk factors than men. For women, all but one psychosocial risk factor was associated with poorer quality of life. Poorer eating disorder-specific quality of life was predicted by higher levels of objectified body consciousness, internalization of sociocultural ideals, and restrained eating. The relationship between objectified body consciousness and quality of life was moderated by gender, but gender did not significantly influence the relationship between other psychosocial risk factors and quality of life. Thus, only body objectification predicted eating disorder-specific quality of life for both women and men. The eating disorder-specific quality of life scale was shown to have higher sensitivity for use in a college student population.

The findings of this study have important implications for research and practice. They support that even women without eating disorders may have impaired health-related quality of life if they have higher levels of psychosocial risk factors. Therapists and counselors should assess quality of life in women who place a high worth on sociocultural standards of beauty and thinness. These findings also inform clinicians that interventions aimed at reducing levels of psychosocial risk factors may enhance quality of life in these women. Further research is recommended to investigate the developmental trajectory of psychosocial risk factors such as restrained eating and internalization of sociocultural ideals and their potential impact on quality of life. Evaluation of quality of life may benefit prevention programs, as quality of life becomes more impaired as an individual's attitudes and behaviors approach a clinical eating disorder.

Chapter Summary Points

- Eating disorders are serious mental illnesses and mainly include anorexia nervosa, bulimia nervosa, binge eating disorder, and other specified or unspecified feeding and eating disorders.
- In the United States, the prevalence of eating disorders is widespread and it is estimated that as many as 10 million females and 1 million males suffer from eating disorders such as anorexia nervosa or bulimia nervosa. Eating disorders have the highest mortality rate of any mental illness.
- Eating disorders commonly develop in adolescent girls and young women and are prevalent in industrialized societies in which there is an abundance of food, and thinness among women is considered attractive.
- Eating disorders are manifested by a variety of unhealthy eating and weight control habits that become obsessive, compulsive, and/or impulsive in nature.

- Numerous biological, social, cultural, and environmental factors are believed to contribute to the development of eating disorders, and these factors are inextricably linked.
- Beneficial measures for prevention of eating disorders include increasing public awareness, targeting those most at risk, addressing cultural support for eating disorders, and increasing protective factors against eating disorders.
- Specific gender differences exist in disorder prevalence, certain symptomatology, and rates of diagnosis and treatment.
- Adequate nutrition, reducing excessive exercise, and eliminating purging behaviors are the foundations of treatment for eating disorders. An interdisciplinary team approach involving a physician, nutritionist, and therapist is recommended.
- A treatment plan must be individualized to a patient's needs and can include individual, group, or family psychotherapy, medical care and monitoring, nutritional counseling, and medications.
- Quality of life issues and concerns associated with eating disorders are commonly multidimensional and encompass health and physical functioning, psychological and spiritual well-being, socioeconomic integrity, and family well-being.
- Healthcare providers who treat individuals with eating disorders need to obtain disorder-specific training in the course and outcomes of the disorders as well as in treatment models with the strongest evidence base.
- The inclusion of family caregivers in the treatment process is of primary importance in the maintenance of quality of life. Collaboration is especially important for communication and improved outcomes.
- Healthcare providers need to be mindful of the vital role of social support in the treatment plan, especially with respect to family caregivers. Social support is a significant moderator of family caregiver distress, an important predictor of care burden, a predictor of changes in burden and depression, and a buffer against the negative impact of care-giving.
- Although not as prevalent, eating disorders do occur in older women. Healthcare providers may be less likely to suspect an eating disorder in an older woman, especially if the individual has been functional for most of her adult life.
- Because symptoms of an eating disorder may be dismissed in an older woman, persistence in finding help and treatment with a qualified eating disorder professional is vital.
- Women of ethnic minority groups tend to be reluctant to seek treatment for eating disorders. Consequently, eating disorders have largely gone underdetected and undertreated in this cohort.

Critical Thinking Exercise

Case Study

M.G. is an 18-year-old female whose life has spun out of control over the past 2 years. She dropped out of school, dyed her hair orange, stole her parents' credit cards, and has gotten several tattoos and piercings. She was recently involved in a car accident in which she had been driving while under the influence of chemical substances. She has withdrawn from her friends and is involved with drinking, taking drugs, and risky behavior with a rough crowd in the community.

M.G. had an older brother who was killed 2 years ago in Afghanistan when his Marine unit was ambushed. She has a younger sister to whom she hardly speaks. When at home, M.G. keeps to herself and barely interacts with the rest of the family. She avoids mealtimes with her family, which inevitably became a battleground over her appearance and behavior. Her parents are devastated and beside themselves with worry and distress. M.G.'s family is so upset by her behavior that they can't bear the scrutiny and judgmental comments of others. They rarely attend church and family functions, and feel alone and abandoned.

Since her brother died, M.G. would lock herself in her room several times a week, eat a large amount of food and then purge afterward by self-induced vomiting and use of laxatives. Eating was soothing, and purging kept her from gaining weight. As a result, M.G. developed severe reflux and dental erosion. Her voice became raspy from smoking cigarettes and vomiting. M.G. had been to outpatient treatment and has seen a few therapists and psychiatrists but felt they were angry with her and judged her by her appearance. She left previous treatment too early and subsequently had not been helped. Both her parents are employed. The family health insurance provides limited mental health coverage and some degree of coverage for outpatient treatment of eating disorders that meet DSM-V diagnostic criteria for anorexia nervosa and bulimia nervosa. Her parents want M.G. to re-enter treatment but she refuses.

One day M.G. passed out in the bathroom and was taken to the emergency room by her parents. She was admitted to a medical unit with severe fluid and electrolyte imbalances and metabolic alkalosis. During her medical treatment, M.G. was again evaluated by a psychiatrist, but this time one who specialized in treating eating disorders. This psychiatrist helped M.G. to realize that she was seriously ill and if she didn't get her life under control quickly she might die. M.G. admitted that she didn't want to die. She was tired of the pain she felt and wanted to get better. When her medical condition was stabilized, M.G. entered a residential treatment facility that specialized in treating women her age for eating disorders.

Questions for Seminar Discussion

1. Discuss the eating disorder that M.G. likely had and factors that may have contributed to its development.
2. Discuss the physical and psychological symptoms that M.G. exhibited. What comorbid conditions did M.G. likely have?
3. What barriers did M.G. encounter in receiving treatment?

4. What treatment options seem to be more effective in treating M.G.'s eating disorder?
5. What is residential treatment and what kind of treatment approaches might M.G. experience in this facility?
6. Discuss the importance of a multidisciplinary approach to M.G.'s treatment, rehabilitation, and quality of life.
7. Discuss the physical, psychological/spiritual, socioeconomic, and family issues that influenced M.G.'s quality of life.
8. Discuss objective and subjective burden of care on the family caregivers and how this affected family quality of life.
9. What strengths and weaknesses were present that factor into the ability of M.G. and her family to manage illness and quality of life demands?
10. Discuss resources that are available to help M.G. manage her illness and improve her quality of life.

Internet Resources

Academy for Eating Disorders: a global professional association committed to leadership in eating disorders research, education, treatment, and prevention. http://www.aedweb.org/

Eating Disorders Coalition for Research, Policy, & Action: promotes education, research, resources, advocacy, and public policy. http://www.eatingdisorderscoalition.org

International Association of Eating Disorders Professionals: education and certification for multidisciplinary healthcare providers. http://www.iaedp.com

National Association of Anorexia Nervosa and Associated Disorders: provides information and resources for patients, families, and professionals. http://www.anad.org

National Eating Disorders Association (NEDA): provides information and resources for patients, family, and professionals. http://www.NationalEatingDisorders.org

National Institute of Mental Health: provides information and resources for patients, families, and professionals. http://www.nimh.nih.gov/health/topics/eating-disorders/index.shtml

References

Academy for Eating Disorders. (2011). Eating disorders: Critical points for early recognition and medical risk management in the care of individuals with eating disorders. Retrieved from http://www.aedweb.org

American Psychiatric Association. (2010). *Practice guideline for the treatment of patients with eating disorders* (3rd ed.). Retrieved from http://psychiatryonline.org/pb/assets/raw/sitewide/practice_guidelines/guidelines/eatingdisorders.pdf

American Psychiatric Association. (2013). *Diagnostic and statistical manual of mental disorders* (5th ed.). Arlington, VA: American Psychiatric Association.

Berrett, M., Hardman, R., O'Grady, K., & Richards, S. (2007). The role of spirituality in the treatment of trauma and eating disorders: Recommendations for clinical practice. *Eating Disorders, 15,* 373–389.

Björkman, T., Angelman, T., & Jönsson, M. (2008). Attitudes towards people with mental illness: A cross-sectional study among nursing staff in psychiatric and somatic care. *Scandinavian Journal of Caring Sciences, 22,* 170–177.

Brown, M., Cachelin, F., & Dohm, F. (2009). Eating disorders in ethnic minority women: A review of the emerging literature. *Current Psychiatry Reviews, 5,* 182–193.

Cachelin, F., Rebeck, R., Veisel, C., & Striegel-Moore, R. (2001). Barriers to treatment for eating disorders among ethnically diverse women. *Eating Disorders, 30,* 269–278.

Crow, S., Peterson, C., Swanson, S., Raymond, N., Specker, S., Eckert, E., & Mitchell, J. (2009). Increased mortality in bulimia nervosa and other eating disorders. *American Journal of Psychiatry, 166,* 1342–1346.

de la Rie, S., van Furth, E., de Koning, A., Noordenbos, G., & Donker, M. (2005). The quality of life of family caregivers of eating disorder patients. *Eating Disorders, 13,* 345–351.

Eating Disorders Coalition for Research, Policy, & Action. (2008). Why people with eating disorders need mental health parity now: A matter of life and death. Retrieved from http://www.eatingdisorderscoalition.org/documents/talkingpointsparity.pdf

Franco, K. (2012). Cleveland Clinic Center for Continuing Education: Eating disorders. Retrieved from http://www.clevelandclinicmeded.com/medicalpubs/diseasemanagement/psychiatry-psychology/eating-disorders/

Gadalla, T. (2009). Eating disorders in men: A community-based study. *International Journal of Men's Health, 8*(1), 72–81.

Genetic factors have a role in the development and treatment of eating disorders. (2005). *Drugs and Therapy Perspectives, 21*(4), 23–25.

Highet, N., Thompson, M., & King, R. (2005). The experience of living with a person with an eating disorder: The impact on carers. *Eating Disorders, 13,* 327–344.

Hillege, S., Beale, B., & McMaster, R. (2006). Impact of eating disorders on family life: Individual parents' stories. *Journal of Clinical Nursing, 15,* 1016–1022.

Hudson, J., Hiripi, E., Pope, H., & Kessler, R. (2007). The prevalence and correlates of eating disorders in the National Comorbidity Survey Replication. *Biological Psychiatry, 61,* 348–358.

Jones, A., Evans, M., Bamford, B., & Ford, H. (2008). Exploring quality of life for eating-disordered patients. *European Eating Disorders Review, 16,* 276–286.

Katzman, D., & Golden, N. (2008). Anorexia nervosa and bulimia nervosa. In L. Neinstein, C. Gordon, D. Katzman, D. Rosen, E. Woods (Eds.), *Adolescent health care* (5th ed., pp. 477–489). Philadelphia PA: Lippincott Williams & Wilkins.

Levine, M., & Smolak, L. (2005). *The prevention of eating problems and eating disorders: Theory, research, and practice.* Mahwah, NJ: Erlbaum.

Lock, J., Couturier, J., & Agras, W. (2008). Costs of remission and recovery using family therapy for adolescent anorexia nervosa: A descriptive report. *Eating Disorders, 16,* 322–330.

Marsden, P., Karagianni, E., & Morgan, J. (2007). Spirituality and clinical care in eating disorders: A qualitative study. *International Journal of Eating Disorders, 40,* 7–12.

Matusek, J., & Knudson, R. (2009). Rethinking recovery from eating disorders: Spiritual and political dimensions. *Qualitative Health Research, 19*(5), 697–707.

McMaster, R., Beale, B., Hillege, S., & Nagy, S. (2004). The parent experience of eating disorders: Interactions with health professionals. *International Journal of Mental Health Nursing, 13,* 67–73.

National Association of Anorexia Nervosa and Associated Disorders. (2015). Eating disorders statistics. Retrieved from http://www.anad.org/get-information/about-eating-disorders/eating-disorders-statistics/

National Eating Disorders Association. (2015a). Eating disorders in women of color: Explanations and implications. Retrieved from http://www.nationaleatingdisorders.org/eating-disorders-women-color-explanations-and-implications

National Eating Disorders Association. (2015b). Get the facts on eating disorders: What are eating disorders? http://www.nationaleatingdisorders.org/get-facts-eating-disorders

National Eating Disorders Association. (2015c). Statistics on males and eating disorders: Prevalence in men. Retrieved from https://www.nationaleatingdisorders.org/statistics-males-and-eating-disorders

Padierna, A., Quintana, J., Arostegui, I., Gonzalez, N., & Horcajo, J. (2000). The health-related quality of life in eating disorders. *Quality of Life Research, 9,* 667–674.

Richards, P.S., Berrett, M., Hardman, R., & Eggett, D. (2006). Comparative efficacy of spirituality, cognitive, and emotional support groups for treating eating disorder inpatients. *Eating Disorders, 14,* 401–415.

Sanftner, J. (2011). Quality of life in relation to psychosocial risk variables for eating disorders in women and men. *Eating Behaviors, 12,* 136–142.

Sargent, J., Stein, K., & Rosen, D. (2009). Eating disorders. In J. Urbancic, & C. Grob, (Eds.), *Women's mental health: A clinical guide for primary care providers* (pp. 181–224). Philadelphia, PA: Lippincott Williams & Wilkins.

Shapiro, J., Berkman, N., Brownley, K., Sedway, J., Lohr, K., & Bulik, C. (2007). Bulimia nervosa treatment: A systematic review of randomized controlled trials. *International Journal of Eating Disorders, 40*(4), 321–336.

Simon, J., Schmidt, U., & Pilling, S. (2005). The health service use and cost of eating disorders. *Psychological Medicine, 35,* 1543–1551.

Steiner, H., Kwan, W., Shaffer, T., Walker, S., Miller, S., Sagar, A., & Lock, J. (2003). Risk and protective factors for juvenile eating disorders. *European Child and Adolescent Psychiatry, 12*(Suppl. 1), 38–46.

Stewart, M., Schiavo, R., Herzog, D., & Franko, D. (2008). Stereotypes, prejudices, and discrimination of women with anorexia nervosa. *European Eating Disorders Review, 16,* 311–318.

Striegel-Moore, R., & Bulik, C. (2007). Risk factors for eating disorders. *American Psychologist, 62*(3), 181–198.

Striegel-Moore, R., Rosselli, F., Perrin, N., DeBar, L., Wilson, G., May, A., & Kraemer, H. (2009). Gender differences in the prevalence of eating disorder symptoms. *International Journal of Eating Disorders, 42*(5), 471–474.

Tantillo, M., MacDowell, S., Anson, E., Taillie, E., & Cole, R. (2009). Combining supported housing and partial hospitalization to improve eating disorder symptoms, perceived health status, and health related quality of life for women with eating disorders. *Eating Disorders, 17,* 385–399.

U.S. Department of Labor. (2014). 2014 report to congress compliance with the Mental Health Parity and Addiction Equity Act of 2008. Retrieved from http://www.dol.gov/ebsa/publications/mhpaeareporttocongress2014.html

Walker, S., & Lloyd, C. (2011). Barriers and attitudes health professionals working in eating disorders experience. *International Journal of Therapy and Rehabilitation, 18*(7), 383–391.

Weltzin, T. (2012). Gender differences: Part 2. Eating disorders in males. *Psychiatric Times* (October, 2012), *29*(10), 32–34.

Wilson, G., Grilo, C., & Vitousek, K. (2007). Psychological treatment of eating disorders. *American Psychologist, 62*(3), 199–216.

Winn, S., Perkins, S., Murray, J., Murphy, R., & Schmidt, U. (2004). A qualitative study of the experience of caring for a person with bulimia nervosa. Part 2: Carers' needs and experiences of services and other support. *International Journal of Eating Disorders, 36,* 269–279.

Yager, J., Devlin, M., Halmi, K., Herzog, D., Mitchell, J., Powers, P., & Zerbe, K. (2012). Guideline watch (August 2012): Practice guideline for the treatment of patients with eating disorders, 3rd ed. Retrieved from http://psychiatryonline.org/pb/assets/raw/sitewide/practice_guidelines/guidelines/eatingdisorders-watch.pdf

Bipolar Disorder

Introduction

Bipolar disorder, a type of mood disorder also known as manic-depressive disorder, is a serious mental illness characterized by shifts of emotion. In bipolar disorder, individuals experience episodes of both mania and depression that are associated with unusual swings of mood and energy that affect the ability to function. Bipolar disorder is a major public health problem that frequently coexists with anxiety disorders and substance use disorder. Even though bipolar disorder is equally prevalent among women and men, evidence indicates that significant gender differences exist in the presentation, course, treatment, and outcomes of the disorder. This chapter explores the issues of

bipolar disorder that affect young women. The significant impact of bipolar disorders on the quality of life of young women and their families is also discussed.

Incidence

Bipolar disorder comprises a spectrum of symptom categories, including bipolar I, bipolar II, cyclothymic disorder, and other specified bipolar and related disorder (OSBRD). Bipolar disorder affects about 5.7 million adult Americans, or roughly 2.6% of the U.S. population aged 18 and older, every year. Of these cases, approximately 82.9%, or 2.2% of the adult population, is considered severely afflicted (National Institute of

Mental Health [NIMH], 2015). The overall lifetime prevalence of bipolar disorder considered in total (bipolar, I, II, and subthreshold together) is 4.0%, with a yearly prevalence of 2.8% (Harvard School of Medicine, 2007). When considering estimates of specific subcategories of bipolar disorder, the lifetime prevalence of bipolar I is 1.0%, and 1.1% for bipolar II. Bipolar I prevalence is estimated at 1.1% in females and 0.8% in males. Bipolar II prevalence is estimated at 1.3% in females and 0.9% including males (Merikangas et al., 2007).

Bipolar disorder affects women and men equally, and is found in all ages, races, ethnic groups, and social classes. Women often develop bipolar disorder in the late teens or early adult years. The age of onset for all bipolar disorders ranges from late adolescence to early adulthood (Merikangas et al., 2007), at about 18 to 25 years old, and at least one-half to two-thirds of all patients experience onset before age 18 (Podawiltz, 2011a). Some individuals may experience their first symptoms earlier during childhood, and others late in life (NIMH, 2012a).

The average age of onset for the first manic, hypomanic, or major depressive episode is approximately 18 years. Even though bipolar II disorder can begin in late adolescence and throughout adulthood, average age of onset is the mid-20s. Cyclothymic disorder usually begins in adolescence or early adulthood, and carries a 15% to 50% risk that a person with cyclothymic disorder will subsequently develop bipolar I or bipolar II disorder. Among children who develop cyclothymic disorder, the average age at onset is 6.5 years (American Psychiatric Association, 2013).

Evidence suggests that patients with bipolar disorder are at higher risk of premature death from general medical disorders. This may be attributed to coexisting unhealthy lifestyle behaviors such as smoking, obesity, binge eating, sedentary lifestyle, social isolation, healthcare disparities, and substance abuse. Biologic factors associated with increased risk of mortality among patients with bipolar disorder include stress-related effects on the immune system and hypothalamic-pituitary axis, increased sympathetic nervous system activity, and metabolic side effects of pharmacologic treatments (Roshanaei-Moghaddam & Katon, 2009).

Individuals with bipolar disorder are at high risk for suicide, and have a suicide rate 15 times higher than the general population (Dennehy et al., 2011). It is estimated that 25% to 50% of individuals with bipolar disorder attempt suicide at least once in their lifetime (Fountoulakis, Gonda, Siamouli, & Rihmer, 2009). Bipolar I and bipolar II both have a lifetime risk of approximately 26% for completed suicide (Hoes, 2009). Approximately 10% to 15% of those with bipolar I disorder commit suicide. Patients are at highest risk during episodes of depression or mixed mania (in which depression and mania occur simultaneously). Patients with bipolar II disorder have a higher risk for suicide compared to bipolar I or major depressive disorder (University of Maryland Medical Center [UMMC], 2013). Individuals with bipolar II disorder tend to have much higher completed and attempted suicide rates. Their completed suicides may account for approximately 44% of all suicides (Hoes, 2009). Rapid cycling—a severe variation of bipolar disorder—increases the risk of suicide, especially in conjunction with earlier age onset of depression, bipolar I subtype, being female, being single, and having a history of drug abuse, panic disorder, sexual abuse, or psychosis during depression (Gao et al., 2009).

Etiology and Risk Factors

Bipolar disorder is a serious chronic psychiatric illness typically distinguished by repeated episodes of depression and mania. The exact cause remains unknown and the mechanism of the illness is poorly understood. It is believed that numerous genetic, biologic, and environmental factors act together to generate and maintain the chemical imbalances in the brain that shape this complicated disorder. Risk factors can be categorized as those that may impart lifetime vulnerability to bipolar disorder (such as genetic or biologic factors) and those that increase the likelihood for the onset of an episode of depression or mania (such as stressful life events or stimulant/antidepressant use) (Puri & Gilmore, 2011).

Genetic Factors

Evidence suggests that genetic transmission of bipolar disorder occurs; however, efforts to identify specific genes associated with bipolar disorder have yet to be successful. The genetic inheritance is complex and is most likely polygenic rather than attributed to genes of major effect. It is believed that susceptibility genes combined with neurobiologic trait abnormalities of structure or functioning may contribute to clinical expression of the disorder (Fusar-Poli, Howes, Bechdolf, & Borgwardt, 2012). Family studies indicate that having first-degree relatives with bipolar disorder or major depressive disorder significantly increases the risk for developing the illness as compared to the occurrence of bipolar disorder in the general population (McNamara, Nandagopal, Strakowski, & DelBello, 2010).

Recent findings from genomic studies revealed that abnormal sequences of DNA may increase the risk of developing early-onset bipolar disorder. The abnormal DNA sequences are known as rare *copy number variants* (CNVs). These CNVs are spontaneously occurring (de novo) genetic mutations that are not inherited from parents. In a genome-wide analysis of de novo CNVs, findings indicated a significantly higher frequency of de novo CNVs in persons with bipolar disorder, with particular enrichment of CNVs among persons with age of onset younger than 18. Researchers concluded that rare spontaneous genetic mutations are an important contributor to the risk for bipolar disorder (Malhotra et al., 2011).

Neurobiologic Abnormalities

Preliminary evidence from longitudinal and cross-sectional neuroimaging studies indicates that bipolar disorder is associated with dynamic and excessive loss of gray matter in the prefrontal cortex of the brain. The deficits in prefrontal cortex gray matter are commonly found in young adults with bipolar disorder, but not in first-episode or adolescent individuals with bipolar disorder. In concurrence with the progressive loss of gray matter density, adolescent and adult individuals with bipolar disorder reveal significantly smaller frontal white matter tracks, as compared to healthy control subjects (McNamara et al., 2010). Evidence from twin studies suggests that white matter pathology in the frontal lobe may be associated with genetic risk for bipolar disorder, whereas most of the widespread abnormalities of gray matter may be associated with environmental effects and the illness itself (Fusar-Poli et al., 2012).

Stressful Life Events

Stressful life events have long been acknowledged as distal and proximal precursors of bipolar disorder. Severe trauma or abuse during childhood likely occurs in nearly half of the persons with bipolar disorder and contributes to earlier age at onset of illness as well as worsening of the course of illness (McNamara et al., 2010). Stressful life events may precipitate manic and hypomanic episodes as well as depression (Proudfoot, Doran, Manicavasagar, & Parker, 2011). Prior stressful life events may increase vulnerability to subsequent stressors proximal to the onset of mania through a sensitization mechanism—a progressive intensification of a response following repetitive exposures. Stressful life events may increase the risk for developing bipolar disorder independent of familial risk (McNamara et al., 2010).

Substance Use

Substance use is prevalent among individuals with bipolar disorder. It is considered a co-occurring condition in that up to 60% of persons with bipolar disorder develop substance use or dependence at some point in their lives (UMMC, 2013). Evidence indicates that 40% of clinically referred adolescents with bipolar disorder also have co-occurring substance use disorder, which suggests that bipolar adolescents have a five- to sixfold increased risk of substance use as compared to adolescents without major psychopathology (McNamara et al., 2010). High rates of bipolar disorder have also been observed in persons with substance use disorder and it is suggested that substance use may be a risk factor for developing bipolar disorder in that it may directly cause symptoms that resemble those of primary bipolar disorder, such as idiopathic mania following use of psychostimulants. Substance use may precipitate symptoms of bipolar disorder in vulnerable persons through a mechanism of sensitization (McNamara et al., 2010). Although many adolescents with bipolar disorder develop substance use disorder subsequent to the onset of bipolar disorder, approximately one-third develop bipolar disorder following the development of substance use disorder. Further investigation is needed that systematically and prospectively assesses substance use and substance use disorder in the role of precipitating or accelerating the development of bipolar disorder (McNamara et al., 2010).

Stimulant and Antidepressant Medications

Epidemiological evidence suggests that the high rate of stimulant and antidepressant use in this country may be associated with higher prevalence rates and lower age at onset of bipolar disorder. In the last decade, a 40-fold increase in diagnosis of childhood and adolescent bipolar disorder in office-based medical settings has occurred. Treatment with stimulants and antidepressants over the long term may trigger or exacerbate manic symptoms as well as hasten the age at which mania occurs. Persons with bipolar disorder who also

have substance use disorder are at greater risk for antidepressant-induced mania. Additionally, offspring of bipolar parents who went on to develop bipolar disorder have a significantly higher prevalence of stimulant and antidepressant exposure as compared to counterparts who did not develop the illness (McNamara et al., 2010).

Evidence has emerged indicating that certain common medications may trigger mania. These medications include steroids, pseudoephedrine, dopamine agonists, interferon, and bronchodilators. Further research is needed to confirm the potential mood-destabilizing effects of these drugs (Proudfoot et al., 2011).

Omega-3 Fatty Acid Deficiency

A significant presence of deficiency in omega-3 fatty acids in persons with bipolar disorder and in those with ultra-high risk for the illness, as compared to healthy control subjects, has been found. It is presently unclear whether the omega-3 fatty acid deficiency observed in persons with bipolar disorder as well as those with ultra-high risk for developing the disorder is related to dietary deficiency, genetic factors, or both. Omega-3 fatty acid deficiency may also influence behavioral sensitization and dopamine levels in the brain (McNamara et al., 2010).

Circadian Rhythms and Seasonality

Disrupted circadian rhythms are likely associated with the onset of manic symptoms in persons with bipolar disorder. Sleep deprivation tends to shift bipolar individuals toward episodes of mania or hypomania, while increased sleep tends to shift bipolar individuals toward increased depressive symptoms. Sleep deprivation may be a final common pathway through which a variety of external factors trigger episodes of bipolar mania or hypomania (Proudfoot et al., 2011).

Research supports the existence of a seasonal pattern of bipolar mania in which seasonal factors have a potential to precipitate episodes of mania. Bipolar individuals tend to experience more manic episodes during spring and summer months, and it is purported that the rapidly increasing photoperiod (duration of sunlight) of the spring, and the rapidly decreasing photoperiod later in summer may influence a higher prevalence of manic bipolar episodes (Proudfoot et al., 2011). More research is needed to further clarify the role that disrupted circadian rhythms and seasonality play in influencing the occurrence of manic episodes in persons with bipolar disorder.

Degree of Risk of Bipolar Disorder

The literature has been consistent in identifying a substantial risk of bipolar disorder in offspring and siblings of parents who have bipolar disorder. Children who have a first-degree relative (parent or sibling) affected with bipolar disorder have a 10-fold risk of developing the illness as compared to children without a family history of bipolar disorder (Fusar-Poli et al., 2012). Offspring of one parent with bipolar disorder have a 15% to 30% chance of developing bipolar disorder, and that risk increases to 70% to 75% if the second parent is also affected (Fusar-Poli et al., 2012; McNamara et al., 2010). The concordance rate of bipolar disorder between identical twins is approximately 70% (Fusar-Poli et al., 2012). Although evidence points to high heritability of bipolar disorder among persons with first-degree relatives with bipolar disorder, and is therefore a robust risk factor, not all offspring of bipolar parents or siblings develop the illness (Goldstein et al., 2010; McNamara et al., 2010). Nevertheless, the high rates of heritability for bipolar disorder indicate that offspring of parents with bipolar disorder should be considered as appropriate candidates for evaluating the efficacy of early intervention strategies in prospective longitudinal studies (McNamara et al., 2010).

The hallmark feature of bipolar disorder is mania/hypomania. The degree of risk associated with factors that increase the likelihood for the onset of bipolar mania is unclear. However, some factors may not trigger bipolar mania in isolation but in certain circumstances where the factors likely coalesce in a way that precipitates bipolar mania/hypomania in susceptible individuals. Evidence is, for the most part, preliminary and tentative, and further research is needed to discern why certain factors bring on mania in some persons with bipolar disorder but not in others (Proudfoot et al., 2011).

Risk Reduction

Bipolar disorder carries with it considerable functional impairment. Thus, early identification and intervention is essential to avert occurrence of the illness. To this end, researchers have examined the concept of illness prodrome within the context of psychosis. Illness prodrome is the phase of first dynamic changes in behavior and mental state that is positioned between stable, premorbid abnormalities and the first syndromal episode of a disorder (Correll et al., 2007). In other words, the prodrome presents signs or symptoms of an approaching illness or condition. In the arena of psychosis prevention, recognition of a specific clinical prodrome of a mental illness enables subsequent development of specific psychosis prodrome rating scales for individuals at high risk for the illness. Focus on the clinical prodrome, which has emerged with schizophrenia research, has produced promising results concerning the potential to reduce pre-illness symptom manifestations and progression to the full disorder (Correll et al., 2007). However, the presence of an identifiable prodromal state in bipolar disorder and the subsequent possibility of early prevention remain problematic, owing to the paucity of information concerning the presence and duration of specific signs and symptoms that precede the first mania episode. Also, the characteristics of bipolar disorder, which consists of depression and mania, and the current classification system, which uses a combination of symptom clusters for the defining mania episode, makes determination of a prodromal onset more difficult than in psychosis (Correll, 2007). Nonetheless, evidence has begun to emerge that explicates prodromal clinical features presented by children and adolescents prior to the first onset of mania. These features include common mood symptoms that are subsyndromal (that is, symptoms that fall just short of the requirements for a diagnosis of that disorder) as well as syndromal of major depressive disorder. Prodromal features also include episodic subsyndromal manic symptoms, such as deficits in concentration/attention, sleep disturbances, anger, irritability, mood swings, and increased energy (McNamara et al., 2010).

Even though progress in the identification of risk factors and prodromal clinical features has been made, there is currently scarce evidence concerning interventions that may be protective against the onset of mania when administered in the prodromal period. Consequently, numerous uncertainties have emerged, including whether persons with robust risk factors and prodromal clinical features will develop mania, the existence of a 10-year lag between onset of prodromal mood symptoms and onset of mania, and the fact that risk factors and prodromal clinical features lack specificity for mania. These uncertainties represent limitations in the clinical staging model for bipolar disorder and have hindered progress in evaluating efficacy of early interventions in clinical trials (McNamara et al., 2010).

Clinical trials that have investigated pharmacological interventions in children and adolescents with familial risk for developing bipolar disorder found that mood stabilizers and antipsychotic medications had limited efficacy in treatment of those at risk for mania and depression, and are likely not well suited as first-line treatment for at risk youth. However, omega-3 fatty acid deficiency may represent a preventable risk factor for the development of bipolar disorder. Long-term dietary omega-3 fatty acid supplementation may be efficacious and well tolerated as monotherapy for the treatment of prodromal mood symptoms (that is, depression) in youth at high risk for transitioning to mania (McNamara et al., 2010).

Gender Similarities and Differences

The prevalence of bipolar disorder is approximately equal in women and men (Altshuler et al., 2010). The average age of onset of bipolar disorder tends to be at the age of 25, and women tend to have a later age of onset than men. For women, age of onset of bipolar disorder is about 3.2 years later than men. Women tend to experience midlife onset of bipolar disorder more commonly than men, with onset during the fifth decade of life occurring more frequently (Arnold, 2003). Women are more likely to be misdiagnosed with unipolar depression and face substantial delays in treatment for bipolar disorder due to misdiagnosis, whereas men have a lesser tendency to be misdiagnosed and are apt to face shorter treatment delays. Women with bipolar II are especially vulnerable to delayed diagnosis and treatment (Arnold, 2003; Sit, 2004).

Gender differences have been identified in certain characteristics and in the course of bipolar disorder. Presence of triggering events are more likely to be found in women than men (Yazla, Inanç, Billci, & Dusenen, 2012). Women are more likely than men to experience rapid cycling, in which manic and depressive episodes alternate at least four times in a year (UMMC, 2013). Women tend to initially present with depression and have more frequent depressive episodes than men, whereas men tend to have more frequent and more severe episodes of mania. Women are more likely than men to present seasonality patterns of bipolar disorder, where depression occurs more frequently in fall and winter than in spring and summer.

Women experience bipolar II disorder and mixed mania (simultaneous depression and mania) more frequently than men. The fact that bipolar women experience more severe and recurrent depressive episodes than men may contribute to their perceiving worse overall health and well-being than bipolar men. Specifically, bipolar women tend to perceive poorer overall functioning and well-being with substantially greater pain and worse physical health (Arnold, 2003). Among men and women with bipolar disorder, evidence indicates that women experience poorer quality of life than men (de la Cruz, Lai, Goodrich, & Kilbourne, 2013; Vornik & Hirschfeld, 2005).

Although comorbidity of medical and psychiatric disorders occurs in both women and men, it tends to be more common in women, and adversely affects recovery from mania more frequently in women. Comorbid medical disorders commonly seen in women include thyroid disease, migraine headaches, and obesity. Women also tend to experience comorbid bulimia, post traumatic stress disorder, social phobia, and obsessive-compulsive disorder more frequently than men (Arnold, 2003; Baldassano, 2006). Bipolar men are more likely to be employed, less likely to be married, have a higher incidence of lifetime alcohol abuse, are more likely to have a history of violence, and more likely to have legal problems than bipolar women (Baldassano, 2006; Yazla et al., 2012). While both men and women with bipolar disorder are at similar risk of suicide (Arnold, 2003), evidence suggests that more bipolar women than bipolar men are likely to have a history of suicide attempts (Baldassano, 2006).

Diagnosing Bipolar Disorder

Bipolar disorder is a lifelong recurrent, cyclical, and relapsing illness that can take years to correctly diagnose. The symptom constellations of bipolar disorder are distinguished by episodes of depression, mania, and hypomania; can occur in mixed states; are changeable; and can range from mild to severe. Bipolar disorder can be debilitating, with an increasing risk for suicide, medical and psychiatric comorbid disorders, frequent hospitalizations, and substantial disability (Hoes, 2009). The symptoms of bipolar I, bipolar II, cyclothymia disorder, and other specified bipolar and related disorder categories are discussed below.

Bipolar I Disorder

Individuals with bipolar I disorder are described as having one manic episode or mixed episode and one or more depressive episodes, lasting for at least one week. Characteristically, a regular pattern is established in which manic episodes precede or follow depressive episodes. Hypomanic episodes that last at least four consecutive days may commonly occur but are not required diagnostic criteria for bipolar I disorder (American Psychiatric Association, 2013). Hypomania is a form of mania in which symptoms, typically euphoria, are less severe, do not last as long, and tend not to cause impairment in social or occupational functioning. In bipolar I disorder, episodes are more acute and severe than in bipolar II and cyclothymic disorder. A manic episode causes marked impairment in social and occupational functioning and frequently requires hospitalization (American Psychiatric Association, 2013). If left untreated, patients may average four episodes of dysregulated mood per year (Hirschfeld, 2007; UMMC, 2009).

Bipolar II Disorder

Individuals with bipolar II disorder experience predominantly major depressive episodes with occasional episodes of hypomania. The hypomania usually lasts about 4 days, and is not severe enough to cause marked impairment in social or occupational functioning, or to require hospitalization (American Psychiatric Association, 2013). Full-blown manic episodes or mixed episodes do not occur in bipolar II. Although most bipolar II patients return to fully functional levels between episodes, the course of the illness tends to be chronic in nature, and they experience significantly more depressive episodes. Depressive episodes tend to cause clinically significant distress or impairment in social, occupational, or other important areas of functioning (American Psychiatric Association, 2013) Patients with bipolar II disorder tend to have shorter periods of well-being between episodes than bipolar I patients. Bipolar II tends to be highly associated with the risk for suicide (Hirschfeld, 2007; UMMC, 2009).

Cyclothymic Disorder

Individuals with cyclothymic disorder experience mood cycles that are less severe than those experienced in bipolar I and bipolar II disorders. Cyclothymic disorder is characterized by at least 2 years of frequent mood cycles of hypomanic episodes that shift back and forth with mild depression, but symptoms do not meet the criteria for bipolar I or II in severity, number, duration, or pervasiveness (American Psychitric Association, 2013; Hirschfeld, 2007). The hypomanic symptoms tend toward irritability, in comparison to the more euphoric presentation in bipolar II. The course of cyclothymia is more chronic and tends to last about 2 years, with single episodes that persist for more than 2 months. Cyclothymic disorder may be a precursor to full-blown bipolar disorder, or it may continue as a low-grade chronic condition (Hoes, 2009; UMMC, 2009).

Other Specified Bipolar and Related Disorder

In this category, individuals display symptoms of illness that do not meet the full criteria for bipolar I, bipolar II, or cyclothymic disorder. These individuals present with symptoms that do not last long enough, or symptoms that are too few, to be diagnosed with bipolar I or bipolar II disorder. However, patients in this category exhibit

symptoms that are clearly out of the normal range of behavior for the individual and cause clinically significant distress or impairment in social, occupational, or other important areas of functioning (American Psychiatric Association, 2013). Presentations that may be classified in this category include short duration hypomanic episodes (2-3 days) and major depressive episodes, hypomanic episodes with insufficient symptoms and major depressive episodes, hypomanic episodes without prior major depressive episodes, and short-duration cyclothymic episodes (less than 24 months) (American Psychiatric Association, 2013).

Clinical Features of Mania and Depression

Mania

Mania is a distinct period of abnormally and persistently elevated, expansive, or irritable mood lasting at least 1 week, or any duration if hospitalization is necessary. During mania, patients experience three or more unrelenting symptoms to a significant degree. Symptoms include inflated self-esteem or grandiosity, excessive speech or pressured speech, racing thoughts, distractibility, and increase in goal-directed activity (either socially, at work or school, or sexually) or psychomotor agitation. Patients may exhibit a decreased need for sleep and feel rested after only a few hours of sleep. They may exhibit excessive involvement in pleasurable activities that have a high potential for painful consequences, such as engaging in unrestrained buying sprees, sexual indiscretions, or foolish business investments (American Psychiatric Association, 2013). During manic episodes, patients may experience marked impairment in occupational functioning, in usual social activities, or in relationships with others. Hospitalization may be necessary to prevent harm to themselves or others. Psychotic features such as delusions, hallucinations, or disorganized speech or behavior may be present. It is important to note that mania is not the result of direct effects of drugs, illness, or antidepressant treatments (American Psychiatric Association, 2013; Hoes, 2009).

Hypomania

Hypomania is characterized by persistently elevated, expansive, or irritable mood usually of shorter duration than mania (lasting at least four consecutive days). Hypomanic patients, to a significant degree, experience three or more of the symptoms described under mania. Hypomanic mood is noticeably different from the patient's usual depressed mood and often manifests as increased creativity, productivity, and sociability. Hypomania may also be distinguished by increased irritability that is noticeable to family and coworkers (American Psychiatric Association, 2013). A hypomanic episode is an unmistakable change in functioning that is uncharacteristic of the person when not symptomatic. However, hypomania is not severe enough to cause marked impairment in social or occupational functioning or to warrant hospitalization. Psychotic features are not present in hypomania (American Psychiatric Association, 2013; Hoes, 2009; Sit, 2004).

Bipolar Depression

Bipolar depression is characterized by low mood or diminished interest or enthusiasm that persists for at least 2 weeks, and a considerable decrease in numerous areas of functioning is apparent. Bipolar depression is also characterized by neurovegetative changes, cognitive impairment, and altered functioning (Sit, 2004). During bipolar depressive episodes, individuals lose interest in life or pleasurable activities. They may experience feelings of sadness, worthlessness, guilt, and hopelessness. Decision making and concentration are difficult and delusional ideation may be exhibited (American Psychiatric Association). Patients may

experience agitation or lethargy and inertia, as well as social withdrawal and isolation. They may experience physical symptoms such as pain, fatigue, decreased libido, along with appetite, weight, and sleep changes. Depressed mood may also be accompanied by thoughts of death and dying, and suicidal ideation and attempts (American Psychiatric Association, 2013; Hoes, 2009).

Symptoms of bipolar depression are almost identical to those of major depression, the primary form of unipolar depressive disorder. It is frequently difficult to distinguish between unipolar and bipolar depression, particularly in persons with bipolar II disorder. Patients more likely to have unipolar depression are apt to suffer longer depressive episodes, have a later onset of symptoms, and have no family history of bipolar disorder. Patients with unipolar depression tend to exhibit more "typical" depressive features, such as insomnia, decreased appetite, physical agitation, and somatic complaints. People with major depression can experience a variety of other moods, but none meet the criteria for a manic state. In contrast, patients with bipolar depression tend to have more prior episodes of depression of shorter duration, usually 2 to 3 months, which is commonly not as long as major depression lasts. The depressive symptoms in people who are bipolar tend to vary in that some may experience increased sleep, weight gain, and feel heaviness or slowness in their bodies, whereas others may experience impaired sleep. However, unlike those with unipolar depression, persons with bipolar depression do not feel sleepy the next day. In comparison to major depressive episodes, bipolar depression tends to develop more gradually, and psychotic features while depressed may be more common (Hirschfeld, 2007; UMMC, 2009).

Mixed Mania

Mixed mania, also known as mixed episodes, is characterized by symptoms of mania and depression that occur daily for a week. Patients with mixed mania exhibit agitation, refractory anxiety, intractable insomnia, suicidality, obsessions and impulses, and hypersexuality. There is also a higher frequency of psychosis and suicidality in mixed mania as compared to pure mania (Sit, 2004).

Rapid Cycling

Rapid cycling is a pattern in which distinct manic and depressive episodes alternate four or more times yearly. Mood episodes are separated by a mood switch to an opposite pole or by remission for 8 or more weeks. In severe cases, the mood switches can progress to several cycles a day. Typically, rapid cycling begins in the depressive phase, and is followed by mania. Rapid cycling is seen in both bipolar I and bipolar II disorder, and is associated with treatment resistance, poor long-term prognosis, and higher risk for suicide. Rapid cycling occurs in 15% to 20% of all cases of bipolar disorder, and women account for 70% to 90% of rapid cycling cases. Rapid cycling in women is associated with increased rates of hypothyroidism, depression, suicidality, substance abuse, anxiety, and increased use of antidepressants (Hoes, 2009; Sit, 2004; UMMC, 2009).

Comorbidity

Comorbid psychiatric and physical disorders are commonly found in persons with bipolar disorder. Comorbid medical conditions that bipolar women develop include heart disease, asthma and other lung problems, gastrointestinal disorders, skin infections, hypertension, diabetes, migraine headaches, hypothyroidism, obesity, and cancer. Although some of these conditions are associated with pharmacological therapy, research is ongoing in attempting to identify the direction of causal relationships between comorbidities and social, cultural, and biological factors (Hoes, 2009).

Comorbid psychiatric disorders are also common in bipolar disorder, and occur in higher rates in women than men. Alcohol and substance use disorder is noted to occur in over half of individuals with bipolar disorder, with up to 90% lifetime prevalence. Anxiety disorders such as panic disorder, social phobia, obsessive-compulsive disorder, and posttraumatic stress disorder frequently coexist with bipolar disorder, and may worsen the course of the illness. In addition, personality disorders and eating disorders, most notably bulimia, are more commonly seen in bipolar women (Hoes, 2009; Sit, 2004).

Treatment

Presently, there is no cure for bipolar disorder. Treatment is aimed at decreasing the associated morbidity and mortality of the disorder. The psychiatrist initially performs a diagnostic evaluation and assesses the safety and functioning level of the patient in order to determine the optimum treatment setting. The psychiatrist and patient are guided in choosing from among the various possible treatment options and settings by the cross-sectional (i.e., current clinical status) and longitudinal (i.e., frequency, severity, and consequences of past episodes) circumstances of the treatment decisions. Such treatment decisions must be based on awareness of the possible favorable and unfavorable effects of available options along with information about patient preferences. Treatment decisions must be repeatedly reassessed as new information becomes available, the patient's clinical status changes, or both. Lack of insight or minimization is often a major part of bipolar disorder and may hinder the ability of the patient to make sound treatment decisions. Consequently, from the outset, diagnosis and treatment options should be discussed with the patient, and the patient and family/significant others should be engaged in the treatment plan (Podawiltz, 2011b). The increasing evidence of gender differences in a number of clinical features of bipolar disorder informs the need for individualized and collaborative treatment strategies for bipolar women, especially in consideration of different phases of the reproductive cycle, pregnancy, and the postpartum period (Barnes & Mitchell, 2005).

Pharmacological Therapy

Mood stabilizing drugs form the basis of treatment for women with bipolar disorder. Lithium has been used for many years for the treatment of bipolar disorder and is very effective for treating mania and for suicide prevention (NIMH, 2012b). Lithium may produce adverse side effects that can be especially troublesome and can contribute to drug noncompliance **(Table 6–1)**. Dosage adjustment may help to reduce side effects; however, side effects that persist despite dosage adjustment may be managed with other medications. Administering lithium with meals or changing lithium preparations may also be helpful in reducing adverse side effects. Serum levels of lithium must be monitored closely to maintain a therapeutic range and avoid toxicity (NIMH, 2012b). Lithium has been known to cause hypothyroidism, especially in women. Suboptimal thyroid function may trigger rapid-cycling or depressive episodes. Thus, close monitoring of thyroid function is imperative during lithium treatment.

Anticonvulsant drugs such as valproate, carbamazepine, and lamotrigine are also widely used as mood stabilizers in bipolar disorder (NIMH, 2012b). In contrast to lithium, valproate has a wide therapeutic window. Consequently, inadvertent overdose is not common, and purposeful overdose is less likely to be lethal as compared to lithium. Women with past or current hepatic disease may have increased risk for hepatotoxicity. Anticonvulsant drugs may also produce adverse side effects that can be distressing to women and contribute to treatment nonadherence (Table 6–1).

Atypical antipsychotic (AAP) drugs used in the treatment of schizophrenia also have mood stabilizing properties that are applicable to bipolar disorder. AAP drugs may be used as monotherapy or in combination with lithium or valproate (UMMC, 2013). AAP drugs include clozapine, olanzapine, risperidone, ziprasidone, quetiapine, and ariprazole (NIMH, 2012b). AAP drugs may produce adverse side effects that can be distressing to women and contribute to treatment nonadherence. Evidence suggests that treatment with AAP drugs is associated with weight gain. Women who are prescribed AAP drugs should have their weight, BMI, and waist circumference recorded before the medication is initiated and monitored at least quarterly (or more often if individuals are overweight) when stabilized. Nutritional counseling, weight reduction interventions, or change of medication is recommended if a gain of one BMI unit in normal or overweight women occurs (Üçok & Gaebel, 2008). AAP drugs are also associated with an increased risk for developing type-2 diabetes and hyperlipidemia. Women may be particularly at risk for metabolic syndrome, and close monitoring of glucose metabolism and serum lipid levels is recommended when AAP drugs are prescribed for bipolar disorder treatment (Hoes, 2009; Üçok & Gaebel, 2008).

Certain AAP drugs may increase the risk for cardiac problems. Ziprasidone is associated with increased risk for QTc interval prolongation, which can subsequently increase the risk for cardiac dysrhythmias. A baseline electrocardiogram (EKG) should be done prior to initiating this drug, especially if cardiac risk factors such as known heart disease, history of syncope, family history of sudden death under age 40, or congenital prolonged QTc interval are present. Furthermore, clozapine use has been associated with increased risk of myocarditis. Thus, women who receive clozapine should be monitored for symptoms of myocarditis. If myocarditis develops, clozapine should be discontinued and the patient urgently evaluated by a primary healthcare provider (Üçok & Gaebel, 2008).

Somatic Therapy

Electroconvulsive therapy (ECT), the oldest somatic treatment in psychiatry, is a safe and effective

Table 6–1 ADVERSE SIDE EFFECTS OF PHARMACOLOGICAL THERAPY OF BIPOLAR DISORDER

Drug	Adverse Side Effect	Recommendations
Lithium	Polyuria Polydipsia Weight gain Dulling, impaired memory Poor concentration Confusion Mental slowness Tremor Sedation or lethargy Impaired coordination Nausea Vomiting Dyspepsia Diarrhea Hair loss Benign leukocytosis Acne Edema Hypothyroidism	Dosage adjustment may help to reduce side effects. Beta blockers may be given for tremor. Diuretics may be given for polyuria, polydipsia, or edema. Topical antibiotics or retinoic acid may be given for acne. Taking lithium with meals or changing lithium preparations (especially to lithium citrate) may reduce gastrointestinal distress. Monitor thyroid and kidney function.
Valproate	Benign hepatic transaminase elevations Osteoporosis Tremor Sedation Anorexia Nausea Dyspepsia Vomiting Diarrhea Mild, asymptomatic leukopenia and thrombocytopenia Hair loss Increased appetite Weight gain	Dosage adjustment may help to reduce side effects. Women with past or current hepatic disease may have increased risk for hepatotoxicity. Monitor liver function. Leukopenia and thrombocytopenia are less common and are reversible when the drug is discontinued. Persistent gastrointestinal distress may be relieved by dose reduction, change of preparation (use of divalproex sodium rather than valproic acid), or by administration of a histamine-2 antagonist (e.g., famotidine or cimetidine).

Table 6–1 ADVERSE SIDE EFFECTS OF PHARMACOLOGICAL THERAPY OF BIPOLAR DISORDER (*continued*)

Drug	Adverse Side Effect	Recommendations
Carbamazepine	Diplopia Blurred vision Fatigue Nausea Ataxia Skin rashes Mild leukopenia Mild thrombocytopenia Hyponatremia Hypo-osmolality	Side effects are usually temporary and often reversible with reduction of dosage.
Lamotrigine	Headache Nausea Infection Xerostomia Stevens–Johnson Syndrome	Drug must be started at a low dose and slowly titrated up over a 6-week period to reduce risk of Stevens–Johnson Syndrome.
Atypical Antipsychotics: clozapine olanzapine risperidone ziprasidone ariprazole quetiapine	Drowsiness Dizziness when changing positions Blurred vision Rapid heartbeat Sensitivity to the sun Skin rashes Hyperprolactinemia and associated menstrual dysfunction (risperidone) Weight gain Diabetes mellitus (clozapine, olanzapine) Hyperlipidemia (clozapine, olanzapine) Prolongation of QTc interval (ziprasidone) Myocarditis (clozapine) Extrapyramidal symptoms (risperidone and olanzapine) Cataracts (quetiapine)	Avoid driving or operating machinery until adjusted to drug. Record BMI and weight before initiating drug and at least quarterly thereafter. Baseline EKG should be taken before initiating ziprasidone when cardiac risk factors are present. Monitor closely for signs of prolonged QTc interval. Monitor for signs of myocarditis in clozapine-treated patients. Periodic ophthalmalogical exams with the use of quetiapine.

treatment option for bipolar disorder, particularly when the symptoms are severe or the patient poses a substantial risk to themselves or others (Malhi, Adams, Cahill, Dodd, & Berk, 2009). Robust evidence from studies investigating the effectiveness of ECT in patients with unipolar depression as compared to patients with bipolar depression has shown comparable efficacy (Malhi et al., 2009; Sienaert, 2011). Evidence also confirms that ECT is highly effective in treating mania and mixed episodes, producing remission comparable to that of depression (Loo, Katalinic, Mitchell, & Greenberg, 2011; Sienaert, 2011). ECT has demonstrated clinically meaningful efficacy, particularly in bipolar patients who are resistant to pharmacological therapy (Loo et al., 2011). ECT is generally well tolerated.

Headache and nausea are reported as the most common immediate side effects, and these can be treated preventatively with analgesic and anti-emetic drugs. Typically, general disorientation in the postictal phase is experienced but tends to be self-limiting. Anterograde memory impairment, manifested by difficulty in acquiring and retaining new information, is common but resolves in approximately 1 month. Retrograde amnesia, which is the inability to remember past events and information learned prior to the treatment, is generally short lived, and resolves in about 6 months. ECT has traditionally been recommended as a "last resort" in present treatment algorithms; however, more recent evidence of efficacy and safety suggest that ECT should be considered earlier in the treatment course, especially when psychotic symptoms, suicidal thoughts and acts, or catatonia are present (Sienaert, 2011).

Psychosocial Treatment

A number of specific psychosocial interventions can be effective when utilized in conjunction with pharmacological therapy and psychiatric management. The specific objectives of psychosocial treatment are to lessen distress, improve the patient's functioning between episodes, and decrease the likelihood and severity of future episodes. Psychosocial treatment also improves mood, adherence to treatment, and restoration of social rhythms (Sit, 2004). Psychosocial interventions can provide support, education, and guidance to patients with bipolar disorder and their families (NIMH, 2012a).

Evidence-based treatment approaches have been derived from cognitive behavior therapy, interpersonal therapy, family-focused therapy, and psychoeducation therapy. Psychodynamic and other forms of therapy may be indicated for some patients. Psychiatrists usually employ a combination or synthesis of different approaches according to their training and the needs and preferences of the patients.

Specific aims for each of the psychosocial interventions used in bipolar disorder are:

- **Cognitive behavioral therapy:** helps bipolar women to recognize and change harmful thought patterns and behaviors associated with the disorder.
- **Interpersonal and social rhythm therapy:** helps bipolar women improve their personal interactions and establish regular daily routines. Regular daily routines and sleep schedules may be protective against manic episodes.
- **Family-focused therapy:** concentrates on improving family relationships to mend harmful relationships or patterns of interaction that contribute to or result from the patient's symptoms. Family coping strategies are enhanced, as well as communication and problem-solving ability.
- **Psychoeducation:** teaches bipolar women and their relatives or loved ones about the effects, treatment, and management of bipolar disorder. This therapy helps them to recognize signs of relapse so that early treatment may be sought before a full-blown relapse occurs (NIMH, 2012a).

Quality of Life Issues Associated With Bipolar Disorder

Bipolar disorder is a serious, chronic mental illness that is prevalent in the community, in primary care clinics, and in psychiatric clinics. The pernicious nature of bipolar disorder, which is marked by painful symptoms, disturbed family and social relations, disrupted work function, and suicide, has an enormous impact on quality of life. Misdiagnosis and consequent delay in obtaining effective treatment leads to a variety of negative consequences that substantially influence quality of life. Quality of life issues and concerns associated with bipolar disorder are commonly multidimensional and encompass health and physical functioning, psychological and spiritual well-being, socioeconomic integrity, and family well-being.

Poorer quality of life is experienced in bipolar individuals who have early onset, longer duration of illness, delayed diagnosis, bipolar II or cyclothymic disorder, substance dependence, and depressive symptoms. Poor quality of life also may persist in clinically euthymic patients (i.e., those with mood within normal range, neither elevated nor depressed) (Gutiérrez-Rojas et al., 2008; Singh, Matoo, Sharan, & Basu, 2005). Although manic and hypomanic patients tend to have significantly poorer quality of life than euthymic patients, evidence suggests that bipolar depression, not mania, predicts greater illness burden and chronicity (Vornik & Hirschfeld, 2005). Hence, depressive symptoms play a crucial role in determining quality of life in bipolar patients. The depressive episode appears to predominate in the evaluation of quality of life, particularly in patients in mixed episode. Bipolar women, who are apt to present with more severe and debilitating forms of the disorder, as well as more severe and recurrent depressive episodes, bipolar II disorder and mixed mania, are particularly vulnerable to poor quality of life (Vornik & Hirschfeld, 2005).

Issues Affecting Health and Physical Functioning

Many women with bipolar disorder experience poor health and physical functioning, particularly when the illness is untreated, misdiagnosed, or accompanied by comorbid conditions. Bipolar women experience a greater degree of disability, and consequently, poorer quality of life (Sajatovic, 2005).

MEDICAL COMORBIDITY

As noted earlier, women with bipolar disorder frequently develop comorbid medical conditions, including heart disease, asthma and other lung problems, gastrointestinal disorders, skin infections, hypertension, diabetes, migraine headaches, hypothyroidism, obesity, and cancer. Women with bipolar disorder are less likely to receive medical care as compared to those without mental illness. Substance abuse, including smoking and alcohol and drug use, contributes to the development of a number of comorbid medical problems and reduces access to effective medical care. The presence of comorbid conditions in bipolar women may be associated with biological, social, and cultural factors, as well as effects of pharmacological therapy (Hoes, 2009; Sit, 2004; UMMC, 2009). Bipolar women must be monitored closely and referred for appropriate treatment if serious life-threatening medical problems develop.

REPRODUCTIVE CYCLE ISSUES

Evidence that explains the impact of the female reproductive cycle on the clinical course of bipolar disorder is scarce. Consequently this area remains poorly understood. It is purported that estrogen and progesterone fluctuations during the reproductive cycle may lead to symptom exacerbation (Barnes & Mitchell, 2005). Women with bipolar disorder commonly report premenstrual exacerbation of symptoms, and there is a high prevalence of self-reported premenstrual exacerbation of manic or hypomanic symptoms. In spite of this, evidence of mood changes associated with the menstrual cycle phase has been inconsistent (Payne, 2011; Shivakumar, Bernstein, Suppes, & The Stanley Foundation Bipolar Network, 2008). Nonetheless, research has shown that women reporting premenstrual exacerbation have more frequent illness episodes, relapse more rapidly, and have greater symptom severity. Furthermore, reports of premenstrual exacerbation could be a potential marker for a more severe clinical phenotype in reproductive-age women with bipolar disorder (Dias et al., 2011).

Drug therapy can adversely affect the menstrual cycle. Antiepileptic drugs, particularly valproate, may contribute to an increased risk of polycystic ovarian syndrome, with associated hyperandrogenism and menstrual disturbances in reproductive-aged women. However, only limited data specifically addresses this issue for bipolar women, and results appear inconclusive (Freeman & Gelenberg, 2005). Risperidone has been linked with menstrual dysfunction that is associated with prolactinemia. Elevated prolactin levels can cause galactorrhea, irregular menses, amenorrhea, annovulation, sexual dysfunction, and increased risk of osteoporosis. Other AAP drugs such as ziprasidone, clozapine, and quetiapine can also cause menstrual dysfunction but at a much lower rate than risperidone (Barnes & Mitchell, 2005; Freeman & Gelenberg, 2005).

Oral contraceptive use is a major concern for bipolar women of childbearing age because certain drugs used in treatment of bipolar disorder can alter the efficacy of oral contraceptives. Evidence obtained in studies of epileptic populations indicates that carbamazepine, oxcarbazepine, and topiramate can cause a decrease in serum levels of oral contraceptives, most likely from enhanced liver metabolism that increases the metabolism of ethinyl estradiol (Reddy, 2010). Thus, women who are prescribed these drugs for treatment of bipolar disorder in concurrence with use of oral contraceptives should be advised to use barrier methods of birth control, monitor for spotting, or consult with their gynecologist to increase the dosage of the oral contraceptive pill (Burt & Rasgon, 2004; Marangell, 2008; Reddy, 2010). On the other hand, oral contraceptives may likewise alter the efficacy of drugs used for bipolar treatment. Evidence from research of epileptic women indicates that lamotrigine plasma levels were substantially reduced in women taking oral contraceptives. Thus, women prescribed lamotrigine concurrently with oral contraceptives may require increased lamotrigine doses. (Burt & Rasgon, 2004; Marangell, 2008; Reddy, 2010).

PREGNANCY ISSUES

Pregnancy was previously considered a time during which bipolar women were less likely to experience episodes of affective illness. However, evidence suggests that pregnancy is a period of substantial risk for recurrence of mood episodes in bipolar women (Kushkituah, 2014). The rate of recurrence is estimated to be as high as 50% (Viguera et al., 2007). In view of the risk for teratogenicity associated with drug therapy, many bipolar women elect to discontinue medications during pregnancy and while trying to conceive (Marangell, 2008; Kushkituah, 2014). High risk of illness recurrence, especially of depressive and dysphoric mixed states, is significantly associated with abrupt cessation of mood stabilizing medication. The risk of recurrence is markedly reduced by continuation of mood stabilizer treatment during pregnancy (Viguera et al., 2007). Alternatively, many women who discontinue medications may elect to restart pharmacologic therapy once the high risk associated with first trimester exposure has passed. Whether medications should be resumed automatically or when early signs of potential relapse manifest is unclear. However, women with history of self-harm, protracted recovery from previous episodes, impaired insight, or a strained support system should resume drug therapy to reduce overall maternal and fetal risk (Marangell, 2008).

Lithium is teratogenic and its use during pregnancy increases the risk for fetal birth defects such as Ebstein's anomaly, a severe congenital heart defect. Many women who are pregnant may decide to stop taking the drug during pregnancy. Abrupt discontinuation of lithium can increase the risk of mood episodes. Thus, discontinuation of lithium should be accomplished by gradual taper, over a period of 15 to 30 days, to decrease the risk of relapse. Women who continue lithium therapy during pregnancy must be monitored closely (Kushkituah, 2014). Screening with high-resolution ultrasound and fetal electrocardiography, as well as maternal serum alpha-fetoprotein screening, is highly recommended (Freeman & Gelenberg, 2005; Kushkituah, 2014; Marangell, 2008).

Antiepileptic drugs are human teratogens. Valproate and carbamazepine use during pregnancy increases the risk of the child developing spina bifida and other fetal neural tube defects in the first trimester, as well as other birth defects (Burt & Rasgon, 2004; Kushkituah, 2014). Pregnant women may also experience vitamin K-dependent clotting deficiencies that increase the risk of cerebral hemorrhage in the infant. Women should avoid using valproate or carbamazepine during pregnancy if clinically feasible, especially during the first trimester. However, if treatment is pursued during pregnancy, the minimally effective dose must be used, especially during the first trimester when the risk of teratogenicity is increased. Folate administration while attempting conception and during the first trimester is highly recommended, as well as vitamin K supplementation in the last month of pregnancy (Burt & Rasgon, 2004). Lamotrigine use during the first trimester of pregnancy has been associated with increased risk for cleft palate malformation. Although evidence suggests that the teratogenic risk of lamotrigine is less than that of valproate or carbamazepine, data regarding reproductive safety of lamotrigine is sparse (Nonacs, 2009).

The effects of AAP drugs in pregnancy have been largely understudied. Evidence suggests that there was no significant increase in risks of spontaneous abortion, stillbirths, teratogenicity, or prematurity when compared to controls not exposed to the medication. Data regarding the effects of other AAP drugs in pregnancy is scarce. In view of the absence of data that precludes the use of AAP drugs during pregnancy, patients are likely to be maintained on AAP drugs if they are clearly needed or the potential benefit justifies the potential risk to the fetus. Close follow-up for safety issues such as weight gain, diabetes, and hypertension during pregnancy is strongly recommended (Burt & Rasgon, 2004, Cohen, 2008; Freeman & Gelenberg, 2005; Kushkituah, 2014).

ECT has been shown to be relatively safe during pregnancy, especially early in pregnancy when use of medications is most constrained. ECT is recommended as an alternative to drug therapy during pregnancy, particularly if psychotic decompensation or suicidal ideation has occurred. No teratogenicity has been associated with ECT, but uterine contractions, spontaneous labor, and fetal compromise have been known to occur in more advanced stages of pregnancy, when the fetus was fully formed. Special precautions should be taken to reduce potential risks (Burt & Rasgon, 2004; Swann, 2004).

All bipolar women of childbearing potential must be given accurate and balanced information about potential risks and benefits of pregnancy. More than one-third of such women, when so advised, choose not to pursue pregnancy (Marangell, 2008). Prenatal counseling should cover possible risks of pharmacological therapy during pregnancy, risks to the mother and child of escalating or uncontrolled symptoms of bipolar disorder, and the risk of genetic transmission of bipolar disorder to the child. During pregnancy, pharmacological therapy must be appraised in terms of adverse fetal and neonatal effects as well as usual concerns for effectiveness, tolerability, and maternal safety. Prior to pregnancy, a detailed plan of potential interventions should be formulated in case of relapse or exacerbations of mood episodes (Kushkituah, 2014; Marangell, 2008).

POSTPARTUM ISSUES

During the postpartum period, bipolar women sustain substantial risk for bipolar recurrence—as high as 25% to 40% in the immediate postpartum period. The rate of relapse in women with bipolar disorder in the 3 to 6 month postpartum period is between 67% and 82%. It is likely that bipolar women commonly experience mixed states rather than pure mania or depressive episodes in the postpartum period (Barnes & Mitchell, 2005). Overall, bipolar women have a 100-fold higher risk of developing postpartum psychosis than women without a history of psychiatric illness (Marangell, 2008). The risk of first time hospitalization for bipolar disorder is seven times greater in the first month postpartum than in women who have not given birth (Sit, 2004). Bipolar depression that develops during the postpartum period is often misdiagnosed as unipolar major depressive disorder. Misdiagnosis may lead to delayed initiation of appropriate treatment, and the consequences can be especially serious. Inappropriate prescription of antidepressants in this situation might trigger mania, rapid-cycling, or a mixed state, any of which increase the risk for psychiatric hospitalization (Sharma, Burt, & Ritchie, 2009).

Hypomanic symptoms may also appear after delivery, with a 9% to 20% occurrence rate. It has been suggested that postpartum hypomania does not merely indicate happiness at having a baby, but is a manifestation of bipolar disorder. Although postpartum hypomania does not impair social or occupational functioning, it is clinically significant in its association with bipolar depression later in the postpartum period (Sharma et al., 2009).

Plans for postpartum interventions, including prophylactic drug therapy, should be made well in advance by the physician and patient during pregnancy. Prophylaxis is an option to reduce risk of postpartum recurrence. Although there is no consensus as to when prophylaxis should begin, some experts suggest initiating prophylaxis in the second or third trimester, when the risk of teratogenicity is lessened. Although mixed results have been obtained in studies investigating the benefits of prophylaxis started in the third trimester or immediately postpartum, prophylaxis may be helpful for women at high risk for postpartum recurrence (Marangell, 2008).

LACTATION

Although breastfeeding is healthy for the mother and is important for the health and well-being of the newborn, it is an issue of concern in bipolar women. Medications taken by the mother pass into the breast milk and can affect the nursing infant (Kushkituah, 2014). Limited data is available regarding the effects of lithium, antiepileptic drugs, and atypical antipsychotic drugs in infants. However,

the American Academy of Pediatrics Committee on Drugs has issued breastfeeding guidelines that caution against giving lithium to nursing mothers because high concentrations of the drug can accumulate in the nursing infant and cause detrimental effects. Lamotrigine can also accumulate in nursing infants in substantial concentrations and can alter short-term and long-term central nervous system function. Although adverse effects of clozapine in the nursing infant have not been observed, concentrations in human milk are relative to simultaneous maternal plasma concentrations, and can be of concern. Carbamazepine and valproate are considered compatible with breastfeeding (American Academy of Pediatrics Committee on Drugs [AAPCD], 2001). Gabapentin, topiramate, olanzapine, and respiridone are not addressed in these guidelines.

Decisions regarding medication use in the postpartum period should be based on the clinical status of the mother and the previous course of the illness, regardless of breastfeeding status (Burt & Rasgon, 2004). Thus, the health and stability of the mother should take priority over the feeding method of the infant. Although breastfeeding provides many probable benefits to both the mother and infant, the sleep disruption associated with breastfeeding as the sole source of food for the infant is contraindicated for many women with bipolar disorder due to the increased risk for psychiatric instability that sleep deprivation can cause (Marangell, 2008). If breastfeeding is chosen, options for ensuring adequate sleep should be considered, such as arranging for other adults to feed the infant, and expressing breast milk earlier in the day for night feedings. The mother and her partner should be educated regarding the potential risks associated with breastfeeding while taking medication. The pediatrician or family physician responsible for the care of the infant should be advised about the medications to which the infant is exposed and should monitor the infant as needed for potential adverse effects. Polypharmacy should be avoided. Monotherapy at the lowest possible dose to maintain psychiatric stability should be used. Options that minimize exposure of the infant while providing breastfeeding benefits include supplementation of breastfeeding with formula feeding, and having the mother take the medication just after she has breastfed the infant or just before the infant is due to have a lengthy sleep period (AAPCD, 2001; Burt & Rasgon, 2004; Marangell, 2008).

MENOPAUSE ISSUES

Evidence that describes the impact of perimenopause on the course of bipolar disorder is scarce (Marsh, Ketter, & Rasgon, 2009). Preceding the end of menses is the perimenopause, a period that marks the beginning of menstrual irregularity and transitions to complete amenorrhea of menopause. Both perimenopause and menopause have been associated with bipolar exacerbations, agitated depression, and psychotic mood episodes. However, the association between gonadal hormones and bipolar mood symptoms remains unclear (Sit, 2004). Evidence suggests that the perimenopausal and postmenopausal periods of women with bipolar disorder are generally a time of worsening mood symptoms, mostly depression (Barnes & Mitchell, 2005; Freeman & Gelenberg, 2005; Marsh et al., 2009; Marsh, Templeton, Ketter, & Rasgon, 2008). Bipolar women who never used hormone replacement therapy at menopause tend to have significantly increased risk of worsening mood symptoms (Freeman & Gelenberg, 2005). Although not conclusive, the literature indicates that the rapid decline of reproductive hormones conferred by surgical menopause may place bipolar women at greater risk for mood instability, especially risk of mania (Marsh, Brown, & Rothschild, 2012).

Issues Affecting Psychological and Spiritual Functioning

PSYCHIATRIC COMORBIDITY

Psychiatric comorbidity occurs at a high rate in bipolar women. Alcohol and substance abuse,

anxiety disorders, personality disorders, and eating disorders are the comorbidities most prevalent in bipolar women. Psychiatric comorbidities have profound clinical implications and are frequently associated with poorer outcomes and poorer response to treatment. These factors significantly contribute to diminished quality of life (Hoes, 2009; Sajatovic, 2005). Psychiatric comorbidities are particularly problematic because they often mask an underlying bipolar condition, and contribute to misdiagnosis and delay of effective treatment.

DEPRESSIVE SYMPTOMS

Evidence indicates that depressive symptoms dominate the longitudinal course of bipolar illness (Keck, McIntyre, & Shelton, 2007) and are another major factor in non-recognition and misdiagnosis of bipolar disorder. Bipolar disorder may go unrecognized for years. Lack of recognition and lack of attention to this condition often results in considerable delay in determination of an accurate diagnosis. This delay has substantial adverse effects (Hirschfeld, 2007). Depressive episodes are commonly misdiagnosed as unipolar depression, and manic episodes with psychotic features may be misdiagnosed as schizophrenia (Johnson, 2007). Failure to correctly diagnose bipolar disorder contributes to delay in receiving proper treatment (Hirschfeld, 2007). One of the foremost challenges that women with bipolar disorder face is obtaining an accurate, early diagnosis. Because women are more likely to present with an initial depressive episode, the likelihood for receiving the misdiagnosis of unipolar major depressive disorder is great (Freeman & Gelenberg, 2005).

The misdiagnosis is often associated with a short-term management focus on relief of presenting symptoms, rather than a lifetime syndrome-based approach which is essential for treating bipolar disorder effectively. The short-term management focus on acute presenting symptoms can result in accumulation of medications for such symptoms as anxiety, insomnia, cycling, and depression (Keck et al., 2007).

The use of antidepressants has substantial clinical implications when misdiagnosis has occurred. In particular, antidepressant therapy can destabilize the clinical course of bipolar disorder. Antidepressants may precipitate mania, induce rapid cycling, and worsen the course of illness (Hirschfeld, 2007; Sajatovic, 2005). Antidepressants are less effective than mood stabilizers for preventing depressive relapse in bipolar disorder. Additionally, therapy with mood stabilizing medication may be less efficacious after such unsuccessful treatment for depressive episodes (Sajatovic, 2005).

SUICIDALITY

Suicidal behavior is a major concern of bipolar disorder. The risk of suicide in patients with bipolar disorder is the highest of any psychiatric illness. Suicidal ideation, suicide attempts, and suicide completion are strongly related to both bipolar I and bipolar II subtypes (de Abreu et al., 2012). Suicide is a complicated behavior associated with an interaction of psychological, social, and genetic factors. In bipolar disorder, risk factors for suicidal behavior include white race, delayed diagnosis, early onset of illness, childhood adversity, impulsivity, psychiatric comorbidities, impaired decision making, previous suicide attempts, family history of completed suicide, and predominance of depressive episodes (Cassidy, 2011; Neves et al., 2010). Bipolar individuals with alcohol and substance abuse comorbidity are also at higher risk for suicidal behavior (Cassidy, 2011; de Abreu et al., 2012). Evidence suggests that patients with bipolar disorder and a history of suicidal attempts experience poor quality of life. Diminished quality of life could be reflective of poor coping skills and inadequate social support, and therefore might also contribute to the risk for suicidal behavior (de Abreu et al., 2012).

Individuals who report suicidal ideation are at greater likelihood to subsequently attempt suicide,

and those who have attempted suicide are at high risk to reattempt suicide and complete the act. Although the exact interrelationship among those who contemplate suicide, those who attempt suicide, and those who complete the act has not been fully clarified, these three groups are related either by overlapping membership, or as advancing steps of a common underlying process. Consequently, the boundaries between these three groups are connected as well as assailable and subject to the fluid effects of intervention and treatment. Thus, identification of bipolar patients at risk for suicide is essential and clinically relevant (Cassidy, 2011). Over the past two decades, a decline in suicide rates has been observed in the United States, Europe, and Canada, especially for women. This may be attributed to better recognition and availability of treatment, as well as increased efficacy of treatment (Fountoulakis et al., 2009).

TREATMENT ADHERENCE

A crucial element of treatment efficacy is treatment adherence, and so it is essential to elucidate the treatment trajectory of bipolar disorder and its underlying goals. Because bipolar disorder is chronic, episodic, and complex in nature, lifelong treatment is necessary. The treatment trajectory for bipolar patients consists of three phases, each with specific goals and strategies. In the first phase, the goal of treatment for an acute episode of bipolar disorder is to achieve symptomatic recovery. When symptomatic recovery is achieved, treatment progresses into the continuation phase. In this phase, drug therapies that helped to achieve mood stability are adjusted in dosage and timing of doses so that tolerability is increased. Poorly tolerated medications or adjunctive medications determined to be nonessential are gradually withdrawn. However, these may be reinstated or replaced if the patient displays early signs of relapse (Swann, 2010).

In the continuation phase, the main goal is for the patient to achieve functional recovery, such that she can manage normal living and working conditions. The patient and physician determine structured routines that help the patient to maintain long-term mood stability. Routines may include regular physical and social activity, regular patterns of sleep, and maintaining a regular medication schedule. Patients are taught to recognize prodromal symptoms that may signal relapse, and to record their daily activities and sleep patterns to help in recognizing trends that affect mood. Additionally, the patient is assisted in developing a support network comprised of family, friends, support groups, therapists, and physicians (Swann, 2010).

When functional recovery has been achieved, the patient transitions to the maintenance phase of treatment. In this phase, the main goals are to prevent relapse of acute episodes and to enhance adaptive functioning of the patient (Swann, 2010). The prevention of relapse during this phase is associated with two essential elements—managing sub-syndromal or prodromal symptoms and addressing treatment nonadherence. Because pharmacological therapy is the primary treatment for bipolar disorder, symptom management requires continual re-evaluation of medications that are successful in achieving syndromal and functional recovery. Particular attention to effectiveness, correct dosage, and adverse effects is essential (Swann, 2010).

Treatment nonadherence is a major problem for bipolar patients and has serious clinical implications. Evidence suggests that the extent of nonadherence may range from 20% to 60%. Treatment nonadherence can increase the risk of relapse, hospitalization, suicide attempts, and completed suicides, as well as decrease the time spent in remission. Furthermore, sudden discontinuation of medication can cause abrupt onset of relapse (Busby & Sajatovic, 2010; Thase, 2011). Some typical predictors of treatment nonadherence are the following:

Patient-related factors. Predictors of nonadherence that are patient-related include younger age, male gender, single status, and denial of diagnosis or chronic nature of the illness. Patient attitudes and beliefs about treatment, such as stigmatization regarding taking psychotropic drugs, fear of drug dependency, and fear of adverse side effects can also contribute to treatment nonadherence (Busby & Sajatovic, 2010; Colom, 2010; Thase, 2011).

Illness-related factors. Predictors of nonadherence that are illness-related include history of manic episodes, early-onset illness, recent bipolar diagnosis, having fewer episodes, and being in the first year of lithium therapy. Past suicide attempts, severe symptoms, cognitive impairments, and the presence of psychiatric comorbidities, such as personality disorder, anxiety disorder, and substance use disorder are also associated with treatment nonadherence (Busby & Sajatovic, 2010; Colom, 2010; Thase, 2011).

Treatment-related factors. Predictors of nonadherence that are treatment-related include intolerable side effects, especially weight gain and drowsiness, perceiving that too many drugs were prescribed, multiple and complicated drug regimens, and concerns about long-term drug regimens. Lack of access to drugs, such as cost and transportation, can also contribute to treatment nonadherence (Busby & Sajatovic, 2010; Thase, 2011).

Treatment adherence is a crucial facet of treatment efficacy, attainment of positive long-term outcomes, and managing an acceptable quality of life. Strategies that can enhance treatment adherence include building a strong therapeutic alliance between healthcare providers and patients, especially emphasizing effective communication and patient education (Thase, 2011). Treatment adherence should be monitored closely in a nonjudgmental manner, with particular attention to events that prompt nonadherence and patient responses to stopping medications. These conversations should be used as an opportunity to teach patients about the importance of long-term treatment (Thase, 2011). Medication regimens should be simplified, and medications that can be discontinued should be slowly withdrawn. Adverse side effects should be proactively addressed and monitored closely. Comorbid disorders including substance use disorders, and interepisode symptoms, such as sleep disturbances, can adversely affect neurocognitive and psychosocial functioning, and thus impact adherence. These conditions need to be treated as well (Thase, 2011).

Psychosocial interventions in conjunction with pharmacological therapy, especially in the maintenance phase, can enhance long-term outcomes by addressing several problems that impede recovery. Psychoeducation in particular can help patients improve medication adherence, develop relapse prevention skills, and improve lifestyle regularity (Colom, 2013). Psychoeducation can enhance quality of life for both patients and significant others who are coping with bipolar disorder (Sajatovic, Chen, Dines, & Shirley, 2007).

SPIRITUALITY

Although bipolar disorder has been the subject of extensive research inquiry, research that has investigated the relationship of spirituality or religion with bipolar disorder is very sparse. It is particularly important to examine this relationship in its varied aspects. Spirituality and religion are important to many bipolar patients as a source of coping and support. Bipolar women likely consider their spiritual beliefs as a more important positive aspect in their lives and in the course of their illness as compared to men (Galvez, Thommi, & Ghaemi, 2011). Engagement in religious activities could be helpful to the day-to-day management of the disorder. However, excessive engagement could be a sign of a worsening condition. Hyper-religiosity might manifest during manic episodes in which psychotic symptoms appear as mystical experiences with religious themes or religious delusions (Persut, Clark, Maxwell, & Michalak, 2011). Patients struggle to disentangle "real" spiritual experience

from the hyper-religiosity experienced as a symptom of mania/hypomania, where the level of preoccupation, conviction, and extent of thinking becomes extreme (Michalak, Yatham, Kolesar, & Lam, 2006). They may be reluctant to turn to healthcare providers for assistance because of the fear that religious thinking might be perceived as a symptom rather than a coping strategy. Spirituality/religion might then become a hidden personal resource or, conversely, a hidden symptom, if the preoccupation is actually a delusion (Persut et al., 2011; Raab, 2007).

Another issue that arises is that spiritual/religious beliefs may create potential barriers between patients and healthcare providers. Spiritual/religious meanings can influence the coping ability of some patients as well as healthcare decisions. To discount or refute these meanings in clinical encounters may unintentionally encourage alienation from treatment regimes. Conflict between spiritual/religious beliefs and attitudes towards pharmacological and therapeutic interventions might contribute to treatment nonadherence. Thus, clinicians should endeavor to include attention to spiritual/religious concerns in therapeutic clinical encounters with bipolar patients (Persut et al., 2011).

Of the little evidence that exists, findings indicate that spirituality and religion are factors among a wide range of psychosocial variables that are influential in determining outcomes in bipolar disorder. It is important to understand that spirituality and religion are relevant as both adverse manifestations of bipolar disorder and as having potentially protective effects (Persut et al., 2011). Further research that explores spirituality and religion as pathology and resource is needed, especially in examining the usefulness of spiritual/religious interventions in the treatment regimen of bipolar disorder. Further research is needed to study how spiritual/religious evidence-based interventions can ethically and effectively be incorporated into therapeutic treatment regimens (Persut et al., 2011).

Issues Affecting Socioeconomic Integrity

Bipolar disorder affects nearly every aspect of a woman's life, and consequently inflicts a huge cost burden on the individual, family, and society. The total economic burden to society of bipolar I and II disorder is staggering, and combined direct and indirect costs estimated in 2009 were $151 billion. The economic burden of bipolar I and II disorder is a major public health problem of underrecognized fiscal importance. When the entire array of bipolar spectrum disorders is considered, the total economic burden is thought to greatly exceed $151 billion (Dilsaver, 2011).

Direct costs of bipolar disorder are comprised of direct medical expenditures, such as the cost of hospitalization, emergency department services, psychiatric visits, and medications. Indirect costs of bipolar disorder include reduced productivity, work loss, unemployment, social welfare costs, and criminal justice costs. A greater part of the per annum total is attributed to indirect costs (Bowden, 2005; Hirschfeld & Vornik, 2005).

Bipolar disorder commonly develops during adolescence and early adulthood, which impedes the achievement of academic and occupational ambitions. The disorder continues for the remainder of the working life of a woman. Functional impairment may remain for many bipolar women even though symptoms diminish during remission (Laxman, Lovibond, & Hassan, 2008). Many aspects of women's lives are affected, which in turn leads to increased indirect costs of the disorder. Family discord, problems with the justice system, and workplace problems are common (Hirschfeld & Vornik, 2005).

Bipolar disorder is associated with high rates of unemployment and job-related difficulties (Bowden, 2005). Employees with bipolar disorder tend to have increased absenteeism due to illness, as well as increased presenteeism, that is, coming to work despite illness or injury, resulting in reduced productivity. They are also more likely to exhaust their sick leave and go on short-term disability. Employers experience significant economic burden in terms of lost productivity and substantial costs of expensive healthcare benefits (Bowden, 2005; Laxman et al., 2008).

Bipolar disorder imposes an immense burden on women and the healthcare system. Bipolar women are more likely to have decreased health-related quality of life and more costs related to medical care, especially when misdiagnosis has occurred. Bipolar women tend to use healthcare services more than those with depression or chronic medical conditions, with inpatient costs being the largest contributor to the cost of care. Evidence suggests that treatment to prevent relapse is the most effective method to reduce costs. Evidence further indicates that proper management of bipolar disorder is likely to improve functioning, reduce costs, and enhance health-related quality of life (Sajatovic, 2005).

In bipolar disorder, impairment in social functioning is common. Along with occupational impairment, bipolar disorder is associated with substantial psychosocial, marital, and interpersonal impairment. Women with bipolar disorder often struggle with social withdrawal, household relations, participation in social activities, participation in daily activities and hobbies, taking initiative and self-sufficiency, among others. Depressive symptoms, even at the subsyndromal level, may be significantly associated with persistent functional impairment after symptomatic recovery from a manic episode, and severity of depression is predictive of impaired social functioning in bipolar disorder (Cerit, Filizer, Tural, & Tufan, 2012).

Stigma is reflective of people's responses to others who have uncommon or disagreeable characteristics. Stigma may be expressed as mild intolerance or through blatantly prejudicial and discriminatory practices. Even though laws have been established that ban discriminatory practices, substantial barriers continue to exist that distance individuals with mental illness from mainstream society

(Vázquez et al., 2011). The intricate social process of stigma involves the co-occurrence of labeling, stereotyping, discrimination, loss of status, and separation in a power differential (Michalak et al., 2011). Stigma may be expressed in three levels: public, structural, and internalized. Public stigma is embedded within the context of large social groups that endorse stereotypes regarding mental illness. Structural stigma occurs within the context of institutional policies and practices that create inequalities through restricting opportunities for mentally ill individuals. Internalized stigma, rooted within a sociocultural context, is a subjective process expressed as negative feelings about the self, maladaptive behavior, identity transformation, or stereotype endorsement. These behaviors result from the individual's perceptions, experiences, or anticipation of negative social reaction related to their mental illness (Michalak et al., 2011).

Stigma is of particular concern to bipolar patients. Evidence suggests that stigma plays a core role in predicting impaired social functioning. Mental illness, particularly bipolar disorder, engenders negative attitudes in society and in patients themselves. Perceived stigma may be of central importance to bipolar patients in how they experience their illness and its consequences and whether they engage available healthcare services (Vázquez et al., 2011). Healthcare system pressures can contribute to significant treatment delays. When combined with the propensity of healthcare professionals to involve police and emergency services for crisis intervention, this situation can reinforce stigmatizing ideas that bipolar individuals are dangerous, unpredictable, or reluctant to seek care (Proudfoot et al., 2009). Family, friends, and the community often lack understanding about the illness, which further contributes to social distance. Consequently, a downward spiral is produced in which stereotypes are internalized diminishing the self-esteem and self-efficacy of the bipolar individual labeled mentally ill, and this gives rise to unintended changes in behavior, such as social withdrawal and decreased engagement with services (Proudfoot et al., 2009). Many individuals with bipolar disorder are therefore likely to keep the illness a secret or avoid contact with people who might reject them (Galvez et al., 2011). Social stigma experienced by bipolar patients can contribute to their distress, disability, and poor quality of life, as well as their ability to self-manage their illness (Michalak et al., 2011).

Perceived social support is a strong predictor of social functioning and is influential in enhancing social functioning and mitigating the effects of internalized stigma. Interventions that oppose stigma and enhance perceived social support can have positive effects on the social functioning of bipolar patients (Cerit et al., 2012). Women in particular appear to rely on strong social support as a coping mechanism for bipolar disorder. It is essential to involve significant and supportive others in the social network of bipolar women as part of their treatment plan (Kriegshauser et al., 2010).

Issues Affecting Family Well-Being

Bipolar disorder imposes great burden on the family caring for an afflicted family member and greatly impacts family quality of life (Perlick et al., 2008). Women make up the majority of family caregivers and are vulnerable to deleterious effects of shouldering the burden of care (Zauszniewski, Bekhet, & Suresky, 2008).

The burden of caring for a bipolar family member, particularly when the patient has long-standing recurrent illness requiring numerous hospitalizations, is considerable and can be categorized as objective and subjective burden. Objective burden refers to any observable and verifiable disruption to family or household life, consequential to the behavioral changes of the ill family member and its social effects (Dore & Romans, 2001; Ganguly, Chadda, & Singh, 2010). Financial problems frequently develop and are associated with cost of care or out-of-control spending by the patient when symptomatic. Relational discord between the patient and spouse/partner often occurs, and separation is common. When patients become symptomatic, they may incur legal difficulties or police involvement that imposes on the family. Moreover, aggressive or violent behaviors that may manifest during manic episodes, as well as suicidality that may manifest during depressive episodes, are dangerous, disruptive, and distressing. The illness of a family member is often disruptive to social and leisure activities of the family and can cause social distancing from friends and other relatives due to shame, embarrassment, and stigma (Dore & Romans, 2001; Ganguly et al., 2010). In addition, difficulties may exist with gaining access to psychiatric health care and obtaining clear information about the diagnosis, care, and treatment (Rusner, Brunt, & Nyström, 2012).

Subjective burden is comprised of the feelings experienced by family caregivers in response to carrying the burden of care. These feelings commonly manifest as distress, emotional reactions, perception of strain, reduced morale, anxiety, depression, anger, and guilt (Dore & Romans, 2001; Ganguly et al., 2010). Often family members may feel responsible for contributing to the illness. They may manifest feelings of rejection toward the patient and anger that the illness has spoiled the lives of the family members. Family members may also feel grief and a sense of loss from contrasting the present state of the ill loved one with the person they knew before the onset of illness. The chronic nature of bipolar disorder is such that the burden of care is a persistent source of stress and strain for family caregivers and family members, because of the difficult task of caring for the ill family member. Subjective burden of care has been associated with the development of affective symptoms in family members, such as depression, that may affect both the physical and mental health of the family and lead to a high level of engagement with mental health services (Dore & Romans, 2001; Ganguly et al., 2010; Rusner et al., 2012).

Objective and subjective burden of care that is present in families of bipolar patients should be addressed by mental health professionals in the treatment plan of these patients. Coping capabilities should be assessed as well as supportive resources. Implementing psychosocial interventions that include family, such as family-focused therapy and family psychoeducation, can address issues of caring burden, reduce stressors, strengthen coping mechanisms, increase supportive resources, and enhance the protective qualities of family relationships (Miklowitz, 2007).

Implications for Healthcare Providers

Bipolar disorder has been acknowledged as a leading cause of disability worldwide, as well as a major public health problem in this country (Miklowitz, 2007). Without a doubt, effective diagnosis and treatment of bipolar disorder is a challenging and complicated process. The wide variety of clinical presentations characteristic of bipolar disorder may contribute to this illness being frequently unrecognized, and consequently subject to inadequate or absent treatment (Hirschfeld, 2007). It is crucial, therefore, that healthcare providers in both primary care and psychiatric care take steps to improve recognition and increase accurate diagnosis of the disorder. Women who present with mood symptoms, especially depression, should be evaluated for bipolar disorder. A history of mood elevation, problems controlling drinking or drug abuse, or a history of suicidality should alert healthcare professionals to the possibility of bipolar disorder. The inclusion of family members or significant others in the evaluation process can be very helpful and provide the insight into patient behavior that those with bipolar disorder often lack (Hirschfeld, 2007). Employing an evidence-based screening instrument, such as the Mood Disorder Questionnaire (MDQ), can be helpful in identifying patients who may have bipolar disorder. The MDQ has been validated in several studies and it has been shown to be an excellent tool for identifying patients who are likely to have bipolar disorder. The instrument screens for a lifetime and concurrent history of manic or hypomanic syndrome, as well as level of functional impairment resulting from these symptoms (Hirschfeld, 2007).

In order to effectively treat patients with bipolar disorder, mental healthcare providers need to address complicating factors of the disorder, such as treatment non-adherence, comorbidities, and cognitive impairment, and core symptoms of dysregulated mood. Thus the inclusion of psychosocial interventions as adjunctive treatments to pharmacological therapy is essential as a prophylactic measure against relapse, especially in the maintenance phase of treatment (Colom, 2013). It is important to recognize that women with more previous affective episodes may not respond to psychosocial interventions as well as women in the early stages of bipolar disorder. This may be due to poor cognitive functioning in terms of memory, learning, executive functioning, and attention that occurs in long-time patients. In addition, long-time patients may have difficulty with changing lifestyle patterns, and may have issues with kindling (the triggering of seizures related to substance withdrawal) and sensitization. Women in advanced stages of bipolar disorder may benefit greatly from tailored treatment interventions that address cognitive rehabilitation, focusing in particular on problem-solving and nonverbal working memory, social care, family support for the patient, and external support for the patient's family. The added treatment challenges that develop with illness progression emphasize the importance of early integrated treatment for women with bipolar disorder (Colom, 2013).

Special Concerns of Age and Ethnicity

It has been noted that while the most common time for the development of bipolar disorder is late adolescence or early adulthood, new onset of bipolar disorder can occur across the life span. As such, the very young and the elderly are both at risk for under-recognition and misdiagnosis, difficulties in accessing appropriate services, and poorer quality care than young or middle-aged adults. For the very young and elderly, poorer long-term outcomes are the likely result (Kupfer, Frank, Grochocinski, Houck, & Brown, 2005).

Symptoms of bipolar disorder in adults differ from those in children and adolescents. Bipolar adults tend to have distinct and persistent episodes of depression and mania, whereas children and adolescents with bipolar disorder tend to fluctuate rapidly in their moods and behavior. Mania in adults usually presents as euphoria, whereas mania in children is often characterized by irritability and belligerence. Bipolar depression in children and adolescents is usually characterized by anger and restlessness. Bipolar children and adolescents may have additional mood and behavioral disorders such as attention deficit hyperactivity disorder, anxiety, conduct disorder, and substance abuse problems. The frequency of childhood bipolar disorder persisting into adulthood remains unclear. Also, it is not known if treating childhood bipolar disorder will prevent future illness (UMMC, 2013).

Although bipolar disorder tends to be diagnosed at similar rates across racial and ethnic groups when structured clinical assessments are used, African-Americans and other disadvantaged groups likely suffer a high degree of health disparity apropos to recognition of bipolar disease, appropriate treatment, and access to that treatment (Gonzalez et al., 2007; Minsky, Vega, Miskimen, Gara, & Escobar, 2003). African-American and Hispanic bipolar patients are at elevated risk of their bipolar disorder being under-recognized or misdiagnosed, especially if the patients are young and exhibit psychotic features (Kennedy, Boydell, van Os, & Murray, 2004; Kilbourne, Haas, Mulsant, Bauer, & Pincus, 2004; Kupfer et al., 2005). Racial and ethnic differences in bipolar diagnosis might be attributed to bias in clinical misinterpretation of symptoms, as well as clinician bias (Kilbourne et al., 2004; Perron Fries, Kilbourne, Vaughn, & Bauer, 2010). Socioeconomic and cultural differences between patients and clinicians, which lead to fundamentally different expressions in communicating symptoms, may also contribute to misdiagnosis in ethnic groups such as African-Americans and Hispanics (Perron et al., 2010).

Research findings indicate that systematic racial and ethnic variations exist in the expression of psychopathology of bipolar disorder. African-Americans tend to present with more severe psychotic symptoms, such as auditory hallucinations, persecutory delusions, and delusions of inference as compared with white persons. Psychotic symptoms in African-American patients are often perceived as more chronic and persistent than affective symptoms (Strakowski et al., 2003). Such racial and ethnic differences in symptom presentation, accompanied by increased levels of functional impairments, may be a key source of diagnostic errors (Perron et al., 2010). African-Americans are more likely to have earlier onset of mania than whites, while whites are more likely to present with depressive episodes before mania (Kennedy et al., 2004). Hispanics are more likely to present with depressive symptoms than whites, and often have higher levels of impairment, likely attributed to delays in seeking treatment. Cultural factors and Spanish language variations that influence symptomatic expressions and cultural idioms of distress, as well as language barriers, lack of cultural competency on the part of healthcare professionals diagnosing Hispanic patients, and difficulty in applying diagnostic criteria to this ethnic group can lead to diagnostic inaccuracies and treatment disparities in Hispanics (Minsky et al., 2003).

Ethnic minority patients constitute a highly vulnerable population within the bipolar community in that they have a tendency toward higher rates of homelessness, higher rates of involuntary commitment, and likely shorter treatment duration with their current psychiatric clinician. Minority bipolar patients may be especially burdened by comorbid substance use disorder and poor adherence to treatment. These factors contribute to placing minority bipolar patients at increased risk for adverse treatment outcomes (Kilbourne et al, 2005; Zeber et al., 2011).

The disparities in diagnosis and treatment of bipolar disorder in older, younger, and ethnic minority patients calls for specific community and mental health service delivery efforts to reduce barriers to early accurate diagnosis and appropriate ambulatory treatment. Such efforts should be employed in a multipronged approach that includes the following (Kilbourne et al., 2005; Kupfer et al., 2005):

- Education of the community that encompasses specific efforts to reduce stigma associated with mental illness, especially bipolar disorder
- Promotion of outreach and coordination of care by policymakers and healthcare professionals for bipolar women, particularly of ethnic minorities, and especially those who have substance use comorbidity and who are homeless
- Education of healthcare professionals designed to increase accuracy of diagnosis once bipolar women, particularly of ethnic minorities, come to clinical attention
- Improvement of efforts to build better treatment alliances with bipolar communities of women
- Adequate continuity of care for all bipolar women, particularly those of ethnic minorities

Research Review

Can aggregate caregivers at risk for adverse health effects be identified by measures of stress, coping, and service use?

Perlick, D., Rosenheck, R., Miklowitz, D., Kaczynski, R., Link, B., Ketter, T., ... Sachs, G. STEP-BD Family Experience Collaborative Study Group. (2008). Caregiver burden and health in bipolar disorder: A cluster analytic approach. *The Journal of Nervous and Mental Diseases, 196*(6), 484–491.

The purpose of this study was to test the following hypotheses using longitudinal data from a large-scale study of family stress and coping in bipolar disorder:

- Measures of caregiver stress and coping can be aggregated to form distinctive burden/adaptation typologies comprised of different subgroups of caregivers.
- Membership in these subgroups will be associated with significant differences on subjective measures of physical and mental health and health behavior.

This study used a cluster analytic approach to identify caregivers with differing stress appraisal and coping profiles, and evaluated group differences in health and mental health outcomes. A sample of 500 primary caregivers who were parents, spouses, or spouse equivalents of patients with bipolar disorder were interviewed on measures of stress, coping, health, and mental health at baseline, and were reassessed 6 and 12 months later. Patients were also assessed for clinical status and functional level over time. K-means cluster analysis and analysis of variance identified and characterized caregiver groups with differing baseline/stress profiles. Mixed effects models examined the effects of cluster, time, and covariates on health outcomes. Factor and cluster analysis revealed three groups of caregivers with different patterns of stress appraisal, coping, and health outcomes over time, controlling for patient clinical and functional status. Effective caregivers had low stress appraisal, used adaptive coping, practiced good health behavior, and had superior health outcomes. Stigmatized caregivers had high stress appraisal associated with perceived stigma, had low mastery and inadequate self-care, but used effective coping and had good health outcomes. Burdened caregivers had high stress appraisal associated with the patient's problem behavior, exercised less adaptive coping and self-care, and had the poorest health outcomes.

The findings of this study suggest that caregivers of bipolar patients can be prospectively identified as being at risk for adverse health outcomes associated with caregiving burden and also identified for prevention-focused intervention. Family caregivers who have high burden profiles may be offered a variety of peer- and clinician-administered interventions, as well as other effective family interventions to improve family health outcomes.

Chapter Summary Points

- Bipolar disorder is a chronic condition that affects women and men equally and is found in all ages, races, ethnic groups, and social classes.
- Women often develop bipolar disorder in the late teens or early adult years, with peak average age of onset ranging from about 18 to 25 years old. At least one-half to two-thirds of all patients experience onset before age 18.
- Risk factors for bipolar disorder can be categorized as those that may impart lifetime vulnerability to bipolar disorder (such as genetic or biologic factors) and those that increase the likelihood for the onset of an episode of depression or mania (such as stressful life events or stimulant/antidepressant use).
- Children who have a first-degree relative (parent or sibling) with bipolar disorder have a tenfold risk of developing the illness as compared to children without a family history of bipolar disorder.
- Women are more likely to be misdiagnosed with unipolar depression and face substantial delays in treatment for bipolar disorder.
- Women are more likely than men to experience bipolar II disorder, mixed mania, rapid cycling, seasonality patterns of the disorder, and more frequent depressive episodes.
- Psychiatric and medical comorbidity tends to be more common in women and adversely affects recovery from mania more frequently in women.
- Mood stabilizing drugs form the basis of treatment for women with bipolar disorder. Specific psychosocial interventions can also be effective when utilized in conjunction with pharmacological therapy and psychiatric management.
- The pernicious nature of bipolar disorder, which is marked by painful symptoms, disturbed family and social relations, disrupted work function, and suicide, has enormous impact on quality of life.
- Misdiagnosis and consequent delay in obtaining effective treatment leads to a variety of negative consequences that substantially influence quality of life.
- Treatment nonadherence has serious clinical implications and the extent may range from 20% to 60%.
- Treatment nonadherence can increase the risk of relapse, hospitalization, suicide attempts, and completed suicides, and decrease the time spent in remission. Abrupt discontinuation of medication can cause sudden onset of relapse.
- It is crucial that healthcare providers in both primary care and psychiatric care take steps to improve recognition and increase accurate diagnosis of bipolar disorder.
- The very young, elderly, and ethnic minority patients are at increased risk for under-recognition and misdiagnosis, difficulties in accessing appropriate services, and poorer quality of care.
- The disparities in diagnosis and treatment of bipolar disorder in older, younger, and ethnic minority women calls for specific community and mental health service delivery efforts to reduce barriers to early accurate diagnosis and appropriate ambulatory treatment.

Critical Thinking Exercise

Case Study

L.R. is a 23-year-old female graduate student working on a master's degree in communications. She suspended her studies when she developed major depression. L.R. had been sexually abused during her adolescence by a family acquaintance, and she lost her parents a year ago in a car accident caused by a drunk driver. Her history reveals alcohol and drug use that she does to deaden her sad memories, as well as feelings of hopelessness and guilt. She was prescribed SSRI antidepressants, and after a few weeks she felt her mood lift and was able to function. However, over time L.R. began experiencing insomnia, anxiety, and feeling wound up. She became unable to concentrate on school assignments or complete classwork, and she experienced terrible migraine headaches. Her functioning was erratic, and she experienced marked agitation, racing thoughts, pressured speech, and reckless behavior. She was admitted to acute psychiatric inpatient services for treatment.

L.R. was diagnosed with bipolar I disorder and was started on lithium therapy. After mood stabilization, she was discharged and treated as an outpatient. She also agreed to attend an outpatient chemical dependency group that met four times a week, which helped her to abstain from substance use. L.R. resides with her older sister Carol. Carol is a financial analyst and her earnings, along with a comfortable inheritance from their deceased parents, enable her to meet the cost of care for her sister. However, the worry and strain of caring for L.R. has made Carol anxious, distressed, and depressed. Some of their relatives distanced themselves from L.R. and Carol when they discovered that L.R. was diagnosed with bipolar disorder.

During lithium treatment L.R. experienced weight gain, acne, and gastrointestinal distress. Even after dosage adjustment, L.R. continued to gain weight and experience distressing side effects. The side effects became intolerable and L.R. stopped taking her medication. She also resumed drinking and taking drugs. Over time, L.R. relapsed with a major depressive episode and was hospitalized after a failed suicide attempt. During hospitalization, L.R. was switched to valproate and also started on low-dose quetiapine. Once her mood was stabilized, she was discharged to outpatient care. L.R. began psychoeducation and cognitive behavioral therapy. She also resumed her chemical dependency group and recognized the need to abstain from alcohol and drugs. She was assessed at each visit for suicidal thoughts, and after 3 months of treatment, L.R. no longer had suicidal thoughts. She was also closely assessed for tolerability of her drug therapy, liver function, and development of side effects. L.R. received nutritional counseling to better manage her weight and prevent weight gain. Valproate therapy was better tolerated with a minor dosage adjustment to manage mild nausea. Quetiapine dosage was lowered due to daytime sleepiness. L.R. worked on maintaining a routine of regular physical and social activity, regular sleep pattern, and a regular medication schedule. Carol accompanied L.R. to psychoeducation and cognitive behavioral therapy sessions. Carol was better able to help L.R. in managing her regular schedules and in building a network of supportive family and friends. Carol also learned how to better cope with caring for her sister.

Questions for Seminar Discussion

1. Discuss the type of bipolar disorder that L.R. exhibited and factors that may have contributed to its development.
2. Discuss the physical and psychological symptoms that L.R. exhibited. Why was L.R. misdiagnosed?
3. What comorbid condition did L.R. have and how might it have contributed to misdiagnosis of bipolar disorder?
4. What might have been done initially to obtain a more accurate diagnosis of L.R.'s illness?
5. Discuss L.R.'s response to SSRI antidepressants. What did she experience?
6. Discuss the phases of treatment that L.R. underwent. What goals were accomplished at each phase?
7. What health and physical functioning, psychological/spiritual, socioeconomic, and family issues influenced L.R.'s quality of life?
8. Discuss objective and subjective burden of care experienced by Carol and how these affected her quality of life.
9. What strengths and weaknesses were present that factor into the ability of L.R. and her sister to manage illness and quality of life demands?
10. Discuss resources that are available to help L.R. manage her illness and improve her quality of life.

Internet Resources

American Psychiatric Association: largest global association of psychiatrists committed to promoting education, research, and highest quality of care for individuals with mental illness and substance use disorders, and their families. http://www.psych.org/

American Psychological Association: the largest national professional association that advances the creation, communication, and application of psychological knowledge to benefit society and improve people's lives. http://www.apa.org/

Depression and Bipolar Support Alliance: provides hope, help, support, and education to improve the lives of individuals with bipolar disorder. http://www.dbsalliance.org/

National Institute of Mental Health: provides information about mental illnesses, promotes research, and disseminates the latest scientific findings in the field of mental health. http://www.nimh.nih.gov/index.shtml

Substance Abuse and Mental Health Services Administration (SAMHSA): provides leadership and resources committed to reducing the impact of substance abuse and mental illness on America's communities. http://www.samhsa.gov/

References

Altshuler, L., Kupka, R., Hellemann, G., Frye, M., Sugar, C., McElroy, S., ... Zermeno, M. (2010). Gender and depressive symptoms in 711 patients with bipolar disorder evaluated prospectively in the Stanley Foundation Bipolar Treatment Outcome Network. *The American Journal of Psychiatry*, 167(6), 708–715.

American Academy of Pediatrics Committee on Drugs. (2001). The transfer of drugs and other chemicals into human milk. *Pediatrics*, 108, 776–789.

American Psychiatric Association. (2013). *Diagnostic and statistical manual of mental disorders* (5th ed.). Arlington, VA: American Psychiatric Association.

Arnold, L. (2003). Gender differences in bipolar disorder. *Psychiatric Clinics of North America*, 26, 595–620.

Baldassano, C. (2006). Illness course, comorbidity, gender, and suicidality in patients with bipolar disorder. *Journal of Clinical Psychiatry*, 67(Suppl. 11), 8–11.

Barnes, C., & Mitchell, P. (2005). Considerations in the management of bipolar disorder in women. *Australian and New Zealand Journal of Psychiatry*, 39, 662–673.

Bowden, C. (2005). Bipolar disorder and work loss. *The American Journal of Managed Care*, 11(Suppl. 3), S91–S94.

Burt, V., & Rasgon, N. (2004). Special considerations in treating bipolar disorder in women. *Bipolar Disorder*, 6, 2–13.

Busby, K., & Sajatovic, M. (2010). Patient, treatment, and systems-level factors in bipolar disorder nonadherence: A summary of the literature. *CNS Neuroscience and Therapeutics*, 16, 308–315.

Cassidy, F. (2011). Risk factors of attempted suicide in bipolar disorder. *Suicide and Life-Threatening Behavior*, 41(1), 6–11.

Cerit, C., Filizer, A., Tural, U., & Tufan, A. (2012). Stigma: A core factor on predicting functionality in bipolar disorder. *Comprehensive Psychiatry*, 53, 484–489.

Cohen, L. (2008). Atypical antipsychotics in pregnancy. Retrieved from http://womensmentalhealth.org/mcm_obgyn/atypical-antipsychotics-in-pregnancy/

Colom, F. (2013). Achieving remission and recovery in bipolar disorder. Retrieved from https://depressiontribunegrel.wordpress.com/2013/05/25/improving-outcomes-in-bipolar-disorder-2/

Correll, C., Penzner, J., Lencz, T., Auther, A., Smith, C., Malhotra, A., ... Cornblatt, B. (2007). Early identification and high-risk strategies for bipolar disorder. *Bipolar Disorders*, 9, 324–338.

de Abreu, L., Nery, F., Harkavy-Friedman, J., de Almeida, K., Gomes, B., Oquendo, M., & Lafer, B. (2012). Suicide attempts are associated with worse quality of life in patients with bipolar disorder type I. *Comprehensive Psychiatry*, 53, 125–129.

De la Cruz, M., Lai, Z., Goodrich, D., & Kilbourne, A. (2013). Gender differences in health-related quality of life in patients with bipolar disorder. *Archives of Women's Mental Health*, 16, 317-323.

Dennehy, E., Marangell, L., Allen, M., Chessick, C., Wisniewski, S., & Thase, M. (2011). Suicide and suicide attempts in the Systematic Treatment Enhancement Program for Bipolar Disorder (STEP-BD). *Journal of Affective Disorders*, 133, 423–427.

Dias, R., Lafer, B., Russo, C., Del Debbio, A., Nierenberg, A., Sachs, G., & Joffe, N. (2011). Longitudinal follow-up of bipolar disorder in women with premenstrual exacerbation: Findings from STEP-BD. *American Journal of Psychiatry*, 168(4), 386–394.

Dilsaver, S. (2011). An estimate of the minimum economic burden of bipolar I and bipolar II disorders in the United States: 2009. *Journal of Affective Disorders*, 129, 79–83.

Dore, G., & Romans, S. (2001). Impact of bipolar affective disorder on family and partners. *Journal of Affective Disorders*, 67, 147–158.

Fountoulakis, K., Gonda, X., Siamouli, M., & Rihmer, Z. (2009). Psychotherapeutic intervention and suicide risk reduction in bipolar disorder: A review of the evidence. *Journal of Affective Disorders*, 113, 21–29.

Freeman, M., & Gelenberg, A. (2005). Bipolar disorder in women: Reproductive events and treatment considerations. *Acta Psychiatrica Scandinavica*, 112, 88–96.

Fusar-Poli, P., Howes, O., Bechdolf, A., & Borgwardt, S. (2012). Mapping vulnerability to bipolar disorder: A systematic review and meta-analysis of neuroimaging studies. *Journal of Psychiatry & Neuroscience*, 37(3), 170–184.

Galvez, J., Thommi, S., & Ghaemi, S. (2011). Positive aspects of mental illness: A review in bipolar disorder. *Journal of Affective Disorders*, 128, 185–190.

Ganguly, K., Chadda, R., & Singh, T. (2010). Caregiver burden and coping in schizophrenia and bipolar disorder: A qualitative study. *American Journal of Psychiatric Rehabilitation*, 13, 126–142.

Gao, K., Tolliver, B., Kemp, D., Ganocy, S., Bilali, S., Brady, K., ... Calabrese, J. (2009). Correlates of historical suicide attempt in rapid-cycling bipolar disorder: A cross-sectional assessment. *Journal of Clinical Psychiatry*, 70(7), 1032–1040.

Goldstein, B., Shamseddeen, W., Axelson, D., Kalas, C., Monk, K., Brent, D., ... Birmaher, B. (2010). Clinical, demographic, and familial correlates of bipolar spectrum disorders among offspring of parents with bipolar disorder. *Journal of the American Academy of Child & Adolescent Psychiatry, 49*(4), 388–396.

Gonzalez, J., Thompson, P., Escamilla, M., Araga, M., Singh, V., Farrelly, N., … Bowden, C. (2007). Treatment characteristics and illness burden among European Americans, African Americans, and Latinos in the first 2,000 patients of the Systematic Treatment Enhancement Program for Bipolar Disorder. *Psychopharmacology Bulletin, 40*(1), 31–46.

Gutiérrez-Rojas, L., Gurpegui, M., Ayuso-Mateos, J., Gutiérrez-Ariza, J., Ruiz-Veguilla, M., & Juardo, D. (2008). Quality of life in bipolar disorder patients: A comparison with a general population sample. *Bipolar Disorders, 10*, 625–634.

Harvard School of Medicine. (2007). National Comorbidity Survey (NCS). Retrieved from http://www.hcp.med.harvard.edu/ncs/

Hirschfeld, R. (2007). Screening for bipolar disorder. *The American Journal of Managed Care, 13*(7 Suppl.), S164–S169.

Hirschfeld, R., & Vornik, L. (2005). Bipolar disorder: Costs and comorbidity. *The American Journal of Managed Care, 11*(3 Suppl.), S85–S90.

Hoes, M. (2009). Bipolar disorder. In J. Urbancic, & C. Grob (Eds.), *Women's mental health: A clinical guide for primary care providers* (pp. 58–86). Philadelphia, PA: Lippincott Williams & Wilkins.

Johnson, R. (2007). Mental illness in primary women's health care. In B. Hackley, J. Kriebs, & ME Rousseau (Eds.), *Primary care of women: A guide for midwives and women's health providers.* Sudbury, MA: Jones & Bartlett.

Keck, P., McIntyre, R., & Shelton, R. (2007). Bipolar depression: Best practices for the outpatient. *CNS Spectrums: The International Journal of Neuropsychiatric Medicine, 12*(12 Suppl. 20), 1–15.

Kennedy, N., Boydell, J., van Os, J., & Murray, R. (2004). Ethnic differences in first clinical presentation of bipolar disorder: Results from an epidemiological study. *Journal of Affective Disorders, 83*, 161–168.

Kilbourne, A., Bauer, M., Pincus, H., Williford, W., Kirk, G., & Beresford, T. for the Veterans Administration (VA) Cooperative Study # 430 Team. (2005). Clinical, psychosocial, and treatment differences in minority patients with bipolar disorder. *Bipolar Disorder, 7*, 89–97.

Kilbourne, A., Haas, G., Mulsant, B., Bauer, M., & Pincus, H. (2004). Concurrent psychiatric diagnoses by age and race among persons with bipolar disorder. *Psychiatric Services, 55*(8), 931–933.

Kriegshauser, K., Sajatovic, M., Jenkins, J., Cassidy, K., Muzina, D., Fattal, O., … Singer, B. (2010).

The Journal of Nervous and Mental Disease, 198(5), 370–372.

Kupfer, D., Frank, E., Grochocinski, V., Houck, V., & Brown, C. (2005). African American participants in bipolar disorder registry: Clinical and treatment characteristics. *Bipolar Disorder, 7*, 82–88.

Kushkituah, Y. (2014). What should be known about bipolar disorder and pregnancy. *International Journal of Childbirth Education, 29*(2), 78–84.

Laxman, K., Lovibond, K., & Hassan, M. (2008). Impact of bipolar disorder in employed populations. *The American Journal of Managed Care, 14*(11), 757–764.

Loo, C., Katalinic, N., Mitchell, P., & Greenberg, B. (2011). Physical treatments for bipolar disorder: A review of electroconvulsive therapy, stereotactic surgery, and other brain simulation techniques. *Journal of Affective Disorders, 132*, 1–13.

Malhi, G., Adams, D., Cahill, C., Dodd, S., & Berk, M. (2009). The management of individuals with bipolar disorder: A review of the evidence and its integration into clinical practice. *Drugs, 69*(15), 2063–2101.

Malhotra, D., McCarthy, S., Michaelson, J., Vacic, V., Burdick, K., Yoon, S., … Sebat, J. (2011). High frequencies of de novo CNVs in bipolar disorder and schizophrenia. *Neuron, 72*(6), 951–963.

Marangell, L. (2008). Current issues: Women and bipolar disorder. *Dialogues in Clinical Neuroscience, 10*(2), 229–238.

Marsh, W., Brown, A., & Rothschild, A. (2012). Manic episode after total abdominal hysterectomy with bilateral salpingo-oopherectomy: A case report. *Menopause: The Journal of The North American Menopause Society, 19*(4), 476–478.

Marsh, W., Ketter, T., & Rasgon, N. (2009). Increased depressive symptoms in menopausal age women with bipolar disorder: Age and gender comparison. *Journal of Psychiatric Research, 43*, 798–802.

Marsh, W., Templeton, A., Ketter, T., & Rasgon, N. (2008). Increased frequency of depressive episodes during the menopausal transition in women with bipolar disorder: Preliminary report. *Journal of Psychiatric Research, 42*, 247–251.

McNamara, R., Nandagopal, J., Strakowski, S., & DelBello, M. (2010). Preventative strategies for early-onset bipolar disorder: Towards a clinical staging model. *CNS Drugs, 24*(12), 983–996.

Merikangas, K., Akiskal, H., Angst, J., Greenberg, P., Hirschfeld, R., Petukhova, M., & Kessler, R. (2007). Lifetime and 12-month prevalence of bipolar spectrum disorder in the National Comorbidity Survey Replication. *Archives of General Psychiatry, 64*, 543–552.

Michalak, E., Livingston, J., Hole, R., Suto, M., Hale, S., & Haddock, C. (2011). 'It's something that I manage but it is not who I am': Reflections on internalized stigma in individuals with bipolar disorder. *Chronic Illness, 7*(3), 209–224.

Michalak, E., Yatham, L., Kolesar, S., & Lam, R. (2006). Bipolar disorder and quality of life: A patient-centered perspective. *Quality of Life Research, 15*, 25–37.

Miklowitz, D. (2007). The role of the family in the course and treatment of bipolar disorder. *Current Directions in Psychological Science, 16*(4), 192–195.

Minsky, S., Vega, W., Miskimen, T., Gara, M., & Escobar, J. (2003). Diagnostic patterns in Latino, African American, and European American psychiatric patients. *Archives of General Psychiatry, 60*, 637–644.

National Institute of Mental Health. (2012a). Bipolar disorder (Publication No. 12-3679). Retrieved from http://www.nimh.nih.gov/health/publications/bipolar-disorder-in-adults/Bipolar_Disorder_Adults_CL508_144295.pdf

National Institute of Mental Health. (2012b). Mental health medications (Publication No. 12-3929). Retrieved from http://www.nimh.nih.gov/health/publications/mental-health-medications/NIMH-Mental-Health-Medications_45027.pdf

National Institute of Mental Health. (2015). Bipolar disorder among adults. Retrieved from http://www.nimh.nih.gov/health/statistics/prevalence/bipolar-disorder-among-adults.shtml

Neves, F., Malloy-Diniz, L., Romano-Silva, M., Aguiar, G., de Matos, L., & Correa, H. (2010). Is the serotonin transporter polymorphism (5-HTTLPR) a potential marker for suicidal behavior in bipolar disorder patients? *Journal of Affective Disorders, 125*, 98–102.

Nonacs, R. (2009). Lamotrigine and pregnancy: An update. Retrieved from http://womensmentalhealth.org/posts/lamotrigine-and-pregnancy-an-update/

Payne, J. (2011). Bipolar disorder in women with premenstrual exacerbation. *American Journal of Psychiatry, 168*(4), 344–346.

Perlick, D., Rosenheck, R., Miklowitz, D., Kaczynski, R., Link, B., Ketter, T., … Sachs, G. STEP-BD Family Experience Collaborative Study Group. (2008). Caregiver burden and health in bipolar disorder: A cluster analytic approach. *The Journal of Nervous and Mental Diseases, 196*(6), 484–491.

Perron, B., Fries, L., Kilbourne, A., Vaughn, M., & Bauer, M. (2010). Racial/ethnic group differences in bipolar symptomatology in a community sample of persons with bipolar I disorder. *The Journal of Nervous and Mental Disease, 198*(1), 16–21.

Persut, B., Clark, N., Maxwell, V., & Michalak, E. Religion and spirituality in the context of bipolar disorder: A literature review. *Mental Health, Religion, & Culture, 14*(8), 785–796.

Podawiltz, A. (2011a). Bipolar disorder: Lessons for rural physicians: Adjunctive interventions for maintaining remission. Diagnosing bipolar disorder: Signs and symptoms. Retrieved from http://www.cmeinstitute.com/Psychlopedia/Pages/BipolarDisorder/6lrp/default.aspx

Podawiltz, A. (2011b). Bipolar disorder: Lessons for rural physicians: Adjunctive interventions for maintaining remission. A review of current bipolar disorder treatment guidelines. Retrieved from http://www.cmeinstitute.com/Psychlopedia/Pages/BipolarDisorder/6lrp/sec2/section.aspx

Proudfoot, J., Doran, J., Manicavasagar, V., & Parker, G. (2011). The precipitants of manic/hypomanic episodes in the context of bipolar disorder: A review. *Journal of Affective Disorders, 133*, 381–387.

Proudfoot, J., Parker, G., Benoit, M., Manicavasgar, V., Smith, M., & MCrim, A. (2009). What happens after diagnosis? Understanding the experiences of patients with newly-diagnosed bipolar disorder. *Health Expectations, 12*, 120–129.

Puri, R., & Gilmore, M. (2011). Understanding bipolar disorder and the role of support workers. *British Journal of Healthcare Assistants, 5*(8), 372–376.

Raab, K. (2007). Manic depression and religious experience: The use of religion in therapy. *Mental Health, Religion, & Culture, 10*(5), 473–487.

Reddy, D. (2010). Clinical pharmacokinetic interactions between antiepileptic drugs and hormonal contraceptives. *Expert Review of Clinical Pharmacology, 3*(2), 183–192.

Roshanaei-Moghaddam, B., & Katon, W. (2009). Premature mortality from general medical illnesses among persons with bipolar disorder: A review. *Psychiatric Services, 60*, 147–156.

Rusner, M., Brunt, D., & Nyström, M. (2012). The paradox of being both needed and rejected: Existential meaning of being closely related to a person with bipolar disorder. *Issues in Mental Health Nursing, 33*, 200–208.

Sajatovic, M. (2005). Bipolar disorder: Disease burden. *The American Journal of Managed Care, 11*(Suppl. 3), S80–S84.

Sajatovic, M., Chen, P., Dines, P., & Shirley, E. (2007). Psychoeducational approaches to medication adherence in patients with bipolar disorder. *Disease Management & Health Outcomes, 15*(3), 181–192.

Sharma, V., Burt, V., & Ritchie, H. (2009). Bipolar II postpartum depression: Detection, diagnosis, and treatment. *American Journal of Psychiatry, 166*, 1217–1221.

Shivakumar, G., Bernstein, I., Suppes, T., & The Stanley Foundation Bipolar Network. (2008). Are bipolar mood symptoms affected by the phase of the menstrual cycle? *Journal of Women's Health, 17*(3), 473–478.

Sienaert, P. (2011). What have we learned about electroconvulsive therapy and its relevance for the practicing psychiatrist? *The Canadian Journal of Psychiatry, 56*(1), 5–12.

Singh, J., Matoo, S., Sharan, P., & Basu, D. (2005). Quality of life and its correlates in patients with dual diagnosis of bipolar affective disorder and substance dependence. *Bipolar Disorders, 7*, 187–191.

Sit, D. (2004). Women and bipolar disorder across the lifespan. *Journal of the American Medical Women's Association, 59*, 91–100.

Strakowski, S., Keck, P., Arnold, L., Collins, J., Wilson, R., Fleck, D., … Adebimpe, V. (2003). Ethnicity and diagnosis in patients with affective disorders. *Journal of Clinical Psychiatry, 64*, 747–754.

Swann, A. (2004, August). CME Certified Symposium Monograph. Special needs of women with bipolar disorder. *International Journal of Neuropsychiatric Medicine, 9*(8), 1–10.

Swann, A. (2010). Improving outcomes in bipolar disorder: From early recognition and treatment to remission. Approaches to preventing relapse in bipolar disorder: Addressing nonadherence and prodromal symptoms. Retrieved from http://www.cmeinstitute.com/Psychlopedia/Pages/BipolarDisorder/2iobd/default.aspx

Thase, M. (2011). Bipolar disorder: Lessons for rural physicians: Adjunctive interventions for maintaining remission. Strategies for increasing treatment adherence in bipolar disorder. Retrieved from http://www.cmeinstitute.com/Psychlopedia/Pages/Bipolar Disorder/6lrp/default.aspx

Üçok, A., & Gaebel, W. (2008). Side effects of atypical antipsychotics: A brief overview. *World Psychiatry, 7*, 58–62.

University of Maryland Medical Center. (2013). Bipolar disorder. Retrieved from http://www.umm.edu/patiented/articles/how_serious_bipolar_disorder_000066_4.htm

Vázquez, G., Kapczinski, F., Magalhaes, P., Córdoba, R., Lopez Jaramillo, C., Rosa, A., … Tohen, M. The Ibero-American Network on Bipolar Disorder (IAN-BD) Group. (2011). Stigma and functioning in patients with bipolar disorder. *Journal of Affective Disorders, 130*, 323–327.

Viguera, A., Whitfield, T., Baldessarini, R., Newport, D., Stowe, Z., Reminick, A., … Cohen, L. (2007). Risk of recurrence in women with bipolar disorder during pregnancy: Prospective study of mood stabilizer discontinuation. *American Journal of Psychiatry, 164*, 1817–1824.

Vornik, L., & Hirschfeld, R. (2005). Bipolar disorder: Quality of life and the impact of atypical antipsychotics. *The American Journal of Managed Care, 11*(9 Suppl.), S275–S280.

Yazla, E., Inanç, L., Bilici, M., & Dusunen, A. (2012). Relationship of sociododemographic features, clinical symptoms and functioning level among bipolar patients with manic episode and difference between these variables according to gender. *Journal of Psychiatry & Neurological Sciences, 25*(3), 221–229.

Zauszniewski, J., Bekhet, A., & Suresky, M. (2008). Factors associated with perceived burden, resourcefulness, and quality of life in female family members of adults with serious mental illness. *Journal of the American Psychiatric Nurses Association, 14*(2), 125–135.

Zeber, J., Miller, A., Copeland, L., McCarthy, J., Zivin, K., Valenstein, M., … Kilbourne, A. (2011). Medication adherence, ethnicity, and the influence of multiple psychosocial and financial barriers. *Administration and Policy in Mental Health, 38*, 86–95.

Chapter 7

Substance Abuse

LEARNING OUTCOMES

On completion of this chapter, the learner will be able to:

1. Explain the incidence, etiology, and legal implications of substance abuse in young women.
2. Describe risk factors and effects of substance abuse in young women.
3. Discuss how differences in gender and genetic makeup influence physiological and psychological responses to substance use and abuse.
4. Analyze current treatment practices associated with substance abuse.
5. Discuss the impact of substance abuse on the quality of life of young women.
6. Explore implications for enhancing quality of life outcomes in young women with substance use disorder.

Introduction

Substance abuse encompasses the overuse of, misuse of, or addiction to any chemical substance such as tobacco, alcohol, or drugs, including over-the-counter (OTC) drugs, prescription drugs, and illicit drugs. Substance abuse and problems related to substance abuse are among the most pervasive health and social concerns of society. Most notably, tobacco use is the single most preventable cause of death and disability in the United States and it significantly contributes to mortality from cardiovascular disease and cancer. Alcohol use is associated with personal health consequences as well as alcohol-related injuries, fatalities, and crime. OTC and prescription drug abuse and misuse affects individuals of all ages and is especially hazardous when combined with other medications or alcohol. In the United States, illicit drug use greatly influences the health of people of all ages. Drug abuse is markedly associated with cardiac illness and death, neurological damage, fetal and infant morbidity and mortality, and infection with HIV and hepatitis.

Substance use disorders are complex illnesses that present unique threats to women's health. Contrary to the mistaken belief that substance abuse is predominantly a men's problem, women are substantially affected by the entire spectrum of substance issues. In fact, women who use alcohol, tobacco, or other drugs may develop substance use disorders and/or substance-related health problems faster than men (Savage, 2010). This chapter explores the issues of substance abuse that affect young women. The significant impact of substance abuse on the quality of life of young women and their families is also discussed.

Incidence and Prevalence

A drug is any chemical substance other than food that is purposely taken into the body to affect body processes. People have used natural and manufactured drugs throughout history to alter their moods and serve as health aids. Drugs are currently consumed for legitimate health reasons in the prevention and treatment of diseases, as well as maintenance of health. However, drugs are also taken for illegal reasons, such as for pleasure, as in recreational drug usage. Presently, legal drugs in the United States include alcohol, nicotine, caffeine, OTC drugs, and drugs obtained with a medical prescription. Although recreational drugs are often associated with illegal substances, alcohol, tobacco, caffeine, and many prescription drugs, such as amphetamines and tranquilizers, are also sometimes used as recreational drugs.

Drugs that are used for a purpose other than that for which they were legally intended constitutes drug misuse. Drug misuse includes taking more or less of a prescribed or OTC medication, using an outdated medication, or using a medication prescribed for someone else. Excessive drug use that is inconsistent with accepted medical practices constitutes drug abuse. The dangers of misusing or abusing a drug are frequently associated with the ability of that drug to cause addiction or physical dependence. Many legally prescribed drugs, such as barbiturates, tranquilizers, analgesics, opiates, and legal substances such as alcohol and tobacco, can be addictive. The addictive

characteristic of such drugs can create physical as well as psychological dependence, known as *habituation*. Habituation is the repeated use of a drug because it engenders an increase in pleasurable feelings or a decrease in stress or anxiety with each use. Habituation becomes detrimental when the need for the drugged state of consciousness becomes so consuming that all energies are directed to compulsive, drug-seeking behavior.

Substance abuse is widely prevalent in the United States, yet incidence has remained relatively constant between 2002 and 2010, ranging from 21.6 to 22.7 million people, but the rate was lower in 2011. According to the 2011 National Survey of Drug Use and Health (NSDUH), an estimated 20.6 million people aged 12 or older have been categorized with substance dependence or abuse (8.0% of the population aged 12 or older). Of these, 3.9 million had dependence or abuse of illicit drugs but not alcohol, 2.6 million had dependence or abuse of both alcohol and illicit drugs, and 14.1 million had dependence or abuse of alcohol but not illicit drugs. The rate of substance dependence or abuse was 6.9% among youths aged 12 to 17, 18.6% among young adults aged 18 to 25, and 6.3% among adults aged 26 or older (Substance Abuse and Mental Health Services Administration [SAMHSA], 2012).

In the 2011 NSDUH, the rate of substance dependence or abuse among females aged 12 or older was 5.7% as compared to10.4% in males of that age. Among youths aged 12 to 17, the rate of substance dependence or abuse for females and males was 6.9%. The rate of substance dependence or abuse among racial and ethnic groups was estimated at 8.2% for whites, 7.2% for African-Americans, 8.7% for Hispanics, 16.8% for American Indians or Alaska Natives, and 9.0% for persons reporting two or more races. The rate of substance dependence or abuse among Asians was 3.3% and Native Hawaiians or Other Pacific Islanders was 10.6.6 % (SAMHSA, 2012). The rate of substance involvement among women aged 18 or older, who are non-Hispanic American Indian/ Alaska Native, non-Hispanic Native Hawaiian/ Other Pacific Islander and non-Hispanic women of multiple races (17.5%, 17.6 %, and 17.7 %, respectively) is more than triple the rate of substance use among non-Hispanic Asian women (5.4 %). The rate of substance use among women aged 18 or older is estimated at 11.9% among non-Hispanic white women, 12.2% among African-American women, and 9.4% among Hispanic women (U.S. Department of Health and Human Services [USDHHS], 2011).

Evidence suggests that the risk of death is eight times higher among substance using women as compared to women in the general population. Women who die of substance-related causes tend to be relatively young. The most common cause of death is overdose, followed by cardiovascular disease, alcohol/drug disorders, cancer, liver disease, motor vehicle accidents, homicide, and complications of HIV/AIDS and hepatitis (Hser, Kagihara, Huang, Evans, & Messina, 2011).

Etiology and Risk Factors

Initiation of substance use and progression to substance abuse and dependence is influenced by a number of factors. The following discussion examines risk factors that increase the likelihood of initiation of substance use, ongoing substance involvement, and substance abuse and dependence.

Age

Evidence indicates that the initiation of drug use prior to adulthood increases the risk of adolescents for developing clinical features associated with drug dependence (Chen, Storr, & Anthony, 2009). It is posited that early onset drug use may prolong exposure to environmental or contextual factors that increase or reinforce a progression toward more advanced drug involvement, such as family drug-taking habits or socioeconomic status,

or drug availability in the larger community or local neighborhood. From a developmental psychopathology perspective, the excess risk associated with early-onset drug use may be explained by drug-induced disruption of processes of adolescent brain development or possibly the development of a higher threshold for reinforcement in neurochemical reward systems (Chen et al., 2009).

Genetic Factors

Substance use disorders aggregate in families such that individuals with relatives who have substance use disorders are more likely to develop a disorder. Both genetic and environmental factors play important and interconnected roles in the development of substance use disorders, with heritability estimates ranging from 50% to 60% (Wermier et al., 2010). Investigations into genetic linkages and associations in addiction have been ongoing for decades. Results have pointed to possible genetic involvement in substance dependence as well as in protection against dependence (Ball, 2007). Genes may play a direct role in affecting the metabolism of substances in the body or an indirect role in influencing an individual's temperament or personality in such a way as to increase the risk for substance dependence (Malliarakis & Lucey, 2007). The interaction of genetic predisposition with conflict or psychopathology commonly present in the environment of parental substance abuse likely increases the probability of substance abuse in the offspring (Center for Substance Abuse Treatment [CSAT], 2009).

Family Characteristics

Major environmental risk factors for substance initiation and dependence across ethnic and cultural populations of women include growing up in households that are chaotic, argumentative, violent, and blame-oriented (CSAT, 2009). Women who grow up in families in which they have assumed adult responsibilities as a child—including household duties, parenting of younger children, and emotional support of parents—are more likely to initiate drug and alcohol use. Women who have a history of over-responsibility with their family of origin are also more likely to be dependent on substances. Adverse childhood experiences, characterized by childhood abuse and various forms of dysfunctional households, especially in households of parental substance abuse, significantly increase early initiation of use on or before the age of 14 (CSAT, 2009).

Marital Status

Marital status is a substantial risk factor for drug involvement among women. Women who are married tend to have a lower rate of substance use or dependence as compared to women who are divorced, separated, or who have never been married (CSAT, 2009). Evidence suggests that divorce is positively associated with drug use. Conflicts arising from women's drug use within a marriage can cause marital problems and possibly lead to divorce. Conversely, stress and depression arising from marital discord and/or dissolution may lead women to drug use (Agrawal, Gardener, Prescott, & Kendler, 2005).

Partner Influence

A major factor in substance use and abuse among women is the interaction, assistance, and encouragement of other people. To a certain extent, partners can be influential with patterns of substance use. Women are more likely to have been introduced to substance use by their partners and women who are substance dependent are more likely to have partners who use substances or are substance dependent. Some women persist with substance use in order to have an activity in common with their partner or to maintain their relationship. The partner frequently may be the substance supplier. This dynamic of partner as supplier and the other being the substance user to

maintain the relationship is present in heterosexual as well as same-sex relationships (CSAT, 2009).

Women who share needles with partners who inject drugs or participate in non-monogamous unsafe sexual activity are at high risk for contracting HIV/AIDS and hepatitis. Some women are reluctant to demand safe sex practices for fear of consequences from partners. Issues such as fear of partner alienation, intimate partner violence, or relationship dissolution can cause psychological distress that can increase substance use and related problems. The presence of children in the relationship further complicates matters and the woman may feel unable to leave her partner for emotional or financial reasons. Furthermore, a partner may hinder or prevent a woman from entering or staying in treatment, or the partner's support while a woman is in treatment may be passive or inconsistent (CSAT, 2009).

Personality Factors

Evidence suggests that certain personality factors are associated with substance use and abuse. Novelty seeking, which is characterized by risk-taking behavior that anticipates a rewarding sensation, is significantly associated with substance use—more so with initiation of use than progression from use to abuse/dependence (Agrawal et al., 2005). The initial stimulus to try a drug may be dependent on the ability of the individual to overcome social, religious, and cultural inhibitions and ignore legal ramifications (Agrawal et al., 2005).

Evidence suggests that extroversion is associated with substance initiation. Extroverted individuals are more apt to have an extensive peer network through which drugs can be obtained. Another personality factor, locus of control, is associated with progression to substance abuse and dependence (Agrawal et al., 2005). Deterioration of voluntary control over a drug habit is a characteristic of substance abuse and dependence. As drug tolerance increases, increased drug consumption is required to satiate the need and experience pleasurable effects of the drug, constituting a loss of self-control (Agrawal et al., 2005).

Certain premorbid personality factors often provide a basis for substance abuse. These include obsessiveness and anxiety, difficulty in regulating affect and behavior (such as temper tantrums and frequent tearfulness), and low self-esteem and ego integration. A negative self-perception of physical attractiveness is associated with increased substance use (CSAT, 2009).

Sexual Orientation

Evidence suggests that sexual minority women (i.e., women who have sex with women) experience higher rates of substance use, abuse, and dependence as compared to women who are exclusively heterosexual (CSAT, 2009; Hughes, Szalacha, & McNair, 2010). The heightened risk among sexual minority women may be explained by perceived social stress associated with stigmatization, prejudice, and discrimination (Hughes et al., 2010). Adolescent females and women who are struggling with issues or prejudice surrounding sexual orientation are at greater risk for initiating and maintaining drug and alcohol use. Furthermore, lesbians who have a history of childhood sexual abuse may be at heightened risk for lifetime substance abuse as compared to lesbians who do not have a comparable history (CSAT, 2009).

Traumatic Life Events

Research findings consistently indicate that women, especially young women, who have experienced traumatic events such as sexual and physical assaults, childhood sexual and physical abuse, and intimate partner violence, are at high risk for initiation of substance use and the subsequent progression from use to the pathological states of abuse and dependence (Agrawal et al., 2005; Danielson et al., 2009). It is posited that some women with history of sexual and/or physical abuse may use

substances to self-medicate their depression or the anxiety that results from the abuse. Another explanation suggests that women with history of sexual and/or physical abuse who primarily use cocaine and amphetamines may be trying to increase their vigilance against further victimization. Abuse victims with low self-esteem may attempt to increase their sociability by using alcohol (CSAT, 2009).

Substance use and abuse can increase vulnerability to additional trauma. It can diminish the ability to defend oneself, alter judgment, and draw one into unsafe environments. Women may be drawn into a "vicious cycle" of substance abuse and violence. As such, violence becomes both a risk factor and a consequence of substance abuse (CSAT, 2009). Research findings indicate that intimate partner violence (IPV; also known as domestic violence), is significantly related to substance initiation, abuse, and dependence (CSAT, 2009). IPV is a pattern of coercive behavior used by a current or former intimate partner—such as a cohabitating or non-cohabitating sexual or romantic partner, or opposite or same-sex partner—to achieve power and control over another person. Coercive behaviors often include use of physical and sexual violence, verbal and emotional abuse, stalking, economic abuse, and sexual, emotional, and psychological intimidation (Black et al., 2011). The introduction to substances by an intimate partner can be a way of gaining control and establishing power (CSAT, 2009). By continuing to supply drugs to their substance abusing women, abusive partners can sustain their power and control (Taylor, 2011). Women who have experienced IPV may engage in substance use as a means of coping with domestic violence (CSAT, 2009).

Co-occurring Psychiatric Disorders

Substance abuse is acknowledged to occur concurrently with several mental illnesses. Addicted women are noted to be particularly affected by mental health comorbidity. For women, substance use, abuse, and dependence have been strongly associated with anxiety and depressive disorders, eating disorders, and post-traumatic stress disorders (Agrawal et al., 2005; Carlson, 2006; CSAT, 2009; Greenfield, Back, Lawson, & Brady, 2010). Findings from the National Epidemiological Survey on Alcohol and Related Conditions (NESARC) indicated that associations between substance use disorders and obsessive-compulsive, histrionic, schizoid, and antisocial personality disorders were significantly stronger among women (Grant et al., 2006).

Various patterns of associations have been recognized. One such pattern is that substance use may mask the presence of mental health problems. When a woman stops using and enters treatment, psychiatric problems may emerge full force and complicate the course of substance abuse and recovery (Carlson, 2006). Another pattern acknowledges that the association between psychiatric disorders and substance involvement increases as the relative pathology of the stage in the drug habit increases (Agrawal et al., 2005). Self-medication with substances may be an attempt to reduce painful or disturbing psychiatric symptoms (Harris & Edlund, 2005). Psychiatric symptomatology can induce further substance abuse, which can in turn lead to further symptomatology (Agrawal, 2005). Nonetheless, while mental disorders may be influential in initiating substance use to gain symptom relief, psychiatric disorders may also arise as an outcome of substance use. Mental disorders may also develop independently of—and concurrently with—the existing pattern of substance use (CSAT, 2009).

Discrimination

Acts of discrimination can range from minor slights to harmful acts of violence. Various levels of discrimination, based on gender, age, race, ethnicity, language, culture, socioeconomic level, sexual orientation, and disability, can influence substance use and recovery. For some women, substance abuse is a way of coping with the social stresses of discrimination. The influence of discrimination on substance abuse may be multiplied when women experience more than one type of discrimination (CSAT, 2009).

Acculturation

As immigrants become increasingly acculturated into American society, evidence suggests that substance use increases (CSAT, 2009). Acculturation is a process of cultural modification through adoption of cultural traits and social patterns by means of prolonged and continuous interaction with a different culture than one's native culture. Acculturation may bring about intergenerational conflict and feelings of disconnection. Individuals may experience a struggle for cultural identity, and feelings of grief and loss in response to the life left behind. The conflicts and distress experienced through acculturation may put a woman at risk for substance abuse (CSAT, 2009).

Socioeconomic Status

Women who have lower incomes, less education, and less likelihood of employment tend to be more prone to substance use disorders. Unemployment seems to be a factor associated with substance abuse and dependence, as incidence of substance abuse and dependence is greater among women who are unemployed. The temporal association between unemployment and the development of substance use disorders tends to be complex and not well understood at this time (CSAT, 2009).

In the United States, socioeconomic status associated with race and ethnicity often results in disadvantaged life circumstances and increased social vulnerability for African-American and Hispanic women. This increased social vulnerability is noticeable in decreased levels of educational accomplishment, lower employment opportunities, fewer job skills, limited financial resources, and susceptibility to racial discrimination.

Although evidence indicates that the rate of substance involvement among African-American and Hispanic women is fairly consistent with that of white women, the disparity in social vulnerability and disadvantaged life circumstances may increase environmental risk factors for proximal and distal substance involvement (Amaro et al., 2005).

Degree of Risk of Substance Abuse

Drug involvement is a complex multistage process that starts with a proximal stage of initiation of drug use and progresses to a distal stage of drug abuse and dependence (Agrawal et al., 2005). For women, the path on this continuum toward drug abuse is complicated, yet it is patterned. The typical pattern begins with a disintegration of protective factors—characteristics that have a protective influence against the development of substance use, such as having parental warmth, parental caring, religiosity, effective coping skills, and having supportive communication in a satisfying relationship or happy marriage (Agrawal et al., 2005; CSAT, 2009). When protective factors break down, a subsequent proliferation of fears, anxieties, phobias, and failed relationships can establish an environment conducive to initiation of substance use and abuse.

No single biological, psychological, or social factor is solely responsible for substance initiation, abuse, or dependence. Reasons attributed to initiation of substance use differ among women and are often associated with a variety of issues such as marital discord, stress, a desire to lose weight or have more energy, or thrill-seeking behavior (Agrawal et al., 2005; CSAT, 2009). The reasons women progress from proximal substance use to distal substance abuse and dependence are not entirely clear. The causes of substance use disorders are complex and interrelated, and involve the interaction of numerous factors (Agrawal et al., 2005).

Definitive patterns of substance involvement, however, have emerged from empirical evidence. Although evidence suggests a greater prevalence of substance use and dependence among men, the gender gap is narrowing for substance involvement across ethnicities, particularly among young women (CSAT, 2009). Like men, women tend to initiate use based on, but not limited to, substance availability, level of ease in obtaining the substances, cost of substances, the ratio between perceived benefit versus perceived risk associated with use, and general viewpoint toward substance use. However, women are more apt to temporarily change their pattern of substance use in response to caregiver responsibilities (CSAT, 2009).

Significant relationships are substantially influential in initiation of use and subsequent progression to substance abuse and dependence. Women tend to accelerate to injecting drugs at a faster rate than men, and the high-risk behaviors and rituals associated with drug injection are directly influenced by significant relationships (CSAT, 2009). A positive association exists between women's earlier patterns of use (inclusive of earlier age of initiation, amount, and frequency of use) and a higher risk for dependency and negative drug-related occupational outcomes. The tendency to advance more quickly from initiation of use to the development of substance-related harmful consequences is greater in women (CSAT, 2009; Griffin, Bang, & Botvin, 2010).

Risk Reduction

The reduction of risk of substance use and abuse in women entails a multifaceted approach involving individual, family, community, and societal commitment to prevention of use of tobacco, inappropriate use of alcohol and pharmaceuticals, and use of illicit drugs. The issues surrounding substance abuse are multidimensional and interdependent, with no immediate or simple solution for prevention.

TOBACCO USE

For women who smoke, the single most significant step that can be made to improve well-being is to stop smoking. Although the rate of smoking has declined in this country over the past 50 years, tobacco use continues in epidemic proportions and is the leading cause of preventable death in the United States (USDHHS, 2012). Women's risk of dying from smoking has more than tripled and is now equal to men's risk. In the United States, more than 20 million women and girls currently smoke cigarettes (National Prevention Council [NPC], 2014b).

Living tobacco-free brings serious health benefits, decreases the risk of developing acute and chronic diseases such as heart disease, cancer, pulmonary disease, and strokes, and reduces the risk of premature death (NPC, 2014b). To live tobacco-free requires avoidance of all types of tobacco products, including cigarettes, cigars, smokeless tobacco, pipes, and hookahs. A tobacco-free life also necessitates freedom from exposure to secondhand smoke. Efforts must target young people to prevent initiation of tobacco usage, assist those who want to quit, and protect people from exposure to secondhand smoke (NPC, 2014a). Effective, comprehensive tobacco control measures reduce tobacco use. Helpful strategies for reduction of tobacco use include the enforcement of comprehensive smoke-free laws, employment of mass media and countermarketing campaigns, improvement of accessibility and affordability of options that help people quit, and implementation of evidence-based strategies to reduce tobacco use by children and youth (USDHHS, 2012).

Comprehensive tobacco-free and other evidence-based tobacco control policies are essential aspects of an effective prevention strategy. Evidence indicates that there is no safe level of secondhand smoke exposure. Policies that advocate smoke-free and tobacco-free environments improve indoor air quality, decrease adverse health outcomes among nonsmokers, reduce cigarette consumption, and encourage quitting among those who smoke. Comprehensive policies that ban smoking and all forms of tobacco use are needed in workplaces, healthcare and educational facilities, and multi-unit housing (USDHHS, 2012). The regulation of manufacturing, marketing, and distribution of tobacco products by the U.S. Food and Drug Administration, as well as enforcement by federal, state, tribal, local, and territorial governments is an important aspect of prevention efforts (USDHHS, 2012).

Evidence suggests that more than seven in ten smokers want to quit. An essential strategy for quitting smoking is expansion of tobacco cessation services. Services that include counseling and medications are valuable in assisting people to quit tobacco use. Utilizing counseling and medication strategies together has been found to be more efficacious than employing either strategy alone. Promoting the use of tobacco cessation benefits through health plans enhances the use of these services (USDHHS, 2012).

Another effective prevention strategy is the enlistment of sustained mass-media advertising and countermarketing campaigns. When combined with other tobacco control strategies, a reduction in tobacco use occurs. Media campaigns through traditional modalities (e.g., television, radio, billboard, print) as well as Internet and social media outlets can effectively convey the health risks of tobacco use, promote cessation, decrease social acceptability of tobacco use, and build public support for tobacco control policies. Additionally, reducing depictions of tobacco use in entertainment media (e.g., movies, music videos) can reduce tobacco use in young people (USDHHS, 2012).

DRUG AND ALCOHOL ABUSE

Prevention of drug and alcohol abuse increases the chances of women for living long, healthy, and productive lives. Binge drinking, underage drinking, drinking or using drugs while pregnant, substance-impaired driving, inappropriate use of pharmaceuticals (both prescription and over-the counter), and use of illicit drugs is dangerous and constitutes excessive use of substances. Substance use and abuse can impede judgment and lead to harmful risk-taking behavior. Prevention of substance abuse can improve quality of life, academic performance, workplace productivity, and military preparedness. Prevention also reduces crime and criminal justice expenses, decreases motor vehicle crashes and fatalities, and lessens the cost of health care for acute and chronic conditions. Strategies that can be effective in local prevention of substance abuse include implementation of policies to increase access, early screening and treatment of women with substance abuse, and altering the attitudes of people toward substance use and abuse (NIDA, 2003).

Strategies of prevention of alcohol abuse begin with the support of state, tribal, local, and territorial implementation and enforcement of alcohol control policies. Evidence suggests that states with more rigorous alcohol control policies tend to have lower rates of binge drinking among adults and college students (National Institute on Alcohol Abuse and Alcoholism [NIAAA], 2015). Evidence-based policies such as prohibiting the sale of alcohol to minors and intoxicated persons, reducing days and hours of the sale of alcohol, and restricting the number of places that legally sell alcohol have been effective in reducing excessive alcohol use and related problems (NIAAA, 2015). Laws that restrict the minimum legal drinking age to 21 and the adoption of campus-based policies and practices such as alcohol-free late-night student activities, restrictions of alcohol marketing to primarily underage audiences, and supporting and enforcing the minimum legal drinking age are valuable in reducing high-risk alcohol use among college students (NIAAA, 2015).

The creation of environments or social conditions that empower young people to avoid substance use is another valuable prevention strategy. Decreasing the exposure of young people to alcohol marketing and increasing exposure to anti-drug campaigns can effect change in attitudes toward drinking and drug use. Positive social environments that afford meaningful alternative youth activities, enhance family relationships, develop self esteem, and dispel myths about substance use can assist young people in making healthy decisions (NIDA, 2003).

Early identification and treatment is essential and offers hope to individuals involved with substance abuse. The Screening, Brief Intervention, and Referral to Treatment (SBIRT) services implemented in primary care and trauma centers is a valuable strategy for early recognition and treatment (SAMHSA, 2011). SBIRT is a comprehensive integrated public health approach to the provision of early intervention and treatment services for individuals with substance use disorders. It is a useful early identification and treatment approach for those at heightened risk of developing these disorders. Opportunities for early intervention with at-risk substance users are provided in primary care centers, hospital emergency rooms, trauma centers, and other community settings before more severe consequences can occur. Screening rapidly determines the severity of substance use and identifies the appropriate level of treatment. Brief intervention then concentrates on developing insight and awareness concerning substance use and motivation toward behavioral change. Referral to treatment makes available access to specialty care for those identified as needing more extensive treatment (SAMHSA, 2011).

Another important strategy involves the reduction of inappropriate access to and use of prescription drugs. A comprehensive approach should be employed to deal with prescription drug abuse that focuses on reducing abuse while guaranteeing legitimate access for pain management. The use of prescription drug monitoring programs, in association with implementation and enforcement of laws that reduce inappropriate access, can decrease misuse of prescription drugs. Safe management of prescription drugs can be augmented by consumer and prescriber education about appropriate and safe medication use and disposal practices (Executive Office of the President of the United States, 2011).

Understanding the short- and long-term negative effects that drugs can have, in addition to development of personal strengths and self-confidence, is an important foundation that enables women to effectively resist drugs. The development of healthy ways to cope with stress can minimize the likelihood that women will turn to drugs as a coping mechanism. Enhancement of self-esteem is another significant personal strength that provides an underpinning for drug avoidance.

Gender Similarities and Differences

Women and men differ with respect to numerous aspects of substance use and abuse. The rates of drug use and abuse among men are higher than that of women, and the rates steadily increase throughout adolescence to peak in young adulthood. Substance dependency in men tends to be attributed to heritability with little or no environmental contribution, whereas substance dependency in women tends to be influenced by both heritability and significant environmental influence. In addition, social persuasion from sexual and/or social relationships with young injection drug users can increase women's risk of sharing injection equipment and related high-risk behaviors (Kloos, Weller, Chan, & Weller, 2009, NIDA, 2015b).

Social and cultural norms may contribute to gender differences in substance abuse, especially regarding alcohol. Women tend to restrict drinking out of concern for loss of social control and sexual inhibition. Because women tend to experience more social disapproval and stigmatization for using substances, it is likely that fear of stigma may also contribute to their lower rates of substance use and abuse. It is also possible that fear of stigma and social disapproval might cause women

to underreport use and abuse, making differences between men and women not as dramatic as originally perceived (Kloos et al., 2009).

Women and men differ with respect to physical responses to substances. For example, higher concentrations of body fat, lower volume of body water, slower rate of alcohol metabolism, and lower levels of alcohol dehydrogenase make women more vulnerable to higher blood alcohol concentrations and intoxication after ingesting smaller quantities of alcohol as compared to men (CSAT, 2009; Greenfield et al., 2010; NIDA, 2015b). Changes in the levels of ovarian steroidal hormones such as estrogen and progesterone that occur during the menstrual cycle likely influence the behavioral effects of drugs in women. Moreover, sex differences in neuroendocrine adaptation to stress and reward systems may influence women's susceptibility to drug abuse and relapse (Greenfield et al., 2010; NIDA, 2015b).

Women typically have a quicker progression from initial use to the onset of dependency and first admission to treatment. Female substance abusers experience a more rapid onset of physical and social consequences. This phenomenon is known as telescoping, and has been consistently observed in research on gender and substance abuse. Accelerated progression among women has been typically noted with opioids, cannabis, and alcohol (Greenfield et al., 2010; Kloos et al., 2009). Furthermore, women tend to present a graver clinical profile consisting of more medical, behavioral, psychological, and social problems when entering treatment, despite having used a lesser amount of substances over a shorter period of time in comparison to men. Women tend to enter treatment through social service referral as compared to men, who tend to enter treatment via employer referrals or criminal justice agencies (Greenfield et al., 2010; Kloos et al., 2009). Once in treatment, women had lower 30-day retention and were less likely to complete treatment as compared to men. Lower mean income, greater number of previous treatments, and increased likelihood of crack cocaine usage tended to intensify the problems faced by women in treatment. On the other hand, men are more apt to have poorer coping skills, more negative social influences, and increased exposure to substances when entering treatment (Kloos et al., 2009). Overall, women are less likely than men to seek treatment and are more likely to face gender–specific treatment barriers, such as childcare responsibilities, transportation issues, financial issues, and social stigma (Greenfield et al., 2010). Evidence suggests that women have treatment outcomes that are just as good as, or better, than men's treatment outcomes (Green, 2006). In some cases, such as with smoking cessation, women tend to have better treatment response than men. Although both men and women are vulnerable to relapse soon after discharge from inpatient treatment, women tend to engage in aftercare more than men (Kloos et al., 2009).

Women with substance use disorder are more vulnerable to and have earlier onset of serious medical problems and disorders. For example, women tend to develop alcohol-related physical health problems at lower doses and over a shorter period of time than men. Although less evidence is available regarding gender differences in health problems resulting from illicit drugs, women may also have more health consequences resulting from other substances. Evidence suggests that moderate to heavy alcohol and drug consumption substantially increases the risk for cervical, breast, and other cancers, premenopausal osteoporosis, peripheral neuropathy, and cognitive impairments. In comparison to men, women can develop more rapid onset of cirrhosis, heart damage, and nerve damage with fewer years of heavy drinking. Moreover, with illicit drug use, women have greater risk of liver and kidney diseases, bacterial infections, and opportunistic diseases. Substance abuse also increases the risk of HIV/AIDS in women and has significantly harmful effects on reproductive processes (CSAT, 2009).

Female substance abusers are more likely than men to have family histories of violence and alcoholism. They are also more likely to have experienced a traumatic event before the onset of substance abuse. Women tend to have a higher incidence of post-traumatic stress disorder and more frequent histories of physical and sexual trauma. Female substance abusers are also more likely to have co-occurring depression, eating disorders, anxiety disorders, and borderline personality disorders. Male substance abusers, on the other hand, are more likely to exhibit co-occurring antisocial personality disorder and conduct disorder (Greenfield et al., 2010; Kloos et al., 2009).

Diagnosing Substance Abuse

Smoking Addiction

Smoking addiction is the dependence on tobacco such that cessation of smoking results in withdrawal symptoms. Withdrawal is an adverse reaction characterized by unpleasant symptoms and an intense psychological and physiological demand for nicotine. Symptoms of nicotine withdrawal are presented in **Box 7–1**. Smoking is undeniably an addictive behavior, with nicotine being the primary addictive pharmacological component. Nicotine may have several different effects, sometimes acting as a relaxant and sometimes as a stimulant. This compound in itself reinforces and strengthens the desire to smoke. It may also facilitate short-term memory, help in performing certain tasks, reduce anxiety, negate hunger symptoms, increase blood pressure and heart rate, temporarily relieve feelings of depression, and increase pain tolerance. Many women—even pregnant women and teenage girls—report that they smoke to avoid weight gain. Although there is no scientific consensus yet on the physiological or biochemical mechanism responsible for this association between weight regulation and smoking behavior, some evidence suggests that nicotine elevates the basal metabolic rate.

The physical and psychological withdrawal symptoms that occur with cessation of cigarette smoking differ considerably in duration and intensity. For heavy smokers, withdrawal

---

Box 7–1: Symptoms of Nicotine Withdrawal

- Cigarette craving
- Irritability
- Restlessness
- Depression
- Anxiety
- Difficulty in concentrating
- Troubled sleep
- Tiredness
- Headache
- Drowsiness
- Increased appetite
- Gastrointestinal disturbances such as diarrhea and constipation

---

symptoms may occur within 2 hours of the last cigarette. The peak period of physiological symptoms from smoking cessation is usually 24 to 48 hours into abstinence, but many smokers report "craving" cigarettes for as long as a year.

Alcohol Consumption and Alcoholism

Alcohol functions as a central nervous system depressant that effectively impairs all major body systems. When consumed in small quantities, it has a mild, relaxing effect. Consumption of larger quantities results in compromised sensory motor coordination, judgment, emotional control, and reasoning capabilities. Because alcohol circulates throughout the body, nearly all bodily functions can be affected by increased alcohol consumption. It usually takes about 15 minutes for alcohol to reach the bloodstream, and the peak effect occurs in one hour. Once in the bloodstream, alcohol is quickly carried to the liver, heart, and brain. Alcohol is especially dangerous when combined with other drugs, such as depressants and anti-anxiety medications

(see **Table 7–1**). Combining alcohol with drugs can produce an effect greater than that expected with either substance taken alone.

Chronic alcohol abuse commonly reveals itself as a pattern. Manifestations of alcohol abuse include daily consumption of large amounts of alcohol, regular heavy drinking on weekends, and visible as periods of sobriety between binges of daily heavy drinking that may last for weeks or months. Alcoholism generally appears between ages 20 and 40 but can also present in childhood or early adolescence. Alcohol becomes a problem when an individual is no longer able to control when and how much drinking takes place. Clinical diagnosis of alcoholism is based on the presence of at least three of the following symptoms, persisting for a month or more, or occurring repeatedly over a longer period of time:

- Alcohol taken in large amounts (five or more drinks per day)
- Persistent desire to quit drinking or one or more unsuccessful attempts to cut down or quit alcohol

Table 7–1 ALCOHOL AND DRUG INTERACTIONS

Type of Drug	Examples	Possible Effects
Analgesics (narcotic)	Codeine, opioids	Increased central nervous system (CNS) depression, possibly leading to respiratory arrest, death
Analgesics (non-narcotic)	Ibuprophen, acetaminophen	Gastric irritation and bleeding, increased risk of liver damage
Antidepressants	Tofranil, tricyclics	CNS depression, decreased alertness
Anti-anxiety drugs	Valium, Librium, Xanax, Ativan	CNS depression, decreased alertness
Antihistamines	Actifed, Dimetapp, cold medications (prescribed and over-the-counter)	Increased drowsiness
Antibiotics	Penicillin, erythromycin	Nausea, vomiting, headache; some antibiotics are rendered less effective
CNS stimulants	Dexedrine, Ritalin, Adderall, caffeine	Some counter the depressant effects of alcohol but do not influence level of intoxication
Diuretics	Lasix, Diuril, Hydromox	Reduction in blood pressure, possible lightheadedness
Psychotropics	Tindal, Mellaril, Thorazine	Increased CNS depression, possibly leading to respiratory arrest
Sedatives	Dalmane, Nembutal, Quaalude	Increased CNS depression, possibly leading to respiratory arrest
Tranquilizers	Valium, Miltown, Librium	Increased CNS depression, decreased alertness and judgment

- Considerable time spent obtaining, using, or recovering from alcohol
- Continued drinking despite social, psychological, or physical symptoms such as ulcers, that are worsened by alcohol
- Withdrawal symptoms, such as physical trembling, sweating, high blood pressure, delusions, and hallucinations when alcohol intake is curbed (see **Box 7–2**)
- Avoidance or relief of withdrawal symptoms by drinking
- Desire or need for a drink to start the day
- Denial of an alcohol problem
- Sleep problems
- Attempts to control drinking by changing brands or going "on the wagon"
- Depression and paranoia
- Failure to recall what happened during a drinking episode

Box 7–2: Symptoms of Alcohol Withdrawal

- Depression
- Irritability
- Agitation
- Lack of concentration
- Body tremors
- Nausea and vomiting
- Generalized weakness, achiness
- Sweating
- Fever
- Dry mouth
- Elevated blood pressure
- Headache
- Anxiety
- Puffy, blotchy skin
- Fitful sleep with nightmares
- Brief hallucinations
- Delirium tremens (DTs)

- Dramatic mood swings
- Participation in behaviors or activities while drinking that are regretted afterward
- Experience of the following symptoms after drinking: headaches, nausea, stomach pain, heartburn, gas, fatigue, weakness, muscle cramps, irregular or rapid heart rate

Drug Use and Abuse

No drug use is completely benign. At the very least, all psychoactive drugs affect the central nervous system. Often habitual drug users end up in the emergency room because of overdosing, injury due to an accident, or injury related to the drug use. In addition to the direct physiological effects and risks of drug use, women are likely exposed to additional risks associated with the administration of drugs to the body, such as HIV and hepatitis that can be transmitted through sharing needles to inject drugs. Indications of drug use are presented in **Box 7–3**.

STIMULANTS

Stimulants affect the central nervous system and increase heart rate, blood pressure, body temperature, and metabolism. Stimulants can create a feeling of exhilaration, increased energy, and mental alertness. They can also produce tremors, reduced appetite, weight loss, irritability, anxiety,

Box 7–3: Indications of Drug Use

- Abrupt change in attitude, including lack of interest in previously enjoyed activities
- Frequent vague and withdrawn moods
- Sudden decline in work or school performance
- Sudden resistance to discipline or criticism
- Secret telephone calls and meetings, with a demand for greater personal privacy
- Increased frustration levels
- Decreased tolerance for others
- Change in eating and sleeping habits
- Sudden weight loss
- Frequent borrowing of money
- Stealing
- Disregard for personal appearance
- Impaired relationships with family and friends
- Disregard for deadlines, curfews, or other regulations
- Unusual temper flare-ups
- New friends, especially known drug dealers, and strong allegiance to these friends

Modified from National Institute on Drug Abuse. (2014d). What are the signs of drug use in adolescents and what role can parents play in getting treatment? Retrieved from http://www.drugabuse.gov/publications/principles -adolescent-substance-use-disorder-treatment-research-based-guide/frequently-asked-questions/what-are-signs-drug -use-in-adolescents-what-role-can-parents-play-in-getting-treatment

insomnia, panic attacks, paranoia, violent behavior, and psychosis. Stimulants are addictive and can trigger cardiovascular complications, stroke, and seizures.

Caffeine is one of the most widely used stimulants in the world and is found in many sources. The effects of caffeine include relief of drowsiness, help in the performance of repetitive tasks, improved mental capacity for work, and increased basal metabolic rate. Caffeine also triggers anxiety, insomnia, irregular heartbeat, faster breathing, upset stomach and bowels, dizziness, and headache in some women. Women who consume large amounts of caffeine and stop their intake may experience headaches, irritability, and fatigue.

Cocaine (street names include "coke," "blow," "snow," "bump," "toot") is a popular stimulant drug in the United States. It is commonly inhaled through the nose (snorted) in powder form but can also be smoked or injected. The drug is rapidly metabolized by the liver. The risk of developing tolerance is high with repeated use and users will need increasing amounts to achieve its effects. *Crack* is a mixture of cocaine and baking soda that can be smoked. Crack sets off rapid ups and downs and consequently produces a powerful chemical and psychological dependence. Crack users frequently need another "hit" within minutes of the previous one. Smoking cocaine in its freebase form, that is, cocaine that has been converted from its salt to its base form by heating with ether or boiling with sodium bicarbonate, also delivers a concentrated high that can disappear within seconds.

Amphetamines (street names include "bennies," "black beauties," "truck drivers," "uppers") are manufactured chemicals sold under various names. Generally found in pill form, the drugs may be ground and sniffed or made into a solution for injection. Amphetamines were once widely prescribed for weight control because they suppress the appetite and stimulate the central nervous system. *Methamphetamine*, which is a form of amphetamine (street names include "speed," "meth," "crank," "chalk," "ice"), has become less expensive and widely available, hence use has skyrocketed.

DEPRESSANTS AND ANTI-ANXIETY DRUGS

Depressants, sedatives, or hypnotics relax the central nervous system. *Alcohol* is the most widely used depressant. *Depressants* have a synergistic effect when mixed together. As the user builds up tolerance, the likelihood of a potentially fatal overdose increases.

Barbiturates (street names include "barbs," "reds," "yellows," "phennies," "tooies") are depressants that are used medically for inducing relaxation and sleep, relieving tension, and treating seizures. Barbiturates may also be administered intravenously for general anesthesia. In low doses, barbiturates cause mild intoxication, euphoria, decreased alertness, and decreased muscle coordination. Higher doses may result in slurred speech, decreased respirations, cold skin, weak and rapid heartbeat, and unconsciousness. Side effects of barbiturates include drowsiness, impaired judgment

and performance, and a hangover that may last for hours or days.

Anti-anxiety drugs such as *benzodiazepines* (street names include "candy," "downers," "tranks") are primarily prescribed to treat tension and muscular strain. The most commonly used benzodiazepines are alprazolam (Xanax) and diazepam (Valium). Benzodiazepines are relatively fast-acting medications that create effects in less than an hour. The most common side effects are drowsiness and loss of coordination. When combined with other substances such as alcohol, benzodiazepines can cause serious, life-threatening complications. When taken with benzodiazepines, medications such as anesthetics, antihistamines, sedatives, muscle relaxants, and some prescription painkillers may increase central nervous system depression. Similar to barbiturates, high doses of benzodiazepines result in slurred speech, drowsiness, and stupor.

CANNABIS (MARIJUANA)

Cannabis, also known as marijuana, pot, or weed, is made up of a mixture of crushed leaves and flower buds of the *Cannabis sativa* plant. This drug is usually ingested by smoking. *Hashish* is an extract of cannabis, but is two to ten times as concentrated as marijuana. The primary psychoactive ingredient of both marijuana and hashish is tetrahydrocannabinol (THC). Marijuana abuse and dependence typically occurs in conjunction with abuse of other drugs such as alcohol and cocaine (NIDA, 2015c).

When taken in low to moderate doses, the effects of marijuana are similar to the effects of alcohol and some tranquilizers. In contrast to alcohol, however, marijuana at low doses does not dull sensation. Rather, marijuana may cause slight alterations in perception. The acute physical effects of marijuana include increased heart rate; bloodshot eyes; dry mouth and throat; increased appetite; impaired short-term memory, attention, judgment and other cognitive functions; and impaired coordination and balance. High doses cause sensory distortion and diminish the ability to perceive and react (NIDA, 2015c).

Marijuana for medical use has been a controversial subject for many years. Research has confirmed that cannabis contains active ingredients with therapeutic potential for relieving pain, controlling nausea, stimulating appetite, and decreasing ocular pressure. Marijuana-based medications have been approved by the FDA for the treatment of nausea in patients undergoing cancer chemotherapy and to stimulate appetite in patients with wasting syndrome due to AIDS, cancer, and anorexia (NIDA, 2015c).

PSYCHEDELICS AND HALLUCINOGENS

Hallucinogenic drugs create changes in perception and thought processes. A common feature of the hallucinogenic experience is suspension of normal psychic mechanisms that integrate the self with the environment. Some of the more common effects induced by hallucinogenic drugs include changes in mood, sensation, and perception. Four common types of hallucinogens and their street names are *peyote* ("buttons," "mesc," "cactus"), *psilocybin* ("magic mushrooms," "purple passion"), *lysergic acid diethylamide* (LSD, "acid," "cubes," "yellow sunshine"), and *phencyclidine* (PCP, "angel dust," "hog," "love boat," "peace pill"). Peyote is derived from the peyote cactus and the active ingredient is mescaline. Peyote has been used by natives in northern Mexico and the southwestern United States as a part of traditional religious ceremonies for centuries and can be ingested or smoked. Psilocybin is derived from particular types of mushrooms indigenous to tropical and subtropical regions of South America, Mexico, and the United States, and can be ingested. LSD is manufactured from lysergic acid, which is found in ergot, a fungus that grows on rye and other grains and can be ingested. PCP was developed in the 1950s as

an anesthetic agent but such use has since been discontinued due to harmful adverse effects. PCP can be swallowed, smoked, or ingested (NIDA, 2014c).

Hallucinogenic drugs can also cause other unpleasant or adverse effects. Depending on the amount ingested, LSD can cause dilated pupils, elevated body temperature, increased heart rate and blood pressure, profuse sweating, loss of appetite, sleeplessness, dry mouth, and tremors. LSD may also produce a delayed reaction, known as a *flashback*. The effects of peyote are similar to those of LSD as well as uncoordinated movements (ataxia) and flushing. Psilocybin can cause muscle relaxation or weakness, ataxia, excessive papillary dilation, nausea, vomiting, and drowsiness (NIDA, 2014c). The effects of PCP are also dosage related. At low to moderate doses, PCP can cause increased heart rate, respirations, and blood pressure as well as shallow breathing, flushing, generalized numbness in the extremities, and loss of muscular coordination. At high doses, PCP can cause a drop in blood pressure, pulse, and respirations, nausea, vomiting, blurred vision, flicking up and down of the eyes, drooling, dizziness, loss of balance, and can also bring about violent or suicidal behavior, seizures, and coma. Death may result from accidental injury or suicide. The sedative effects of PCP can be enhanced by interaction with other central nervous system depressants such as alcohol or benzodiazepines, and produce coma (NIDA, 2014c).

OPIOIDS

Opioids are drugs derived from opium, and include morphine, codeine, heroin, methadone, fentanyl, oxycodone, hydrocodone, oxymorphone, meperidine, and propoxyphene. Opioid drugs have sleep-inducing and pain-relieving properties. Numerous opioid drugs are used medically for pain relief and are manufactured in injectable and oral preparations. However, opioids possess a high potential for abuse. Opioids relax the user, and when injected may produce an immediate "rush." The user may experience euphoria, drowsiness, impaired coordination, confusion, dizziness, a feeling of heaviness in the body, constipation, and nausea (NIDA, 2015a). With large doses of opioids, the skin becomes moist, cold, and bluish, and pupils become smaller. Respirations slow and the user may become unresponsive.

Heroin (street names include "smack," "skag," "horse," "junk") is an opioid drug that is synthesized from morphine. It can be smoked, sniffed, or injected. Chronic use of heroin can lead to addiction and severe health consequences. Approximately 23% of heroin users develop dependency on the drug. Reduction or abrupt cessation of the drug may trigger symptoms of withdrawal, which include restlessness, insomnia, diarrhea, vomiting, muscle and bone pain, cold flashes with goose bumps, and kicking movements. Symptoms are also accompanied by a severe craving for the drug, which can precipitate continued abuse and/or relapse. Craving for heroin can persist for years after drug cessation, especially when the user is exposed to circumstances and environments associated with drug use. Withdrawal symptoms usually subside after one week; however, some individuals may experience persistent withdrawal symptoms that linger for months. Although heroin withdrawal is thought to be less hazardous than barbiturate or alcohol withdrawal, abrupt withdrawal by heavily dependent users who are in poor health might at times be fatal (NIDA, 2014b).

Inhalants

Inhalants (street names include "laughing gas," "poppers," "snappers," "whippets") are chemicals that produce vapors that have psychoactive effects and are predominantly abused by preadolescents and young adults. The chemicals that are used as inhalants are not meant for inhalation, such as solvents, aerosols, cleaning fluids, and petroleum products. Although the effects of inhalants vary by chemical, users tend to experience stimulation and loss of inhibitions. Adverse side effects include headache, nausea and vomiting, slurred speech, loss of motor coordination, wheezing, cramps, muscle weakness, depression, and memory impairment (NIDA, 2015a). Abusers frequently have chemical odors on the breath or clothing, paint or other stains on the face or clothing, and hidden empty solvent containers or chemical soaked rags may be in their possession. Regular use of inhalants leads to tolerance, so increasingly higher doses are needed to achieve the desired effects. Because many inhalants are widely available household products, they are often tried by young people or those who cannot afford or do not have access to more illicit drugs.

Club Drugs

Club drugs, also known as designer drugs, are a group of pharmacologically heterogeneous psychoactive drugs, produced in chemical laboratories, and are frequently abused by teens and young adults at bars, nightclubs, concerts, and parties. They include *MDMA* (methylenedioxymethamphetamine), *GHB* (gamma-hydroxybutyrate), *Rohypnol* (flunitrazepam), and *Ketamine*.

MDMA (street names include "ecstasy," "Adam," "Eve," "lover's speed," "peace") is a synthetic psychoactive drug that is similar in chemical composition to methamphetamine and mescaline. MDMA is usually taken as a pill or capsule but can also be ground to a powder and snorted or injected. The drug produces feelings of euphoria, emotional warmth, increased energy, increased tactile sensitivity, and lowered inhibitions. Adverse side effects include anxiety, chills, sweating, teeth clenching, muscle cramping, sleep disturbances, depression, impaired memory, hyperthermia, and addiction (NIDA, 2015a).

Rohypnol (street names include "forget-me pill," "Mexican valium," "R2," "roach," "roofies," "rope") is a benzodiazepine chemically similar to sedative-hypnotic drugs such as Valium and Xanax. Rohypnol is not approved for medical use in the United States and its importation is banned. Rohypnol causes sedation and muscle relaxation, confusion, memory loss, dizziness, impaired coordination, dependence, and addiction. It can be ingested orally in pill form and can also be ground to a powder and snorted (NIDA, 2015a).

GHB (street names include "G," Georgia," "homeboy," "liquid ecstasy," "liquid X, "soap," "scoop," "goop") is a central nervous system depressant that was approved by FDA in 2002 strictly for the treatment of narcolepsy. GHB causes drowsiness, nausea, headache, disorientation, loss of concentration, memory loss, unconsciousness, seizures, and coma. Repeated use can lead to dependence, whereupon cessation can produce symptoms of withdrawal such as insomnia, sweating, anxiety, and tremors. More severe withdrawal symptoms may occur with overdose of GHB or related compounds, particularly if other drugs or alcohol are involved (NIDA, 2015a). GHB is usually ingested orally in either liquid or powder form.

Ketamine (street names include "SV," "cat Valium," "Special K," "vitamin K") is a dissociative anesthetic agent that is mostly used in veterinary practice. The drug is usually snorted or injected intramuscularly. Ketamine produces feelings of being separate from one's body and environment. It can cause impaired motor function, anxiety, tremors, numbness, impaired memory, nausea, delirium, respiratory depression and arrest, and death. Binging has been reported with ketamine, and users can develop tolerance and craving for the drug (NIDA, 2015a).

PRESCRIPTION DRUGS

After marijuana, prescription and over-the-counter drugs are the most frequently abused substances by Americans aged 14 and over. Prescription drugs are considered abused when they are taken without a prescription, used in ways other than prescribed, or for the feelings or experience elicited by the medication (NIDA, 2014c). The three classes of prescription drugs most commonly abused are *opioids* (prescribed for pain, such as codeine, morphine, oxycodone, hydrocodone, and oxymorphone), *central nervous system depressants* (prescribed for anxiety and sleep disorders, such as benzodiazepines and barbiturates), and *stimulants* (prescribed for narcolepsy and attention–deficit hyperactivity disorders, such as methylphenidate [Ritalin] and dextroamphetamine [Dexedrine]). *Over-the-counter drugs* commonly abused include certain cough suppressants, antihistamines, and sleep aids. Cough syrup and cold medications that contain dextromethorphan can produce euphoria, and at high doses have PCP-like or Ketamine-like dissociative effects. Most of these drugs can cause addiction and place abusers at high risk for adverse health effects, including overdose, especially when taken with other drugs or alcohol (NIDA, 2014c).

Drug Dependency

Drug dependency refers to the physical attachment, psychological attachment, or both that a person may develop to a drug. Physical dependence occurs through normal adaptation of body cells to chronic exposure to a drug. These physiological changes produce an overpowering constant need for the drug. Physical dependence on a drug will cause the individual to experience withdrawal symptoms such as intense anxiety, extreme nausea, and deep craving for the drug when the drug is abruptly reduced or stopped. Physical dependency can be caused by tranquilizers, barbiturates, and opioids. Dependence is frequently accompanied by drug tolerance. Tolerance requires that the individual take higher doses of the drug in order to achieve the same effect (NIDA, 2014c). Cross-tolerance can also develop with drug dependence.

In this condition, the tolerance of one drug leads to tolerance of other drugs that are chemically related or that have similar effects.

Physical dependence of a drug is not the same as addiction, although the two are closely associated. Addiction can include physical dependence, and is distinguished by compulsive drug seeking behavior and use, despite devastating consequences (NIDA, 2014c). With psychological dependence, habituation creates strong cravings for a drug because the drug produces pleasurable feelings or relieves stress or anxiety. Physical and psychological dependence do not always co-exist. For example, marijuana and LSD may not create physical dependence; however, their continued use can cause psychological dependence.

Screening for Substance Abuse

The extent and nature of the substance use disorder and its interaction with other life areas must be understood in order to achieve careful diagnosis, appropriate case management, and successful treatment of women. The screening and assessment process is the starting point for gaining this understanding and for matching women with suitable treatment services (CSAT, 2009). To ensure that important information is obtained, healthcare providers should utilize evidence-based standardized screening and assessment instruments and interview protocols that are accurate, valid, and sensitive in identifying problems with women. Numerous specific instruments are available to assist counselors in determining if further assessment is needed, the nature and extent of a woman's substance use disorder, if a co-occurring psychiatric disorder is present, if a woman has had traumatic experiences and if particular consequences exist, and treatment-related factors that may influence the woman's response to interventions (CSAT, 2009).

Substance abuse screening is performed to detect women who have or are developing alcohol- or drug-related problems. Characteristically, substance abuse problems are more likely identified in men than in women. However, women are more likely to present significant health problems associated with consuming fewer substances in a shorter period of time (CSAT, 2009). The screening process, which is typically the first contact between a woman and the treatment system, enables the woman to develop an initial impression of treatment. Women enter the treatment system most frequently through obstetric and primary care; hospital emergency rooms; social service agencies in connection with housing, child care, disabilities, and domestic violence; community mental health services; and correctional facilities. Screening can be done by nurses, nurse practitioners, physicians, physicians' assistants, and social service professionals to determine whether women use or abuse alcohol, drugs, or tobacco. Because *how* screening is conducted sets the tone of treatment and initiates the relationship with the woman, it can be as important as the actual information that is gathered. Although a screening can outline a woman's involvement with alcohol, drugs, or both, it does not provide a diagnosis or give particulars regarding how substances have affected the woman's life (CSAT, 2009). **Box 7–4** presents the most important domains that should be included in the screening process.

An interview or a short written questionnaire is used to screen for substance use disorders. Numerous screening instruments exist for alcohol consumption, and several tools have been adapted to screen for specific drugs. However, evidence that supports reliability and validity of these instruments specifically for use with women is limited. Instruments frequently used to screen for substance abuse in women include the Alcohol Use Disorder Identification Test (AUDIT), Texas Christian University Drug Screen II (TCUDS II), and the CAGE Questionnaire. The AUDIT is noted to be

Box 7–4: Essential Domains of Screening for Substance Use Disorder

The screening of women for substance use disorder should include the following essential areas:

- Substance abuse

- Pregnancy considerations

- Immediate risks related to serious intoxication or withdrawal

- Immediate risks for self-harm, suicide, and violence

- Past and present mental disorders, such as PTSD, other anxiety disorders, mood disorders, and eating disorders

- Past and present history of violence and trauma, including sexual victimization and interpersonal violence

- Health screenings, including for HIV/AIDS, hepatitis, tuberculosis, and STDs

Modified from Center for Substance Abuse Treatment. (2009). *Substance abuse treatment: Addressing the specific needs of women.* (Treatment Improvement Protocol (TIP) Series 51. HHS Publication No. (SMA) 09-4426). Rockville, MD: Substance Abuse and Mental Health Services Administration.

effective in screening for heavy alcohol consumption among nonpregnant women. The TCUDS II is used widely in criminal justice settings and has good reliability among female populations. The CAGE Questionnaire screens for lifetime drug or alcohol consumption; however, there is criticism that the CAGE lacks gender sensitivity. Women with alcohol use problems are more likely to receive false negative scores on the CAGE Questionnaire—that is, the likelihood for some women who are at risk for substance problems to screen negative (CSAT, 2009).

Although up to 40% of people seeing physicians and/or reporting to hospital emergency departments for care likely have an alcohol use disorder (CSAT, 2009), physicians frequently refrain from screening, referring, or intervening with these patients (Kuehn, 2008). Even healthcare professionals who use screening tools for some patients are less likely to screen women, particularly older women, women of Asian descent, and those from middle and upper socioeconomic levels, because substance abuse in these populations is not an expected occurrence. Moreover, women are less likely to be admonished about their alcohol consumption or counseled to modify or stop their drinking. Without a doubt, in order to be worthwhile, screening must bring about suitable referrals for further evaluation and treatment. Missed opportunities can be ill-fated, especially during prenatal care, in light of the consequences of substance use for maternal and infant health (CSAT, 2009).

In response to the disengagement that starts with lack of identification of substance-related problems of the patient and extends to the failure of appropriate referrals and brief interventions, the SBIRT was developed and implemented across healthcare settings. To date, substantial evidence indicates that the SBIRT program has been effective in reducing risky alcohol consumption. The evidence for the effectiveness of SBIRT in reducing risky drug use is accumulating and shows promising results. The effectiveness of SBIRT approaches for all forms of tobacco use, especially smoking, has been endorsed by the U.S. Preventative Services Task Force. SBIRT approaches for screening adults, particularly pregnant women, for tobacco use, have been effective in increasing the proportion of smokers who successfully quit smoking and remain abstinent after 1 year (SAMHSA, 2011).

Treatment of Substance Abuse

Substance addictions are complex conditions distinguished by intense and sometimes uncontrollable drug craving, as well as compulsive drug seeking behavior and persistent use even in the face of devastating consequences. Although the route to drug addiction is initiated with the voluntary act of taking drugs, eventually the ability of an a woman to decide to refrain from taking drugs becomes compromised, resulting in compulsion to seek and consume the drug.

This behavior is mainly the consequence of prolonged drug exposure on brain functioning. The disease of addiction affects numerous brain pathways, including those engaged in reward and motivation, learning and memory, and inhibitory control over behavior (NIDA, 2009). Treatment is not a simple process, due to the many dimensions of drug abuse and addiction as well as the disruption it causes in various aspects of life. Many components are incorporated into effective treatment programs, and each is focused on a particular aspect of the illness and its consequences. Treatment of substance addiction must assist the woman to stop using drugs, sustain a drug-free lifestyle, and attain productive functioning in the family, at work, and in society. Addiction is typically a chronic disease. As such, women cannot simply stop using drugs for a few days and be cured. Long-term or repeated episodes of care are required to attain the crucial goal of sustained abstinence and recovery of their lives (NIDA, 2009). Key principles of effective treatment of substance abuse are summarized in **Box 7–5**.

Medication and behavioral therapy are indispensable elements of an overall therapeutic treatment process, particularly when combined. The treatment process often begins with detoxification, which is followed by treatment and relapse prevention. An important focus at the initiation of treatment is the easing of withdrawal symptoms, and preventing relapse is essential for sustaining treatment effectiveness. As with other chronic conditions, relapse may occur, and this requires revisiting prior treatment components. A continuum of care approach is needed in which a customized treatment regimen addresses all aspects of a woman's life. This approach should include medical and mental health services, and follow-up options such as community- or family-based recovery support systems. Such an approach to treatment is crucial to a woman's success in achieving and maintaining a substance free lifestyle (NIDA, 2009).

Smoking Cessation

Smoking cessation is the most significant personal behavior a woman can undertake to improve her health. Although the recovery from smoking takes time, smoking cessation results in a gradual decrease in risk for cancer and cardiovascular disease. The same is not true for risk of chronic obstructive pulmonary disease. Although cessation of smoking decreases the rate of loss of pulmonary function, lost function cannot be regained. Timely cessation of cigarette smoking is the best prevention of symptomatic pulmonary disease.

Smoking cessation is not an easy process. Women who desire to stop smoking on their own may either choose gradual reduction or abrupt cessation (going "cold turkey"). The process of gradual reduction

Box 7–5: Principles of Effective Treatment for Substance Abuse

The key principles that should form the basis of any effective treatment program are:

- Addiction is a complex but treatable disease that affects brain function and behavior.
- No single treatment is appropriate for everyone.
- Treatment needs to be readily available.
- Effective treatment attends to multiple needs of the individual, not just his or her drug abuse. Many drug-addicted individuals also have other mental disorders.
- Remaining in treatment for an adequate period of time is critical.
- Counseling—individual and/or group—and other behavioral therapies are the most commonly used forms of substance abuse treatment.
- Medications are an important element of treatment for many patients, especially when combined with counseling and other behavioral therapies.
- An individual's treatment and services plan must be assessed continually and modified as necessary to ensure that it meets her changing needs.
- Medically assisted detoxification is only the first stage of addiction treatment and by itself does little to change long-term drug abuse.
- Treatment does not need to be voluntary to be effective.
- Drug use during treatment must be monitored continuously, as lapses during treatment do occur.
- Treatment programs should assess patients for the presence infectious diseases such as HIV/AIDS, hepatitis B and C, tuberculosis, and should provide targeted risk-reduction counseling to help patients modify or change behaviors that place them at risk of contracting or spreading infectious diseases.

Modified from National Institute on Drug Abuse. (2012a). *Principles of drug abuse treatment: A research-based guide* 3rd ed. (NIH Publication No. 12–4180). Retrieved from http://www.drugabuse.gov/sites/default/files/podat_1.pdf

involves gently tapering the number of cigarettes smoked per day and also reducing the relative amount of tar and nicotine exposure by changing to brands of cigarettes with progressively lower and lower levels of these substances. Many strategies can be used in the process of gradual reduction, all of which serve to modify traditional smoking behavior and reinforce progress toward total cessation.

The abrupt cessation, or "cold turkey," approach requires making a sudden decisive break from cigarettes. Some people find that they are able to use this approach if they do it one day at a time. They promise themselves to be smoke free for 24 hours; at the end of that day they reaffirm their commitment to another smoke-free day. It may take several weeks or months for a former heavy smoker to become confident about the newly acquired nonsmoking status.

Smoking cessation programs have evolved since 1964, when the first Surgeon General's Report on Smoking and Health was published. Intervention strategies for smoking cessation now include a variety of treatment modalities. These modalities may be individualized or group based, formal or informal in design. Multicomponent, behaviorally oriented programs seem to elicit the most favorable results for short- and long-term smoking cessation. These programs frequently incorporate several treatment modalities, including aversive conditioning, contracting, self-control, stimulus control, group support, and cessation maintenance. These strategies help individuals to recognize high-risk smoking situations, develop alternative coping strategies, improve problem-solving skills, manage stress, and utilize social support (NIDA, 2012c).

Pharmacological agents, such as nicotine gum and transdermal nicotine patches, are often used with multicomponent treatment programs as well. Although the evidence is not consistent, a number of studies have found that the use of nicotine gum in conjunction with sessions of counseling to manage psychological issues can be effective in helping some people stop smoking. Transdermal nicotine patches are showing greater efficacy as an alternative to nicotine gums. Other forms of treatment for smoking cessation that are available by prescription include nasal sprays, lozenges, and a special inhaler (NIDA, 2012c). Two medications have also been used for smoking cessation. Varenicline (Chantix) is a smoking cessation aid that blocks the pleasant effects of nicotine on the brain. The drug is used in conjunction with education and counseling to help individuals to stop smoking. Another drug that aids in smoking cessation is the antidepressant bupropion (Zyban), which reduces cravings for nicotine and other effects of nicotine withdrawal (NIDA, 2012c). Both varenicline and bupropion must be used cautiously because behavior changes, agitation, depressed mood, suicide ideation, and actual suicide behavior can develop with either drug, and thus treatment must be closely monitored by the healthcare provider.

Other treatment strategies for smoking cessation that some people have found helpful include hypnosis and acupuncture. In addition, a vaccine for the prevention and treatment of tobacco addiction is currently under investigation. This vaccine is designed to stimulate the production of antibodies that would block access of nicotine to the brain (NIDA, 2012c).

Alcoholism

The most difficult and significant step for an alcoholic is admitting to an alcohol problem. Often, well-intended friends or family members, out of fear, embarrassment, loyalty, or hope, shield the alcoholic from the truth. Confrontation, either personal or via a motor vehicle accident or drunk driving conviction, that makes the individual acknowledge the alcohol problem, is often a turning point in seeking assistance. Recovery from alcoholism is enhanced when the person has a strong emotional support system, including concerned family, friends, and employer.

Alcoholism is a complex problem, and each case must be treated with sensitivity and recognition of its unique situation and contributing factors. Standard treatment programs focus on the relief of physiological dependence but do not eliminate the underlying disease. Individual personality, psychological, and sociocultural factors must be addressed to help the alcoholic woman regain control of her life. Alcohol treatment programs often follow three steps in the treatment of alcoholism:

- Managing acute intoxication episodes
- Correcting chronic health problems associated with alcoholism
- Changing long-term behavior

The most successful treatment modalities combine multiple approaches and provide ongoing support for people who are learning to live without alcohol, and help them to deal with their withdrawal symptoms through detoxification programs. Detoxification programs are generally available in medical or psychiatric facilities. Psychological addiction is usually addressed immediately after the detoxification process is completed. Programs such as Alcoholics Anonymous, which is entirely run by volunteers who are recovering alcoholics, provide support for people trying to maintain their abstinence from alcohol.

Three medications have been approved by the FDA for treatment of alcohol dependence and are currently available. Naltrexone blocks opioid receptors in the brain that are associated with the rewarding effects of drinking and the craving for alcohol. Naltrexone is highly effective in reducing relapse to heavy drinking in some but not all patients. This disparity may be associated with genetic differences. Acamprosate is a medication that helps modulate and regulate brain activity and reduces symptoms of protracted (post-acute) withdrawal, such as insomnia, anxiety, restlessness, and dysphoria. Disulfiram interferes with the degradation of alcohol, resulting in the accumulation of acetaldehyde. The acetaldehyde can cause a very unpleasant reaction that includes flushing, nausea, and palpitations. Compliance may be problematic, but in highly motivated patients, disulfiram can be very effective. Topiramate, an anticonvulsive medication, has been under investigation for treatment of alcohol dependence, and results from clinical trials have been encouraging (NIDA, 2009).

Drug Dependency

There are three basic approaches to drug abuse treatment: detoxification, behavioral treatment therapies, and outpatient or residential programs. Different forms of intervention are available to meet the needs of different women and are applicable to diverse dependencies.

DETOXIFICATION

Detoxification is supervised withdrawal from drug dependence. It is a process designed to manage the acute and potentially dangerous physiological effects of stopping drug use. Detoxification is commonly regarded as a precursor to treatment or a first stage of treatment. It can be done either with or without medication, and in a hospital or outpatient setting. Medically assisted detoxification is the first step in the treatment process. Detoxification alone is rarely adequate to help women attain long-term abstinence. Patients who do not receive further treatment beyond detoxification may revert to drug abuse patterns similar to those who were never treated (NIDA, 2009, 2012a).

Medications assist in the suppression of withdrawal symptoms during detoxification. The medications used in detoxification help to reestablish normal brain function, prevent relapse, and diminish cravings. Presently, medication is available for use in opioid addiction, and work is underway in developing medications for the treatment of stimulant (cocaine, methamphetamine) and cannabis (marijuana) addictions. In reality, most people with severe addiction problems are users of more than one drug. Thus individuals with polydrug habits will require treatment for all of the substances that they abuse (NIDA, 2009).

The medications used to treat opioid addiction include methadone, buprenorhine, and naltrexone. Methadone and buprenorphine are used to suppress withdrawal symptoms and relieve cravings. These medications are used for both detoxification and short- and long-term maintenance treatment. Naltrexone blocks the effects of heroin or other opioids at their receptor sites and is used in patients who have already been through detoxification (NIDA, 2009). Naltrexone is not as widely used as the other medications due to compliance issues. Overall, the medications help patients disengage from drug-seeking and associated criminal behavior and become more receptive to behavioral treatment modalities (NIDA, 2009). Once the detoxification process is completed, formal assessment and referral to subsequent drug addiction treatment should follow (NIDA, 2012a).

Behavioral Treatment

Behavioral treatment approaches are available to help patients participate in the treatment process, change their attitudes and behaviors associated with drug abuse, and enhance healthy life skills. These approaches can augment the efficacy of medication therapy as well as assist women to stay in treatment longer. Because behavioral treatment therapies focus on different facets of addiction, combinations of behavioral therapies and medications (when available) are likely to be more successful than either approach used by itself (NIDA, 2009, 2012a). Behavioral treatment therapies that may be offered include:

- *Cognitive-behavioral therapy.* This approach focuses on helping women to recognize, avoid, and cope with situations in which they are most likely to abuse drugs.
- *Mulitdimensional family therapy.* This approach was developed for adolescents with drug abuse problems and their families, and focuses on a wide range of influences on their drug abuse patterns. It is designed to improve family functioning on the whole.
- *Motivational interviewing.* This approach makes the most of the readiness of women to change their behavior and enter treatment.
- *Motivational incentives.* This approach, also known as contingency management, utilizes positive reinforcement to encourage drug abstinence (NIDA, 2009).

Outpatient or Residential Programs

Treatment for drug abuse and addiction can be provided in a variety of diverse settings and employ an array of behavioral approaches. Outpatient behavioral treatment offers a wide assortment of programs for women who attend a clinic at regular intervals. Most outpatient programs offer individual or group drug counseling. Outpatient treatment is less costly than residential or inpatient treatment and is frequently more suitable for employed individuals or those who have extensive social support. It is important to note that low-intensity programs may provide little more than drug education, and their efficacy could be questionable. On the other hand, other models of outpatient programs, such as intensive day treatment, could be similar to residential programs with respect to services and effectiveness, depending on the characteristics and needs of the individual patient. Some outpatient treatment programs are designed to also treat the patients' medical or mental health problems along with their drug disorders (NIDA, 2012a).

For women who experience more severe problems, particularly those with long histories of substance addiction, involvement in serious criminal activity, and severely impaired social functioning, long-term residential treatment programs, such as therapeutic communities, can be very helpful. Therapeutic communities are highly structured, drug-free environments in which patients remain at a residence typically for 6 to 12 months. While in residence, patients live under strict rules and participate in individual and group therapy. Therapeutic communities are different from other treatment approaches. In therapeutic communities the entire community, which includes treatment staff and residents, as well as the social context, are utilized as active components of treatment to achieve change in patients' attitudes, perceptions, and behaviors related to drug use. Addiction is considered within the context of the social and psychological deficits of an individual. The focus of treatment is on building personal accountability and responsibility and developing socially productive lives. Treatment can at times be confrontational, and it provides activities that help residents scrutinize damaging beliefs, self-concepts, and destructive behavior patterns. Residents develop more harmonious and constructive ways to interact with others.

Many therapeutic communities offer additional services such as employment training and other supportive services. Therapeutic communities can be modified to accommodate pregnant women or women who have children (NIDA, 2009, 2012a).

Short-term residential treatment is another option. These programs make available relatively brief but intensive treatment based on a modified 12-step approach. The short-term residential treatment program is comprised of a 3- to 6-week hospital-based inpatient treatment phase followed by extended outpatient therapy and participation in a self-help group, such as Alcoholics Anonymous. After completion of a residential treatment program, it is essential that patients remain engaged in outpatient treatment programs and/or aftercare programs. These programs facilitate recovery by decreasing the risk of relapse once a patient leaves the residential setting (NIDA, 2012a).

Criminal justice sanctions united with drug treatment have been effective in decreasing crime associated with drug abuse. Individuals under legal coercion are likely to stay in treatment longer and have treatment outcomes that are just as good as or better than those not under legal pressure. Frequently, drug abusers interface with the criminal justice system earlier than they do with health or other social systems. Consequently, they are often presented with opportunities for intervention and treatment prior to, during, after, or instead of incarceration. This may in due course interrupt and shorten a career of drug use (NIDA, 2012a).

Quality of Life Issues Associated With Substance Abuse

Substance abuse is a chronic condition that frequently leads to severe impairment or distress. The substance abuser characteristically experiences painful symptoms, disrupted physical and psychological functioning, threatened personal safety, disturbed family and social relations, criminal activity,

and disrupted school and work roles and obligations. Without a doubt, substance abuse greatly impacts the quality of life of women. Quality of life issues and concerns associated with substance abuse are complex, multidimensional, and commonly involve the domains of health and physical functioning, psychological and spiritual well-being, socioeconomic integrity, and family well-being.

In comparison to other mental health and biomedical disciplines, research that systematically presents quality of life as an essential outcome has been lagging in the field of substance addiction, despite the impact of substance abuse on patients, families, and society (Laudet, 2011; Tracy et al., 2012). Although a growing body of evidence focuses largely on the quality of life of alcohol dependent populations, research directed toward quality of life in drug abusing populations remains sparse. Research in drug abusing populations tends to spotlight populations with opioid dependency and/or dual diagnoses of substance abuse and mental illnesses or dual diagnoses of substance abuse and HIV or hepatitis C (Laudet, 2011). Research has also yielded evidence on some domains of quality of life, such as health and physical functioning or psychological functioning with respect to achieving recovery goals (Laudet, 2011). Evidence that focuses solely on quality of life of women with substance abuse is particularly limited (Robinson, 2006). Nonetheless, existing evidence suggests that women with substance abuse tend to experience poorer quality of life than male substance abusers and non-substance abusing populations (Domingo-Salvany et al., 2010; Tracy et al., 2012). Evidence also suggests that quality of life remains poor during active addiction, improves significantly with abstinence, and deteriorates among individuals who relapse (Laudet, Becker, & White, 2009).

Effective treatment approaches that sustain remission and decrease risk of relapse are essential for maintaining acceptable quality of life among female substance abusers. However, women may experience numerous obstacles and barriers that impede them from achieving long-standing stable recovery. Although treatment barriers may not be exclusive to women, the myriad demands associated with women's various caregiver roles, the intrinsic socioeconomic and health conditions particularly related to substance use disorders, and the societal bias and stigma related to substance abuse likely generate treatment barriers for women more frequently (CSAT, 2009). Such barriers exist on the individual, relational, sociocultural, structural, and system levels. They obstruct treatment entry, engagement in and continuous use of treatment services across the spectrum of care, and maintenance of connections with community services and self-help groups that support recovery over the long term.

Treatment engagement approaches that support the initiation of treatment and address the diverse challenges that frequently impede treatment involvement have become essential to the stable recovery of women from substance dependency. Engagement services are comprised of an assortment of strategies aimed at promoting suitable access to treatment, increasing treatment utilization, promoting treatment retention, and enhancing treatment outcome. The strategies range from formal approaches such as comprehensive case management and incentive programs that promote engagement to less formal specific services such as transportation and escorts to appointments, phone calls to initiate services and remind patients of appointments, and child care during scheduled appointments or sessions. Of particular benefit to women are outreach services, pretreatment intervention groups, and comprehensive case management (CSAT, 2009).

Issues Affecting Health and Physical Functioning

HEALTH EFFECTS OF TOBACCO ADDICTION

Women who use tobacco often develop considerable health consequences that impact the health and physical functioning domain of quality of life. Health risks to smokers depend not only on smoking status but also on specific smoking behaviors and duration of such behaviors, such as amount smoked, inhalation patterns, and the content of tar and nicotine in cigarettes. Women who smoke substantially increase their risk for cancer of the lung, bladder, cervix, pancreas, kidney, larynx, esophagus, liver, and colon. Smoking increases the risk of cardiovascular disease, stroke, premature decline in pulmonary function, and chronic obstructive pulmonary disease. Smoking also imparts an increased risk of peptic ulcer disease and Crohn's disease (CSAT, 2009). Moreover, women who smoke often experience premature signs of aging such as wrinkles, blotchy skin, and discolored teeth.

Reproductive health is affected by smoking. Women who smoke may experience an increased risk of estrogen deficiency, menstrual irregularities, dysmenorrhea, and amenorrhea. They may be at risk for early menopause as well as osteoporosis. Smoking can cause delayed conception and infertility, and increases the risk of adverse effects on pregnancy and fetal growth, such as spontaneous abortion, premature delivery, stillbirths, and babies with low birthweight. Furthermore, the effects of smoking can be transmitted to infants via breast milk after the baby is born.

HEALTH EFFECTS OF ALCOHOL CONSUMPTION AND ALCOHOLISM

Research findings have acknowledged that women are more susceptible to the consumption and long-term effects of alcohol and drugs than men. As discussed earlier, differences in absorption to metabolic processes make it more difficult for women to physically manage the consequences of substance abuse. The tendency to have higher levels of alcohol and drugs in the system for longer periods of time increases women's vulnerability to diseases and organ damage associated with substance abuse (CSAT, 2009).

Heavy alcohol consumption can cause considerable health consequences that impact the health and physical functioning domain of quality of life. In alcohol consumption, the body organ most vulnerable to the effects of alcohol is the liver, as it metabolizes alcohol. Heavy drinking can result in alcoholic hepatitis, which is characterized by inflammation and destruction of liver cells. Heavy drinking can also lead to cirrhosis, which produces progressive scarring and dysfunction of liver tissue. In comparison to men, women develop liver disease in a shorter period of time and after consuming less alcohol (CSAT, 2009). Chronic heavy alcohol consumption is also associated with cardiovascular damage, stroke, and cardiovascular disease. Although light consumption (less than one drink per day) may be a protective factor for older women at risk for coronary heart disease, women who are alcohol dependent or consume heavier amounts of alcohol are more likely to die prematurely of cardiac-related conditions (CSAT, 2009). Evidence indicates that alcohol significantly increases the risk of cancers in the breast, cervix, ovaries, oral cavity, pharynx, esophagus, larynx, stomach, colon, rectum, and liver. Chronic heavy alcohol consumption can also produce several nutritional and gastrointestinal problems, such as nutritional and vitamin deficiencies, osteoporosis, gastritis, stomach ulcers, and intestinal lesions (CSAT, 2009).

The most dramatic effects of alcohol are on the brain and behavior. As a central nervous system depressant, alcohol alters the activity of brain neurons, impairing sensory, motor, and cognitive function. Moderate amounts of alcohol also have disturbing effects on perception, judgment, and psychomotor skills. The anesthetic effect of alcohol may cause diminished perception of pain and temperature, possibly leading to serious injury or exposure to extreme temperatures. Chronic alcohol consumption can also lead to progressive reduction in behavioral activity, general anesthesia, coma, and even death (CSAT, 2009).

Although drinking may decrease judgment, increase interest, and reduce inhibitions in sex, it also impairs a woman's ability to achieve orgasm. Alcohol also plays an indirect role in many unwanted pregnancies and sexually transmitted infections. Because of impaired judgment and reasoning due to intoxication, contraception and safe sex practices may be forgotten or ignored. Alcohol is often a factor in episodes of acquaintance rape and incidents of pressured sex (CSAT, 2009).

Alcohol can harm reproductive health and pregnancy. Chronic heavy drinking may be associated with menstrual disorders, infertility, and possibly early menopause. Alcohol crosses the placental barrier and has varying effects on the developing fetus, depending on degree and timing of exposure, genetic differences in maternal metabolism of alcohol, maternal nutritional status, and possible interaction with other drug compounds. Heavy alcohol consumption during pregnancy increases risk of spontaneous abortion. A direct effect of alcohol in pregnant women is fetal alcohol syndrome, which is characterized by specific mental and physical abnormalities in infants born to mothers who consumed alcohol during pregnancy. Symptoms of fetal alcohol syndrome include small body weight and size, slower than normal development and failure to catch up, skeletal and organ deformities, facial abnormalities, and central nervous system handicaps (Bertrand et al., 2004). In addition, alcohol consumption may inhibit the release of the hormones oxytocin and prolactin, which are necessary for initiation and maintenance of lactation.

HEALTH EFFECTS OF DRUG USE AND ABUSE

The use and abuse of drugs can seriously impair the health and physical functioning domain of quality of life. The effects of drug abuse on health and physical functioning vary and are dependent on numerous factors such as amount and duration of use, patterns of use, and mono- or polydrug usage. As previously noted, across substance use, women who are substance abusers are more vulnerable to physical complications and experience more symptoms than men (CSAT, 2009).

Stimulants such as cocaine and amphetamines can produce cardiovascular damage due to the substantial strain placed on the cardiovascular system. Methamphetamine use can cause severe dental decay. Cocaine and crack are dangerous for both pregnant women and their unborn babies. These drugs can cause miscarriage, premature labor, low birthweight babies, and babies with small head circumference. Women who use cocaine while pregnant are more likely to miscarry in the first trimester than other groups of women, including women who do not use drugs and women who use heroin or other narcotics. Infants born to cocaine and crack users suffer major complications, including drug withdrawal and permanent disabilities. Because cocaine affects blood pressure, it can deprive the fetal brain of oxygen or cause rupture of fetal cerebral blood vessels that can result in the prenatal equivalent of a stroke and permanent physical and mental damage. Cocaine babies may also experience respiratory and kidney problems, visual problems, low birthweight, seizures, depression, lack of coordination, and developmental retardation.

Regular use of depressants such as barbiturates and antianxiety drugs can lead to physical dependence. Furthermore, using depressants in combination with alcohol can have serious, life-threatening effects. Barbiturates are highly addictive, and addicts tend to be sleepy, confused, or irritable. Withdrawal from barbiturate dependence is a time-consuming process and is difficult to manage. Withdrawal symptoms include anxiety, insomnia, delirium, and convulsions. Systemic dependence is so critical that occasionally abrupt cessation of barbiturate use can lead to death. Physiological and physical dependence on anti-anxiety drugs can occur within 2 to 4 weeks. Withdrawal symptoms from anti-anxiety drugs may include coma, psychosis, and death. Use of depressants during pregnancy can be problematic. Barbiturates easily cross the placenta and can cause birth defects and behavioral problems. Babies born to mothers who abused sedatives during pregnancy may be physically dependent on the drugs and are more prone to respiratory problems, feeding difficulties, disturbed sleep, sweating, irritability, and fever.

Marijuana and hashish abuse can lead to impaired sleep, impaired memory, and impaired learning skills. These effects may not be permanent. Frequent marijuana use has the potential to promote cancer of the lungs and other parts of the respiratory system. Over the long term, chronic marijuana abuse may lead to addiction, increased risk of cough and bronchitis, increased heart rate and hypertension, compromised immunity, and increased risk of developing comorbid mental disorders and psychosis (NIDA, 2015c). Chronic use of marijuana may suppress ovulation and alter hormone levels in women. Frequent use of marijuana during pregnancy may result in lower birthweight infants and appears to be associated with altered responses to visual stimuli, increased tremulousness, and a high-pitched cry in infants, which could be indicative of problems with neurological development. Evidence suggests that marijuana-exposed children are more likely to demonstrate gaps in problem solving skills, memory, and the ability to remain attentive (NIDA, 2015c).

Hallucinogenic drugs can cause users to be unpredictably violent. PCP, in particular, can increase the risk of violent or suicidal behavior, seizures, and coma. Hallucinogenic drugs increase the risk of developing flashbacks, stupor, coma, convulsions, heart and lung failure, and brain damage. Hallucinogenic drugs produce tolerance to their psychedelic effects but do not create physical dependence or produce symptoms of withdrawal, even after long-term use. As with most psychoactive drugs, however, there is danger of psychological dependence. It is unknown whether use of hallucinogenic drugs during pregnancy affects the fetus.

Opioid drugs use can lead to physical dependence, and death is possible from a fatal drug overdose. Over time, opioid users may develop malnutrition, compromised immunity, heart infections, skin abscesses, and congested lungs. Abuse of opioids, especially heroin, is associated with increased risk of transmission of HIV, hepatitis B and C, sexually transmitted diseases, and other blood-borne diseases through use of unsterile drug equipment and risky behavior brought about by drug abuse (NIDA, 2012d). The risk of contracting HIV and hepatitis is especially high among women who inject drugs as well as have sexual intercourse with partners who inject drugs (CSAT, 2009). Use of heroin during pregnancy, coupled with poor nutrition and inadequate prenatal care, is associated with adverse consequences such as low birthweight that likely contributes to developmental delay. Consistent abuse of heroin during pregnancy may cause the infant to be born physically dependent on heroin and suffer severe withdrawal symptoms after birth (NIDA, 2012d).

Inhalants may cause serious medical complications such as hepatitis with liver failure, kidney failure, respiratory impairment, cardiovascular and nervous system damage, destruction of bone marrow, blood abnormalities, skeletal muscle damage, unconsciousness, and sudden death. The abuse of inhalants during pregnancy may be hazardous to infants and children, placing them at high risk of developmental harm. Although research is scarce, evidence suggests that prenatal exposure to toluene (found in paint thinners, gasoline, and correction fluid) may result in infants with low birthweight, occasional skeletal abnormalities, delayed neurobehavioral development, and altered regulation of body composition in males, as well as weight gain in both males and females (NIDA, 2012b).

The club drugs GHB and Rohypnol are often implicated in sexual assault. Because these drugs are available in an odorless, tasteless, and colorless form, they are commonly combined with alcohol or other beverages for ingestion. Women who ingest these drugs, whether knowingly or unknowingly, place themselves at risk for "date rape" (also known as drug-assisted sexual assault). The drugs can sedate and incapacitate unsuspecting victims and prevent them from resisting sexual assault perpetrated by an assailant (NIDA, 2014a, 2015a). Chronic use of MDMA can cause brain damage. Heavy use can also cause significant impairments in visual and verbal memory.

Health issues, in particular, create powerful treatment barriers for women. The nature and severity of health issues and substance abuse influence the difficulties women encounter in accessing treatment, securing appropriate services, and coordinating medical and substance abuse treatment needs. While actively using substances, women are often neglectful of their own health. Women involved with substance abuse often place substance use above all other concerns of their lives including health care. Substance use and activities necessary to acquire drugs frequently place women on the outer fringes of society. This causes women to avoid contact with healthcare systems, thus making them unreachable or difficult to follow for needed health care. Consequently, entry into treatment is likely delayed or difficult to coordinate because of the added burden imposed by health issues such as HIV/AIDS, hepatitis, other infectious diseases, mental disorders, and gynecological and obstetric conditions (CSAT, 2009).

Comprehensive case management can be effective in closing the gap between service and agencies. The premise of case management is to match services with a patient's need rather than make the patient fit into the particular services offered by the agency. Comprehensive case management that includes medical and social case management is an indispensable part of the wide spectrum of services frequently required for most women, particularly those who are pregnant or who have children. The various services and functions provided by case management include outreach, needs assessment, planning and resource identification, service linkages, monitoring and ongoing reassessment, and patient advocacy. Since the inception of case management, communities have advanced in developing formal connections, procedures, and integrated care systems. Case management services have become essential to overseeing the correct referral and utilization of services (CSAT, 2009). Evidence suggests that substance-dependent women who receive intensive case management are likely to access a greater variety of services (Jansson, Svikis, Breon, & Cieslak, 2005). They also have significantly higher levels of substance abuse treatment initiation, engagement, and retention as compared to women who receive routine screening and referral. Furthermore, rates of abstinence from alcohol and drugs tend to be higher with longer length of abstinence among women involved in case management (Jansson et al., 2005; Morgenstern et al., 2006).

Issues Affecting Psychological and Spiritual Functioning

PSYCHOLOGICAL FUNCTIONING

As previously acknowledged, women involved with substance abuse tend to have a high co-occurrence of mental disorders such as anxiety, major depression, post-traumatic stress disorder, and eating disorders. In fact, women are more likely to have three or more psychiatric diagnoses concurrently with a substance use disorder. Mental illness may precede substance abuse, where self-medication is employed to manage painful or distressing symptoms of mental illness. On the other hand, mental illness may develop as a consequence of substance abuse. Mental illness may also develop independently of and concurrently with the present pattern of substance use (CSAT, 2009).

The presence of co-occurring mental illnesses impairs quality of life, often entails enormous suffering, and indicates substantial need for help in several areas. Evidence suggests that increased severity of substance use and having more psychiatric and psychological symptoms are associated with poorer quality of life (Schaar & Öjehagen, 2003). In particular, women involved with substance abuse and who have co-occurring symptoms of trauma and sexual violence are likely to experience substantial impact on quality of life (Tracy et al., 2012). Improvement in psychiatric and psychological symptoms usually predicts improvement in quality of life in substance abusers with co-occurring mental illness (Schaar & Öjehagen, 2003).

Treatment is especially important for improving the psychological functioning domain of quality of life. However, women who have co-occurring mental illness frequently experience difficulties with adherence to health-related treatment recommendations, such as treatment attendance, diet restrictions, or medication compliance (CSAT, 2009). Numerous personal issues can obstruct a woman's interest in and commitment to entering treatment. Women may anticipate being unable to cope with stress, manage weight, or cope with symptoms associated with other mental illnesses, and this generates substantial apprehension in making a commitment to treatment (CSAT, 2009). Motivation is an essential factor to behavioral change processes, and thus can influence commitment to treatment (Laudet et al., 2009). Consequently, having a low level of motivation as well as low degree of readiness for treatment can be obstructive to treatment entry and progress. Other personal issues that can create barriers to treatment include feelings associated with previous treatment failures, feelings of guilt and shame associated with substance use, feelings of helplessness, belief that change is not possible, and fear of losing custody of children in response to admitting substance use and seeking treatment (CSAT, 2009).

Outreach services are a key component in enabling women to become aware of substance abuse treatment and can be effective in augmenting the likelihood of treatment entry, especially for women facing various obstacles. Effective outreach programs serve to connect women to substance abuse treatment regardless of their point of entry. Outreach must identify and address a woman's most urgent concerns first, provide empathy regarding her fears and resistances, and assist her in navigating the human service system. This is especially important when the decision to seek alcohol or drug treatment is stymied by overwhelming challenges such as lack of adequate, appropriate, or accessible programs or alienation from institutional connections due to relapse. Outreach offers substantial benefit in helping women to initiate contact with treatment providers; however, their response to outreach is likely influenced by level of readiness, history of trauma, and degree of support (CSAT, 2009).

At entry to substance abuse treatment, all women should undergo screening for co-occurring mental illness. Women with the possible existence of mental illness should be referred for a comprehensive mental health assessment and receive appropriate treatment for the co-occurring condition. It is important to note that drugs as well as withdrawal symptoms often mimic symptoms of mental illness. Thus it is vital that continual reassessment of mental illness symptoms takes place in order to ascertain diagnostic accuracy and plan appropriate treatment (CSAT, 2009).

Certain factors specific to women may destabilize recovery and increase the risk of substance abuse relapse. Women who have interpersonal problems and conflicts, negative affect, low self-worth especially associated with intimate relationships, more symptoms of depression, or severe untreated childhood trauma are vulnerable to relapse. Moreover, women who lack skills to prevent relapse, have greater difficulty in severing ties with other people who use substances, and fail to establish a new network of friends are at greater risk for relapse. It is important that treatment programs include relapse prevention education that will help women recognize triggers that lead to relapse and enhance abstinence (CSAT, 2009).

Evidence suggests that social support is an essential resource of recovery from substance abuse and improvement of quality of life. Social support helps to promotes physical and mental health, and provides assistance, emotional support, and a sense of belonging that may reduce or buffer stress and improve quality of life. Among persons involved with substance abuse, diminished social support is predictive of relapse and an increased level of social support is predictive of reduced substance use. Furthermore, among substance users with mental illness, social support is associated with better quality of life (Laudet, Morgen, & White, 2006).

Spirituality

Spirituality or religiousness is associated with mental health symptoms in substance-abusing women. Increased manifestation of depression and post-traumatic stress disorder is often associated with negative religious coping whereby women with substance abuse and co-occurring mental illness increasingly struggle with their faith and experience extensive emotional difficulties. They may feel alienated from their faith, punished by God, or perceive negative religious social interaction such as criticism or judgmental attitudes from others (Connors, Whiteside-Mansell, & Sherman, 2006).

On the other hand, in terms of being a relevant resource for maintaining a stable recovery from substance abuse, spirituality has been recognized as a key external resource that helps to buffer stress, sustain recovery from addiction, and enhance quality of life (Laudet et al., 2006). During screening and assessment, sensitivity to positive and negative dimensions of spirituality and religiousness, and the impact imparted on quality of life is necessary to help women explore their own perceptions and coping mechanisms and utilize spirituality and religiousness in the recovery process. Resources that include social support, spirituality, and religiousness likely contribute substantially to the overall recovery experience and should be made an integral part of the resources offered to the recovering community (Laudet et al., 2006).

Issues Affecting Socioeconomic Integrity

Nearly every dimension of women's lives is impacted by substance abuse. Accordingly, substance abuse imposes a massive burden of cost on society, family, and the individual. The total economic burden of substance abuse to society is staggering, with combined direct and indirect costs estimated in 2007 as $193 billion (National Drug Intelligence Center, 2011). These costs attributed to substance abuse are estimated in three principle areas: health, crime, and productivity. In the area of health, costs include direct medical expenditures, such as the cost of hospitalization, emergency department services, specialty treatment, insurance costs, and medications. The costs of crime are comprised of costs attributed to the criminal justice system such as police, adjudication, the prison system, costs associated with crime victims and property, and other related costs. Costs associated with productivity include costs associated with work loss, unemployment, premature mortality, social welfare costs, as well as costs of incarceration (National Drug Intelligence Center, 2011). It is apparent that the societal burden of substance abuse cannot be measured only in terms of dollars because substance abuse contributes significantly to morbidity, mortality, deterioration of social and family structure and has long-reaching effects on the health, well-being, and social development of subsequent generations of offspring.

Women in general experience unique challenges related to disparity in employment opportunities, income, health insurance, and childcare support. These issues significantly impact women with substance abuse and those seeking treatment. Consequently these issues create substantial threats to the socioeconomic integrity of quality of life and make women vulnerable to numerous social and economic barriers associated with substance abuse

and treatment. The social and economic barriers frequently obstruct treatment entry, impede treatment adherence, and may affect the likelihood for relapse. Women involved with substance abuse commonly face obstacles of financial constraint such as employment barriers, unemployment, poverty, lack of access to health insurance, dependent children, and co-occurring health and psychiatric conditions. They are less likely to be able to afford out-of-pocket treatment costs and are less likely to support themselves while in treatment. Accessibility of treatment also becomes an obstacle because many women may not be able to afford a car, or lack other means of transportation to treatment (CSAT, 2009).

Another substantial obstacle to treatment and recovery is stigma. Societal attitudes toward women with substance abuse are influenced by ascribed roles and gender expectations across cultures. As such, societal stigma toward women who abuse substances is likely more pronounced than that toward men. Women who abuse substances are frequently characterized as being morally lax, sexually promiscuous, and as irresponsible, neglectful mothers. Women with children are often fearful that admitting to substance abuse may cause them to lose custody of their children. Social stigma is acknowledged as a major reason for which women avoid seeking treatment. Fear and stereotype compound the shame and guilt women suffer about substance use, and this subsequently interferes with help-seeking behavior. The engagement approach of pretreatment intervention groups involves providing individual or structured feedback to women regarding their substance use, available treatment services and processes, and approaches to enhance motivation and decrease substance use. For women in particular, this strategy focuses on certain psychosocial barriers, such as stigma. Used as an initial step in treatment, pretreatment intervention groups can help women overcome reluctance or suspicions about treatment services (CSAT, 2009).

Cultural and ethnic issues may also create obstacles to treatment. The cultural values, gender roles and expectations of some cultural groups may cause women of these groups to experience more negative attitudes toward their substance use and they may have more difficulty engaging in help-seeking behavior and treatment services. Furthermore, women of certain ethnic groups may experience discrimination on the part of treatment staff that creates a barrier to engaging in treatment services. Language and cultural barriers can generate obstacles that may impede treatment entry and retention. Women from ethnic, cultural, or sexual minorities may face social indifference, lack of culturally appropriate programming, and limited cultural competence among staff (CSAT, 2009).

Women often experience obstacles when trying to negotiate multiple social service systems that have different expectations and purposes. The requirements of multiple systems such as substance abuse treatment, child welfare, and welfare reform services are frequently not integrated, and services may be fragmented. Thus a woman is required to navigate through a maze of service agencies to gain aid for housing, transportation, child care, substance abuse treatment, education, vocational training, and medical care. Furthermore, many agencies have conflicting requirements or use repetitive intake processes such as different forms that gather the same information. These complicated repetitive requirements can be daunting, discouraging, and obstructive to treatment and early recovery (CSAT, 2009).

Women with substance abuse problems may become involved with the criminal justice system. They may be victims or perpetrators of criminal activity and drug offenses, especially minority women. In addition to self-referral and social service agencies, the criminal justice system is a main source of referral to treatment for women. Evidence suggests that women referred to treatment through the criminal justice system tend to have better treatment outcomes (CSAT, 2009). On the other hand, for women already incarcerated, it is questionable whether those who are in state and federal prisons receive effective drug treatment. Women who are incarcerated for drug offenses tend to have more health problems and co-occurring disorders, more issues related to pregnancy and need for prenatal care, greater likelihood of issues concerning violence and abuse, and greater likelihood of issues concerning parenting, child care, and child custody (CSAT, 2009).

Issues Affecting Family Well-Being

The impact of substance abuse on marital and familial relationships is substantial and complicated. Substance abuse commonly causes family distress, disruption of family roles and relationships, violence, and abuse. Family history of substance abuse has profound effects on the development of substance abuse problems in women. Women who use substances tend to have parents and other family members who use substances and also have dysfunctional family patterns. Substance use in the family likely contributes to the development of substance abuse in the woman. Many women who are involved with substance abuse grew up in families in which they were exposed to substance abuse, sexual abuse, violence, and other relational dysfunction. Women who were raised in a substance-using family environment often develop relationships that mimic such broken family dynamics. As such, many women with family members who abused substances are likely to involve themselves with partners, spouses, or friends who also abuse substances. Consequently, relationships centered on substance use, as well as those that include physically or emotionally harmful behaviors, may be influential in enabling a woman's ongoing substance use (CSAT, 2009; Ripley, Cunion, & Noble, 2006).

Women who are involved with substance abuse are often the primary caregivers of children and other family members. This can make women reluctant or unable to enter and remain in treatment. Family members and friends who are involved in substance use frequently discourage women from entering and sustaining treatment and recovery. Women may also fear family or partner opposition or reactions to seeking help outside the family. Fear of losing one's partner is a common deterrent to treatment as well (CSAT, 2009).

Women who are pregnant or have children face substantial barriers to treatment. Few programs are equipped to address prenatal, postpartum, or childcare needs. Programs that accept mothers with children often impose restrictions and age limits. In addition, resources for pregnant women are scarce. Issues of child custody and fear of prosecution and incarceration may also deter pregnant women and women with children from seeking treatment (Jackson & Shannon, 2012). Pregnancy, nonetheless, offers a unique opportunity for intervention. The concern for the well-being of the fetus, the desire to care for the new child or existing children, and desire to avoid risks to one's own health are strong motivating factors for pregnant and parenting women to enter substance abuse treatment (Hankin, McCaul, & Heussner, 2000; Jackson & Shannon, 2012). Treatment engagement services, particularly case management, are important strategies to assist women in overcoming barriers to treatment, enhance abstinence, and improve family and social relationships (McLellan et al., 2003). Family therapy and teaching skills that can help repair family relationships, such as communication, stress management, assertiveness, and problem solving, are essential treatment approaches to help women achieve stable recovery. As women achieve stable recovery through treatment and developing positive relationships as well as establishing other resources of support, they will need to reevaluate relationships that are detrimental to their well-being. Decisions to end detrimental relationships must be supported. It is also important to realize that some women may choose to continue their participation in or may be

unable to escape destructive relationships (CSAT, 2009).

Codependency is an important factor for many women who become embroiled within the chaos of another person's life. Codependence refers to a person obsessed, tormented, or dominated by the behavior of others. The premise of codependency is that everyone in the family of a substance user or abuser is diseased. Consciously or unconsciously, and to their lifelong detriment, codependents interact with the user and enable this person to partake in his or her addiction. Codependents often feel miserable, hopeless, and angry as they accept the role of victim. A woman may be codependent in a relationship with a lover, spouse, parent, child, or friend. A codependent typically feels responsible for the behavior and mood of the other.

The codependent must learn how to separate her own life from the life of an addicted person. The recovery from codependence is similar to recovery from substance dependence in that only the codependent can take the necessary steps toward her recovery. A codependent must learn not to try to control another's life and must learn to relinquish the role of victim. Treatment programs and 12-step self-help groups are helpful in providing support and encouragement for codependent recovery.

Implications for Healthcare Providers

Drug dependency treatment programs must address the spectrum of physical and psychosocial issues that confront the female substance abuser. These challenges are especially difficult for women who have concerns such as contraception, pregnancy, motherhood, childbearing, and health problems in addition to drug dependency. Women are less likely to seek treatment for drug abuse, and respond differently to drug treatment in comparison to men. Female substance abusers are often caregivers and are less likely to seek care for themselves because of the needs of others. Women frequently need specialty treatment such as prenatal care, mental health services, domestic violence counseling, and childcare assistance. In addition, the treatment needs of women cannot be evaluated within a context of homogeneity. As substance abusers, women constitute heterogeneous subgroups that span the lifecycle.

Psychosocial and behavioral treatment programs that emphasize increased self-esteem and choosing positive life options may be more successful with certain women. Treatment programs must focus on the special needs of women and acknowledge the barriers that women must overcome to obtain treatment. The utilization of treatment engagement approaches such as outreach, pre-intervention groups, and comprehensive case management are key components of treatment for women and assist women to achieve a sustaining recovery.

Special Concerns of Age and Ethnicity

For older women, alcohol dependence and prescription drug abuse are chief issues of concern; however, the problem of substance abuse in this population remains, for the most part, underreported, undiagnosed, or ignored (Boyle & Davis, 2006). Older women are vulnerable to developing substance-related problems. Age-related risk factors include losses or deaths, financial problems, changes in metabolism related to age, health problems, changing social roles, and synergistic effects of combining alcohol and other drugs. Women face many adjustments and challenges with aging that may include retirement, widowhood, loss of friends, and financial constraint. Women may turn to substance use to cope with these challenges. Because many older women live alone, the extent

of their substance use is difficult to measure. Furthermore, stigma may cause many older women to hide their substance use and there is less of a tendency for them to engage in activities that might reveal a substance use problem (Boyle & Davis, 2006; CSAT, 2009).

Healthcare professionals often miss detecting substance abuse in older women because signs of substance abuse are frequently attributed incorrectly to consequences of aging or health conditions more prevalent in later life, such as dementia or Parkinson's disease (Martin, 2008). Furthermore, a lack of appropriate diagnostic criteria compounds misdiagnosis of substance abuse in elderly women. The risk of prescription drug abuse is great among the elderly. Older persons commonly do not comply with the recommended use of their medications. They may have difficulty reading a prescription label, or hearing and understanding verbal directions. The elderly frequently are treated for numerous conditions by a variety of physicians, and often have several pharmacies filling prescriptions at the lowest prices. Elderly persons may hoard old or unused medications "just in case" the need arises. They may be more likely to self-medicate to avoid the expense or inconvenience of visiting a physician. These behaviors increase the risk of intentional or unintentional drug abuse (Martin, 2008).

Appropriate treatments adapted for the specific needs of older women with substance abuse problems are essential. Older women will likely present a high prevalence of co-occurring physical and mental health disorders that will require a higher level of service need. The incorporation of both primary and psychiatric care into treatment programs for older women or providing appropriate referral mechanisms to ancillary services can help ensure management of health problems within the context of their treatment programs (Rosen, Smith, & Reynolds, 2008). Older women may particularly benefit from screening, brief interventions, and case management approaches, especially for limiting alcohol abuse in this population. An interdisciplinary treatment team should be part of a well-coordinated treatment approach that should also involve family or significant others in the plan for individualized support services. Residential treatment programs in which the majority of patients are significantly younger will probably not address the needs of older women effectively. Thus treatment of older women may be more effective if provided at senior centers, congregational meal sites, geriatric meal programs, home care programs, or peer outreach (CSAT, 2009).

Substance abuse is prevalent in women of various racial and ethnic groups. As such, racial and ethnic disparities in health result in diverse outcomes and consequences in various groups. The multifaceted interaction of culture and health, along with the influence of distinct ways of thinking toward, definitions of, and beliefs about health and substance use among racial and ethnic groups, are influential in the psychosocial development of women and their substance use and abuse (CSAT, 2009).

The risks, consequences, and treatment processes for substance abuse differ by numerous factors comprised of gender, race, ethnicity, sexual orientation, and age. The risk of women for substance use disorders is best understood within a framework in which the influences of gender, race, ethnicity, culture, education, economic status, age, geographic location, sexual orientation, and other factors come together. Gaining an awareness of group differences across the subdivisions of the population of women is foundational for designing and implementing effective substance abuse treatment programs (CSAT, 2009).

Women of diverse groups encounter unique challenges that affect their substance use or abuse and its treatment. Counselors and treatment staff need to acknowledge women's individual and group strengths and their distinctive capacity for resilience that can facilitate adaptation in the face of adversity, tragedy, and stress. Resiliency resources involve beliefs associated with health care and substance abuse, value placed on family and spirituality by each individual or group, the influence of group history on present behaviors, and both the status of women and the socialization process of women in particular cultures. In addition, resiliency resources may include flexibility of gender norms, communication styles, rituals, the stigma confronted by each individual or group, and the mind-set toward self-disclosure and help-seeking behavior (CSAT, 2009).

Research Review

What are the prospective patterns and predictors of quality of life among women in substance abuse treatment?

Tracy, E., Laudet, A., Min, M., Kim, H., Brown, S., Jun, M., & Singer, L. (2012). Prospective patterns and correlates of quality of life among women in substance abuse treatment. *Drug and Alcohol Dependence, 124,* 242–249.

Quality of life has been increasingly acknowledged as central to recovery in substance abuse services. Research that investigates quality of life is relatively new in the field of addiction. Furthermore, little is known about the role of social support and other correlates as predictors of quality of life among women with substance use disorder. Thus, the purpose of this study was twofold:

- To describe trajectories of quality of life in four domains (physical, psychological, social, and environmental) from treatment intake to 1- and 6-month posttreatment intake periods.
- To identify the role of sociodemographic, clinical, treatment, and social support domains as correlates of quality of life changes at 6 months posttreatment intake, controlling for baseline levels of quality of life.

A sample of 240 women who were diagnosed as substance dependent according to DSM-IV criteria for substance dependence, and in treatment for at least one continuous week consented to participate in this study. Women who had a known diagnosis of schizophrenia or were taking medication for a major thought disorder were excluded from participation. Face-to-face interviews were conducted with study participants at 1 week (T1), 1 month (T2), and 6 months (T3) posttreatment intake. Demographic data and number of co-occurring mental disorders was collected at intake. Symptomatology associated with childhood and adult trauma was measured by The Trauma Symptom Checklist-40 at intake. Social support was measured by The Social Support for Recovery Scale and The Friends Support for Abstinence Scale at T3. Treatment process variables determining extent of drug and alcohol use and 12-step meeting attendance were assessed by The Treatment Services Review at T3. Quality of life domains of physical, psychological, social, and living environment were assessed by the World Health Organization Quality of Life measure at each assessment point. Data was analyzed with descriptive statistics, bivariate correlations, repeated measures of analysis of variance, and hierarchical multiple regression.

Results showed significant improvement in all domains of quality of life across the follow-up time points, although the quality of life scores remained below those of healthy population norms. Trauma symptoms significantly predicted quality of life in the physical and psychological domains. The treatment process variable of alcohol use showed a significant negative relationship with the environmental domain of quality of life. Recovery support and friends support showed consistent significant positive relationships with quality of life across all four domains.

The findings of this study suggest that, although improvement of quality of life was observed, women continued to experience quality of life that was poorer than that of the general population. Quality of life satisfaction at the end of treatment could be predictive of commitment to abstinence. Poor quality of life at intake suggests that women likely start treatment at a disadvantage that may influence their response to treatment services in ways different than their substance use alone. The significant relationship between extent of alcohol use and living environment quality of life suggests that the extent of substance use may not be the most salient factor that determines life satisfaction in this population. It implies the need for services focused on other areas of functioning as well as sobriety and reduction of use, such as trauma symptoms, living conditions, and social support. Moreover, the degree of trauma symptoms substantially impacts quality of life and underscores the need for more trauma informed interventions and services for women. The findings of this study also suggest that social support is essential for recovery and abstinence, and enhancing social support may contribute to improved quality of life for women in substance abuse treatment.

Chapter Summary Points

- Substance abuse encompasses the overuse of, misuse of, or addiction to any chemical substance such as tobacco, alcohol, or drugs, which includes over-the-counter drugs, prescription drugs, and illicit drugs.
- Initiation of substance use and progression to substance abuse and dependence in women is influenced by a number of factors such as age, genetic factors, family history, marital status, partner influence, traumatic life events, personality characteristics, sexual orientation, socioeconomic factors, and co-occurring psychiatric disorders.
- The reduction of risk of substance use and abuse in women entails a multifaceted approach involving individual, family, community, and societal commitment to prevention of use of tobacco, inappropriate use of alcohol and pharmaceuticals, and use of illicit drugs.
- Women and men differ with respect to numerous aspects of substance use and abuse such as rate of use and abuse, physical response to substances, telescoping, sociocultural norms, development of health complications, history of trauma and abuse, and response to treatment.
- The extent and nature of the substance use disorder and its interaction with other life areas must be understood in order to achieve careful diagnosis, appropriate case management, and successful treatment of women.
- The screening and assessment process is the starting point for gaining this understanding and for matching women with suitable treatment services.
- Treatment is a complex process due to the many dimensions of drug abuse and addiction, as well as the disruption it causes in various aspects of life.
- Many components are incorporated into effective treatment programs, and each is focused on a particular aspect of the illness and its consequences.
- Addiction is typically a chronic disease. As such, women cannot simply stop using drugs for a few days and be cured. Long-term or repeated episodes of care are required to attain the crucial goal of sustained abstinence and recovery of their lives.
- The treatment process often begins with detoxification, which is followed by treatment and relapse prevention.
- Women with substance abuse commonly experience poor quality of life that encompasses painful symptoms, disrupted physical and psychological functioning, threatened personal safety, disturbed family and social relations, criminal activity, and disrupted school and work roles and obligations.
- Effective treatment approaches that sustain remission and decrease risk of relapse are essential for maintaining acceptable quality of life among female substance abusers.
- Women frequently experience numerous barriers that impede them from achieving long-standing stable recovery. Barriers involve demands associated with women's various caregiver roles, the intrinsic socioeconomic and health conditions particularly related to substance use disorders, and the societal bias and stigma related to substance abuse.
- Treatment engagement approaches that support the initiation of treatment and address the diverse challenges that impede treatment involvement are essential to the stable recovery of women from substance dependency.

- The problem of substance abuse in older women is substantial yet often remains underreported, undiagnosed, or ignored. Appropriate treatments adapted for the specific needs of older women with substance abuse problems are essential.
- Women of diverse racial and ethnic groups encounter unique challenges that affect their substance use, abuse, and treatment. Counselors and treatment staff need to be culturally competent, acknowledge women's individual and group strengths, and recognize their distinctive capacity for resilience that can facilitate adaptation in the face of adversity, tragedy, and stress.

Critical Thinking Exercise

Case Study

E.K. is a 20-year-old inner city African-American woman who is substance dependent. She had been using alcohol and drugs since she was 13 years old, when she would drink beer and liquor with older school friends and smoke marijuana. E.K.'s father is an alcoholic who was chronically unemployed and on welfare. Her mother is a weak and ineffectual codependent. Her older brother also smokes marijuana and occasionally uses cocaine. Her brother rarely appeared high to E.K., and this made her think she could just as easily handle her substance use. E.K. also has a childhood history of sexual abuse perpetrated by her uncle. Her alcohol and marijuana use helps her to cope with traumatic memories, symptoms of depression, and her chaotic family life.

As E.K.'s alcohol and marijuana abuse escalated, her school performance and social relationships deteriorated. She was expelled from school at age 17 and was subsequently arrested for marijuana possession. At the age of 18, E.K. left home to move in with her 22-year-old boyfriend who also was a substance abuser. E.K.'s boyfriend initiated her into cocaine and barbiturate use and occasional club drugs. Their relationship was dysfunctional and the boyfriend would become physically and verbally abusive when high on cocaine. Recently E.K. discovered she was pregnant and desired to stop using drugs and alcohol for the sake of her baby, "the only good thing in her life." She tried to stop using drugs and alcohol on her own but was not very successful. Her boyfriend "didn't want things to change" and became angry. When he found out about her pregnancy, he denied the baby was his and began pressuring her to have an abortion. On the pretense of going to an abortion clinic, E.K. went instead to a neighborhood outreach center and was referred to treatment.

E.K. entered a residential all women's substance treatment program. Case management services arranged for E.K. to receive prenatal care during detoxification and subsequent behavioral treatment. During her stay in residential treatment, E.K. had individual and group therapy sessions as well as classes in infant care and job training. E.K. believed that her baby was more important than getting high and was motivated to recover. With counseling, she began to realize that her relationship with her boyfriend was harmful and it had to end for her sake and the sake of her baby. Following delivery of a small but apparently healthy baby girl, E.K. was able to transition to a community halfway house. There she was able to reside with her daughter while she continued outpatient treatment. She also joined a 12-step support group that helped her develop new social ties with friends who were sober and substance free.

Questions for Seminar Discussion

1. Discuss the risk factors for substance abuse. What factors made E.K. vulnerable to substance abuse?
2. What gender differences exist in substance abuse?
3. Discuss the condition of telescoping. What makes you think that E.K. is at risk for telescoping to occur?
4. How does substance abuse affect women's health? Discuss complications for which E.K might be at particular risk.
5. How does substance abuse affect pregnancy, especially E.K.'s pregnancy? Discuss complications that can develop in children born of substance abusing mothers.
6. Discuss the various barriers to treatment entry, continuation, and stable recovery. How do these barriers affect quality of life?
7. Discuss the barriers that challenged E.K.'s recovery from substance abuse.
8. Discuss the engagement strategies that helped E.K. enter and continue treatment.
9. Discuss resiliency resources that counselors should use to help women of various racial and ethnic groups facilitate adaptation in the face of adversity, tragedy, and stress.
10. Discuss factors that can destabilize recovery and lead to relapse.

Internet Resources

Alcoholics Anonymous: Alcoholics Anonymous® is a 12-step fellowship program whereby group members support each other in recovery from alcoholism. http://www.aa.org

Centers for Disease Control and Prevention: Provides information and education for healthcare professionals, scientists, students, and general public on issues of substance abuse. http://www.cdc.gov

Narcotics Anonymous: Narcotics Anonymous® is a 12-step fellowship program whereby group members support each other in recovery from the effects of addiction. http://www.na.org

National Inhalant Prevention Coalition: NIPC serves as an inhalant referral and information clearinghouse to educate youth and adults about the debilitating effects of dangerous gateway drugs. http://www.inhalants.org

National Institute on Alcohol Abuse and Alcoholism: NIAAA supports and conducts research on the impact of alcohol use on human health and well-being. http://www.niaaa.nih.gov

National Institute on Drug Abuse: NIDA supports and conducts research and facilitates effective dissemination and use of research results in the prevention, treatment and policy development regarding drug abuse and addiction. http://www.drugabuse.gov

Society for Research on Nicotine and Tobacco: stimulates the generation of new knowledge concerning nicotine in all its manifestations and informs governmental regulatory and other public agencies regarding nicotine and tobacco. http://www.srnt.org

Substance Abuse and Mental Health Services Administration: SAMHSA provides leadership and resources committed to reducing the impact of substance abuse and mental illness on America's communities. http://www.samhsa.gov/

References

Agrawal, A., Gardner, C., Prescott, C., & Kendler, K. (2005). The differential impact of risk factors on illicit drug involvement in females. *Social Psychiatry and Psychiatric Epidemiology 40*(6), 454–466.

Amaro, H., Larson, M., Gampel, J., Richardson, E., Savage, A., & Wagler, D. (2005). Racial/ethnic differences in social vulnerability among women with co-occurring mental health and substance abuse disorders: Implications for treatment services. *Journal of Community Psychology, 33*(4), 495–511.

Ball, D. (2007). Addiction science and its genetics. *Addiction, 103*, 360–367.

Bertrand, J., Floyd, R., Weber, M., O'Connor, M., Riley, E., Johnson, K., … National Task Force on FAS/FAE. (2004). *Fetal alcohol Syndrome: Guidelines for referral and diagnosis.* Atlanta, GA: Centers for Disease Control and Prevention. Retrieved from http://www.cdc.gov/ncbddd/fasd/documents/fas_guidelines_accessible.pdf

Black, M., Basile, K., Breiding, M., Smith, S., Walters, M., Merrick, M., … Stevens, M. (2011). *The national intimate partner and sexual violence survey (NISVS): 2010 summary report.* Atlanta, GA: National Center for Injury Prevention and Control, Centers for Disease Control and Prevention.

Boyle, A., & Davis, H. (2006). Early screening and assessment of alcohol and substance abuse in the elderly: Clinical implications. *Journal of Addictions Nursing, 17*, 95–103.

Carlson, B. (2006). Best practices in the treatment of substance-abusing women in the child welfare system. *Journal of Social Work Practice in the Addictions, 6*(3), 97–115.

Center for Substance Abuse Treatment. (2009). *Substance abuse treatment: Addressing the specific needs of women.* (Treatment Improvement Protocol (TIP) Series 51. HHS Publication No. (SMA) 09-4426). Rockville, MD: Substance Abuse and Mental Health Services Administration.

Chen, C., Storr, C., & Anthony, J. (2009). Early-onset drug use and risk for drug dependence problems. *Addictive Behaviors, 34*, 319–322.

Connors, N., Whiteside-Mansell, L., & Sherman, A. (2006). Dimensions of religious involvement and mental health outcomes among alcohol- and drug dependent women. *Alcoholism Treatment Quarterly, 24*(1-2), 89–108.

Danielson, C., Amstradter, A., Dangelmaier, R., Resnick, H., Saunders, B., & Kilpatrick, D. (2009). Trauma-related risk factors for substance abuse among male versus female young adults. *Addictive Behaviors, 34*, 395–399.

Domingo-Salvany, A., Brugal, M., Bario, G., González-Saiz, F., Bravo, M., del la Fuente, L., & the ITINERE Investigators. (2010). Gender differences in health related quality of life of young heroin users. *Health and Quality of Life Outcomes, 8*, 145.

Executive Office of the President of the United States. (2011). Epidemic: Responding to America's prescription drug abuse crisis. Retrieved from https://www.whitehouse.gov/sites/default/files/ondcp/issues-content/prescription-drugs/rx_abuse_plan.pdf

Grant, B., Stinson, F., Dawson, D., Chou, S., Ruan, W., & Pickering, R. (2006). Co-occurrence of 12-month alcohol and drug use disorders and personality disorders in the United States: Results from the National Epidemiological Survey on Alcohol and Related Conditions. *Alcohol Research & Health, 29*(2), 121–130.

Green, C. (2006). Gender use of substance abuse treatment services. *Alcohol Research and Health, 29*(1), 55–62.

Griffin, K., Bang, H., & Botvin, G. (2010). Age of alcohol and marijuana use onset predicts weekly substance use and related psychosocial problems during young adulthood. *Journal of Substance Use, 15*(3), 174–183.

Greenfield, S., Back, S., Lawson, K., & Brady, K. (2010). Substance abuse in women. *Psychiatric Clinics of North America, 33*, 339–355.

Hankin, J., McCaul, M., & Heussner, J. (2000). Pregnant, alcohol-abusing women. *Alcoholism: Clinical and Experimental Research, 24*(8), 1276–1286.

Harris, K., & Edlund, M. (2005). Self-medication of mental health problems: New evidence from a national survey. *Health Services Research, 40*(1), 117–134.

Hser, Y., Kagihara, J., Huang, D., Evans, E., & Messina, N. (2011). Mortality among substance-using mothers in California: A 10-year prospective study. *Addiction, 107*, 215–222.

Hughes, T., Szalacha, L., & McNair, R. (2010). Substance abuse and mental health disparities: Comparison across sexual identity groups in a national sample of young Australian women. *Social Science and Medicine, 71*, 824–831.

Jackson, A., & Shannon, L. (2012). Examining barriers to and motivations for substance abuse treatment among pregnant women: Does urban-rural residence matter? *Women & Health, 52*, 570–586.

Jansson, L., Svikis, D., Breon, D., & Cieslak, R. (2005). Intensity of case management services: Does more equal better for drug-dependent women and their children? *Social Work in Mental Health, 3*(4), 63–78.

Kloos, A., Weller, R., Chan, R., & Weller, E. (2009). Gender differences in adolescent substance abuse. *Current Psychiatry Reports, 11*, 120–126.

Kuehn, B. (2008). Despite benefit, physicians slow to offer brief advice on harmful alcohol use. *Journal of the American Medical Association 299*(7), 751–753.

Laudet, A. (2011). The case for considering quality of life in addiction research and clinical practice. *Addiction Science and Clinical Practice, 6*, 44–55.

Laudet, A., Becker, J., & White, W. (2009). Don't wanna go through that madness no more: Quality of life satisfaction as predictor of sustained remission from illicit drug misuse. *Substance Use and Misuse, 44*, 227–252.

Laudet, A., Morgen, K., & White, W. (2006). The role of social supports, spirituality, religiousness, life meaning, and affiliation with 12-step fellowships in quality of life satisfaction among individuals in recovery from alcohol and drug problems. *Alcoholism Treatment Quarterly, 24*(1-2), 33–73.

Malliarakis, K., & Lucey, P. (2007). Social discriminates of health: Focus on substance use and abuse. *Nursing Economic$, 25*(6), 368–375.

Martin, C. (2008). Prescription drug abuse in the elderly. *The Consultant Pharmacist, 23*(12), 930–942)

McLellan, A., Gutman, M., Lynch, K., McKay, J., Ketterlinus, R., Morgenstern, J., & Woolis, D. (2003). One-year outcomes from the CASAWORKS for Families intervention for substance-abusing women on welfare. *Evaluation Review, 27*(6), 656–680.

Morgenstern, J., Blanchard, K., McRady, B., McVeigh, K., Morgan, T., & Pandina, R. (2006). Effectiveness of case management for substance-dependent women receiving temporary assistance for needy families. *Research and Practice, 96*(11), 2016–2013.

National Drug Intelligence Center (2011). *The economic impact of illicit drug use on American society.* Washington, DC: United States Department of Justice. Retrieved from http://www.justice.gov/archive/ndic/pubs44/44731/44731p.pdf

National Institute on Alcohol Abuse and Alcoholism. (2015). Planning alcohol interventions Using NIAAA's College AIM. (NIH Publication No. 15-AA-8017). Retrieved from http://www.collegedrinkingprevention.gov/CollegeAIM/Resources/NIAAA_College_Matrix_Booklet.pdf

National Institute on Drug Abuse. (2003). Preventing drug use among children and adolescents: A research-based guide for parents, educators, and community leaders (2nd ed.). https://www.drugabuse.gov/publications/preventing-drug-abuse-among-children-adolescents/acknowledgments

National Institute on Drug Abuse. (2009). NIDA DrugFacts: Treatment approaches for drug addiction. Retrieved from http://www.drugabuse.gov/sites/default/files/drugfacts_treatmentapproaches.pdf

National Institute on Drug Abuse. (2012a). *Principles of drug addiction treatment: A research-based guide* 3rd ed. (NIH Publication No. 12–4180). Retrieved from http://www.drugabuse.gov/sites/default/files/podat_1.pdf

National Institute on Drug Abuse. (2012b). *Research report series: Inhalants.* (NIH Publication Number 12-3818). Retrieved from http://www.drugabuse.gov/sites/default/files/inhalantsrrs.pdf

National Institute on Drug Abuse. (2012c). *Research report series: Tobacco/nicotine.* (NIH Publication Number 12-4342). Retrieved from http://www.drugabuse.gov/sites/default/files/tobaccorrsv3.pdf

National Institute on Drug Abuse. (2012d). Topics in brief: Medication-assisted treatment for opioid addiction. Retrieved from http://www.drugabuse.gov/sites/default/files/tib_mat_opioid.pdf

National Institute on Drug Abuse. (2014a). DrugFacts. Hallucinogens - LSD, peyote, psilocybin, and PCP. Retrieved http://www.drugabuse.gov/sites/default/files/hallucinogens_df_12_2014.pdf

National Institute on Drug Abuse. (2014b). DrugFacts: heroin. Retrieved from http://www.drugabuse.gov/sites/default/files/drugfacts_heroin_10_14.pdf

National Institute on Drug Abuse. (2014c). *Research report series: Prescription drug abuse.* (NIH Publication Number 15-4881). Retrieved from http://www.drugabuse.gov/sites/default/files/prescriptiondrugrrs_11_14.pdf

National Institute on Drug Abuse. (2014d). What are the signs of drug use in adolescents and what role can parents play in getting treatment? Retrieved from http://www.drugabuse.gov/publications/principles-adolescent-substance-use-disorder-treatment-research-based-guide/frequently-asked-questions/what-are-signs-drug-use-in-adolescents-what-role-can-parents-play-in-getting-treatment

National Institute on Drug Abuse. (2015a). Commonly abused drug charts. Retrieved from http://www.drugabuse.gov/drugs-abuse/commonly-abused-drugs-charts

National Institute on Drug Abuse. (2015b). Drug Facts: Substance use in women. Retrieved from http://www.drugabuse.gov/publications/drugfacts/substance-use-in-women

National Institute on Drug Abuse. (2015c). *Research report series: Marijuana.* (NIH Publication Number 15-3859). Retrieved from http://www.drugabuse.gov/sites/default/files/mjrrs_4_15.pdf

National Prevention Council. (2014a). Smoking and youth. Retrieved from http://www.cdc.gov/tobacco/data_statistics/sgr/50th-anniversary/pdfs/fs_smoking_youth_508.pdf

National Prevention Council. (2014b). Women and smoking. Retrieved from http://www.cdc.gov/tobacco/data_statistics/sgr/50th-anniversary/pdfs/fs_women_smoking_508.pdf

Ripley, J., Cunion, A., & Noble, N. (2006). Alcohol abuse in marriage and family contexts: Relational pathways to recovery. *Alcoholism Treatment Quarterly, 24*(1-2), 171–184.

Robinson, R. (2006). Health perceptions and health-related quality of life of substance abusers: A review of the literature. *Journal of Addictions Nursing, 17,* 159-168.

Rosen, D., Smith, M., & Reynolds, C. (2008). The prevalence of mental and physical health disorders among older methadone patients. *American Journal of Geriatric Psychiatry, 16*(6), 488–497.

Savage, C. (2010). Substance abuse. Retrieved from http://healthywomen.org/condition/substance-abuse

Schaar, I., & Öjehagen, A. (2003). Predictors of improvement in quality of life of severely mentally ill substance abusers during 18 months of co-operation between psychiatric and social services. *Social Psychiatry and Psychiatric Epidemiology, 38,* 83–87.

Substance Abuse and Mental Health Services Administration. (2011). White paper on Screening, Brief Intervention and Referral to Treatment (SBIRT) in behavioral healthcare. Retrieved from http://www.samhsa.gov/sites/default/files/sbirtwhitepaper_0.pdf

Substance Abuse and Mental Health Services Administration. (2012). *Results from the 2011 National Survey on Drug Use and Health: Summary of National Findings and Detailed Tables* (NSDUH Series H-44, HHS Publication No. (SMA) 12-4713). Rockville, MD: Substance Abuse and Mental Health Services Administration. Retrieved from http://www.samhsa.gov/data/NSDUH/2011SummNatFindDetTables/Index.aspx

Taylor, O. (2011). The sexual victimization of women: Substance abuse, HIV, prostitution, and intimate partner violence as underlying correlates. *Journal of Human Behavior in the Social Environment, 21,* 834–848.

Tracy, E., Laudet, A., Min, M., Kim, H., Brown, S., Jun, M., & Singer, L. (2012). Prospective patterns and correlates of quality of life among women in substance abuse treatment. *Drug and Alcohol Dependence, 124,* 242–249.

U.S. Department of Health and Human Services, Health Resources and Services Administration, Maternal and Child Health Bureau (2011). *Women's Health USA 2011.* Rockville, Maryland: U.S. Department of Health and Human Services. Retrieved from http://www.mchb.hrsa.gov/whusa11/hstat/hshb/pages/205idu.html

U.S. Department of Health and Human Services. (2012). *Preventing tobacco use among youth and young adults: A report of the Surgeon General.* Atlanta, GA: U.S. Department of Health and Human Services, Centers for Disease Control and Prevention, National Center for Chronic Disease Prevention and Health Promotion, Office on Smoking and Health.

Wermier, A., Laucht, M., Schimmelmann, B., Bannaschweski, T., Sonuga-Barke, E., Rietschel, M., & Becker, K. (2010). From nature versus nurture, via nature and nurture, to gene x environment interaction in mental disorders. *European Child and Adolescent Psychiatry, 19,* 199–210.

Chapter 8

Consequences of Risky Sexual Behavior

Introduction

Engaging in new behaviors is a significant developmental aspect that occurs during the period of adolescence and young adulthood. However, new behaviors often become risky and can lead to negative health outcomes. Sexual experimentation is a common behavior during this period and can subsequently lead to life-altering consequences. Adolescent and young women frequently become sexually active before they develop skills and experience in self-protection and in setting and expressing the kinds of behaviors with which they feel comfortable. Adolescent and young women often become sexually active before acquiring adequate information about sexually transmitted infections and before they have access to health services and supplies that can mitigate risk for untoward health outcomes. Research findings indicate that many young women nationwide are engaged in sexual risk behaviors associated with unintended pregnancies and sexually transmitted infections, including HIV infection (Centers for Disease Control and Prevention [CDC], 2012e). Healthy sexuality and responsible sexual behavior are essential for the overall health of young women. Sexual experiences that are positive or negative can impact overall well-being and quality of life of adolescent and young women. This chapter explores the serious consequences of sexual experimentation in adolescent and young women—sexually transmitted infections and unintended pregnancy. The significant impact of sexually transmitted infections and unintended pregnancy on the quality of life of adolescent and young women and their families is also discussed.

Incidence

Sexually Transmitted Infections

Sexually transmitted infections (STIs) are infections of the reproductive tract that are transmitted by sexual contact. Common STIs include chlamydia, syphilis, gonorrhea, herpes simplex virus type 2 (HSV-2), viral hepatitis, human immunodeficiency virus (HIV), human papillomavirus (HPV), and trichomoniasis. STIs are a major public health problem with incidence and prevalence rates that are startling. The United States has the highest rate of STIs in the industrialized world. Nationwide, it is estimated that there are approximately 110,197,000 STIs among men and women overall. Of this number, approximately 59,569,500 women are infected and 50,627,400 men. Evidence suggests that approximately 26% of the young women in this country who are between the ages of 14 and 19—that is, 3.2 million adolescents—are infected with at least one of the most common sexually transmitted diseases: chlamydia, HSV-2, HPV, and trichomoniasis (CDC, 2008).

It is estimated that over 19.7 million new cases of STIs occur in the United States each year.

Although most of these STIs are not likely to cause harm, some have the potential to cause serious health problems, especially if not diagnosed and treated early (CDC, 2013a). Young women and men between the ages of 15 and 24 are predominantly affected. Although representing only 25% of the sexually experienced population, this age group accounts for approximately 50% of all new STIs. The annual rate of new infections in men and women occurring in this age group is roughly equal, with new infections among young women equal to 51%, and 49% among young men (CDC, 2013a). The majority of newly acquired infections are attributed to HPV. Although approximately 90% of HPV infections tend to resolve on their own within 2 years and cause no harm, some infections will persist and potentially lead to serious diseases such as genital warts and cervical cancer (CDC, 2013a). While exact incidence is not known because HPV is not reportable, the CDC estimates that 79,100,000 new and existing HPV infections existed in the United States in 2008 (CDC, 2013a).

Chlamydia, chancroid, gonorrhea, and syphilis are notifiable conditions. This means that federal law requires healthcare providers to report these STIs to prevent and control their spread. Chlamydia is the most frequently reported notifiable STI in the United States. In 2009, nearly 1.25 million cases were reported to the CDC, with at least that many more estimated to have gone undetected (CDC, 2010a). Chlamydia is among the most prevalent of all STIs, and since 1994 has encompassed the largest proportion of all STIs reported to CDC (CDC, 2012d). Evidence from national surveys conducted between 1999 and 2008 indicates that chlamydia prevalence is 6.8% among sexually active females aged 14–19 years. The highest age-specific rates of reported chlamydia in 2011 were among young women aged 15–19 years (3,416.5 cases per 100,000 females) and 20–24 years (3,722.5 cases per 100,000 females) (CDC, 2012d). Sexually active adolescents and women aged 14 to 24 years of age have nearly three times the prevalence of chlamydia as women aged 25 to 39 years of age (CDC, 2011a). Chancroid, on the other hand, is uncommon in the United States, with only 24 cases reported in 2010. This number may be an underestimate; however, reflecting the fact that the causative organism of chancroid is difficult to culture (CDC, 2011b).

Gonorrhea is the second most frequently reported notifiable STI in this country. In 2011, gonorrhea rates per 100,000 population were highest among adolescents and young adults, with the highest rates observed among young women aged 15–19 years (556.5) and 20–24 years (584.2) (CDC, 2012d). The rate of primary and secondary syphilis, the third most commonly reported notifiable STI, tends to be higher among men than among women, especially among men who have sex with men. In 2011 the rate of syphilis infection was 2.4 per 100,000 among women aged 15–19, and 3.8 per 100,000 among women aged 20–24 (CDC, 2012d). In contrast to other bacterial STIs that affect mostly adolescents and adults younger than 25 years, syphilis persists into the 30s and 40s in both women and men (CDC, 2010a).

Viral hepatitis has multiple routes of transmission, sexual contact being one of them. Although not common, hepatitis A can be transmitted during sexual activity due to fecal-oral contact, and is mostly associated with sex with multiple partners, sex with trauma, or presence of other STIs (CDC, 2010c). In 2010, incidence of hepatitis A in males was 0.6 per 100,000, and roughly similar to the incidence among females of 0.5 per 100,000. Approximately 1.6% of hepatitis A cases were likely attributed to sexual activity (CDC, 2013c). Hepatitis B is transmitted during sexual activity through exchange of bodily fluids with an infected partner. In 2010, the rate of incidence was approximately 1.6 times higher for males than that for females. Incidence among males was 1.36 per 100,000 and for females 0.83 per 100,000. About 8% of hepatitis B cases were likely attributed to

sexual activity (CDC, 2013c). Although not common, hepatitis C can also be transmitted through sexual activity. In 2010, the incidence rate of hepatitis C among 20- to 29-year-olds was 0.8 cases per 100,000, and less than 0.1 case per 100,000 for persons 19 years and younger. The incidence rate for both males and females was 0.3 per 100,000. Approximately 17.9% of hepatitis C cases were likely attributed to sexual activity (CDC, 2013c).

Genital herpes is one of the most common STIs in the United States but its exact prevalence is unknown because herpes simplex virus (HSV) is not a reportable infection. The National Health and Nutrition Examination Survey (NHANES) findings estimated that in 2008, among those aged 15 to 49 years, 15.9 million American women (21.7% prevalence) and 8.2 million men (11.3% prevalence) were infected with HSV-2. Moreover, among 15- to 24-year-olds, 1.69 million young women (8.2% prevalence) and 812,000 men (3.86% prevalence) were infected with HSV-2 (Satterwhite et al., 2013).

Trichomoniasis is considered the most common curable STI. In this country, about 3.7 million people have the infection but only about 30% develop symptoms (CDC, 2012a). The findings of the NHANES study estimated that in 2008, 2.31 million women (3.15% prevalence) aged 15 to 49 years were infected with trichomoniasis nationwide. Among women aged 15 to 24 years, approximately 309,000 young women (1.50% prevalence) were infected (Satterwhite et al., 2013).

The incidence and prevalence of HIV infection among women is substantial. Currently, approximately 1.1 million individuals in the United States are living with HIV. Nearly 280,000, or 24%, are women. In 2010, approximately 9,500 (20%) new infections were diagnosed in women. Young women 13 to 24 years of age account for 22% of those infected, and 29% are young women 25 to 34 years of age. Transmission of HIV in women is predominantly due to heterosexual contact. In 2010, 84% of new HIV infections occurred through heterosexual sex. In 2011, 8102 (25%) new cases of acquired immune deficiency syndrome (AIDS) were diagnosed in women (Kaiser Family Foundation, 2013).

There is substantial morbidity and mortality associated with STIs, yet frequently the connections are difficult to pinpoint. In many cases morbidity and mortality are related to sequelae of STIs, and this is especially the case for women. Pelvic inflammatory disease, ectopic pregnancy, and cervical cancer are complications exclusive to women that can disproportionately increase female mortality. Deaths from pelvic inflammatory disease, ectopic pregnancy, cervical cancer, liver disease, and AIDS tend to be temporally far removed from STI acquisition, thus making the connection less apparent, and mortality rates underestimated (World Health Organization, 2013).

Racial and Ethnic Considerations

Surveillance evidence indicates that some racial or ethnic minority groups have higher rates of reported STIs when compared with rates among whites. Surveillance data suggest that higher rates of reported STIs occur among some racial or ethnic minority groups when compared with rates among whites (CDC, 2012a). For example, the rate of chlamydia is estimated to be six times higher among African-American women aged 15 to 19 years and 4.8 times higher among African-American women aged 20 to 24 years as compared to white women of similar age groups. Incidence rates among American Indian/Alaskan Native women were four times higher than white women, and incidence rates among Hispanic women were twice that of white women. Similar trends for gonorrhea and syphilis are also noted. The incidence rate of gonorrhea is 15.9 times higher among African-American

women aged 15 to 19, and 12.1 times higher among African-American women 20 to 24 years of age as compared to white women of similar age groups. The disparity in gonorrhea incidence rates is 5.2 times higher among American Indian/Alaskan Native women and 2.1 times higher among Hispanic women as compared to white women. The disparity of syphilis is 17 times higher among African-American women, 1.2 times higher among American Indian/Alaskan Native women, and 2.0 times higher among Hispanic women as compared to white women (CDC, 2012a). It is especially noteworthy that women of color, particularly African-American women, are disproportionately affected by HIV. HIV incidence rates are 20 times higher among African-American women and four times higher among Hispanic women as compared to white women. Newly infected African-American and Hispanic women are more likely to be younger than white women (Kaiser Family Foundation, 2013).

Etiology and Risk Factors

A variety of individual characteristics, behaviors, and environmental conditions can increase the risk of women for acquiring an STI (Caple & Schub, 2012).

Biologic Factors

The prevalence rates of many STIs are highest among adolescents, whose lack of immunity and biologic susceptibility are contributing factors to their vulnerability to such infections. Seventy-one percent of all adolescent girls have had vaginal sex by the age of 19 years, with the end result being many young women at risk for STIs (Alan Guttmacher Institute, 2013). The earlier a woman begins to have sexual intercourse, the longer is her period of sexual activity, the greater her number of partners, and the less apt she is to use barrier contraception (Schmid, 2001). Compared to older women prior to menopause, female adolescents and young women are more susceptible to cervical infections, such as chlamydia infections, gonorrhea, and HIV, because of the ectropion of the immature cervix and resulting larger exposed surface area of cells unprotected by cervical mucus. These cells eventually recede into the inner cervix as women age. Women who are postmenopausal are also at increased risk because of the thin vaginal and cervical mucosa that occurs as estrogen levels decline. Women who are pregnant have higher rates of cervical ectropion (Cunningham et al., 2010).

Other biologic factors that may increase a woman's risk of acquiring, transmitting, or developing complications of certain STIs include vaginal douching, risky sexual practices, use of hormonal contraceptives, and bacterial vaginosis. Risk for contracting the infections that can lead to pelvic inflammatory disease (PID) may be increased with vaginal douching, and the risk for PID may also increase with greater frequency of douching (CDC, 2010b). Certain sexual practices such as anal intercourse, sex during menses, and vaginal intercourse without sufficient lubrication (dry sex), may also predispose a woman to acquiring an STI. The bleeding and tissue trauma that results from these practices can facilitate invasion by pathogens. The role of oral contraceptives in the acquisition and transmission of STIs is not fully understood, however. Evidence suggests that combined oral contraceptives may be associated with decreased risk of PID but increased risk of chlamydial infection (Morrison, Turner, & Jones, 2009; Nelson, 2007). Combined oral contraceptives do not increase the risk of HIV infection (Morrison et al., 2009). Bacterial vaginosis is associated with multiple STIs and increases the risk for acquiring genital herpes and HIV (Atashili, Poole, Ndumbe, Adimora, &

Smith, 2008; Cherpes, Meyn, Krohn, Luri, & Hillier, 2003).

Age

An acknowledged risk factor for STIs is younger age. As previously discussed, individuals in the 15- to 24-year-old age group are disproportionately affected and account for approximately 50% of all new STI cases annually. Adolescent and young women in this age group are more likely to engage in risky sexual behaviors. Moreover, they may be uncomfortable in negotiating condom use or in discussing sexual matters with their partners. They may also lack the self-confidence to refuse to engage in unprotected sexual activity. Also, being in an age-discordant relationship—a relationship between an adolescent female and adult male—increases the risk of adolescent STI (Caple & Schub, 2012).

Sexual Behaviors

Specific sexual behaviors increase the risk of acquiring STIs. These behaviors include engaging in unprotected sex without use of condoms, having multiple sex partners, having concurrent sexual relationships, and having anonymous sex partners. Risky sexual behavior also includes prostitution, engaging in anal intercourse (receptive anal sex carries the highest risk for acquiring HIV), engaging in unprotected sex with a partner who has unhealed lesions or known STI, serosorting (selecting partners based on having similar HIV-positive status), and forced sexual intercourse (Caple & Schub, 2012).

Social and Psychological Factors

A number of social and psychological factors increase the risk of acquiring STIs. The use of alcohol and drugs is associated with an increased risk of HIV and STIs (Caple & Schub, 2012).

This association may arise for several reasons, including social factors such as poverty and lack of educational or economic opportunities, as well as individual factors such as low self esteem and propensity for high-risk behavior. Drug and alcohol use lowers inhibitions and undermines cognitive and social skills. This can increase engagement in risky sexual behaviors and make it difficult for substance users to protect themselves. Intravenous drug use and sharing needles can unequivocally increase risk of transmitting HIV and STIs, as can engaging in unprotected sex with an intravenous drug user (Caple & Schub, 2012). Women of lower socioeconomic status have increased risk of acquiring STIs, most likely related to having inadequate preventive care or education regarding STI risk reduction. This is a common problem among the homeless. The homeless are frequently at increased risk for sexual victimization, or engage in survival sex (trading sexual acts for food or shelter), which increases the risk of STI transmission (Caple & Schub, 2012).

Relationships that lack equal distribution of power can decrease women's ability to negotiate for safe sex practices or to refuse to have unprotected intercourse. Notably, gender power imbalances and cultural proscriptions often associated with sexual relationships can make it difficult for women to protect themselves from infection (Caple & Schub, 2012). Some women may be dependent upon an abusive male partner or a partner who places a woman at risk through his own risky behavior. Women who have been exposed to sexual, verbal, and physical abuse experience erosion of their sense of self-efficacy to exercise control over sexual behaviors. They have an increased likelihood for experiencing anxiety, depression, and post-traumatic stress disorder. These issues increase the risk for engaging in unsafe sexual behaviors. Additionally, fear of physical harm and loss of economic support may hamper women's efforts to enact protective practices. Survivors of childhood sexual abuse

tend to have higher rates of engaging in unprotected sex as well as higher rates of engaging in substance abuse, which increases the risk of acquiring STIs (Caple & Schub, 2012).

Risk of acquiring an STI is determined not only by a woman's actions but also by her partner's behaviors. Although prevention counseling customarily includes recommending that women identify any partner who is at high risk, and the nature of their sexual practices, this advice may be unrealistic or culturally inappropriate in many relationships because of the use of drugs and other medical factors. Women who engage in sexual activities only with other women may also be at risk for infection. Many women who identify themselves as lesbians have had intercourse with a man by choice, by force, or by necessity. Their female partners may also have other STI risk factors such as injection drug use.

Women who have mental illnesses such as schizophrenia, bipolar disorder, psychosis, depression, and anxiety disorders are at increased risk for acquiring STIs. This is especially noteworthy among indigent, homeless, publicly insured, and institutionalized populations. Women with mental illnesses frequently display poor judgment and impulsive behavior that can lead to risky sexual behavior. Furthermore, low self esteem that accompanies mental illness is a barrier to accepting responsibility for behavior and personal health (Caple & Schub, 2012).

Cultural Factors

Relationships and sexual behavior are regulated by cultural norms that influence sexual expression in interpersonal relationships. Women are often socialized to please their partners and to place men's needs and desires first; as a consequence they may find it difficult to insist on safer sex behaviors. Traditional cultural values associated with passivity and subordination may diminish the ability of many women to adequately protect themselves.

Power imbalances in relationships are the result of, and contribute to, the continuance of traditional gender roles that identify men as the initiators and decision makers of sexual activities and women as passive gatekeepers (Miller, Exner, Williams, & Ehrhardt, 2000). As long as traditional gender norms characterize the roles in sexual relationships as men having the dominant role in sexual decision making, women will find it difficult to negotiate with their partners about condom use. Furthermore, cultural norms define talking about condoms as implying a lack of trust that runs counter to the traditional gender norm expectations for women (Maman, 2000). Women often do not request condom use because of a need to establish and maintain intimacy with partners. Urging women to insist on condom use may be unrealistic if their cultural norm includes traditional gender roles that do not encourage women to talk about sex, initiate sexual practices, or control intimate encounters.

Various cultural and ethnic groups may adhere to values regarding health care, drug and alcohol use, and sexual behavior that can increase risk for acquiring STIs. Lack of regular health care because of poverty, mental illness, or cultural beliefs may contribute to deficient education regarding safe sex practices. Psychological barriers to STI screening and treatment, such as mistrust of the healthcare system, lack of linguistically appropriate treatment or education, stigma and shame associated with STIs and STI care, and social pressures can increase risk for STIs and can lead to advanced disease progression and death (Caple & Schub, 2012).

Risk Reduction

A strong knowledge base is the first step in protecting against STIs. Every woman should have a thorough understanding of STI risk, symptoms to watch for, and prevention strategies. Prevention is particularly important, especially because a number of STIs are incurable.

Apart from abstinence, the most reliable prevention strategy for STIs is long-term mutual monogamy with a single partner. The most significant risk factor for any STI is the woman's partner(s). The risk of acquiring an STI increases when a woman has more than one sex partner. STIs should be considered a possibility whenever a woman is not in a strictly exclusive monogamous long-term relationship.

If there is any doubt about a partner's or one's own monogamy or HIV status, safer sex practices are important for any sexual relationship. Safe sex entails any form of sex in which semen, blood, or vaginal secretions are not passed from one person to another. Latex condoms with spermicide are the key ingredient of safer sex practices. Latex condoms must be used correctly each time a person has oral, anal, or vaginal intercourse. If a condom breaks or falls off, its protective effect is lost. Data consistently show that latex condoms, when used consistently and correctly, greatly reduce the chances of transmitting HIV and many other STIs. The risk of acquiring an STI increases with the number of partners a person has, but a person only needs to be exposed once to acquire an STI.

STIs are transmitted by sexual activity. Sexual activity includes traditional sexual intercourse in which the male penis is inserted into the female vagina, as well as other forms of skin-to-skin and mucous membrane-to-mucous membrane contact, such as oral and anal sex. STIs can be transmitted by both homosexual and heterosexual encounters; however, many STIs are less common among lesbian women. Although the notion of safe sex is misleading, safer sex practices do exist that reduce the overall risk of acquiring STIs. Consistent and correct use of latex condoms can reduce the risk of STI transmission. A comparison of sexual activities and their relative risk levels are presented in **Table 8–1**.

HIV and many other STIs are acquired when blood or sexual fluids from one person come in

Table 8–1 RELATIVE LEVELS OF RISK FOR SEXUAL ACTIVITIES

Sexual Activity	Level of Risk	Risk Reduction
Anal intercourse without condom use	High	Use a latex condom. Only have sex with a mutually monogamous tested partner.
Vaginal intercourse without condom use	High	Use a latex condom. Only have sex with a mutually monogamous tested partner.
Oral sex	High Likely less risky than vaginal or anal intercourse for some STIs.	Use a latex condom for oral sex with a man. Use a dental dam or other moisture barrier for oral sex with a woman. Only have sex with a mutually monogamous tested partner.
Mutual masturbation (hand-to-genital contact)	Very low if no visible symptoms or cuts in the skin are present.	Refrain from activity when there are symptoms or cuts in the skin.
Kissing (no sores or broken skin)	Very low, slight risk of oral herpes or syphilis infection.	Refrain from kissing when possible symptoms are present.
All sexual activities with a mutually monogamous partner who is free from infection	None, assuming partner is truly negative.	Ascertain that partner has been tested for all STIs and is trustworthy.
Abstaining from all sexual contact	None	

contact with the mucous membranes of another person. Areas that are susceptible include the interior of the vagina, the tip of the penis, and any cuts or nicks in the skin. Although latex condoms are effective at preventing bodily fluid exchange, they provide less protection from STIs that have other modes of transmission. Herpes and HPV, for example, are spread by contact with symptoms or infected genital skin. A condom covers some but not all of the potentially infectious area, thereby making it a less reliable means of protection against these STIs. Some sexual practices are more risky than others for contracting certain STIs. A person is highly unlikely to get HIV from receiving oral sex even without a condom; however, they could easily get syphilis, oral gonorrhea, or herpes

in this way. Consistent condom use can greatly reduce risk but does not guarantee that one will not contract an STI. Viruses that are located at sites other than the penis, such as the scrotum, vulva, anal region, or inner thighs are not covered by condoms, and transmission from these sites can still occur.

Frank, honest communication prior to sexual activity is important. Although it may be difficult to have an honest discussion about infections and previous risk behaviors, the price of not communicating can be high. Honest communication is a mark of personal maturity. If a potential partner is unable or unwilling to discuss infections and intimacy concerns, it may be an indication of other issues that merit evaluation before proceeding with sexual closeness. Sexual activity should be avoided if either partner has any symptoms of infection or if there are any suspicions of infections. Delaying activity for a few days or having symptoms evaluated may prevent lifelong consequences. Many people with STIs do not know they are infected, thus many couples now see a clinician together for examination and STI screening before initiating a sexual relationship.

Talking about incurable STIs such as herpes and HPV is especially difficult. The timing of communication is important. Stigma associated with the disease is a serious issue and establishing some level of trust before informing a potential sex partner may be judicious. Being calm and knowledgeable about an infection aids in communication. Many people are ignorant about the course of infection of STIs or the means by which they are spread. Open and frank discussion benefits both partners and helps people come to healthier and better terms with their infections.

Gender Differences and Dimensions

Although both men and women can acquire STIs, women are biologically more likely to become infected with STIs than men. The risk of a woman contracting gonorrhea from a single act of intercourse is 60% to 90%, while the corresponding risk for a man is 20% to 30%. Men are two to three times more likely to transmit HIV to women than the reverse. The difference arises because the vagina has a larger amount of genital mucous membranes exposed and is an environment more conducive for infections than the penis (Office on Women's Health, 2011). In addition, risk for trauma is greater during vaginal intercourse for women than for men.

STIs are frequently asymptomatic in women, and therefore are more likely to go undetected than the same diseases in men. Additionally, when

or if symptoms develop, they are often confused with those of other diseases not transmitted sexually. This relative frequency of asymptomatic and unrecognized infections in women results in delayed diagnosis and treatment, chronic untreated infections, and complications. It can be more difficult to diagnose STIs in a woman because the anatomy of her genital tract makes clinical examination more difficult. Lesions that occur inside the vagina and on the cervix are not readily visible, and the normal vaginal environment (a warm, moist, enriched medium) is ideal for nurturing an infection. Overall, women experience most of the STI burden and complications, including infertility, perinatal infections, genital tract neoplasia, and death. In women, these diseases are frequently silent and present as asymptomatic, but remain damaging and infectious.

Considerable stigma accompanies an STI diagnosis, regardless of the culprit organism. Many people still equate STIs with immorality, promiscuous behavior, and low social status. Reproductive tract infections may be perceived as dirty, shameful, or as punishment for previous behavior and an infected woman may fear that healthcare providers will not care for her or will be offended by doing so. Women are more vulnerable than men to the stigma of STIs. American society tends to perceive sexual activity via a moral double standard in which it is acceptable for men to have vast sexual experience while similar sexual experience in women is frowned upon and often censured.

Diagnosis and Treatment of Common Sexually Transmitted Infections

Prompt diagnosis and treatment are predicated on the assumption that any person who believes that he or she may have contracted an STI, has symptoms of an STI, has had sexual relations with someone who has symptoms of an STI, or has a partner who has been diagnosed with an STI will seek care. To obtain prompt diagnosis and treatment, patients must know how to recognize the major signs and symptoms of all STIs and must be willing and able to obtain health care if they experience symptoms or have sexual contact with someone who has an STI. Healthcare providers have the responsibility of educating their patients regarding the signs and symptoms of STIs. This may be done when a woman comes in for her annual health examination, seeks contraception, or obtains preconception or prenatal care. Healthcare providers also must ensure that patients know where and how to obtain care if they suspect they might have contracted an STI. Many local health departments have clinics specially designed to treat STIs, with services often available for free or at a reduced cost.

All women who are sexually active should be screened regularly through history, physical exam, and laboratory studies. An assessment of sexual risk should occur during the collection of the health history. Risk assessment depends on a woman's willingness to self-identify risk factors that may be seen as socially unacceptable or stigmatizing. Some women may be reluctant to reveal such risk factors directly to healthcare providers but are willing to do so if asked to fill out a questionnaire that assesses sexual risk history. Pertinent questions that should be included in an assessment of sexual risk history are presented in **Table 8–2**. A woman who is diagnosed with an STI should be screened for other STIs because comorbidity of such infections is high and many STIs can be asymptomatic.

The diagnosis of an STI is made based on the integration of relevant history, physical,

---

Table 8–2 Assessment of Risk for STIs

Part 1: Sexual Risk History

Are you sexually active?
Have you had sex/intercourse with anyone in the past 6 months/year?
- If no, have you had intercourse in the past?
- If yes, have your partners been men, women, or both?
- How many people have you had sex with in the past 6 months/year?
- Presently, how many different people are you having sex with?
- Does your partner have any other partners that you know of?

Have you ever had sex with someone who has been in jail?
Have you ever had sex with someone who has had a blood transfusion or hemophilia?
Have you ever had sex with someone whom you were afraid put you at risk for HIV/STI?
- Someone who had a positive HIV test?
- Someone you think might have HIV/AIDS?
- Someone who uses drugs? IV drugs? Cocaine?
- Someone who might have had sex with a prostitute or with both men and women?

Have you ever been told you had an STI?
- Never?
- Chlamydia?
- Gonorrhea?
- Trichomoniasis?
- Syphilis?
- HPV?
- Other? (please list)

Table 8–2 Assessment of Risk for STIs (*continued*)

Part 1: Sexual Risk History

Have you ever been told you had a pelvic infection or PID?

Many women have sex when they have drunk too much alcohol or have been using drugs. Has this happened to you?

Do you use drugs?

If so, what kinds of drugs do you use?

- Opioids: Types, route of administration, and frequency?
- Stimulants: Types, route of administration, and frequency?
- Crack cocaine: Frequency? Have you ever had sex in a crack house?
- Alcohol: Types and frequency?

Have you ever blacked out from alcohol or drugs, especially during sex?

Have you ever traded sex for drugs, money, food, housing or anything else?

Do you ever have sex when you are high?

Can you tell me the kinds of sex that you have? This will help determine what your risks are:

- Mouth on penis or vulva: Protected? Unprotected?
- Penis in vagina: Protected? Unprotected?
- Penis in the rectum: Protected? Unprotected?
- Mouth on anus: Protected? Unprotected?

If you are sexually active:

- Do you worry about catching a sexually transmitted infection or HIV (the AIDS virus)?
- Do you do anything to prevent catching an infection?
- Have you had sex without a condom?
- When did you start using condoms?
- Have you performed oral sex on a man or woman without using a barrier (dental dam, condom, plastic wrap)?

Part 2: Menstrual Gynecologic History

Do you experience now or have you ever experienced:

- Frequent vaginal infections
- Unusual vaginal discharge/odor
- Vaginal itching/burning/sores/warts
- Sexually transmitted infections (ask about individual infections)
- Abdominal pain
- Pelvic inflammatory disease/infection of the uterus, tubes, ovaries
- Rape
- Physical/emotional/sexual abuse
- Abnormal PAP test
- Pain/bleeding with intercourse
- Severe menstrual cramps occurring at the end of your period
- Ectopic pregnancy

and laboratory data. A history that is accurate, comprehensive, and specific is essential for accurate diagnosis. Generally, the history should be taken first, with the woman dressed. Information should be collected in a nonjudgmental manner, avoiding assumptions of sexual preferences. All partners should be referred to as "partner," rather than by gender. It is helpful to begin with open-ended questions because they often elicit information that might otherwise be missed.

These queries can be followed with symptom-specific questions and relevant history. Specific areas to address include the reason why the woman has sought care and any symptoms she has noticed; a sexual history, including a description of the date and type of sexual activity; number of partners; whether she has had contact with someone who recently had an STI; and potential sites of infection (such as mouth, cervix, urethra, and rectum). Pertinent medical history includes anything that will influence the management plan, such as history of drug allergies, previously diagnosed chronic illnesses, and general health status. A menstrual history, including the date of the woman's last menstrual period, must always be obtained so that pregnancy may be ruled out because certain medications used to treat STIs are contraindicated in pregnancy. When indicated, an HIV-oriented systems review should be conducted. Any positive answers regarding symptoms should be followed up to elicit information about onset, duration, and specific characteristics, such as color, amount, and consistency of discharge.

Before the actual physical examination is performed, the healthcare provider should discuss the procedure to be followed with the woman so that she is prepared. The physical examination begins with careful visualization of the external genitalia, including the perineum. Erythema, edema, distortions, lesions, trauma, and any other abnormalities are noted. Palpation can locate areas of tenderness. During the speculum examination, the vagina and cervix are inspected for edema, thinning, lesions, abnormal coloration, discharge, trauma, and bleeding. Thorough palpation of inguinal area and pelvic organs, milking of the urethra for discharge, and assessment of vaginal secretion odors are essential.

Appropriate laboratory studies will be suggested in part by the results of the history and physical examination. Additional laboratory studies may be performed in female patients because women are often infected with more than one STI simultaneously and because many are asymptomatic. The tests include microscopic examination of vaginal secretions (wet mount), chlamydia and gonorrhea testing, Venereal Disease Research Laboratory (VDRL) or rapid plasma regain (RPR) testing for syphilis, and hepatitis B panel. When an STI is diagnosed, testing for other STIs is essential. The woman should be notified that HIV testing will be performed unless she specifically declines such testing. Other laboratory tests, such as complete blood count, urinalysis, and urine culture and sensitivity should be obtained if indicated. If the history or physical examination indicates pregnancy is possible, a urine human chorionic gonadotropin (hCG) test should be performed.

Accurate identification and timely reporting of STIs are integral components of successful infection control efforts. Healthcare providers are required to report certain STIs to the state public health officials, who in turn report these infection rates to the CDC. Nationally notifiable STIs include chancroid, chlamydia, gonorrhea, hepatitis, HIV, and syphilis (CDC, 2012d). The requirements for reporting other STIs differ from state to state. Women with STIs should be asked to identify and notify all partners who might have been exposed to the infection. Healthcare providers are legally responsible for reporting all cases of those infections identified as reportable and should know the requirements of the state in which they practice. The patient must be informed when a case will be reported and told why. Failure to inform the patient that the case will be reported is considered a serious breach of medical ethics.

Confidentiality is a crucial issue for many patients. When an STI is reportable, women need to be told that they may be contacted by a health department representative. They should be assured that the information reported to and collected by health authorities is maintained in strictest confidence. Reports are protected by statutes of subpoena in most jurisdictions. Every effort, within the limits of one's public health responsibilities, should be made to reassure patients.

Human Papillomavirus and Genital Warts

HPV is now the most common STI in the United States. Although most HPV infections are asymptomatic, subclinical, or unrecognized, and many infections clear spontaneously, HPV can cause genital warts and cervical cancer. Most genital warts are caused by HPV types 6 and 11, which carry a low risk for triggering invasive cancer. However, HPV types 16, 18, 31, 33, and 35 occasionally found in genital warts have been identified as associated with cervical intraepithelial neoplasia (CDC, 2010b). Two high-risk HPV types, 16 and 18, cause 70% of cervical cancers (Munoz et al., 2003).

Genital warts, also known as chondyloma, are frequently seen in the posterior part of the introitus; however, lesions can also be found on the buttocks, vulva, vagina, anus, and cervix. Typically, lesions appear as small (2–3 mm in length and 10–15 mm in height) papillary swellings occurring singularly or in clusters on the genital and anorectal region. Warts are usually flesh colored or slightly darker on Caucasian women, black on African-American women, and brownish on Asian women. Infections of long duration may appear as a cauliflower-like mass. In moist areas, such as the vaginal introitus, the lesions may appear to have multiple fine, fingerlike projections. Vaginal lesions frequently appear as multiple warts. Flat-topped papules 1–4 mm in diameter are sometimes seen on the cervix, and often visualized under magnification. Although they are usually painless, the lesions may sometimes be uncomfortable, particularly when very large, inflamed, or ulcerated. Chronic vaginal discharge, prutitus, dyspareunia, or postcoital bleeding can occur as well.

Diagnosis is made by careful, thorough clinical examination of visible genital warts or by biopsy of cervical lesions and (rarely) of lesions at other sites if the diagnosis is not clear. Screening for other STIs should be done when genital warts are present. Women with genital warts should have cervical cancer screening. Cervical cancer screening should begin within 3 years of the onset of sexual activity or by age 21. The recommended screening test is the Papanicolaou (Pap) smear.

Women who have cervical dysplasia may need to seek aggressive treatment to prevent possible cancer development. Colposcopic examination and biopsy of suspicious areas are indicated. It is also important that women be diligent about personal care, medical follow-up care, and annual Pap smears and pelvic examinations.

Although warts may regress spontaneously, they are frequently symptomatic or psychologically distressing. Treatment is often indicated to remove visible warts for psychological and aesthetic reasons, as well as to reduce (but not eliminate) the likelihood of transmission. HPV infections can be quite persistent and can recur regardless of which treatment method is selected. Treatment is easier and less painful in earlier stages. Although no treatment can "cure" HPV, evidence suggests that the immune systems of most individuals will eventually clear the virus even without treatment. At that point, a person would no longer have HPV, though he or she could be reinfected with a new exposure. Treatment options will be selected based on the extent of HPV infection and its location and include topical agents applied by the patient or healthcare provider, cryotherapy (freezing of warts), laser surgery, electrosurgery, and surgical excision.

Women who are experiencing discomfort associated with genital warts may find bathing the area with an oatmeal solution and drying the area with a hair dryer on a low setting will provide some relief. The area should be kept clean and dry to decrease the growth of warts. Cotton underwear and loose-fitting clothing may help to decrease irritation and discomfort. Women should maintain a healthy lifestyle to strengthen the immune system. Although use of latex condoms may reduce transmission of HPV, condoms do not provide reliable protection against HPV. HPV is spread by genital skin-to-skin contact, not by bodily fluids. Because a latex condom does not cover all of the genital skin, it cannot guarantee prevention of transmission, even if no visible symptoms are present. A female condom may provide more protection than a traditional condom that covers the penis; however, neither type of condom use can guarantee immunity.

The most clinically significant HPV types can now be prevented with vaccination. Both the bivalent vaccine (HPV2, Cervarix), and the quadrivalent vaccine (HPV4, Gardisil) protect against HPV types 16 and 18, which cause the majority of cervical cancers. The quadrivalent vaccine also prevents HPV types 6 and 11, which causes the majority of genital warts, thus providing some protection against vulvar and vaginal cancers and precancers (CDC, 2010b). Routine HPV vaccination is recommended for girls aged 11 to 12 years. HPV vaccines can be given to girls as young as age 9 and are also recommended for adolescent and young women aged 13 to 26 years who were not vaccinated or did not complete the series earlier. Ideally, vaccination should occur before the adolescent or woman becomes sexually active, and therefore has the potential for HPV exposure. Vaccination is also recommended for women who have evidence of existing HPV infection, such as Pap test abnormalities or genital warts, to provide protection against HPV types that have not yet been acquired. Vaccination will not treat existing HPV infection, cervical cytologic abnormalities, or genital warts (American College of Obstetrician and Gynecologists [ACOG], 2010b).

Both vaccines are given in a series of three intramuscular injections. The second dose is given 1–2 months after the first dose. The third dose is given 6 months after the second dose. Ideally, the same vaccine product should be given for the entire three-dose series (CDC, 2010b). The series does not need to be restarted if the second and third doses are delayed. HPV vaccines are not recommended during pregnancy but can be given during lactation. If a woman is found to be pregnant after the first dose is given, the remaining doses in the series should be delayed until after she gives birth. Women who have received HPV vaccine are advised to continue routine cervical cancer screening because 30% of cervical cancers are caused by HPV types other than 16 or 18 (CDC, 2010b).

Genital Herpes

Genital herpes is a recurrent incurable viral infection characterized by painful vesicular eruption of the skin and mucosa of the genitals. Two types of HSV have been identified as causing genital herpes: HSV-1 and HSV-2. HSV-2 is usually transmitted sexually, and HSV-1 is transmitted nonsexually. Even though HSV-1 is more commonly associated with gingivostomatitis and oral ulcers (fever blisters) and HSV-2 with genital lesions, both types are not exclusively associated with those sites. HSV-2 infection increases the risk of women acquiring HIV by at least threefold (Freeman et al., 2006).

Most people who have HSV-2 have never been diagnosed with genital herpes. Despite their mild or unrecognized infections, they intermittently shed the HSV-2 virus in the genital tract. Consequently, most genital herpes infections are transmitted by individuals who do not know they have HSV-2 or who do not have symptoms at the time of transmission (CDC, 2010b).

An initial or primary genital herpes infection characteristically has both systemic and local symptoms and lasts approximately 3 weeks. Women tend to have a more severe clinical course than do men. Flu-like symptoms with fever, malaise, and myalgia first appear about a week after exposure, peak within 4 days, and subside over the next week. Multiple genital lesions develop at the site of infection, usually the vulva. Other commonly affected sites include the perianal area, the vagina, and cervix. The legions begin as small, painful blisters or vesicles that become unroofed, leaving ulcerated lesions. Individuals with primary herpes often develop bilateral tender inguinal lymphadenopathy, vulvar edema, vaginal discharge, and severe dysuria.

Ulcerative lesions last 4 to 5 days before crusting over. New lesions may develop over a period of 10 days during the course of the infection. Cervicitis is also common with initial HSV-2 infections. The cervix may appear normal, or it may be friable, reddened, ulcerated, or necrotic. A heavy, watery to purulent vaginal discharge is common. Extragenital lesions may be present because of autoinoculation. Urinary retention and dysuria may develop secondary to autonomic involvement of the sacral nerve root.

Women experiencing recurrent episodes of genital herpes typically develop only local symptoms that are less severe than those associated with the initial infection. Systemic symptoms are usually absent, although the characteristic prodromal genital tingling is common. Recurrent lesions are unilateral, are less severe than the original lesions, and usually last 7 to 10 days without prolonged viral shedding. Lesions begin as vesicles and progress rapidly to ulcers. Very few women with recurrent disease have cervicitis.

Although a diagnosis of genital herpes infection may be suspected from the history and physical examination, it can be confirmed only by laboratory studies. Isolation of HSV in cell culture or by polymerase chain reaction (PCR) is the preferred test in women who have genital ulcers or other mucocutaneous lesions. Viral culture is less sensitive than PCR. Viral culture is best taken during a primary infection or if the specimen is taken during the vesicular stage of the disease because the sensitivity of a culture declines rapidly as lesions begin to heal.

Genital herpes is a chronic and recurring disease for which there is no known cure. Systemic antiviral drugs partially control the signs and symptoms of HSV infections when used for the primary or recurrent episodes, or when used as daily suppressive therapy. These drugs do not cure the infection, however, nor do they alter subsequent risk, frequency, or rate of recurrence after discontinuation. Three antiviral medications provide clinical benefits for genital herpes: acyclovir, valacyclovir, and famciclovir. Topical antiviral therapy is not recommended due to its minimal benefits (CDC, 2010b).

Measures are also recommended to decrease discomfort and help prevent secondary infection. Lesions should be cleaned twice a day with a saline solution, and coexisting bacterial infections must be treated with appropriate antibiotics. Oral analgesics such as aspirin or ibuprofen may be used to relieve pain and systemic symptoms associated with initial infection. Topical agents should be used cautiously because affected mucous membranes are very sensitive. Ointments containing cortisone should be avoided. Occlusive ointments may prolong the course of the infection.

Complementary measures that may increase comfort for women with active lesions include warm sitz baths with baking soda; keeping lesions warm and dry using a hair dryer set on cool, or patting the area dry with a soft towel; wearing cotton underwear and loose clothing; applying cold milk or witch hazel compresses followed by aloe vera gel or Burrow's solution four times a day for 30 minutes; oatmeal baths; applying cool, wet black tea bags to lesions; and applying compresses with an infusion of cloves or peppermint oil and clove oil to lesions (Collins-Bride & Murphy, 2004; Sinclair, 2004).

Chancroid

Chancroid is a bacterial infection of the genitourinary tract caused by the gram negative bacteria *Haemophilus ducreyi*. Chancroid is a genital ulcer;

thus it is a risk factor for HIV transmission. The major way chancroid is acquired is through sexual contact and trauma. Infection through autoinoculation of fingers or other sites occasionally occurs. The incubation period, though not well established, usually ranges from 4 to 7 days but may be as long as 3 weeks.

Typically the woman presents with a history of a painful macule on the external genitalia that rapidly changes to a pustule and then to an ulcerated lesion. The patient may develop enlarged unilateral or bilateral inguinal nodes, known as buboes. After 1 to 2 weeks, the skin overlying the lymph node becomes erythematous, the center necroses, and the node becomes ulcerated.

A probable diagnosis of chancroid can be made when one or more painful genital ulcers are present and there is no evidence of syphilis (per dark-field examination of ulcer exudates or serological testing at least 7 days after onset of ulcer). The clinical presentation, ulcer appearance, and regional lymphadenopathy must be typical for chancroid, and HSV testing of the exudates is negative. Testing for HIV and syphilis should be performed concurrently at the time of diagnosis and repeated in 3 months.

Chancroid is treated with oral antibiotics, such as azithromycin, ceftriaxone, erythromycin base, or ciprofloxacin. Women who have comorbid HIV infection may require repeated or longer therapy.

Trichomoniasis

Trichomoniasis is caused by *Trichomonas vaginalis*, an anaerobic one-celled protozoan with characteristic flagellae. The organism most commonly lives in the vagina of women and in the urethra of men. Among women presenting with vaginitis symptoms, 4% to 35% will have *T. vaginalis* infection. Trichomoniasis is sexually transmitted during vaginal-penile intercourse or vulva-to-vulva contact. Nonsexual transmission is rare but possible because the organism is capable of surviving outside a host in a wet environment such as wet

towel or swimsuit. Trichomoniasis is believed to facilitate HIV transmission (Sutton et al., 2007).

Although trichomoniasis may be asymptomatic, women commonly experience a characteristically yellow to greenish frothy, mucopurulent, copious, malodorous discharge. Inflammation of the vulva, vagina, or both may be present, and the woman may have irritation, prutitus, dysuria, or dyspareunia. Usually, the discharge worsens during and after menstruation.

Diagnosis is usually made by wet prep visualization of the typical one-celled flagellate trichomonads. This method has a sensitivity of only approximately 60% to 70%. Culture is a sensitive and highly specific method of diagnosis, yet it is not routinely performed. Culture is performed when trichomoniasis is suspected but cannot be confirmed with microscopy. All patients with trichomoniasis should undergo testing for other STIs, such as chlamydia, gonorrhea, syphilis, and HIV.

The only class of drugs useful for oral or parenteral therapy of trichomoniasis is nitroimidazoles. Of the nitroimidazoles, metronidazole and tinidazole are approved by the FDA for treatment of trichomoniasis in this country. Treatment of patients and their sex partners is efficacious in relieving symptoms, achieving microbiologic cure, and reducing transmission (CDC, 2010b). Both the patients and their sex partners should abstain from sex until they have been treated and are asymptomatic.

Chlamydia

Chlamydia is caused by the bacterium *Chlamydia trachomatis*. Chlamydia infection is usually asymptomatic. When present, symptoms may include spotting or postcoital bleeding, mucoid or purulent cervical discharge, urinary frequency, dysuria, lower abdominal pain, or dyspareunia. Bleeding results from inflammation and erosion of the cervical columnar epithelium. Chlamydia can invade the upper reproductive tract, subsequently causing PID.

All sexually active women aged 25 years or younger should be screened for chlamydia annually (CDC, 2010b). Women older than age 25 with known risk factors should also be screened. Chlamydia testing is performed using urine or swab specimens from the endocervix or vagina. Screening procedures for chlamydia infection include nucleic acid amplification tests (NAATs), cell culture, direct immunofluorescence, enzyme immunoassay (EIA), and nucleic acid hybridization tests. NAATs are the preferred technique because they provide the highest sensitivity. Women with a positive urine test should have a pelvic exam to identify complications such as PID. All patients with chlamydia should be tested for other STIs, including gonorrhea, syphilis, and HIV.

Treatment for chlamydia is comprised of antibiotic regimens that cure the infection and usually relieve symptoms. The recommended antibiotic regimens are presented in **Box 8–1**. Treatment of current and recent sexual partners is imperative.

A test of cure (3 to 4 weeks after treatment) is not necessary unless a woman is pregnant, has persistent symptoms, or may have reinfection. A high prevalence of reinfection is observed in women who have chlamydia infections in the preceding several months, usually from reinfection by an untreated partner. Patients should be advised to abstain from sex until their sexual partners are treated. They must wait 7 days after single-dose treatment or until completion of a 7-day regimen before resuming sexual activity. Patients with chlamydia must be advised that they need to be rescreened 3 months after treatment.

Gonorrhea

Gonorrhea is caused by the aerobic gram-negative diplococcus *Neisseria gonorrhoeae*. Gonorrhea is almost exclusively transmitted by sexual activity, primarily through genital-to-genital contact. It is also spread by oral-to-genital and anal-to-genital

---

Box 8–1: Recommended Antibiotic Therapy for the Treatment of Chlamydia

Recommended regimens:

Azithromycin 1 gm orally in a single dose
     Or
Doxycycline 100 mg orally twice a day for 7 days

Alternative regimens:

Erythromycin base 500 mg orally four times a day for 7 days
     Or
Erythromycin ethylsuccinate 800 mg orally four times a day for 7 days
     Or
Levofloxacin 500 mg orally once daily for 7 days
     Or
Ofloxacin 300 mg orally twice a day for 7 days

Reproduced from Centers for Disease Control and Prevention. (2010b). Sexually transmitted diseases treatment guidelines, 2010. *Morbidity and Mortality Weekly Report, 59*(RR-12), 1–110. Retrieved from http://www.cdc.gov /mmwr /pdf/rr/rr5912.pdf

contact. Sites of infection in females include the cervix, urethra, oropharynx, Skene's glands, and Bartholin's glands. In addition to young age, early onset of sexual activity and having multiple sex partners increase the risk of women for contracting this STI.

Women with gonorrhea often remain asymptomatic. When symptoms are present, they are often less specific than the symptoms in men. Women may report dyspareunia, unusual vaginal discharge or bleeding, postcoital bleeding, unilateral labia pain and swelling, and pelvic pain or tenderness. Later in the course of the infection, women may develop purulent, irritating vaginal discharge, rectal pain and discharge, menstrual irregularities with longer, more painful menses, and chronic or acute lower abdominal pain. A gonococcal anal infection following anal intercourse may present as perfuse purulent anal discharge, rectal pain, and blood in the stool. Rectal itching, fullness, pressure, and pain may also be present. Women with gonococcal pharyngitis may present with a red, swollen uvula and pustule vesicles on the soft palate and tonsils similar to streptococcal infections.

The main complication of gonorrheal infection is PID. Women may also develop a pelvic abscess or Bartholin's abscess. Disseminated gonococcal infections (DGIs) are a rare complication and can occur in 0.5% to 3% of untreated cases. DGI occurs in two stages. The first stage is characterized by bacteremia with chills, fever, and skin lesions. This is followed by the second stage, during which the patient develops acute septic arthritis with characteristic effusions, most commonly of the elbows, wrists, knees, and ankles (Miller, 2006).

Gonorrhea testing can be performed by culture, nucleic acid hybridization tests, and NAATs. NAATs can be performed using urine or swab specimens from the endocervix or vagina. All patients with gonorrhea should be tested for other STIs, including chlamydia, syphilis, and HIV.

Treatment for gonorrhea is complicated by the fact that *N. gonorrhoeae* has the ability to develop resistance to antimicrobial therapies. Current recommended antibiotic regimens are presented in **Box 8–2**. Quinolones are no longer used to treat gonorrhea due to the development of a high rate of quinolone-resistant strains of *N. gonorrhoeae* throughout the United States as well as globally. Patients treated for gonorrhea are also concomitantly treated for chlamydia because co-infection rates are high, and dual therapy may hinder the

---

Box 8–2: Recommended Treatment Regimens for Uncomplicated Gonorrhea

Ceftriaxone 250 mg IM in a single dose
OR, IF NOT AN OPTION
Cefixime 400 mg orally in a single dose
OR
Single-dose injectible cephalosporin regimens
PLUS
Azithromycin 1 g orally in a single dose
OR
Doxycycline 100 mg a day for 7 days

Reproduced from Centers for Disease Control and Prevention. (2010b). Sexually transmitted diseases treatment guidelines, 2010. *Morbidity and Mortality Weekly Report, 59*(RR-12), 1–110. Retrieved from http://www.cdc.gov/mmwr/pdf/rr/rr5912.pdf

development of resistant strains. A test of cure (3 to 4 weeks after treatment) is not necessary (CDC, 2010b). Decreased susceptibility of the infectious organism to cefixime has been reported, which has raised concerns about the potential development of cephalosporin-resistant strains.

Syphilis

Syphilis is a systemic disease caused by *Treponema pallidum*, a motile spirochete. Syphilis is characterized by periods of active symptoms and periods of asymptomatic latency. This disease can affect any tissue or organ in the body. Transmission is thought to be by entry into the subcutaneous tissue through microscopic abrasions that can occur during sexual intercourse. The infection can also be transmitted through kissing, biting, or oral-genital sex. Syphilis is a complex infection that can lead to serious systemic disease and even death when untreated. Infection manifests itself in distinct stages with different symptoms and clinical manifestations.

PRIMARY SYPHILIS

Primary syphilis may develop about 3 to 12 weeks after sexual contact with an infected individual. It is characterized by a primary lesion, or chancre, which often begins as a painless papule at the site of inoculation and then erodes to form a nontender, shallow, indurated clean ulcer that is several millimeters to a few centimeters in size. The chancre is loaded with spirochetes and is most commonly found on the genitalia, although it may also occur on the cervix, perianal area, or mouth. The chancre heals within 2 to 6 weeks with or without treatment.

SECONDARY SYPHILIS

Secondary syphilis may occur within 1 week to 6 months after primary syphilis and is characterized by a widespread symmetrical maculopapular rash on the palms and soles, as well as generalized lymphadenopathy. The woman may also experience fever, headache, and malaise. Wart-like lesions known as condylomata lata may develop on the vulva, perineum, or anus. If the patient is untreated, she enters a latent phase that is asymptomatic for the majority of individuals. At this point, if the disease is still not treated, approximately one-third of patients will develop tertiary syphilis.

TERTIARY SYPHILIS

Tertiary syphilis may appear 10 to 20 years after initial exposure and is characterized by symptoms that manifest according to the involved organ systems. Cardiovascular (chest pain, cough), dermatologic (multiple nodules or ulcers), skeletal (arthritis, myalgia, myositis), and neurologic (headache, irritability, impaired balance, memory loss, tremors) symptoms can develop in this stage. Neurologic complications are not limited to tertiary syphilis; rather, a variety of syndromes (e.g., meningitis, meningovascular syphilis, general paresis, and tabes dorsalis) may span all stages of the disease.

Dark-field examination and direct fluorescent antibody for *T. pallidum* (DFS-TP) of lesion exudates or tissue will provide a definitive diagnosis of early syphilis. The availability of these tests is limited and their sensitivity is low. Thus, they are rarely used (Kent & Romanelli, 2008). The ability to confirm the diagnosis of syphilis depends on serology results obtained during the latency and late infection phases of the disease. Any test for antibodies may not be reactive in the presence of active infection, as it takes time for the immune system to develop antibodies to any antigens. A presumptive diagnosis of syphilis is possible with the use of two serological tests: nontreponemal and treponemal. Nontreponemal tests such as the VDRL and RPR are used as screening tests and are relatively inexpensive, sensitive, moderately non-specific, and fast. The treponemal tests—the fluorescent treponemal antibody absorbed (FTA-ABS) test and the *T. pallidum* passive particle agglutination (TP-PA) assay—are used to confirm positive nontreponemal test results.

The preferred treatment for patients with all stages of syphilis is parenteral penicillin G. It is the only proven therapy that has been widely used for patients with neurosyphilis, congenital syphilis, and syphilis during pregnancy. Single-dose therapy is used to treat primary, secondary, and early latent syphilis. Women who have late latent, tertiary, or unknown-duration syphilis require weekly treatment for 3 weeks. Women who have primary or secondary syphilis should have repeat clinical evaluation and serological testing at 6 and 12 months after treatment. Information on follow-up of patients with tertiary syphilis is limited. Partner treatment is imperative and management depends on the stage of the patient's infection and the timing of the partner's exposure (CDC, 2010b).

Hepatitis

Hepatitis is an inflammation of the liver caused by infection with one of several viruses, A, B, C, D, E, F, and G. The virus types associated with sexual transmission are hepatitis A, B, and C. Of these, hepatitis B is transmitted primarily through sexual contact. When present, symptoms may include fever, fatigue, loss of appetite, nausea, vomiting, abdominal pain, dark urine, clay-colored stools, joint pain, and jaundice. Symptoms may appear 2 to 6 weeks after exposure and develop over a period of several days. Symptoms may last as long as 2 months, although some individuals may experience symptoms for as long as 6 months. Diagnosis of hepatitis is based on clinical symptoms and laboratory blood tests, which confirm the type of virus involved. Diagnosis is often difficult because any form of hepatitis can be present without symptoms.

Hepatitis A

Hepatitis A (HAV) transmission during sexual activity occurs during fecal-oral contact with an infected person. HAV is generally a mild illness that resolves within a few weeks. Some individuals may be asymptomatic. Most people recover completely without lasting liver damage.

Hepatitis B

Hepatitis B (HBV) is a blood-borne pathogen transmitted by percutaneous or mucosal exposure to infectious blood or body fluids such as semen and saliva. HBV is more infectious than HIV and hepatitis C (HCV), with HBV being able to survive outside the body for at least 7 days (CDC, 2010b; 2012c). HBV infection may be transmitted both parenterally and through sexual contact. In particular, hepatitis B surface antigen (HBsAg) has been found in blood, saliva, sweat, tears, vaginal secretions, and semen. Perinatal transmission does occur, but the fetus is not at risk for contracting the infection until the child makes contact with contaminated blood at birth. HBV has also been transmitted by artificial insemination.

HBV infection is a disease that affects the liver. It remains asymptomatic in as many as half of the persons with the infection. When symptoms occur, they begin an average of 90 days after HBV exposure and symptoms usually last for several weeks. About 5% of adults with HBV infection become chronically infected, and 15% to 25% of individuals with chronic infection will die prematurely from liver cancer or cirrhosis (CDC, 2010b; 2012c).

Hepatitis C

Hepatitis C (HCV) is the most common cause of chronic liver disease and the most common blood-borne disease in the United States. HCV is mostly transmitted through contact with infected blood, intravenous drug use, or contaminated blood transfusion. Sexual transmission accounts for about 15% to 20% of HCV infections in the absence of other risk factors. Perinatal transmission of HCV from mother to child is much less frequent (CDC, 2013b). About 60% to 70% of individuals who are newly infected with HCV are usually asymptomatic or have a mild clinical illness. Within 1 to 3 weeks after exposure, HCV ribonucleic acid (RNA) can be detected in blood. Anti-HCV antigens can be detected in the blood at about 8 to 9 weeks after exposure, and anti-HCV antigens can be detected in more than 97% of persons by 6 months after exposure. Approximately 70% to 85% of HCV-infected persons develop chronic HCV infection and 60% to 70% of chronically infected persons have evidence of active liver disease. The majority of persons infected with HCV may not be aware of their infection because they are not clinically ill. However, infected persons are a source of transmission of HCV to others and are at risk for chronic liver disease or other HCV-related chronic diseases decades after infection (CDC, 2013b).

There is no cure for hepatitis. Symptoms are treated and rest and supportive care are recommended. A healthy diet is important and alcohol should be avoided until liver function tests indicate that the liver is functioning normally. Although most individuals with hepatitis recover within a few weeks, 10% to 30% of infected individuals develop a persistent hepatitis infection, either with or without symptoms. Chronic hepatitis may lead to severe liver impairment and is associated with the later development of liver cancer. Chronic infections may be treated with alpha-interferon to relieve symptoms and improve liver function. However, this treatment regimen is expensive, may cause severe side effects, and in the majority of cases is not effective in eliminating infection.

Hepatitis A and B may be prevented by vaccination or by treatment with immune globulin within two weeks of exposure. Vaccination is recommended for all individuals who have had more than one sex partner within the past 6 months as well as for anyone being evaluated or treated for an STI. In addition, all children younger than 19 years of age, injection drug users, residents and staff of facilities for the developmentally disabled, individuals who have a sexual partner or household contact who is HBsAG positive, individuals with end-stage renal disease, chronic liver disease, or HIV, persons whose occupations expose them to blood and body fluids, travelers to areas with high rates of HBV infection, and anyone who wants protection from HBV infection should be vaccinated (CDC, 2010b). Numerous vaccine preparations are available, including one that protects against both HAV and HBV. HAV vaccination is usually administered by intramuscular injection in the deltoid muscle, in a series of two injections at 0, and 6 to 12 months. HBV vaccination is usually administered in a three-dose series at 0, 1, and 6 months, via intramuscular injection in the deltoid muscle. Other dosage schedules for both HBV and HAV vaccinations are also available, depending on patient age and product formulation (CDC, 2010b).

Immunoglobulin may be used to impart temporary (that is, 3 to 6 months) immunity to persons exposed to hepatitis A or B. Immunoglobulin is commonly administered as an adjunct to vaccination. There is no vaccine available for hepatitis C. Prophylaxis with immunoglobulin is not effective in preventing HCV infection after exposure (CDC, 2010b).

Human Immunodeficiency Virus

HIV is a retrovirus—a virus that incorporates its genetic material into the genome of the cell it attacks. When HIV (also known as the AIDS [acquired immunodeficiency syndrome] virus) enters the bloodstream, it attacks specific white blood cells called CD4 or T lymphocytes. The virus also replicates. The CD4 cells are no longer able to stimulate a cellular defense response, and the immune system is compromised. The number of CD4 cells in the body of an infected person decreases as the number of HIV-infected cells increases. AIDS is the final stage of HIV; it is diagnosed when a person has a positive test for antibodies to HIV and a low T-lymphocyte count. An HIV-positive person may also be diagnosed with AIDS when one of 26 known infections, called opportunistic infections, is present. Opportunistic infections present a potentially fatal risk to individuals with AIDS.

HIV is transmitted through sexual intercourse, shared needle use, or contaminated blood or blood products. It is not spread by casual, social, or family contact. Although a lethal organism inside the body, the HIV virus quickly dies when exposed to open air. An individual with HIV may have no physical symptoms so it is impossible to tell whether a person is infected without a blood test. HIV-infected individuals are capable of transmitting the virus to others even in the absence of symptoms. The HIV incubation period ranges from months to years. No individuals or groups of individuals are immune from HIV/AIDS.

As noted earlier, several factors increase women's risk for acquiring HIV. In addition to the anatomically driven susceptibility of the female genitalia, the integrity of the tissues of the lower genital tract influence HIV transmission risk. Trauma during intercourse, STI-related cervicitis, and an STI lesion (such as HSV ulcer or syphilis chancre) increase susceptibility to HIV infection. Overall, any activity or condition that disrupts the tissues of the vagina will increase HIV susceptibility. HIV can also be transmitted through receptive oral sex with ejaculation. Any condition that disrupts the integrity of the oral tissues, including periodontal disease, increases the risk of HIV in this manner. Women who have sex with women have a small risk of transmission, especially in sexual activities that result in some level of vaginal trauma.

However, healthcare providers must be careful not to assume that a woman is at low risk for HIV just because she has expressed a sexual preference for women. Lesbians may have a history of sexual intercourse with men or other risk factors for HIV infection.

The CDC recommends that HIV screening be a routine part of clinical care for patients aged 13 to 64 years in all healthcare settings (Branson et al., 2006). Patients presenting for STI treatment should be screened for HIV at each visit where they have new symptoms. Individuals at high risk for HIV should be tested for the presence of the virus at least once per year. Patients must be informed orally or in writing that HIV testing will be performed unless they decline (opt-out screening). Consent for HIV testing should be incorporated into the general consent for care. A separate consent form specific for HIV screening is not required or recommended (Branson et al., 2006).

HIV infection is diagnosed by testing for the HIV antibodies in a person's blood or oral fluid. HIV screening is conducted with standard enzyme-linked immunosorbent assay (ELISA) or EIA tests that are sent to a laboratory. Testing can also be performed at the point of care with newer rapid HIV tests that yield results in minutes (Greenwald, Burstein, Pincus, & Branson, 2006). If the screening test is reactive, then a more specific confirmatory test such as the Western blot (WB) or an immunofluorescence assay (IFA) is conducted. Although a negative antibody test usually indicates that a person is not infected, these tests cannot detect a recent infection. A patient with a negative test who has known or suspected exposure to HIV should be retested at 3 months after exposure. Prevention counseling is strongly encouraged for patients who are seronegative for HIV but at risk for infection. Women who are at high risk for HIV or who have known or suspected exposure to the virus should also be counseled about the need for repeat testing.

If a screening test is positive for HIV, the healthcare provider must explain the need for confirmatory testing. If confirmatory testing is positive for HIV, the woman must be given time to react emotionally. She must assimilate a great deal of information at the time of this visit. Allowing her to express her feelings prior to discussing issues related to partner notification, treatments, and other issues may allow her to better incorporate important information that must be conveyed at this time. Women with HIV must understand that although they may exhibit no signs or symptoms of HIV disease they are still infectious and will remain so for life. Basic information regarding minimizing transmission risk must be relayed to the patient at the time of diagnosis.

A plan for treatment must be established, which includes prompt referral to a healthcare provider with HIV expertise. Unless the patient is clearly immunocompromised and in need of immediate treatment for opportunistic infection, there is likely to be an interval between diagnosis and treatment decisions. This time can be used by the woman to begin to adapt emotionally and psychologically to her diagnosis. She can make decisions about who must be told about her infection and institute behaviors that are required of her to minimize the risk of transmitting the virus to others. Sensitive and nonjudgmental care at this time can assist the woman in making healthy accommodations in the face of her HIV diagnosis.

Effective management and treatment of the patient with HIV involves the use of antiretroviral therapy (ART) to decrease HIV-related morbidity and prolong the duration and quality of survival. ART will also restore and preserve immunologic function, maximally and durably suppress plasma HIV viral load, and prevent HIV transmission. Six classes of HIV ARTs exist, and combination therapy with multiple ARTs is recommended (Panel on Antiretroviral Guidelines for Adults and Adolescents [PAGAA], 2011, p. 24). The ART classes include:

- Nucleoside reverse transcriptase inhibitors (NRTIs)
- Nonnucleoside reverse transcriptase inhibitors (NNRTIs)
- Protease inhibitors (PIs)
- Fusion inhibitors (FIs)
- CCR5 antagonists
- Integrase strand transfer inhibitors (INSTIs)

Healthcare providers who give gynecologic care to women with HIV must be aware that the infection may necessitate adjustments to the usual standards of care (ACOG, 2010a). HIV, for example, affects the recommendations for cervical cancer screening and management of abnormal Pap test results (ACOG, 2010a; Wright et al., 2007). Women with HIV who develop vaginal infections and STIs may require different treatment regimens and follow-up (CDC, 2010b).

Unintended Pregnancy

Incidence and Prevalence

An unintended pregnancy is a pregnancy that is unplanned, mistimed, or unwanted at the time of conception (Mosher, Jones, & Abma, 2012). It is estimated that 49% of all pregnancies in the United States are unintended (Finer & Zolna, 2011). Unintended pregnancies occur among women of all ages and socioeconomic groups (Finer & Henshaw, 2006). It is estimated that more than half of women in this country will experience an unintended pregnancy by the age of 45 (Jones, Singh, Finer, & Frohwirth, 2006). Unintended pregnancy occurs most frequently among women who are between the ages of 18 and 24, are unmarried, are poor, are members of minority groups, or have not completed high school. Poor and low-income women tend to experience some of the highest rates of unintended pregnancy. Evidence suggests that economic disadvantage is likely to be associated with higher risk for unintended pregnancy due to risky sexual behavior and less vigilance in contraceptive use (Finer & Zolna, 2011). These characteristics signal significant disparities in this aspect of reproductive health (Finer & Henshaw, 2006; Mosher et al., 2012).

Approximately 51% of pregnancies in 2008 were unintended, and 40% ended in abortion. An estimated 1.1 million abortions took place in the United States in 2011, which represents a 13% decline since 2008 (Jones & Jerman, 2014). Women who choose to carry the unintended pregnancy to term will either keep the infant or place the infant for adoption. Comprehensive adoption statistics have not been collected in the United States for many years; thus current information regarding how frequently adoption is chosen as the outcome for unintended pregnancy is limited. However, estimates from the 2002 National Survey of Family Growth indicate that 1% of infants born to never-married women younger than 45 years of age were relinquished for adoption between 1996 and 2002 (Jones, 2008).

Ethnic Considerations

The rate of unintended pregnancy in the United States is significantly higher than the rates in many other developed countries. Unintended pregnancy has been shown to occur disproportionately among minority women, unmarried women, and women who are poor and less educated. Minority women tend to have unintended birth rates that are twice that of white women. African-American and Hispanic women tend to have the highest rates of unintended pregnancy among all racial and ethnic subgroups (Finer & Zolna, 2011). Unintended pregnancy rates among Hispanic women tend to be greater than three times higher than the national average (Finer & Henshaw, 2006). African-American women are more likely to end an unintended pregnancy by abortion, whereas Hispanic women are more likely to carry an unintended pregnancy to completion (Finer & Zolna, 2011).

Risk of Unintended Pregnancy

Women who are at risk for unintended pregnancy are those who have sexual intercourse and are fertile (that is, neither they nor their partner have been contraceptively sterilized). Women at highest risk for unintended pregnancy are likely to be between the ages of 18 and 24 years of age, are economically disadvantaged, and tend to be of African-American ethnicity (Mosher et al., 2012). Inconsistent or incorrect use of contraceptives is the most common reason that unintended pregnancies occur. Contraceptive nonuse or misuse may result from numerous causes, such as lack of knowledge, barriers to access, and complex personal, interpersonal, socioeconomic, and cultural factors. Inconsistent contraceptive use is an important factor that increases the risk for unintended pregnancy. Even perfect contraceptive use does not guarantee avoiding pregnancy, because inherent method failures are possible. Preventing pregnancy requires prolonged and concerted effort.

Prevention of Unintended Pregnancy

The primary way to prevent unintended pregnancy is for couples to use contraception with every act of intercourse during which they do not want to get pregnant. Improving contraception education and counseling, eliminating practice routines that impede obtaining timely service (such as long waits for appointments for contraceptive services), and removing financial and social barriers to contraceptive access are important strategies to reduce unintended pregnancies (Moos, 2003).

Because perfect contraceptive use is unrealistic, emergency contraception (EC) has emerged as an important method for the prevention of unintended pregnancy. EC entails the use of contraceptive methods after intercourse to prevent pregnancy. It works by preventing or delaying ovulation, preventing fertilization, and/or preventing implantation. EC does not cause abortion, has no effect on an established pregnancy, and does not offer any protection from STIs. Access to EC has the potential to reduce the incidence of unintended pregnancies, which would have a tremendous positive impact on the lives of women, men, and their families by decreasing the need for abortion and minimizing the social costs associated with unintended pregnancy and childbearing. EC is the only contraceptive method that can be used after intercourse. It cannot be used as an ongoing method of contraception. Access to EC remains limited because only one of four available methods is obtainable without prescription, and then only to women 17 years of age and older. Removing barriers to EC is an important measure that will help to reduce the rate of unintended pregnancies. Strategies to increase access to EC include making available advance prescriptions to women 16 and younger and providing EC prescriptions over the phone as needed.

Gender Dimensions

Even though women bear most of the physical, psychological, and social burdens related to unplanned pregnancy, gender differences may be observed regarding the issue of contraception. Historically, contraceptive options have been largely for women. This may be due in part to the reality that women, not men, get pregnant, or the fact that family planning research and contraceptive services have focused disproportionately on women. The female reproductive system has been extensively studied for centuries. Studies on male contraceptives have been limited. Currently, options for the male range from mildly effective (withdrawal) to highly effective (vasectomy). It could be argued that the remarkable effectiveness of modern hormonal contraceptives for women has given women high levels of protection but has absolved men from participating in contraceptive protection and

decision making. Men are often silent partners in preventing unwanted pregnancies.

Several factors contribute to the dominant role women play in contraceptive decision making and the availability of services for them. Modern medical care services provide ready access to contraceptive information and options for women. Women are taught and encouraged to see a gynecologist in their teens. There is not a parallel system for men. Society emphasizes to girls and young women early that the penalty of unprotected sex will be an unwanted pregnancy, shame, and economic hardship. The societal message to boys and young men is not the same. Nonetheless, legal issues surrounding paternity and child support in recent years have introduced the penalty concept to an unwanted pregnancy.

Evidence obtained from multicultural surveys indicates that men are willing to participate in contraception and their female partners trust them to do so (Page, Amory, & Bremmer, 2008). Male contraceptive research includes hormonal and nonhormonal methods. Currently, the most significant barriers for expanded use include limited delivery methods and perceived regulatory obstacles. New reversible hormone advances in oral, implant, and injectable androgen methods are promising options for men (Mommers et al., 2008). Evidence also demonstrates that male hormonal contraceptive methods have a 90% to 95% efficacy rate (Page et al., 2008). Nonhormonal male contraceptives include products that target sperm motility. Although considerable progress has been made in clinical research on male contraception, no new product is currently available or likely to be so in the near future.

Options for Women Facing Unintended Pregnancy

Continuing the Pregnancy

The decision to continue the pregnancy involves a long-term commitment to parenting that carries immense responsibility. Women who choose to parent need to have the time and ability to care for the child, adequate financial resources, and support from spouses/partners, family members, and friends. Continuing an unintended pregnancy is especially challenging for women who lack any of these needed requirements. Support and resources are available for women with unintended pregnancies. Healthcare providers can supply pregnant women with information about state and local programs that give social and financial support to pregnant women and their children. Such information may prove vital in their decision-making process. Women who decide to continue a pregnancy should begin prenatal care, either in the setting where options counseling occurred, if those services are provided, or by referral to a prenatal care provider.

ADOPTION

Arrangements for adoption vary according to state law. Children may be placed for adoption through private agencies, independently using an adoption lawyer or facilitator, or directly between the birth and adoptive parents. Adoptions may be closed or open. In closed, or confidential, adoptions, parents do not know each other or have any contact, but adoptive parents are given relevant information about the birth parents, such as health histories. Open adoption encompasses options along a broad continuum that may range from birth parents reading about families and selecting one, to ongoing contact between the families (Smith & Brandon, 2008).

ABORTION

Current options for induced abortion in the United States include aspiration, medication, surgical, and labor induction methods. The decision regarding which method is employed depends on several factors, including the gestational age of the pregnancy, preference of the patient, and the

availability and training of the healthcare provider. Healthcare providers need to be familiar with which abortion options are available for women in their care in order to provide accurate counseling and referrals.

The risks associated with early abortion, including death, are relatively low when procedures are carried out under modern medical conditions. Legality is an important prerequisite for such conditions to be manifest. In places where abortion is illegal or restricted, associated morbidity and mortality rates remain high. In the United States, abortion mortality rates have decreased considerably since the 1970s, largely as a result of advances in technique and elimination of many legal restrictions (Shah & Ahman, 2009).

Quality of Life Issues Associated With Sexually Transmitted Infections and Unintended Pregnancy

STIs and unintended pregnancy produce substantial impact on the quality of life of women, especially for adolescent and young women who are most notably at risk. Quality of life issues and concerns associated with STIs and unintended pregnancies are multidimensional and encompass health and physical functioning, psychological and spiritual well-being, socioeconomic integrity, and family well-being. Research inquiry into the quality of life of young women who experience curable STIs is notably sparse, which is troubling considering the prevalence of STIs in this country.

Most women experience at least one and often several STIs in their lifetime. Sexually transmitted organisms know no class, racial, ethnic, or social barriers. All individuals are vulnerable if exposed to an infectious organism. STIs pose significant health risks for women. Women are not only at higher risk for acquiring STIs than men, but also suffer more significant sequelae from these conditions that threaten quality of life. Moreover, STIs have substantial psychological and interpersonal implications in women's lives.

Adolescent and young women disproportionately experience unintended pregnancy and are vulnerable to physical complications as well as psychosocial, socioeconomic, and family sequelae. Children of unintended pregnancies tend to experience health-related problems as well as abuse, neglect, and poor school performance. Adolescent and young women with unintended pregnancies are less likely to have completed high school or career preparation and are more likely to be single parents (National Campaign to Prevent Teen and Unplanned Pregnancy, 2009). Abortion is a more common outcome of unintended pregnancy among this age group than among women in general. The complex sequelae of unintended pregnancy influence a poorer quality of life.

Issues Affecting Health and Physical Functioning

SEXUALLY TRANSMITTED INFECTION

The issues affecting health and physical functioning of women with STIs depend on the organism causing the infection. Gonorrhea and chlamydia may lead to permanent damage of the reproductive system, even in the absence of symptoms. Genital herpes is an incurable disease with painful and often emotionally devastating symptoms, but generally without posing a long-term health risk. HIV/AIDS, and in some cases syphilis and hepatitis, can be life-threatening. Some diseases attack single structures, such as labia and cervix, while others ascend upward from the vagina, through the cervical canal, and ultimately encompass the pelvic organs.

Women who are infected with chlamydia or gonorrhea maintain high risk for developing PID. PID can subsequently result in reproductive system morbidity such as ectopic pregnancy and tubal factor infertility. Without adequate treatment, approximately 10% to 20% of women with chlamydia or gonorrhea may develop PID. It is also estimated that, among women with PID, subsequent tubal scarring can lead to infertility in 20% of women, ectopic pregnancy in 9%, and chronic pelvic pain in 18% (CDC, 2012d).

Nearly 80% of gonorrhea infections and 80% to 90% of chlamydia infections in women are asymptomatic. Gonorrhea and chlamydia infections are detected mainly through screening. Thus, the symptoms associated with PID are indistinct such that 85% of women with PID defer seeking medical care, thereby increasing the risk for infertility and ectopic pregnancy. Evidence suggests that conscientious screening programs for chlamydia may reduce PID incidence by 60% (CDC, 2012 d).

There is considerable variability with PID symptoms. Some women may experience insidious symptoms, including vaginal discharge, mild but persistent abdominal pain or back pain, or pain during intercourse. Other women may experience sudden and severe pelvic pain, fever, shaking chills, or heavy vaginal discharge or bleeding. PID resulting from chlamydia infection is more likely to present with the former, more subtle symptoms. PID resulting from gonorrhea infection is more likely to present with the latter, more severe set of symptoms.

Clinical evaluation is necessary for PID diagnosis. The first step in confirming the presence of PID is eliminating the possibility of other serious conditions that may manifest in a similar manner. Although uterine tenderness and discharge indicate possible infection, bacterial culture is necessary to identify the causative bacterium and determine the most appropriate treatment course.

If PID is limited to the uterus, antibiotic treatment is usually sufficient to resolve the problem with little likelihood of permanent damage or future complications. Infection in the fallopian tubes, ovaries, or abdominal cavity is a cause for significant concern. Permanent damage from PID is more likely if the infection has invaded the fallopian tubes, because the tubes are fragile and easily damaged by an infectious process. Infection causes swelling and scarring of the tubes, which can lead to blockage and distortion, impairing future fertility.

Pelvic abscess is another serious consequence of PID. Pus and live bacteria may leak from the open end of a fallopian tube and result in peritonitis and abdominal abscess. A sonogram may be performed if an abscess is suspected. If an abscess is present, the sonogram can help determine whether laparoscopy is indicated to drain the abscess.

Women who have had PID must take elaborate precautions to avoid reinfection. Present and previous sexual partners must be treated with the same antimicrobial regimen as the infected woman, whether or not the partners have symptoms.

Perinatal Impact of Sexually Transmitted Infections   Perinatal outcomes can be affected by various STIs because pregnant women may transmit the infection to their fetus, newborn, or infant through vertical transmission (via the placenta, during vaginal birth, or after birth through breastfeeding) or horizontal transmission (close physical or household contact). Some STIs (such as syphilis) cross the placenta and infect the fetus in utero. Other STIs (such as chlamydia, gonorrhea, hepatitis B, and genital herpes) can be transmitted as the baby passes through the birth canal. HIV can cross the placenta during pregnancy, be transmitted during the birth process, and, unlike most other STIs, can infect the infant during breastfeeding. The harmful effects of STIs may include stillbirth, low birth weight, conjunctivitis, pneumonia, neonatal sepsis, neurologic damage, blindness, deafness, acute hepatitis, meningitis, chronic liver disease, and cirrhosis. Many of these problems can be prevented if the woman is screened and treated for STIs during pregnancy.

All pregnant women should be screened for HIV, syphilis, hepatitis B surface antigen, and *C. trachomatis* at the first prenatal visit. Women at risk for gonorrhea or hepatitis C should be screened for these infections. Repeat testing for STIs later in pregnancy is warranted for some women. Because many STI treatment regimens are different for women who are pregnant than for women who are not pregnant, healthcare providers should consult the most current CDC treatment guidelines when caring for pregnant women.

Unintended Pregnancy

Consequences of the decision to continue an unintended pregnancy and parent the child may include potentially adverse effects for both women and their children. Unintended pregnancy is associated with later entry into prenatal care, a lower number of total prenatal visits, substance use and risky sexual behaviors during pregnancy, low birth weight, infant mortality, maternal morbidity and mortality, child abuse, increased medical costs, and insufficient resources for child development (Maxson & Miranda, 2011). Unintended pregnancy often precludes the opportunity to receive preconception care that may otherwise improve pregnancy outcomes. Women with unintended pregnancies are also at greater risk for depression and physical abuse. Couples experiencing unintended pregnancy are more likely to end their relationships and they may forfeit their educational and professional aspirations.

Although the risk of maternal death from abortion increases with advancing gestational age, death from abortion after the first trimester, particularly after 20 weeks gestation, is relatively rare in this country. Serious and minor complications following legal aspiration and dilatation and evacuation abortions are infrequent, but have the potential for affecting the health and physical functioning domain of quality of life. Possible complications include infection, missed or incomplete abortion, cervical tear, uterine perforation, hemorrhage requiring transfusion, and hematometra (a collection or retention of blood in the uterine cavity). Although women who undergo medication abortions, which are induced by the administration of abortifacients such as mifepristone and misoprostol, may avoid complications attributable to instrumentation, other complications such as incomplete abortion, hemorrhage, and infection may also affect women's health and physical functioning.

Issues Affecting Psychological and Spiritual Functioning

SEXUALLY TRANSMITTED INFECTION

PSYCHOLOGICAL FUNCTIONING   A diagnosis of STI can have many psychological implications in women. Physical aspects of STIs frequently influence psychological adjustment, especially when the disease is incurable. Women with genital herpes, for example, may experience symptoms of depression, diminished self-concept, withdrawal from intimate relationships, and diminished quality of life (Barnack-Tavlaris, Reddy, & Ports, 2011).

An STI diagnosis is accompanied by considerable stigma, regardless of the culprit organism. Women are more vulnerable than men to the stigma associated with STIs, owing to entrenched gender norms and stereotypes associated with these infections (East, Jackson, OBrien, & Peters, 2012). For the most part, STIs are viewed by society as dirty diseases associated with deviant, dissolute, and dangerous behavior. Thus, women with STIs are perceived by society as tainted and "vectors of disease" who pass their infections on to men. This perception of women has developed in part from the long historical relationship of STIs with female prostitution and women who engage in sexual behavior outside of socially approved and accepted norms (East et al., 2012). This stereotype paints women as sources of STIs and men as victims of seductive, deviant, immoral women. Accordingly, such stereotypes feed the stigma

and oppression experienced by women with STIs (East et al., 2012). Men who acquire STIs, on the other hand, avoid being subjected to demeaning labels. STIs in men tend to be viewed as a common yet unwelcome outcome of their sexual behavior, as well as a medical/health dilemma, yet STIs are indicative of immorality among women. Even though perceptions of women's sexuality are becoming broader and more accepting, traditional gender norms persist in governing women's sexuality and continue to generate oppressive and demeaning labels (East et al., 2012).

Evidence suggests that women who acquire STIs perceive themselves more negatively as compared to male counterparts. These feelings are reflective of the typical societal norms that sanction women with STIs as shameful, yet these sanctions are not applied to men because of societal approval of male virility. Consequently, the accompanying stigma and shame has enormous impact on the psychological and emotional wellbeing of women (East et al., 2012).

Stigma of STIs is associated with emotional distress, treatment delays, and poor health outcomes. Adverse psychological effects of stigma encompass guilt, embarrassment, isolation, fear, and denial following a diagnosis (Lichtenstein, 2003). Stigma can contribute to feelings of anxiety and depression (Mark, Gilbert, & Nanda, 2009). It can be a factor influencing delays in screening for an STI as well as concealment of an STI, which subsequently increases risk of morbidity or spreading the disease to others. Fear of stigma can reduce women's willingness to identify their sexual partners to health department officials or to disclose to sexual partners that they have been exposed to infection (Lichtenstein, 2003). The stigma and oppression associated with STIs may be experienced when accessing treatment services, which can impede women from obtaining adequate care and treatment (East et al., 2012).

Women may also experience stigma transference, which is the act of deflecting blame for being infected to someone else, such as a sexual partner. Stigma transference is an effort of infected women to salvage self-esteem and maintain a sense of moral dignity, and may serve as a coping mechanism (Lichtenstein, 2003).

SPIRITUALITY   Religious involvement may be influential in attenuating risky sexual behavior. The attenuation of risky sexual behavior is supported by evidence suggesting that greater religious involvement may be protective against risky sexual behavior among young people, which may consequently mitigate risk of adverse outcomes (Kogan et al., 2008). Engagement in religious community, including regular participation in collective worship, may be strongly influential on behavior via a variety of mechanisms (Page, Ellison, & Lee, 2009). Organized religious involvement promotes internalization of religious norms associated with personal contact, encompassing the benefits of devotion, beliefs about divine punishment, and other potentially relevant doctrines. Religious involvement provides positive role models and social reinforcement for adherence to behavioral standards and fosters coreligionist social networks, affording opportunities for wholesome social engagements. Religious congregations may also offer formal programs and other support and resources that can shape and direct wholesome lifestyle choices and healthy behavior (Page et al., 2009).

Aspects of religiousness that are non-organizational may also be associated with health risk behaviors. Religious significance or the frequency of spiritual practices such as prayer or scriptural study may signify a high level of commitment to religious doctrines and teachings. Many of these doctrines persuade against unwholesome behaviors that can have negative health consequences, such as substance use and risky sexual practices. Such spiritual devotion may also involve a close personal relationship with a perceived divine entity, which can offer psychological security and comfort, and moral guidance (Page et al., 2009).

On the other hand, religious involvement can be influential in fostering stigma, particularly in association with conservative judgmental religious teachings that view risky sexual behavior and its consequences as sinful and immoral (Lichtenstein, 2003). Organized religious communities may allow for formal and/or informal sanctions, or the threat of sanctions, against members who deviate from their set of moral standards. Persons for whom religion is especially significant are apt to internalize religious norms and moral standards, making violation of these values unlikely and subsequently guilt producing (Page et al., 2009).

UNINTENDED PREGNANCY

Pregnancy itself is a stressful life event. An unintended pregnancy may impose an additional stressor, which can influence a woman's psychosocial health and contribute to the risk of adverse outcomes. Women with unintended pregnancies may experience high levels of depression, stress, and low levels of support and well-being (Maxson & Miranda, 2011). Unintended pregnancy may lead to perinatal depression because of the stress associated with the situation. Stress can be associated with deciding whether to continue with the pregnancy and determining how the child will fit into the life context of a woman who was not prepared for a child. Stress can also be associated with a decision to place the child for adoption or to terminate the pregnancy, as well as from situational, emotional, and/or financial reasons (Christensen, Stuart, Perry, & Le, 2011). Women who elect to terminate an unintended pregnancy may be at increased risk for emotional distress, depression, suicide, substance abuse, self-harm, and have increased use of mental health services (Thorp, Hartmann, & Shadigian, 2002). Evidence suggests that there is a higher likelihood of postpartum depression among mothers with unintended and unwanted births (Abbasi, Chuang, Dagher, Zhu, & Kjerulff, 2013).

Issues Affecting Socioeconomic Integrity

SEXUALLY TRANSMITTED INFECTION

Long-term socioeconomic consequences of STIs are especially burdensome for women. Social factors such as poverty and access to quality STI services, as well as a woman's inability to negotiate safer sexual practices such as condom use, can significantly affect her sexual health and quality of life. An important predictor of a woman's sexual health has been identified as a woman's relationship status with her male partner. For example, women tend to be more accepting of their partners' concurrent sexual relationships if a perceived shortage of available men exists in a community—and partner concurrency contributes to increased risk for STIs. Significant associations between condom use and sociodemographic characteristics, including age, income, education, and acculturation have been shown. In addition, it may be the behavior of her male partner, rather than the woman's own behavior, that increases a woman's risk for STIs. Even a woman who has only one partner may be obliged to practice safer sex such as using condoms (CDC, 2012d).

STIs impose a considerable economic drain on the healthcare system. Total direct medical costs of the 19.7 million annual cases of STI are estimated to be $15.6 billion per year. This estimate does not include costs of STI prevention, such as screening and vaccination. The indirect costs of STIs, such as loss of wages and productivity; and intangible costs, such as pain and suffering, are thought to be quite high and in some cases, higher than direct medical costs. Factored together, direct and indirect costs of STIs result in substantially higher economic burden on individuals and society (Owusu-Edusei et al., 2013).

UNINTENDED PREGNANCY

The socioeconomic burden of unintended pregnancy is considerable. Nearly half of all pregnancies in the United States are unintended and represent substantial cost to taxpayers. The provision of medical services to women who experience unintended pregnancies and to the infants born as a result of such pregnancies cost taxpayers $9.6–12.6 billion per year (Monea & Thomas, 2011).

The social and economic problems of unintended pregnancy create hardships for women and threaten the health and well-being of their infants. These consequences in turn impact society in areas such as the national economy and the extent of government expenditures (Sonfield, Kost, Gold, & Finer, 2011). Unintended pregnancies are more prevalent among women living in poverty and women with low income. Women who have had unintended pregnancy also tend to have lower levels of educational attainment and labor force participation than women who have had intended pregnancies. Teenage mothers often will drop out of school and claim public assistance. Children who are born from unintended pregnancy are more likely than other children to do poorly in school, live in poverty, claim public assistance, and engage in delinquent and criminal behavior later in life (Monea & Thomas, 2011). The burden of pregnancy-related care presents considerable costs to federal and state governments in the form of public funding such as Medicaid and Children's Health Insurance Program. Half of publicly funded births and their resulting costs are attributed to births resulting from unintended pregnancies. This places a disproportionate burden on public programs (Sonfield et al., 2011).

Issues Affecting Family Well-Being

SEXUALLY TRANSMITTED DISEASE

STIs can greatly compromise family well-being and quality of life. Issues such as asymptomatic infection or fear of stigma that prevents an infected woman from getting screened can affect family well-being. Infection can be transmitted to the spousal or sexual partner in these circumstances and pregnant women can transmit certain infections to the unborn fetus or to the term infant during childbirth. Psychological morbidity commonly associated with STIs can interfere with marital/partner relationships and influence the family role functioning. The economic burden of treatment, loss of wages, and loss of productivity that often accompanies STIs, especially the incurable infections, can present hardships that can impact on family functioning and lead to poor quality of life.

UNINTENDED PREGNANCY

Unintended pregnancy can impact family well-being and quality of life. Unintended pregnancy can cause relational discord among family members, especially in family environments with high levels of conflict and low support. Psychological morbidity, such as depression or emotional distress, can disrupt role functioning. Decisions concerning adoption, abortion, or keeping the baby can cause moral conflict, distress, financial burden, and can cause significant lifestyle alterations of family members.

The nature of family dynamics and communication among family members often influences risky sexual behavior that can lead to unintended pregnancy among young women, especially adolescents. Families with high levels of conflict are likely to experience low levels of parent–child involvement. In such family situations, there is likely to be less parental monitoring, which encourages associations and behaviors that can lead to risky sexual behavior among adolescents (Guiao, Blakemore, & Wise, 2004). Engagement in risky sexual behaviors may also be influenced by lack of parent–adolescent communication about sex-related subjects. Adolescents who communicate less frequently with their parents are at greater risk for engaging in risky sexual behaviors that can lead to STIs and unintended pregnancy. Adolescents

who frequently communicate with their parents about sexual activity are more likely to develop a clear idea of their parents' ideals of sexual behavior for their teenage children, which would give them more confidence in asserting their beliefs to avoid risky sexual acts (Guiao et al., 2004). Adolescents who perceive that there is low parental monitoring of their behavior, who they associate with, and where they go when not at home or in school have a greater likelihood for engaging in risky sexual behavior that could lead to unintended pregnancy (Guiao et al., 2004).

Implications for Healthcare Providers

Sexually Transmitted Infections

Counseling is an indispensable part of caring for a patient with an STI. Women will need support in seeking care at the earliest possible stage of symptoms. Counseling women about STIs is essential in order to prevent new infections or reinfection, to increase compliance with treatment and follow-up, to provide support during treatment, and to assist women with discussions with their partners. Women need to be informed of the serious potential consequences of STIs and of the behaviors that increase their likelihood of infection. Healthcare providers need to make sure that the woman understands which infection she has, how it is transmitted, and why the infection must be treated. Women should be given a brief description of the infection in language they can understand. The discussion must include modes of transmission, incubation period, symptoms, infectious period, and potential complications.

Effective treatment of STIs necessitates a careful, thorough explanation of the treatment regimen and follow-up procedures. Comprehensive and precise instructions about medications must be given, both verbally and in writing. In addition, side effects, benefits, and risks of medications should be discussed. Unpleasant side effects or early relief of symptoms may discourage women from completing their course of medication. All patients should be instructed on the importance of taking their medication until the full regimen is finished, regardless of whether their symptoms diminish or disappear in a few days, in order to prevent development of drug-resistant strains of certain infections or reinfection from inadequate treatment. Comfort measures that decrease distressing symptoms such as pain, nausea, or itching should be suggested. Written information should be provided as this is a time of high anxiety for many women and they may not remember everything they were told. A variety of informational booklets are available, and healthcare providers should offer literature specific to the care setting or patient population they are attending.

Women should be advised to refrain from sexual intercourse until all treatment is completed. After treatment, women should be urged to continue using condoms to prevent recurring infections, especially if they have had PID or continue to have intercourse with new partners. Women may wish to avoid sexual contact with partners who have multiple other sexual partners. All women who have contracted an STI should be taught safer sex practices if this education has not been provided previously. Follow-up appointments should be made as needed.

It is essential that healthcare providers also address the psychosocial component of STIs. Women may be afraid or embarrassed to tell their partners that they need to seek treatment. Confidentiality may be a major concern. The effect of a diagnosis of STI on a committed relationship for the woman, who must now face the necessity of dealing with uncertain monogamy, can be significant. The woman may fear telling her partner about the STI because it may place her in danger of escalating abuse. The potential consequences of informing her partner must be discussed.

In most instances involving STIs, sexual partners should be examined. Thus the woman is asked to identify and notify all partners who might have been exposed (partner notification). This is often difficult to do. Healthcare providers should be empathetic and suggest specific ways of talking with partners that will help decrease women's anxiety and assist in efforts to control infection. It is helpful to remind women that although this is a potentially embarrassing situation, most persons would rather know than not know that they have been exposed to an STI. Healthcare providers who take the time to counsel their patients on how to talk with their partners can improve compliance and case finding. When patient referral may not be effective or possible, health departments should be prepared to assist women, through either contact referral or referral by healthcare provider. With contact referral, a woman agrees to contact her partners by a certain time. If her partners do not obtain medical evaluation or treatment within the given time period, then the healthcare provider referral is implemented. With this referral, partners named by identified patients are notified and counseled by health department clinicians (CDC, 2010b).

Unintended Pregnancy

Healthcare providers may experience complex personal responses when providing care to women with unintended pregnancies. Reactions may range from complete acceptance to deep disturbance about a woman's situation or chosen course of action, with a myriad of emotions possible between these two extremes. No matter what personal feelings are stirred by these clinical encounters, healthcare providers have professional responsibilities when providing patient care. Values clarification is a process that can help healthcare providers to explore the intersection of their personal beliefs and professional responsibilities in order to ultimately uphold patients' rights (Simonds & Likis, 2005). Because unintended pregnancy and its outcomes—including such possibilities as adolescent pregnancy, single parenthood, and abortion—are socially and politically controversial, it is important for healthcare providers who provide care to women of reproductive age to clarify their own values regarding these issues. Ideally, this self-assessment should occur before having a clinical encounter with a woman who is faced with an unintended pregnancy. Because personal beliefs and work environments are dynamic, engaging in a process of ongoing values clarification benefits healthcare providers and the women they care for (Simmonds & Likis, 2005).

Several resources are available to assist healthcare providers to clarify their personal beliefs about pregnancy options and to help them examine the intersection of these beliefs with their responsibilities as professionals. Unexamined personal beliefs about abortion and women's decisions to parent or place a child for adoption can inadvertently affect clinical encounters. Thus, attention to all pregnancy options during the values clarification process is worthwhile. The ultimate goal of values clarification is to ensure that women with unintended pregnancies receive care that is nondirective, free from bias, and nonjudgmental. By engaging in a process of values clarification, healthcare providers can identify situations in which they experience conflict between their personal beliefs and professional responsibilities. Areas of perceived conflict warrant further examination. If after in-depth exploration of personal values healthcare providers discover that conflicts between their personal beliefs and professional responsibilities are irreconcilable, this conflict should be acknowledged. It is the professional obligation of healthcare providers to make a feasible plan to ensure that women who seek care will not be denied their right to comprehensive, respectful pregnancy options counseling.

Fulfilling this responsibility may require referral of patients to other colleagues or different patient care settings. Alternative plans should not create undue hardship for women such as delayed care, long travel distances, or paying out of pocket for services. Women referred to another facility should receive nondirective counseling from that facility that is factual about all available options.

Special Concerns of Age, Race, Ethnicity, and Culture

Race and ethnicity in the United States are population characteristics associated with fundamental determinants of health status (CDC, 2012a). Social and economic conditions such as high rates of poverty, income disparity, unemployment, and low educational attainment can hinder people from protecting their sexual health. People who are financially constrained frequently experience life circumstances that increase their risk for STIs and unintended pregnancy. People who cannot afford basic necessities are unable to access and pay for quality sexual health services (CDC, 2012a). To illustrate, in 2010, the poverty rates, unemployment rates, and high school dropout rates for African-Americans, American Indians/Alaska Natives, and Hispanics were substantially higher than for whites. These disparities are commensurate with observed disparities in STI burden (CDC, 2012a). Furthermore, one-fifth of African-Americans (20.8%) do not have health insurance (CDC, 2012a). Similar challenges are experienced by people of Hispanic ethnicity. For some, problems associated with immigration or undocumented citizenship status creates additional barriers. Even when health care is available, persons of racial and ethnic minority groups may experience fear and distrust of healthcare institutions. Social discrimination, provider bias, or the perception that these factors exist can negatively affect the healthcare-seeking experience for many racial/ethnic minorities (CDC, 2012a). People in communities that have a higher prevalence of STIs may have greater difficulty in reducing their risk for infection. There is higher risk in that each sexual encounter brings a greater chance of coming in contact with an infected partner, as compared to settings with lower prevalence. Recognizing the disparity in STI rates by race or ethnicity is an essential first step in empowering affected communities to organize and focus on this problem (CDC, 2012a).

Sexual risk taking is not confined to young people, so age offers no protection against STIs. Although STIs occur disproportionately in young people between the ages of 15 and 24, the incidence of STIs among older persons is on the rise. Newly-single older women are particularly at risk for contracting STIs (Idso, 2009).

The increased rate of STIs among older women is influenced by several factors. Many women, because of divorce, separation, or death of a spouse or partner, resume dating and enter into new partner sexual relationships. Research findings have indicated that incidence of HPV, genital herpes, chlamydia, and gonorrhea has increased in the population of older women. Women who are menopausal are at particular risk for contracting STIs. During menopause, physiological changes to the vulva and vaginal mucosa occur in that the tissues become thinner. As a result, the mucosal tissue becomes fragile due to decreased vaginal lubrication, and this increased fragility of the mucosa permits easier transmission of viruses and bacteria to invade the tissues and cause infection (Idso, 2009).

Older women generally have not had the benefits of education and counseling about STI prevention. Because this population traditionally has not been considered at risk for STIs, the topic is often overlooked during an annual exam. Evidence suggests that most physicians do not discuss STI prevention with patients older than 50 years. In addition, sexually active divorced, separated, or widowed women may be less likely to use condoms during sexual relations (Idso, 2009). It is vital that healthcare providers recognize the vulnerability of newly single older women and take steps to educate and counsel women regarding their risk for STIs as well as provide strategies for prevention (Idso, 2009).

As previously discussed, notable disparities have been identified concerning unintended pregnancy and abortion in the United States. Women between the ages of 18 and 24, who are unmarried, of low socioeconomic status, Hispanic or African-American, and lacking a high school diploma experience significantly higher rates of both these reproductive events. In spite of this social reality, available data on unintended pregnancy and abortion reveal a complex situation. Although most women who have abortions in this country are unmarried, 25% of married women report that their pregnancies are unintended. Among married women with unintended pregnancies, 27% have an abortion (Finer & Henshaw, 2006). Further research is needed to explore the impact of these reproductive events on the quality of life of women across the various social, cultural, and economic populations.

Research Review

What is the psychosocial well-being and quality of life among women newly diagnosed with symptomatic genital herpes simplex?

Mark, H., Gilbert, L., & Nanda, J. (2009). Psychosocial well-being and quality of life among women newly diagnosed with genital herpes. *Journal of Obstetric, Gynecologic, and Neonatal Nursing, 38,* 320–326.

It is unknown if advances in the understanding of genital HSV infection have affected the reaction of women to a diagnosis and infection of this STI. Thus, the purpose of this study was to assess the psychosocial well-being and quality of life among women newly diagnosed with herpes simplex virus type 2 (HSV-2). This study used a cross-sectional survey design. Women were eligible to participate if they were newly diagnosed with genital HSV, English speaking, and 18 years of age or older. Eighty-three women who were diagnosed with genital herpes simplex virus by culture, visual exam, and/or description of symptoms within the previous 3 months were recruited to participate in the study from primary healthcare clinics. Participants completed a demographic data sheet, the Hospital Anxiety and Depression Scale, and the Recurrent Genital Herpes Quality of Life Scale.

The majority of the sample was white and between the ages of 15 and 34 years old. Most of the sample was diagnosed either by visual exam or culture, and a majority of the women planned to use either daily suppressive or episodic therapy to treat their infection. The results of the study revealed that anxiety and depression were common among the sample. Furthermore, participants reported considerable concern or problems regarding the impact of genital herpes on self esteem, social functioning, sexual functioning, personal relationships, and mental health domains of quality of life. The findings of this study suggest that despite an increased understanding about the frequency of occurrence of HSV-2 and the availability of treatment to limit symptoms and transmission, the impact of a genital herpes diagnosis on women with symptoms is substantial, with psychosocial morbidity and adverse effects on quality of life. Counseling strategies that address both the medical and psychosocial aspects of HSV-2 infection and offer meaningful social support are recommended to enhance psychosocial adjustment and quality of life.

Chapter Summary Points

- Many young women nationwide are engaged in sexual risk behaviors associated with unintended pregnancies and sexually transmitted infections, including HIV infection.
- The prevalence rates of many STIs are highest among adolescents and young adults, who experience numerous biologic, psychosocial, sexual, cultural, and age-related factors that contribute to their vulnerability to such infections.
- Asymptomatic and unrecognized infections occur frequently in women, resulting in delayed diagnosis and treatment, chronic untreated infections, and complications.
- Diagnosing STIs in women is more complicated than in men because the anatomy of the female genital tract makes clinical examination more difficult.

- Considerable stigma accompanies an STI diagnosis, regardless of the culprit organism. Many people still equate STIs with immorality, promiscuous behavior, and low social status.
- To obtain prompt diagnosis and treatment, women must know how to recognize the major signs and symptoms of all STIs and must be willing and able to obtain health care if they experience symptoms or have sexual contact with someone who has an STI.
- Healthcare providers must educate their patients regarding the signs and symptoms of STIs, most especially when a woman comes in for her annual health examination, seeks contraception, or obtains preconception or prenatal care. They must also ensure that patients know where and how to obtain care if they suspect they might have contracted an STI.
- An unintended pregnancy is a pregnancy that is unplanned, mistimed, or unwanted at the time of conception. It is estimated that 49% of all pregnancies in the United States are unintended and occur among women of all ages and socioeconomic groups.
- Women at highest risk for unintended pregnancy are generally between the ages of 18 and 29 years of age, are economically disadvantaged, and tend to be of African-American or Hispanic ethnicity.
- Inconsistent or incorrect use of contraceptives is the most common reason why unintended pregnancies occur.
- Improving contraception education and counseling, eliminating practice routines that impede obtaining timely service, and removing financial and social barriers to contraceptive access are important strategies for reducing unintended pregnancies.
- Options for women facing unintended pregnancy include continuing the pregnancy, placing the baby for adoption, or termination of the pregnancy.
- STIs and unintended pregnancy produce substantial impact on the quality of life of women, especially for adolescent and young women, who are most notably at risk.
- Counseling women about STIs is essential in order to prevent new infections or re-infection, to increase compliance with treatment and follow-up, to provide support during treatment, and to assist women with discussions with their partners.
- Effective treatment of STIs necessitates a careful, thorough explanation of the treatment regimen and follow-up procedures. Comprehensive and precise verbal and written instructions about medications must be given, and the side effects, benefits, and risks of medications should be discussed.
- Although STIs occur disproportionately in young people between the ages of 15 and 24, the incidence of STIs among older persons is on the rise. Newly single older women are particularly at risk for contracting STIs.

Critical Thinking Exercise

Case Study

B.L. is a 22-year-old woman who has been in a relationship with a 25-year-old man for 6 months. She uses birth control pills for contraception. B.L. had been sexually active since she was 17 years old. When she first became sexually active, B.L. thought she was in love with her boyfriend at that time. She doesn't believe in promiscuous behavior and has maintained only monogamous relationships since then. In her present relationship, B.L. and her boyfriend do not use condoms since they agreed to be monogamous.

Lately B.L. developed vague tenderness in her lower abdomen and slight burning on urination. Her symptoms have been occurring for a few weeks. B.L. thought she had a urinary tract infection, which would resolve on its own with over-the-counter medication from the local pharmacy. Over the last week, her symptoms worsened. B.L. went to the emergency room with severe pelvic and abdominal pain and was admitted with a diagnosis of chlamydia and pelvic inflammatory disease. A sonogram revealed an abdominal abscess. B.L. was treated with antibiotics for the infection and a laparoscopy was performed to drain the abscess. Upon learning of the severity of her diagnosis and the likelihood that the pelvic inflammatory disease might make her infertile, B.L. became angry and depressed, and felt ashamed that she had a sexually transmitted infection. The doctor informed B.L. that her sexual partner must also be treated with antibiotics. B.L confronted her boyfriend regarding the source of her infection and he admitted he had been seeing other women. She broke off their relationship. As part of her treatment, B.L. received follow-up therapy and patient education about safe-sex practices, STI screening, and STI prevention. B.L. also sought counseling to deal with her depression and feelings of shame and betrayal.

Questions for Seminar Discussion

1. Discuss the prevalence of chlamydia among young women.
2. Discuss reasons women delay seeking treatment for sexually transmitted infections.
3. Discuss chlamydia infection, its transmission, signs and symptoms, and why it can often be misdiagnosed or underdiagnosed.
4. How is chlamydia treated? Why is it necessary for B.L.'s sexual partner to be treated?
5. What is pelvic inflammatory disease? What problems did PID cause for B.L.?
6. Discuss the possible health consequences for B.L. if PID is left untreated.
7. Why has reinfection with bacterial STIs become common?
8. What information should B.L be taught in order to prevent STIs in the future?
9. How did the chlamydia infection impact on B.L.'s quality of life?
10. Discuss resources that are available to help B.L. manage her infection and improve her quality of life.

Internet Resources

American Sexual Health Association: promotion of sexual health of individuals, families and communities through advocacy and education of the public, professionals and policy makers. http://www.ashastd.org

The Body: The Complete HIV/AIDS Resource: Provides information, education, advocacy, and support for people living with HIV/AIDS. http://www.thebody.com

The Body Pro: The HIV/AIDS Resource for Health Professionals: Provides information, education, and resources for healthcare professionals. http://www.thebodypro.com

Center for Disease Control: Information, statistics, and treatment guidelines. www.cdc.gov/

EngenderHealth: Provides information, advocacy, and programs to advance family planning, gender equality, HIV/AIDS services, and maternal health globally. www.engenderhealth.org

Hepatitis Foundation International: Provides information and education to the public to promote liver health and prevent liver disease. http://www.hepfi.org

Johns Hopkins Center for Sexually Transmitted Disease – Research, Prevention and Training: fosters collaborative interdisciplinary research, education and training of clinicians and scientists, and implementation of public health initiatives. http://www.jhsph.edu/research/centers-and -institutes/center-for-sexually-transmitted-diseases-research-prevention-and-training/resources /index.html

Planned Parenthood: Provides education, advocacy, reproductive and healthcare services and research to promote sexual and reproductive health. www.plannedparenthood.org

Sexuality Information and Education Council of the United States: Provides information, advocacy, and education about sexuality and sexual health. http://www.siecus.org

References

Abbasi, S., Chuang, C., Dagher, R., Zhu, J., & Kjerulff, K. (2013). Unintended pregnancy and postpartum depression among first-time mothers. *Journal of Women's Health, 22*(5), 412–416.

American College of Obstetricians and Gynecologists. (2010a). Gynecologic care for women with human immunodeficiency virus. ACOG Practice Bulletin No. 117. *Obstetrics and Gynecology, 116*, 1492–1509.

American College of Obstetricians and Gynecologists. (2010b). Human papillomavirus vaccination. Committee Opinion No. 467. *Obstetrics and Gynecology, 116*, 800–803.

Atashili, J., Poole, C., Ndumbe, P., Adimora, A., & Smith, J. (2008). Bacterial vaginosis and HIV acquisition: A meta-analysis of published studies. *AIDS, 22*, 1493–1501.

Barnack-Tavlaris, J., Reddy, D., & Ports, K. (2011). Psychological adjustment among women living with genital herpes. *Journal of Health Psychology, 16*(1), 12–21.

Branson, B., Handsfield, H., Lampe, M., Janssen, R., Taylor, A., Lyss, S., & Clark, J. (2006). Revised recommendations for HIV testing of adults, adolescents, and pregnant women in health-care settings. *Morbidity and Mortality Weekly Reports, 55*, 1–17.

Caple, C., & Schub, T. (2012, October 12). Sexually transmitted diseases: Risk factors. [Evidence-based care sheet]. *Cinahl Information Systems, (2p)*.

Centers for Disease Control and Prevention. (2008). Nationally representative CDC study finds 1 in 4 teenage girls has a sexually transmitted disease. Retrieved from http://www.cdc.gov/stdconference/2008/press/release-11march2008.pdf

Centers for Disease Control and Prevention. (2010a). Sexually transmitted disease surveillance 2009. Atlanta, GA: U.S. Department of Health and Human Services. Retrieved from http://www.cdc.gov/std/stats09/surv2009-Complete.pdf

Centers for Disease Control and Prevention. (2010b). Sexually transmitted diseases treatment guidelines, 2010. *Morbidity and Mortality Weekly Report, 59*(RR-12), 1–110. Retrieved from http://www.cdc.gov/mmwr/pdf/rr/rr5912.pdf

Centers for Disease Control and Prevention. (2010c). STDs and viral hepatitis. Retrieved from www.cdc.gov/hepatitis/Populations/STDs.htm

Centers for Disease Control and Prevention (2011a). CDC Grand Rounds: Chlamydia prevention: Challenges and strategies for reducing disease burden and sequelae. *Morbidity and Mortality Weekly Report, 59*, 1–86.

Centers for Disease Control and Prevention (2011b). 2010 Sexually transmitted diseases surveillance: Other sexually transmitted diseases. Retrieved from http://www.cdc.gov/std/stats10/other.htm

Centers for Disease Control and Prevention. (2012a). Trichomoniasis – CDC Fact Sheet. Retrieved from http://www.cdc.gov/std/trichomonas/stdfact-trichomoniasis.htm

Centers for Disease Control and Prevention (2012b). Hepatitis B FAQs for health professionals. Retrieved from http://www.cdc.gov/hepatitis/HBV/HBVfaq.htm

Centers for Disease Control and Prevention. (2012c). National notifiable diseases surveillance system (NNDSS). Retrieved from www.cdc.gov/nndss

Centers for Disease Control and Prevention. (2012d). *Sexually transmitted disease surveillance 2011*. Atlanta, GA: U.S. Department of Health and Human Services.

Centers for Disease Control and Prevention. (2012e). Youth risk behavior surveillance - United States, 2011. *Morbidity and Mortality Weekly Report 61*(4), 1–168.

Centers for Disease Control and Prevention. (2013a). CDC Fact Sheet: Incidence, prevalence, and cost of sexually transmitted infections in the United States. Retrieved from http://www.cdc.gov/std/stats/STI-Estimates-Fact-Sheet-Feb-2013.pdf

Centers for Disease Control and Prevention. (2013b). Viral Hepatitis – Hepatitis C information. http://www.cdc.gov/hepatitis/HCV/index.htm

Centers for Disease Control and Prevention. (2013c). Viral hepatitis surveillance – United States, 2010. Retrieved from http://www.cdc.gov/hepatitis/Statistics/2010Surveillance/

Cherpes, T., Meyn, L., Krohn, M., Lurie, J., & Hillier, S. (2003). Association between acquisition of herpes simplexvirus type 2 in women and bacterial vaginosis. *Clinical Infectious Diseases, 37*, 319–325.

Christensen, A., Stuart, E., Perry, D., & Le, H. (2011). Unintended pregnancy and perinatal depression trajectories in low-income, high risk Hispanic immigrants. *Prevention Science, 12*, 289–299.

Collins-Bride, G., & Murphy, J. (2004). Genital herpes simplex. In W.L. Star, L.L. Lommel, & M.T. Shannon (Eds.) *Women's primary health care* (2nd ed.). San Francisco, CA: UCSF Nursing Press.

Cunningham, F., Leveno, K., Bloom, S., Hauth, J., Rouse, D., & Spong, C. (2010). *Williams obstetrics* (23rd ed.). New York, NY: McGraw Hill.

East, L., Jackson, D., O'Brien, L., & Peters, K. (2012). Stigma and stereotypes: Women and sexually transmitted infections. *Collegian, 19*(1), 15–21.

Finer, L., & Henshaw, S. (2006). Disparities in rates of unintended pregnancy in the United States, 1994 and 2001. *Perspectives on Sexual and Reproductive Health, 38*, 90–96.

Finer, L., & Zolna, M. (2011). Unintended pregnancy in the United States: Incidence and disparities, 2006. *Contraception, 84*(5), 478–485.

Freeman, E., Weiss, H., Glynn, J., Cross, P., Whitworth, J., & Hayes, R. (2006). Herpes simplex virus 2 infection increases HIV acquisition in men and women: Systematic review and meta-analysis of longitudinal studies. *AIDS, 20*, 73–83.

Greenwald, J., Burstein, G., Pincus, J., & Branson, B. (2006). A rapid review of rapid HIV antibody tests. *Current Infectious Diseases Reports, 8*, 125–131.

Guiao, I., Blakemore, N., & Wise, A. (2004). Predictors of teen substance use and risky sexual behaviors: Implications for advanced nursing practice. *Clinical Excellence for Nurse Practitioners, 8*(2), 52–59.

Guttmacher Institute. (2013). Facts on American teens' sexual and reproductive health. Retrieved from http://www.guttmacher.org/pubs/FB-ATSRH.html

Idso, C. (2009). Sexually transmitted infection prevention in newly single older women: A forgotten health promotion need. *The Journal for Nurse Practitioners, 5*(6), 440–446.

Jones, J. (2008). Adoption experiences of women and men and demand for children to adopt by women 18-44 years of age in the United States, 2002. *Vital and Health Statistics 23*(7), 1–36.

Jones, R., & Jerman, J. (2014). Abortion incidence and service availability in the United States, 2011. *Perspectives on Sexual and Reproductive Health, 46*(1), 3–14.

Jones, R., Singh, S., Finer, L., & Frohwirth, L. (2006). *Repeat abortion in the United States* (Occasional Report No. 29). New York, NY: Guttmacher Institute.

Kaiser Family Foundation. (2013). HIV/AIDS policy fact sheet: Women and HIV/AIDS in the United States. Retrieved from www.Kaiserfamilyfoundation.files.wordpress.com/2013/12/6092-11.pdf

Kent, M., & Romanelli, F. (2008). Reexamining syphilis: An update on epidemiology, clinical manifestations, and management. *Annals of Pharmacotherapy*, *42*, 226–236.

Kogan, S., Brody, G., Gibbons, F., Murry, V., Cutrona, C., Simons, R., … DiClemente, R. (2008). The influence of role status on risky sexual behavior among African Americans during the transition to adulthood. *Journal of Black Psychology*, *34*(3), 399–420.

Lichtenstein, B. (2003). Stigma as a barrier to treatment of sexually transmitted infection in the American deep south: Issues of race, gender, and poverty. *Social Science and Medicine*, *57*(12), 2435–2445.

Maman, S. (2000). The intersections of HIV and violence: Directions for future research and interventions. *Social Science & Medicine*, *50*, 459–478.

Mark, H., Gilbert, L., & Nanda, J. (2009). Psychosocial well-being and quality of life among women newly diagnosed with genital herpes. *Journal of Obstetric, Gynecologic, and Neonatal Nursing*, *38*(3), 320–326.

Maxson, P., & Miranda, M. (2011). Pregnancy intention, demographic differences, and psychosocial health. *Journal of Women's Health*, *20*(8), 1215–1223.

Miller, K. (2006). Diagnosis and treatment of *Neisseria gonorrhoeae* infections. *American Family Physician*, *73*(10), 1779–1784.

Miller, S., Exner, T., Williams, S., & Ehrhardt, A. (2000). A gender-specific intervention for at-risk women in the USA. *AIDS Care*, *13*(3), 603–612.

Mommers, E., Kersemaekers, W., Elliesen, J., Kepers, M., Apter, D., Behre, H., … Zitzmann, M. (2008). Male hormonal contraception: A double-blind, placebo-controlled study. *Journal of Clinical Endocrinology and Metabolism*, *93*(7), 2572–2580.

Monea, E., & Thomas, A. (2011). Unintended pregnancy and taxpayer spending. *Perspectives on Sexual and Reproductive Health*, *43*(2), 88–93.

Moos, M. (2003). Unintended pregnancies: A call for nursing action. *The American Journal of Maternal Child Nursing*, *28*, 24–30.

Morrison, C., Turner, A., & Jones, L. (2009). Highly effective contraception and acquisition of HIV and other sexually transmitted infections. *Best Practice and Research: Clinical Obstetrics and Gynaecology*, *23*, 263–284.

Mosher, W., Jones, J., & Abma, J. (2012). Intended and unintended births in the United States: 1982-2010.

National health statistics reports; No 55. Hyattsville, MD: National Center for Health Statistics. Retrieved from http://www.cdc.gov/nchs/data/nhsr/nhsr055.pdf

Munoz, N., Bosch, F., de Sanjose, S., Herrero, R., Castellsaqué, X., Shah, K., … Meljer, C. (2003). Epidemiological classification of human papillomavirus types associated with cervical cancer. *New England Journal of Medicine*, *348*, 518–527.

National Campaign to Prevent Teen and Unplanned Pregnancy. (2009). Why it matters: Teen pregnancy. Retrieved from http://www.thenationalcampaign.org/why-it-matters/wim_teens.aspx

Nelson, A. (2007). Combined oral contraceptives. In R. A. Hatcher, J. Trussell, A. L. Nelson, W. Cates, F. Stewart, & D. Kowal (Eds.), *Contraceptive technology* (19th ed., pp. 193–270). New York, NY: Ardent Media.

Office on Women's Health. (2011). Women who have sex can get HIV. Retrieved from http://www.womenshealth.gov/hiv-aids/women-are-at-risk-of-hiv/women-who-have-sex-can-get-hiv.html

Owusu-Edusei, K., Chesson, H., Gift, T., Tao, G., Mahajan, R., Ocfemia, M., & Kent, C. (2013). The estimated direct medical cost of selected sexually transmitted infections in the United States, 2008. *Sexually Transmitted Diseases*, *40*(3), 197–201.

Page, R., Ellison, C., & Lee, J. (2009). Does religiosity affect health risk behaviors in pregnant and postpartum women? *Journal of Maternal Child Health*, *13*, 621–632.

Page, S., Amory, J., & Bremner, W. (2008). Advances in male contraception. *Endocrinology Review*, *29*(4), 465–493.

Panel on Antiretroviral Guidelines for Adults and Adolescents. (2011). Guidelines for the use of antiretroviral agents in HIV-1-infected adults and adolescents. Retrieved from http://aidsinfo.nih.gov/ContentFiles/AdultandAdolescentGL.pdf

Satterwhite, C., Torrone, E., Meites, E., Dunne, E., Mahajan, R., Ocfemia. M., … Weinstock, H. (2013). Sexually transmitted infections among U.S. women and men: Prevalence and incidence estimates, 2008. *Sexually Transmitted Diseases*, *40*(3), 187–193.

Schmid, G. (2001). Epidemiology of sexually transmitted infections. In S. Faro & D.E. Soper (Eds.), *Infectious diseases in women*. Philadelphia, PA: Saunders.

Shah, I., & Ahman, E. (2009). Unsafe abortion: The global public health challenge. In M. Paul, E. S. Lichtenberg, L. Borgatta, D. Grimes, P. Stubblefield, & M. Creinin (Eds.), *Management of unintended pregnancy and abnormal pregnancy: Comprehensive abortion care* (pp. 10–23). Chichester, UK: Wiley-Blackwell.

Simmonds, K., & Likis, F. (2005). Providing options counseling for women with unintended pregnancies. *Journal of Obstetric, Gynecologic, and Neonatal Nursing, 34*(3), 373–379.

Sinclair, C. (2004). *A midwife's handbook.* St. Louis, MO: Saunders.

Smith, K, & Brandon, D. (2008). The hospital-based adoption process: A primer for perinatal nurses. *The American Journal of Maternal Child Nursing, 33*(6), 382–388.

Sonfield, A., Kost, K., Gold, R., & Finer, L. (2011). The public costs of births resulting from unintended pregnancies: National and state-level estimates. *Perspectives on Sexual and Reproductive Health, 43*(2), 94–102.

Strauss, L., Gamble, S., Parker, W., Cook, D., Zane, S., & Handen, S. (2007). Abortion surveillance-United States, 2004. *Morbidity and Mortality Weekly Report: Surveillance Summaries, 56*(9), 1–33.

Sutton, M., Sternberg, M., Koumans, E., McQuillan, G., Berman, S., & Markowitz, I. (2007). The prevalence of *Trichomonas vaginalis* infection among reproductive-age women in the United States, 2001-2004. *Clinical Infectious Diseases, 45,* 1319–1326.

Thorpe, J., Hartmann, K., & Shadigian, E. (2002). Long-term physical and psychological health consequences of induced abortion: Review of the evidence. *Obstetrical and Gynecological Survey, 58*(1), 67–79.

World Health Organization. (2013). Sexually transmitted infections (STIs). Retrieved from http://www.who.int/mediacentre/factsheets/fs110/en/

Wright, T., Massad, L., Dunton, C., Spitzer, M., Wilkinson, E., & Solomon, D., for the 2006 ASCCP-Sponsored Consensus Conference. (2007). 2006 consensus guidelines for the management of women with abnormal cervical screening tests. *Journal of Lower Genital Tract Diseases, 11*(4), 201–222.

Chapter 9

Violence Against Women

Introduction

Violence is an intentional use of physical force or power, threatened or actual, toward oneself, another person, or against a group or community, which either results in or has a high likelihood of resulting in injury, death, psychological harm, maldevelopment, or deprivation (Krug, Dahlberg, Mercy, Zwi, & Lozano, 2002). Violence takes place throughout modern society and occurs in various forms, which may be categorized according to those committing the violent acts and include self-directed violence, interpersonal violence, and collective violence (Krug et al., 2002). Self-directed violence includes acts of suicide, encompassing ideation, attempted suicide, or completed suicide, as well as acts of self-abuse and self-mutilation. Interpersonal violence includes violence largely occurring between family and intimate partners that usually but not exclusively takes place in the home. It also includes community violence that occurs between persons who are unrelated or may not know each other, and generally takes place outside the home. Collective violence is an act of violence by a group of people in order to attain social, political, or economic objectives. Collective violence may take the form of armed conflicts, genocide, repression and other human rights abuses, terrorism, and organized violent crimes (Krug et al., 2002).

Violence against women is any act of gender-based violence of which the outcome or likely outcome is physical, sexual, or mental harm or suffering to women. This includes threats of such acts and coercion or arbitrary deprivation of liberty, whether occurring in public or in private life (World Health Organization [WHO], 2013). Violence against women impedes the attainment of the goals of equality, development, and peace; and weakens or nullifies the enjoyment by women of their human rights and basic freedoms. Women and girls in all societies, to a greater or lesser extent, experience physical, psychological, and sexual abuse that cuts across the boundaries of income, class, and culture. A cause and consequence of violence is low social and economic standing of women (United Nations, 2010). Many acts of violence against women evolve as a result of the inferior status women hold in a society. The forms of violence that affect women as groups in certain populations of the world include female genital mutilation (also known as female cutting or female circumcision), female infanticide, trafficking of women and girls for sexual exploitation, and acts of rape during war.

Violence against women occurs worldwide throughout the life cycle and is an indication of the historically disparate power relations between men and women. Traditional and customary practices that give women subordinate status in family, workplace, community, and society perpetuate violence. Violence is also intensified by social pressures such as shame that prevents the denouncement of certain acts toward women; women's lack of access to legal aid, information, or protection; a lack of laws that effectively forbid violence against women; insufficient efforts on the part of public authorities to encourage awareness of and enforce existing laws; and the absence of education and other strategies to address the causes and consequences of violence against women. In addition, images in the media of violence against women, especially in the depiction of rape, sexual slavery, or the use of women and girls as sex objects, including pornography, also contribute to the continued prevalence of such violence and adversely influence the community at large, including children and young people (United Nations, 2010).

In the United States, violence against women is a major public health problem. Violence affects women and girls of all ages, from infants to the oldest old. These acts of violence encompass intimate partner violence (domestic violence), sexual assault, sexual abuse, stalking, emotional and verbal abuse, as well as bullying, teen violence, human trafficking, and other forms of trauma and abuse. Violence against women occurs in all types of personal and family relationships and at all economic, educational, cultural, racial, age, and religious levels (Regional Offices on Women's Health, 2010).

In this country, thousands of women are killed each year as a consequence of violence, and many deaths are perpetrated by someone with whom they are involved or were previously involved with intimately. Violence against women not only takes lives but leaves survivors with permanent physical and emotional scars. It erodes families and communities by contributing to family dysfunction, reduced productivity, and disruption of social services. This chapter explores various forms of violence against women as well as the issues that contribute to violence and victimization. The impact of violence on the quality of life of women and their families is also explored.

Incidence and Prevalence

Global Incidence and Prevalence

Violence against women is a worldwide concern of pandemic proportions (UN Women, 2014a). Although the rates of women subjected to violence fluctuate from region to region across the world, evidence indicates that violence against women is a universal phenomenon. Women are exposed to diverse modes of violence—physical, sexual, psychological, and economic—both within and outside the home. Most often, women are subjected to violence by their intimate partners. The rate at which women are abused physically and sexually by their intimate partners differs throughout the world, yet such abuse is a common denominator in all countries or areas without exception (United Nations, 2010).

Women are disproportionately victims of violence throughout the world. Current statistics on violence against women indicate that approximately 35% of women worldwide have experienced either physical and/or sexual intimate partner violence or nonpartner sexual violence. Some national violence studies indicate that as many as 70% of women have experienced physical and/or sexual violence in their lifetime from an intimate partner. Statistics also indicate that intimate partner violence accounts for 40% to 70% of female murders in Australia, Canada, Israel, South Africa, and the United States (UN Women, 2014a).

Female genital mutilation occurs in all parts of the world; however, the practice is mostly prevalent in the western, eastern, and northeastern regions of Africa, some countries in Asia and the Middle East, and among certain immigrant communities in North America and Europe. Highest rates of the practice of female genital mutilation are noted in Djibouti, Guinea, Mali, Egypt, Somalia, and Sudan, and occurrences have been reported among certain populations in India, Indonesia, Iraq, Israel and the Occupied Palestinian Territories, Jordan, Oman, Malaysia, Thailand, and the United Arab Emirates (Sanctuary for Families, 2013). Statistics indicate that an estimated 100 million to 140 million girls and women across the world have been subjected to female genital mutilation. According to the most recent prevalence data, 91.5 million girls and women above 9 years old in Africa are currently living with the consequences of female genital mutilation. It is estimated that annually 3 million girls in Africa are at risk of undergoing female genital mutilation

(WHO, 2008, 2014b). Although the practice has been illegal in the United States since 1996, it was estimated in 1997 by the Centers for Disease Control and Prevention that 150,000 to 200,000 girls were at risk for being forced to undergo female genital mutilation. Since then, anecdotal evidence strongly indicates that the number of girls in this country who are at risk for female genital mutilation has risen steadily since 1997.

Human trafficking is a form of modern-day slavery that ruthlessly exploits women, children, and men for a variety of purposes that include forced labor and sex. Millions of women and girls are trapped in modern-day slavery. Of the estimated 20.9 million victims of trafficking worldwide, women account for up to 60% of all trafficking victims, and women and girls together account for 75%. Twenty-seven percent of all trafficking victims are children, of which two-thirds are girls. Furthermore, 58% of all trafficking cases revealed globally are for the purposes of sexual exploitation, and 98% of the victims forced into sexual exploitation are women and girls. Human trafficking for the objective of sexual exploitation occurs more commonly in Europe, Central Asia, and the Americas, whereas trafficking for forced labor occurs more frequently in Africa, the Middle East, South Asia, East Asia, and the Pacific (United Nations Office on Drugs and Crime [UNDOC], 2012; UN Women, 2014a).

Rape is both an individual act of aggression against a woman and a widespread tactic used in modern wars. The purpose of using rape as a tactic during war is to terrorize the population, break up families, destroy communities, and in some instances, change the ethnic make up of the next generation. Sometimes rape is used to deliberately infect women with HIV or cause women from the targeted community to become incapable of bearing children. During the 1992–1995 war in Bosnia and Herzegovina, an estimated 60,000 women were raped. During the 1991–2001 civil war in Sierra Leone, more than 60,000 women were raped. During the Rwandan genocide of 1994, approximately 250,000 to 500,000 women and girls were raped, and at least 200,000 women in the Democratic Republic of the Congo have been raped since 1998 (United Nations, 2014).

Sexual harassment in the workplace is a serious and pervasive human rights violation that is difficult to quantify due to a lack of universal definition of sexual harassment, differing perceptions among the genders of what constitutes sexual harassment, and reluctance to report the occurrence of sexual harassment. It is likely that the actual number of women who are subjected to sexual harassment far exceeds the number of reported cases. Estimations of approximately 40% to 50% and even up to 81% of women in various countries of the European Union have been subjected to unwanted sexual advances, physical contact, or other forms of sexual harassment at work (Advocates for Human Rights, 2010; UN Women, 2014a).

National Incidence and Prevalence

In the United States, violence against women is pervasive and widespread. According to the results of the National Intimate Partner and Sexual Violence Survey (NIPSVS), it is estimated that in their lifetime, more than 35.6% of women in this country have experienced violence in the form of rape, stalking, or physical violence by an intimate partner. More than 33% of female victims of intimate partner violence have experienced numerous forms of rape, stalking, or physical violence. In their lifetime, approximately 9.4% of women in this country have been raped by an intimate partner and an estimated 16.9% of women have experienced sexual violence other than rape by an intimate partner at some point in their lifetime. Moreover, 24.3% of women, at some point in their lifetime, have been subjected to severe physical violence by an intimate partner, such as being hit with a fist or hard object, beaten, or slammed against something. Additionally, approximately 10.7% of

women in this country have been stalked by an intimate partner during their lifetime. Nearly half of all women in this country have been subjected to psychological aggression by an intimate partner in their lifetime, and 69% of women who are victims of rape, stalking, or physical violence by an intimate partner experienced this violence for the first time before the age of 25 years (Black et al., 2011).

The results of the NIPSVS indicate that over 22 million women in the United States have been raped in their lifetime. An estimated 18.3% of the women in this country have experienced rape that has been comprised of completed forced penetration, attempted forced penetration, or alcohol- or drug-facilitated completed penetration at some time in their lives (Black et al., 2011). It is estimated that 51.1% of the victims were raped by an intimate partner and 40.8% of the victims were raped by an acquaintance. Approximately 13% of women in this country have experienced sexual coercion in their lifetime, consisting of unwanted sexual penetration after being pressured in a non-physical manner, and 27.2% of women have been subjected to unwanted sexual contact. Moreover, nearly 80% of female victims of completed rape experienced their first rape before 25 years of age and 42.2% of rape victims experienced their first completed rape before the age of 18 years. An estimated 12.3% of the victims of rape or attempted rape were younger than 12 years of age when they were first raped and nearly 30% of female rape victims were between 11 and 17 years of age (Black et al., 2011).

Sexual assault is a persistent problem in the U.S. military. In fiscal year 2012 (October 1, 2011–September 30, 2012), it was estimated that 6.1% of active duty women and 1.2% of active duty men have experienced unwanted sexual contact. This translates to approximately 26,000 active duty service members having experienced some form of unwanted sexual contact in one year (Department of Defense Sexual Assault Prevention and Response, 2014). Of the 6.1% of active duty women who experienced unwanted sexual contact, 31% reported completed penetration, 26% reported attempted penetration, 32% reported unwanted sexual touching, and 10% experienced unspecified sexual contact. Of the 1.2% of active duty men who experienced unwanted sexual contact, 10% reported completed penetration, 5% reported attempted penetration, 51% reported unwanted sexual touching, and 34% experienced unspecified sexual contact (Department of Defense Sexual Assault Prevention and Response, 2014). In fiscal year 2013 (October 1, 2012–September 30, 2013), 5,061 reports of alleged sexual assault involving one or more Service members as either the victim or alleged suspect were received by the Department of Defense, which is a 50% increase over the 3,374 reports received in the previous year. Since 2006, the rate of unwanted sexual contact in the U.S. military has been between 4% and 7% for women and between 1% and 2% for men. Since this rate has not changed, it is posited that the increase in reports is likely due to more victims coming forward rather than increased crime (Department of Defense Sexual Assault Prevention and Response, 2014).

NIPSVS results indicate that one in six women (16.2%) in this country has experienced stalking victimization at some point during their lifetime in which they felt very fearful or believed that they or someone close to them would be harmed or killed. It is estimated that 66.2% of stalking episodes were perpetrated by a current or former intimate partner, and the most commonly experienced stalking tactic was repeatedly receiving unwanted telephone calls, voice, or text messages. Over half of the stalking victims were stalked before age 25, and about 20% of the victims experienced stalking between the ages of 11 and 17 years old.

In the United States, human trafficking cases have been reported in all 50 states. The number of trafficking victims is largely unknown due to the covert nature of the crime, invisibility of victims, and high level of underreporting. Nonetheless, it is estimated that hundreds of thousands of minors who are U.S. citizens are at risk of commercial sexual (Polaris Project, 2012). Because few studies have been conducted on human trafficking of U.S. citizens within the United States, statistics are scarce on this issue. However, aggregated data collected by the National Human Trafficking Resource Center revealed that since 2007 to 2015, 103,026 signals via telephone, emails, and online tip reports were received by the human trafficking hotline. A total of 21,434 cases of human trafficking were reported. In 2015, 1,101 calls were received and 2,795 cases of human trafficking were reported. Of the 2,795 cases, 2,085 cases involved sex trafficking, 377 cases involved labor trafficking, 242 cases did not specify type of trafficking, and 90 involved sex and labor. The cases involved 2,340 females, 321 males, 1,757 adults and 877 minors (National Human Trafficking Resource Center, 2015).

In fiscal year 2014 (October 1, 2013 to September 30, 2014) the Department of Justice initiated 208 human trafficking prosecutions charging 355 defendants. Of these human trafficking prosecutions, 190 involved predominantly sex trafficking and 18 involved predominantly labor trafficking, although some involved both. These figures represent an increase from fiscal year 2013, during which the Department of Justice initiated 161 prosecutions charging 253 defendants. Of the 208 human trafficking prosecutions in fiscal year 2014, 184 traffickers were convicted as compared to 174 convictions obtained in fiscal year 2013. Of the 184 convictions, 157 involved predominantly sex trafficking and 27 involved predominantly labor trafficking (Department of State, 2015). Elder abuse, also known as abuse in later life, is a prevalent problem. Millions of elderly adults are abused, neglected, or exploited by family, acquaintances, or those who provide care for them. It is uncertain how many people are subjected to elder abuse but research findings suggest that as many as 11% of adults over age 60 experience abuse, neglect, and exploitation (Brandl & Dawson, 2011). Female elders are abused at a higher rate than males, and the older one is, the more likely one will be abused (National Center on Elder Abuse [NCEA], 2014).

Although each state has mandatory reporting laws for elder abuse and data from the Adult Protective Services agencies of each state indicate a growing trend in reporting the incidence of elder abuse, an overwhelming number of cases of abuse, neglect, and exploitation go undetected and untreated each year. Research evidence suggests that 1 in 14 cases of elder abuse ever comes to the attention of authorities and for every case of elder abuse neglect or exploitation known to programs and agencies, 24 were unknown. Evidence also suggests that major financial exploitation occurs at rates much higher than rates of emotional, physical, and sexual abuse or neglect (NCEA, 2014). Research findings show that of women aged 60 and older who were physically abused, approximately 68% were abused by intimate partners, 20% by other family members, 8% by acquaintances, and 1% by strangers (Brandl & Dawson, 2011).

Cultural and Ethnic Considerations

Women across all racial and ethnic groups are subjected to violence. A woman's experience of intimate partner violence or sexual assault is shaped by her racial and ethnic background. As a result, the occurrence of violence is understood or experienced differently between women of different racial or ethnic groups (UK Center for Research on Violence Against Women [UKCRVAW], 2011). Findings from national studies that have examined the extent of violence against women have been consistent regarding race and ethnicity. Significant differences have been found in rates and types of victimization that women from different racial and ethnic backgrounds have encountered over their lifetimes (Cho, 2012b; Tjaden & Thoennes, 2000). The

most violence is experienced by Native American and African-American women, and the lowest rates of violence are experienced by Asian/Pacific Islander women. White and Hispanic women experience violence at similar rates. Evidence also indicates that 24.8% of white women experience rape, physical assault, and stalking overall as compared to 37.5% Native American women, 29.1% African-American, 23.4% Hispanic women, and 15% Asian/Pacific Islander women (Tjaden & Thoennes, 2000).

Although there are differences in experienced violence among women of various racial and ethnic groups, being a member of a particular racial or ethnic group does not increase a woman's vulnerability to violence, nor does it make men more likely to commit acts of violence. Research findings indicate that socioeconomic characteristics (e.g., poverty), seem to be much more significant as a risk factor for education, marital status, or place of residence (UKCRVAW, 2011). Consequently, numerous sociodemographic characteristics strongly predict rates of violence, and most differences attributed to race disappear when these sociodemographic characteristics are accounted for. In order to understand the meaning of violence perceived by women of different races and cultures, or the unique barriers faced by minority women when they seek help for victimization, it is necessary to first understand the relationships between race, ethnicity, and the experience of physical and/or sexual violence (UKCRVAW, 2011). Evidence indicates that socioeconomic variables almost completely account for racial differences in rates of intimate partner violence and sexual assault. This is likely due to the greater prevalence of social problems such as violence and substance abuse in poor communities, where there are also disproportionately large numbers of women who belong to racial minorities (UKCRVAW, 2011). It stands to reason that the experience of higher rates of violence among minority women is reflective of the number of minority women who live in poverty. Results of studies on violence against women and victimization indicate that sociodemographic and relationship variables almost completely explain the differences between racial groups (Cho, 2012b; Tjaden & Thoennes, 2000). Significant factors that make any woman, regardless of race, more likely to be subjected to intimate partner violence include younger age, being unmarried, having lower income, having lower educational attainment, being unemployed, and having less financial security. Socioeconomic status is a predictor of sexual victimization that cuts across race. Women of low income are more likely to experience higher rates of intimate partner violence and victimization, regardless of race. Overall, it is posited that sociodemographic variables are usually more significant predictors of victimization risk than race (UKCRVAW, 2011).

The characteristics of the neighborhood or community are additional factors that are essential for understanding intimate partner violence and sexual assault. Research findings have indicated that race is a poor predictor of crime and victimization rates when community-level factors are considered (UKCRVAW, 2011). Evidence suggests that racial differences with regard to violent crime victimization and family violence are likely explained by extreme poverty or lack of resources, such as lack of income and social support networks; family disruption, such as occurs with divorce or single-parent households; and social stability, such as occurs with living in one place over time, being married, and having children. Poverty and social instability likely contribute to the vulnerability of women in poor communities. These factors impact a substantial number of minority women who are concentrated in these communities (UKCRVAW, 2011).

Risk Factors

Violence against women, specifically intimate partner violence, is a multifaceted phenomenon consisting of personal, situational, and sociocultural factors. This combination of individual, relational,

community, and societal factors contributes to the risk of becoming a victim or perpetrator of intimate partner violence, yet may or may not be direct causes. Every person identified as "at risk" does not necessarily become involved in violence (CDC, 2013).

Individual Factors

Individual factors point to personal demographics, traits, characteristics, or history of experiences that are associated with a greater likelihood of intimate partner violence victimization or perpetration. Individual demographic and socioeconomic factors include low income, unemployment, low academic achievement, young age, aggressive or delinquent behavior as a youth, and heavy alcohol and drug use (CDC, 2013; Krug et al., 2002). Individual psychosocial characteristics include low self-esteem, depression, anger and hostility, antisocial personality traits, borderline personality traits, emotional dependence and insecurity, having few friends and being isolated from other people, prpetrating psychological aggression, desire for power and control in relationships, and belief in strict gender roles such as male dominance and aggression in relationships (CDC, 2013; Krug et al., 2002). Factors associated with personal history include a prior history of being physically abusive, history of experiencing physical discipline as a child, history of experiencing poor parenting as a child, and being a victim of physical or psychological abuse. It is of particular note that witnessing domestic violence as a child and prior history of victimization are consistently the strongest predictors of perpetration (CDC, 2013; Krug et al., 2002).

Substance use and abuse is consistently associated with all forms of relationship violence. However, it is unclear whether the use of drugs and alcohol has a direct cause-and-effect relationship with violence. It is also unclear whether violence and substance abuse represent two overlapping social epidemics. Intimate partner violence may cause depression and reduced self-esteem, which can lead to an increased use of alcohol or drugs. Conversely, substance abuse may ignite conflicts in interpersonal relationships, which can subsequently lead to violent behavior.

Despite the lack of clarity, the co-occurrence of intimate partner violence and substance abuse is substantial. Evidence suggests that substance use by perpetrators will increase the risk of intimate partner violence in a relationship. On the other hand, evidence suggests that substance use by women will increase their risk of victimization (El-Bassel, Gilbert, Wu, Go, & Hill, 2005). Substance use can induce cognitive disruption and impairment of the ability to process social interactions for the perpetrator and victim of intimate partner violence. Such cognitive disruptions may lead to paranoia, impaired judgment, and distorted cues that increase the likelihood of violent interactions. Conflicts over spending money on and sharing drugs often lead to disputes that can escalate into violence. Drug-dependent women may be perceived by their partners as violating traditional gender norms and therefore their partners may feel justified in perpetrating violence against them (El-Bassel et al., 2005). Intimate partner violence has been shown to lead to the use of illicit drugs, in that women may initiate or increase illicit drug use to cope with the distress of experiencing violence from intimate partners. Thus, these circumstances point to a reciprocal relationship between intimate partner violence and drug abuse such that drug abuse increases the likelihood of intimate partner violence and intimate partner violence increases the likelihood of drug abuse. It must also be considered that, instead of a direct association between intimate partner violence and substance abuse, several psychosocial variables are independently associated with both intimate partner violence and drug abuse. A wide range of psychosocial variables are associated with *both* intimate partner violence and drug use, namely post-traumatic stress disorder (PTSD), lack of social support, childhood sexual abuse, and HIV

risk behavior. These potential confounders must be considered in explaining the association between substance use and intimate partner violence (El-Bassel et al., 2005).

Relationship Factors

Relationship factors point to interpersonal conflicts and direct engagement with others within the immediate context of abuse. These factors include marital conflict—fights, tension, and other struggles, marital instability—divorce or separations, dominance and control of the relationship by one partner over the other, economic dependence, and unhealthy family relationships and interactions. Marital conflict is highly predictive of intimate partner violence (CDC, 2013; Krug et al., 2002).

Community Factors

Community factors are associated with formal and informal social structures that influence the immediate environment in which the individual is found, thereby influencing, delimiting, or determining what occurs in the environment. These community influences are often byproducts of changes that occur in the larger social setting. Community factors include poverty and associated factors such as overcrowding; low social capital such as lack of institutions, relationships, and norms that shape the social interactions of a community; and weak community sanctions against intimate partner violence, such as unwillingness of neighbors to intervene in situations where violence is witnessed (CDC, 2013; Krug et al., 2002).

Societal Factors

Societal factors point to the broad set of cultural values and beliefs that influence the attitudes and views of the public. Societal factors are grounded in traditional gender norms that link manhood to dominance, toughness, and male honor, and promote the attitudes of male entitlement or ownership of women. These attitudes include the opinion that women should stay at home and not enter the workforce, which perpetuates women's economic dependence on the male. Such attitudes promote female submissiveness, women's lack of access to divorce, male economic and decision making control in the household, and acceptance of interpersonal violence and physical chastisement (CDC, 2013; Krug et al., 2002).

Risk Reduction and Prevention

Gender-based discrimination as well as social norms and gender stereotypes that perpetuate violence form the basis for violence against women and girls. Because violence has such destructive consequences on women, intervention efforts have primarily centered on responses and services for survivors. However, the most effective way to stop violence against women and girls is by preventing the occurrence of violence through addressing its root and structural causes (UN Women, 2014b).

Efforts to prevent violence should begin when boys and girls are young. Reaching youths is an effective strategy for faster, sustained progress in preventing and eradicating gender-based violence (UN Women, 2014b). Preventive efforts should focus on educating youths about the promotion of respectful relationships and gender equality. While public policies and interventions often concentrate on victims and perpetrators, targeting youth at a critical time when values and norms regarding gender equality are forged is an essential preventive action (UN Women, 2014b). It is important that educational programs incorporate comprehensive education on sexuality to advance awareness of gender equality, allow women and girls to better protect themselves from violence, to strengthen the responsibility of men for their own sexual and reproductive behavior, and to promote respectful relationships. Education is also an indispensable means for changing

damaging stereotypes and thinking, such as regarding issues of sexual orientation and gender identity (Commission on the Status of Women, 2013).

Preventive efforts should be directed toward the promotion of gender equality, women's empowerment, and women's enjoyment of human rights in communities. Primary interventions are needed to make the home and public spaces safer for women and girls, to ensure women's economic autonomy and security, and increase women's participation and decision-making powers in the home and relationships as well as in public life and politics. Moreover, it is essential to work with men and boys to accelerate progress toward preventing and ending violence against women and girls. Strategies must be implemented that will challenge the deeply rooted inequalities and social norms that perpetuate men's control and power over women and reinforce tolerance for violence against women and girls (UN Women, 2014b).

Risk reduction for rape necessitates that both women and society as a whole take action to eliminate inappropriate use of physical and sexual force. The approach consists of measures to decrease women's susceptibility to physical assault. It is essential that women communicate explicitly their intent or lack thereof in sexual matters. Formalized preparation is imperative in reducing the risk of rape, particularly date rape and marital rape. Any risk reduction program for rape should include the following key components:

- Discussion and understanding of the facts of rape to dispel the myths of rape.
- Training that will develop skills in honest and direct communication about dating, sexual needs, and desires.
- Practical interventions taught through audiovisual presentations, group discussion, and role play.
- Preparation for what to do when rape occurs, including an emphasis on early support and counseling.

Such measures are indispensable in building women's self-esteem and self-confidence. Additionally, these measures provide practical rape intervention strategies and an increased awareness of local supportive resources and services.

The Prevention of Violence against Women and Girls Initiative is a nationwide initiative of the United States Department of Health and Human Services Office on Women's Health. This initiative provides funding for community-level projects that conduct activities and events to educate and bring awareness to aspects of violence against women and girls. Various projects funded by Regional Offices on Women's Health throughout the country have focused on intimate partner violence, domestic violence, sexual assault, sexual abuse, stalking, emotional and verbal abuse, as well as teen violence, bullying, human trafficking, and other forms of trauma or abuse (Regional Offices on Women's Health, 2010).

Gender Similarities and Differences

Intimate Partner Violence

Research on intimate partner violence often focuses on whether there are gender differences in the prevalence, frequency, and severity of violence against intimate partners. Differences in prevalence of intimate partner violence based on gender remains disputed because research in this area has produced mixed results (Chan, 2012). Some findings suggest that intimate partner violence is predominantly perpetrated by men against women (Black et al., 2011; Tjaden & Thoennes, 2000), whereas other findings suggest that men are victimized by intimate partner violence nearly as much as women (Cho, 2012a). Numerous factors have been cited that may explain the inconsistencies in research results. Men and women have been noted to have different reporting patterns of intimate partner violence

that may lead to underreporting of perpetration and victimization. Men's reporting of their violent behavior is influenced by a tendency to blame their partner for provoking violent behavior as well as a fear of criminal consequences and the desire to avoid facing the legal consequences of their own violence. Women also tend to underreport their victimization. Women are likely to discount, downplay, or excuse their partner's violent acts, and are apt to forgive their partner and normalize intimate partner violence, reasoning that their partner really loves them. Women's underreporting may also be influenced by feeling dependent on their abusive partner, having dependent children, shifting attention by blaming themselves, and the need to make themselves better partners (Chan, 2012).

Although findings have been inconclusive, evidence generally supports the claim that men and women may exhibit similar rates of intimate partner violence when no contexts, motivations, and consequences are considered. However, when severity, motives, and impacts of intimate partner violence incidence are considered, evidence supports the claim that men often initiate and perpetrate more severe intimate partner violence, which leads to more severe consequences or injuries (Chan, 2012).

Differences have been noted in the type of violence used by men and women toward their intimate partners. Men are more likely to beat up, choke, or strangle their partners, and women are more likely to throw something at their partner, or slap, kick, bite, punch, or hit with an object (Chan, 2012). Differences in types of violence, however, do not accurately portray the level of severity of violence, because consequences of these types of violence need to be considered. The consequences of a slap can be quite different than the consequences of being strangled. Most studies support the claim that more women are likely to get injured by intimate partner violence than men (Cho & Wilke, 2010).

Intimate partner violence can be distinguished into four major patterns that take into account power dynamics, type and frequency of violence, and perpetrator's motives. The first category is *common couple violence*, which has a lower frequency among couples. Common couple violence is mostly minor, is typically not associated with power and control, and tends to be mutual (Johnson & Ferraro, 2000). Studies that found similar rates of violence between men and women might have captured this type of violence (Cho & Wilke, 2010).

Another category of intimate partner violence is *intimate terrorism*. Intimate terrorism is a tactic whereby violence is motivated by a wish to exert general control over one's partner. Intimate terrorism involves more incidents of violence per couple as compared to common couple violence, and it is less likely to be mutual. Intimate terrorism is more likely to escalate over time and more likely to involve serious injury. What distinguishes intimate terrorism is a pattern of violent and nonviolent behaviors that signifies a general motive to control. The controlling behaviors often involve psychological and emotional abuse (Johnson & Ferraro, 2000). Intimate terrorism is more likely to be perpetrated by men. Research that reported intimate partner violence being perpetrated mostly by men might have captured a preponderance of intimate terrorism (Cho & Wilke, 2010).

A third category of intimate partner violence is *violent resistance*. Violent resistance, which is similar in concept to self-defense, is perpetrated almost entirely by women. Violent resistance often involves severe violence, including killing the male partner. Violent resistance is viewed as an indicator that a woman will soon leave her abusive partner (Johnson & Ferraro, 2000). Although research on this type of violence is scarce, evidence suggests that the majority of female-perpetrated intimate partner violence is self-defensive in nature (Cho & Wilke, 2010).

The last category of intimate partner violence is *mutual violent control*. This is a couple pattern in which both partners are controlling and violent. Mutual violent control has been likened to two intimate terrorists battling for control (Johnson & Ferraro, 2000). It is thought to be a rare phenomenon on which more focused research is needed.

Rape and Sexual Assault

In this country, the incidence and prevalence of rape and sexual assault is higher among women than in men, with nearly 1 in 5 (18.3%) women and 1 in 71 men (1.4%) experiencing rape at some time in their lives. Women are more likely to be raped by intimate partners, family members, acquaintances, or strangers, while men are more likely to be raped by acquaintances or strangers. Both men and women tend to suffer short- and long-term physical and psychological consequences as a result of sexual assault, although women are disproportionately impacted, with 81% of assaulted women as opposed to 35% of assaulted men likely to experience such consequences (Black et al., 2011).

Although women are raped far more frequently than men, the proportion of male to female victimization may be skewed due to gender differences in rates of reporting rape and sexual assault. Although the rates of reporting rape are generally low for women, evidence suggests that men are 1.5 times less likely to report a rape by a male perpetrator than women. This rate might even be lower when factoring in sexual assaults of men committed by women (Chapleau, Oswald, & Russell, 2008).

Gender differences concerning attitudes toward rape lie in rape myths. Rape myths are false or stereotypical beliefs about the blameworthiness of victims, the innocence of rapists, and the illegitimacy of rape as a grave crime (Chapleau et al., 2008). Rape myths of female victims have been identified as: (1) the woman asked for it, (2) the action was not really rape, (3) the male did not mean to do it, (4) the woman wanted it, (5) the woman lied, (6) rape is a trivial event, and (7) rape is a deviant event (Chapleau et al., 2008).

Rape myths about male victims have been identified as: (1) a male being raped by a male is synonymous with loss of masculinity, (2) males raped by males must be homosexual, (3) males are unable to function sexually unless they are sexually aroused, (4) males cannot be forced to have sex against their will, (5) males are less impacted by rape than women, (6) males are always ready to accept any sexual opportunity, and (7) a male should be able to defend himself against sexual assault (Chapleau et al., 2008).

Recognizing Violence

Intimate Partner Violence

Intimate partner violence refers to violence between individuals who have a close personal relationship. An intimate partner can be a current or former spouse (married, common-law, civil union, or domestic partner), boyfriend or girlfriend, a dating partner, or an ongoing sexual partner (Breiding, Basile, Smith, Black, & Mahendra, 2015). Intimate partner violence is also known as domestic violence or battering. It can range from a single episode of violence to ongoing battering, and is often perpetrated as an escalating pattern of abuse whereby one partner controls the other through force, intimidation, or threat of violence. Intimate partner violence occurs across all socioeconomic, educational, and racial and ethnic groups.

Intimate partner violence includes physical violence, sexual violence, psychological aggression (including coercive tactics), and stalking (Breiding et al., 2015). Stalking will be discussed later in this chapter. Each form of abuse, along with manipulation, intimidation, and threats are tactics used by a perpetrator in order to entrap the partner in the relationship (National Network to End Domestic Violence [NNEDV], 2014a).

Physical violence is a powerful method by which a perpetrator maintains control over their partner. The perpetrator creates an environment of constant fear such that even the threat of physical violence is effective in retaining power and control (NNEDV, 2014b). Although physical violence is the most commonly recognized form of intimate partner violence, it may or may not be a part of an abusive relationship. When present early in a relationship, physical violence will usually worsen over time. If physical violence is not present in a relationship it may begin when the woman becomes pregnant, or when she wants to leave the relationship (NNEDV, 2014b). Common forms of physical violence are presented in **Box 9–1**.

Sexual violence is a sexual act that is committed or attempted by another person without freely given consent of the victim or against someone who is unable to consent or refuse (Breiding et al., 2015). Sexual violence in some form is frequently present in abusive relationships, and may be subtle or overt. Sexual violence is seldom discussed, as victims commonly feel shame and humiliation. Sexual violence constitutes forcing the victim to have sex or making the victim afraid to say no to sex. It also includes forcing the victim to participate in degrading or demeaning sexual acts, subjecting the victim to violence or name calling during sex, or denying contraception or protection from sexually transmitted diseases (NNEDV, 2014b). Sexual penetration of the victim may be facilitated by alcohol or drugs. Sexual violence can include forced or alcohol/drug facilitated incidents in which the victim was made to penetrate a perpetrator or other person; non-physically pressured unwanted penetration; intentional sexual touching; or non-contact acts of a sexual nature. Sexual violence can also occur when a perpetrator forces or coerces a victim to engage in sexual acts with a third party (Breiding et al., 2015). Tactics used by perpetrators to coerce victims to engage in or be exposed to a sexual act are presented in **Box 9–2**.

Box 9–1: Forms of Physical Violence

Physical violence includes but is not limited to:

- Scratching
- Grabbing
- Biting
- Shaking
- Hitting
- Slapping
- Choking
- Punching
- Pushing
- Shoving
- Hair-pulling
- Burning
- Throwing
- Using weapons (guns, knives, or other objects)
- Use of restraints or one's body size or strength against another person
- Coercing others to commit any of these acts

Data from Breiding, M., Basile, K., Smith, S., Black, M., & Mahendra, R. (2015). *Intimate partner violence surveillance: Uniform definitions and recommended data elements, Version 2.0.* Atlanta, GA: National Center for Injury Prevention and Control, Centers for Disease Control and Prevention.

Box 9–2: Tactics Used to Perpetrate Sexual Violence

- Use or threat of physical force toward a victim in order to gain the victim's compliance with a sexual act
- Giving alcohol or drugs to a victim in order to gain the victim's compliance with a sexual act
- Taking advantage of a victim who is unable to provide consent due to intoxication or incapacitation from voluntary consumption of alcohol, recreational drugs, or medication
- Exploitation of vulnerability (such as immigration status, disability, undisclosed sexual orientation, age)
- Use of intimidation

(continues)

Box 9–2: Tactics Used to Perpetrate Sexual Violence (*continued*)

- Misuse of authority (such as using one's position of power to coerce or force a person to engage in sexual activity)

- Economic coercion (such as bartering of sex for basic goods, like housing, employment/ wages, immigration papers, or childcare)

- Degradation (such as insulting or humiliating a victim)

- Fraud (such as lies or misrepresentation of the perpetrator's identity)

- Continual verbal pressure (such as wearing down the victim by repeatedly asking for sex)

- False promises by the perpetrator (such as promising marriage, promising to stay in the relationship)

- Nonphysical threats (such as threats to end a relationship or spread rumors)

- Control of a person's sexual behavior/sexuality (such as through threats, reprisals, threat to transmit STD's, threat to force pregnancy)

Modified from Breiding, M., Basile, K., Smith, S., Black, M., & Mahendra, R. (2015). *Intimate partner violence surveillance: Uniform definitions and recommended data elements, Version 2.0.* Atlanta, GA: National Center for Injury Prevention and Control, Centers for Disease Control and Prevention.

Psychological aggression in some form is present in all abusive relationships. Perpetrators use psychological aggression to gain power and control. Psychological aggression involves the use of verbal and non-verbal communication with the intent to harm another person mentally or emotionally and exert control over that person (Breiding et al., 2015). This form of abuse can be severely damaging to the self-esteem of the victim. The damage is so severe that many victims have reported that they would have preferred physical violence rather than endure the ongoing psychological damage from psychological aggression (NNEDV, 2014b). Acts of psychological aggression are not physical acts of violence. In many instances such acts may not be perceived as aggression since they are covert and manipulative in nature. However, psychological aggression is an essential part of intimate partner violence and it frequently co-occurs with other forms of intimate partner violence. Evidence suggests that psychological aggression frequently precedes physical and sexual violence in abusive relationships. Acts of psychological aggression can significantly influence the impact of other forms of intimate partner violence. For example, a victim who is threatened by an intimate partner with physical injury or death before she was subjected to physical violence would likely experience greater amplification of fear. Evidence suggests that the impact of psychological aggression by an intimate partner is as significant as that of physical violence by an intimate partner (Breiding et al., 2015). The common forms of psychological aggression are presented in **Box 9–3**.

The financial tactics of psychological aggression appear to be the most powerful tactics of entrapping a victim in an abusive relationship. In fact, many victims report that it is the main reason they decide to stay in or return to an abusive relationship. Their concern over their ability to provide financially for themselves and their children compels them to

Box 9–3: Forms of Psychological Aggression

Psychological aggression can include but is not limited to:

- Expressive aggression (includes name-calling, humiliating or degrading the victim, or expressing anger in a manner that seems dangerous)

- Coercive control that isolates a person from access to transportation, communication, money, friends, and family (includes monitoring the victim's whereabouts, communications, or threatening to harm self, a loved one, or possessions)

- Threat of physical or sexual violence (includes use of words, gestures, or weapons to communicate the intent to cause death, disability, physical injury, or communicate the intent to compel a victim to engage in sex acts or sexual contact when the victim is either unwilling or unable to consent)

- Control of reproductive or sexual health (includes refusal to use birth control or coercion of victim to terminate pregnancy)

- Exploitation of victim's vulnerability (such as immigration status, disability, undisclosed sexual orientation)

- Perpetrator manipulates his own vulnerability (perpetrator's manipulation of real or perceived disability or immigration status to control a victim's choices or limit a victim's options)

- Gaslighting (includes presenting false information to the victim with the intent of making the victim doubt her own memory and perception)

Modified from Breiding, M., Basile, K., Smith, S., Black, M., & Mahendra, R. (2015). *Intimate partner violence surveillance: Uniform definitions and recommended data elements, Version 2.0*. Atlanta, GA: National Center for Injury Prevention and Control, Centers for Disease Control and Prevention.

remain in an abusive relationship or return to it after leaving (NNEDV, 2014a). The perpetrator gains power and control over the victim. Financial tactics of psychological aggression may be overt or subtle, but will include methods that limit the victim's access to assets, conceal information and accessibility to the family finances, and keep the victim from gaining employment. Financial tactics may be present throughout the relationship, or may manifest when the victim attempts to leave or has left the relationship. Evidence suggests that financial tactics are used in 98% of abusive relationships (NNEDV, 2014a).

Financial tactics can have destructive short- and long-term consequences. A short-term effect concerns the ability of the victim to stay safe through access to assets. Without assets, victims may be unable to acquire safe and affordable housing or the funds to provide for themselves or their children when they leave the relationship. The fear of homelessness often compels victims to return to the abusive relationship. Victims who manage to escape the abuse and survive initially face an overwhelming challenge in obtaining long-term security and safety. Victims often find it extremely difficult to gain independence, safety, and long-term security due to ruined credit scores, sporadic employment histories, and legal issues caused by the violence (NNEDV, 2014a).

Intimate partner violence occurs in both heterosexual and same-sex relationships, and has been shown to occur with the same frequency in both (Center for American Progress, 2011). Lesbian relationships share numerous similarities with heterosexual relationships with respect to intimate partner violence. The pattern of abuse in lesbian relationships similarly includes a vicious cycle of physical, emotional, and psychological mistreatment resulting in feelings of isolation, fear, and guilt in the victim. Perpetrators of intimate partner violence in lesbian relationships often have severe mental illnesses and were abused as children. In lesbian relationships, psychological aggression is the most common form of abuse, and perpetrators of physical violence frequently blackmail their partners into silence. Physical as well as sexual violence often occurs together in the relationship. As in heterosexual relationships, intimate partner violence in lesbian relationships is present across race, ethnicity, and socioeconomic status (Center for American Progress, 2011).

There are notable differences, however between intimate partner violence in lesbian relationships and intimate partner violence in heterosexual relationships. Many lesbians perceive domestic violence as a heterosexual phenomenon and may not recognize the patterns of abuse within their own relationships. In addition, fewer protective measures from the legal system are available to lesbians, and thus lesbian victims may have difficulty seeking assistance from law enforcement and the courts if their relationships are not legally recognized. Most services related to intimate partner violence are designed for heterosexual female victims and male offenders, making it difficult for lesbians to find support. This lack of services is a contributing factor to the lack of recognition of same-sex domestic violence (Center for American Progress, 2011).

Lesbian perpetrators frequently threaten their partners (who are closeted) with revealing their gay orientation to family, friends, and work colleagues. Lesbian victims may perceive this threat as magnified by the sense of isolation resulting from being closeted from friends and family, having fewer civil rights protections, and lacking access to the legal system (Center for American Progress, 2011). Lesbian victims of abuse may experience stigma from their victimization and their sexual orientation, and they may be reluctant to report abuse to legal authorities for fear of revealing their sexual orientation. Reluctance to seek help may also stem from fear of showing a lack of solidarity with the lesbian community and fear of having lesbian relationships perceived by society as inherently dysfunctional (Center for American Progress, 2011). Lesbian victims are more likely to fight back than are heterosexual women. This can lead law enforcement to misconstrue that mutual fighting has occurred in the relationship and fail to notice the larger context of intimate partner violence and the dynamics of power and control that are operating in the relationship (Center for American Progress, 2011). In addition, abusers can threaten to take children away from the victim, especially in states where adoption laws do not allow same-sex parents to adopt each other's children. Victims may not have legal rights, should the couple separate. Children may be used as leverage by the abuser to prevent the victim from leaving the relationship or from seeking help. In instances where the victim is the legally recognized parent, an abuser may threaten to reveal the victim's sexual orientation to social workers hostile to lesbians, which might result in a loss of custody. In extreme situations, the abuser could end up gaining custody of the children (Center for American Progress, 2011).

Rape and Sexual Assault

Rape and sexual assault are crimes of violence and aggression. Rape is forced sexual intercourse that occurs without consent. Rape can include both psychological coercion as well as physical force. Forced sexual intercourse means sexual penetration by the offender(s) of the victim's vagina, mouth, or rectum. Rape can be perpetrated against male as well as female victims, and includes homosexual rape as well as heterosexual rape. The crime of rape also includes attempted rape, which can also include threats of rape (Bureau of Justice Statistics [BJS], 2014). Sexual assault encompasses a wide range of victimizations that are distinguished from rape or attempted rape. Sexual assault includes attacks or attempted attacks that generally involve unwanted sexual contact between the victim and offender. Sexual assault may or may not involve force. It can encompass behaviors such as grabbing, fondling, or verbal threats (BJS, 2014).

Rape may occur among strangers or intimate partners, and among people of opposite sex or same sex. Acquaintance rape is a type of rape in which the victim and the rapist were previously known to each other. They may have interacted in some socially appropriate manner. Acquaintance rape is also known as date rape. It is estimated that nearly 78% of rape victims in this country know their assailant (Planty, Langton, Krebs, Berzofsky, & Smiley-McDonald, 2013).

Rape by anyone an individual knows—coworker, teacher, a husband's friend, boss, or former intimate—is considered acquaintance rape. In many cases of acquaintance rape, the rape has been facilitated by the use of drugs to render the victim unconscious or incapacitated. Flunitrazepam (Rohypnol) is a benzodiazepine that is commonly used to facilitate date rape. This drug is ten times more potent than valium and is tasteless and odorless. Rohypnol is easily dissolved in liquid, takes effect quickly, and produces memory loss for as long as 8 hours. This drug is especially popular on high school and college campuses, as well as in nightclubs. Many women who have consumed a drink with this drug dissolved in it have been raped afterward. The use of Rohypnol is extremely dangerous and can cause death. Other drugs that have been associated with date rape include the central nervous system depressants gamma hydroxybutyrate (GHB) and gamma butyrolactone (GBL). Both are available in liquid form. Abuse of GHB and GBL can cause coma and seizures. Ketamine, a dissociative anesthetic agent that is mostly used in veterinary practice, is another common date rape drug that is snorted or injected intramuscularly. Ketamine can lead to respiratory depression and death.

Rape can occur in a marriage, during legal separation, or after a divorce. Rape in marriage may be called spousal rape or marital rape. Historically, rape within a marriage was not considered a crime because husbands had unlimited sexual access to their wives. However, in 1993, marital rape became a crime in all 50 states. Some states provide exemptions for certain circumstances, such as mental or physical impairment of a woman that makes her unable to consent. In such instances, the rape is considered decriminalized. Marital rape, as distinguished from rape by a stranger, tends to be more traumatic for the victim and may require longer recovery from the trauma. This may be due to a lack of recognition, inability to share the pain, and a profound sense of a betrayal of trust. Marital rape victims may also experience a higher likelihood of repeated assaults than other rape victims. Married perpetrators are more likely to use anal and oral rape to humiliate, punish, and establish full ownership and control over their partners. Victims of marital rape may be pressured to stay in the marital relationship, may be financially dependent on the spouse (especially if they have children or lack outside employment), or they may be pressured by family or friends to remain with the spouse. Children may witness sexual violence or otherwise be adversely affected by it. Moreover, because of cultural reasons, victims of marital rape may have difficulty distinguishing that the spouse's conduct is rape or recognizing that the person they married and love is a rapist (Rape, Abuse, and Incest National Network [RAINN], 2014).

For a variety of reasons, most rapes are unreported. Underreporting of rape may be associated with the tendency of society to blame the victim. Many women fear unwanted publicity from making a formal complaint, or may distrust hospitals and law enforcement agencies. Underreporting may occur because victims may suffer from shame and guilt, fear that they would not be believed, and they may fear reprisal or punishment if the rapist is an acquaintance or employer. Women in prisons and jails are at risk for rape and other forms of sexual violence. Reporting procedures in prisons are often ineffectual and complaints are routinely ignored. To make matters worse, punishment for the crime is rare, and inmates face retaliation from the offender if a report is made.

Stalking

Stalking, like intimate partner violence, is a crime of power and control. Stalking is a course of conduct directed at a specific person that entails repeated (occurring on two or more occasions) physical proximity, nonconsensual communication, verbal written or implied threats, or a combination thereof, that would cause a reasonable person fear or concern for one's safety or the safety of someone else (such as a family member or close friend (Breiding et al., 2015). Stalking behaviors may also be comprised of persistent patterns of sending or leaving unwanted items or gifts that may range from seemingly romantic to bizarre, following or lying in wait for the victim, entering a victim's home or car and leaving evidence of their entry to scare the victim, or damaging or threatening to damage the victim's personal property, pets, or belongings. Stalking behaviors can also include persistently defaming the victim's character, using the Internet to harass the victim, spreading rumors about the victim, or posting personal information (Breiding et al., 2015; National Institute of Justice [NIJ], 2007).

Stalking can be perpetrated in person or by use of electronic media such as phone, fax, Internet, GPS, cameras, or computer spyware. Cyberstalking is the use of technology to stalk victims and shares some characteristics with in-person stalking. Cyberstalking involves initially using email or the Internet to pursue, harass, or contact others in an unsolicited manner. In chat rooms, a perpetrator can intensify cyberstalking by methodically flooding the targeted victim's inbox with obscene, hateful, or threatening messages and images. A cyberstalker may assume the victim's identity by posting fictitious or nonfictitious information to solicit responses from the cybercommunity. The cyberstalker can subsequently use information obtained from the Internet to further intimidate, harass, and threaten the victim through courier mail, phone calls, and appearing at the residence or workplace of the victim (Breiding et al., 2015; NIJ, 2007).

While cyberstalking does not entail physical contact with the victim, it remains a serious crime. The pervasiveness of the Internet and the ease with which personal information is accessible to others from the Internet has made this type of stalking easily done. Potential cyberstalkers may find it easier to stalk via technological means such as the Internet rather than by confronting an actual person. Behaviors that fall short of the legal definition of stalking must be taken seriously since such conduct may be a precursor to stalking. The federal interstate stalking statute has been extended to include cyberstalking (NIJ, 2007).

Human Trafficking

According to the United Nations Trafficking in Persons Protocol, human trafficking is the recruitment, transportation, transfer, harboring, or receipt of persons, accomplished by the threat of or use of force or other forms of coercion. Human trafficking is also accomplished by abduction, fraud, deception, abuse of power or of a position of vulnerability, or by giving or receiving payments or benefits to achieve the consent of a person having control over another person, for the purpose of exploitation (UNODC, 2012). Exploitation encompasses, at a minimum, the exploitation or the prostitution of others, or other forms of sexual exploitation, forced labor or services, slavery or practices similar to slavery and servitude. Human trafficking is a process by which people are recruited in their community and exploited by traffickers who use deception and/or some form of force to entice and control them (UNODC, 2012). Practices that are not considered human trafficking include illegal adoptions, the trade in human organs, child pornography that involves production of sexual images representing children, such as drawings and computer-generated images, and prostitution involving willing adults (Department of State, 2010).

The crime of human trafficking consists of three distinct components: the act, the means, and the purpose. In order to constitute as a trafficking in persons offense, all three components must be present; however, each component has a range of manifestations. The "act" refers to the recruitment, transport, harboring, or receipt of persons intended for trafficking. The "means" is the threat of or use of force, deception, coercion, or abuse of power that is utilized to lure the victims. The "purpose" refers to the manner of exploitation to which traffickers subject the victims, which may be sexual, forced labor, domestic servitude, or other types of exploitation (UNODC, 2012).

The majority of victims of human trafficking that have been detected globally are women. This indicates that being a woman in many parts of the world is associated with the vulnerabilities that lead to victimization through human trafficking. Although many cases of human trafficking begin as individuals attempting to improve the conditions of their lives, circumstances will often transform those attempts into incidences of exploitation and abuse. Victims of human trafficking are often made vulnerable due to deeply rooted social values and practices and thus are easy targets for the intent of criminals on profiting from victims' hopes of a better life. Recruitment and exploitation of vulnerable individuals is relatively easy and frequently carries low risk of detection (UNODC, 2012).

Certain characteristics contribute to the vulnerability of victims. Women are less empowered than men in many societies. Gender inequality is common, as is less access to education and employment opportunities and realization of human and social rights. In terms of becoming victims of trafficking, females can be more physically vulnerable to exploitation through use of force or threats than males (UNODC, 2012).

Children, both boys and girls, lack maturity and are not legally empowered to make their own life decisions. This makes them more vulnerable than adults. Children are dependent on guardians, who may not have their best interest at heart. Also, lack of experience makes children easily trusting of others, which can make them easily exploited by criminals (UNODC, 2012).

Would-be migrants are another group vulnerable to becoming victims of human traffickers. Would-be migrants, who are looking for opportunities abroad, or newly arrived immigrants, are frequently without close family, friends, or other support networks. Would-be migrants eager to find opportunities abroad may not critically assess job advertisements or recruiting firms. Newly arrived immigrants frequently need to find work quickly, and this makes them more vulnerable to accepting dangerous job offers (UNODC, 2012). Some migrants may have irregular immigration status in their country of destination, which may elevate their vulnerability by fearing or being reluctant to contact local authorities. Also, when migrants with restricted access to destination countries seek assistance from traffickers to cross borders with fraudulent documents or through other dishonest measures, their vulnerability to becoming victims of human trafficking is increased (UNODC, 2012).

Other persons potentially vulnerable to human trafficking include adolescents, who may become easy targets for exploitation in the sex industry. Individuals with disabilities may be especially vulnerable to human trafficking (often for begging), as well as albinos in some rural African communities, and refugees fleeing wars or natural disasters (UNODC, 2012).

Factors such as gender, age, migration status, ethnolinguistic background, and poverty are singularly insufficient explanations of vulnerability. However, these characteristics tend to become factors of vulnerability if they marginalize individuals from the rest of the community. Although anyone could become a victim of human trafficking, individuals who lack protection, who are not integrated in the surrounding community, and who are isolated by the national authorities or by the societies where they live are at higher risk of victimization. In these areas of discrimination and marginalization, exploitation by traffickers of the vulnerable situation of potential victims is achievable (UNODC, 2012).

The power of traffickers is grounded in financial and social resources that can be used for profit making. These resources may be amassed from various criminal activities or from business and social networks utilized for criminal purposes. Business networks may include relationships with people who have the means to enlist others, such as owners of recruitment agencies. Business networks may also include those who have the means to transport people, such as taxi or truck drivers, people with the ability to assist with travel documents, such as embassy personnel, and those with the possibility to abuse the services of trafficked persons, such as restaurant or brothel owners. Social networks may also encompass relationships with certain ethnic or family groups or other distinct groups. With the financial resources and social networks, the traffickers can generate those powers that are needed to organize the crime of human trafficking (UNODC, 2012). Human trafficking patterns generally echo these powers and vulnerabilities, regarding both the criminals and the victims. The most common trafficker profile is a male who is a national of the country where the exploitation takes place, although female participation in this crime is higher than for other crimes. The involvement of women in human trafficking is present more frequently in the trafficking of girls. Women commonly occupy low-ranking positions in the trafficking network and their duties are more exposed to the risk of detection and prosecution than male traffickers. On the other hand, most victims of human trafficking are women and children, usually foreign and frequently from backgrounds characterized by economic deprivation and lack of decent employment opportunities (UNODC, 2012).

Female Genital Mutilation

Female genital mutilation is also known as female genital cutting and female circumcision. It is a centuries-old practice that is deeply ingrained in cultural norms and beliefs about the role of women and girls in society. This practice includes all procedures that involve partial or total removal of the external female genitalia, or other injury to the female genital organs for nonmedical reasons. The practice is usually performed on women by traditional circumcisers, who often play other central roles in communities such as attending childbirths. In some communities, female genital mutilation has been medicalized and is performed by medically trained personnel (United Nations Children's Fund, 2013).

For the most part, however, practitioners without medical training perform female genital mutilation as their vocation. Sometimes older women in the family may be responsible for performing the procedure. In most cases the female genital mutilation is performed far from hospitals or clinics. Consequently, most girls and women undergo female genital mutilation without anesthetics, antiseptics, or antibiotics. The manner in which female genital mutilation is performed greatly influences physical and psychological consequences, even when the procedure is done in a medical setting. Women may be deeply impacted by a sense of betrayal, the motivations behind the procedure, loss of sexual sensation and function, and a sense of shame (Sanctuary for Families, 2013).

Female genital mutilation involves a broad range of practices commonly performed on girls before the age of 15 and often in infancy or early childhood. In some communities, it may be performed on a series of young girls, one after the other, as part of a ritual or initiation ceremony. Female genital mutilation may also be performed on adult women, particularly around the time of marriage. In some communities women may be subjected to additional female genital mutilation later in life (Sanctuary for Families, 2013).

The World Health Organization (WHO, 2014a) describes four major categories of female genital mutilation procedures:

Type 1: This type involves performing a clitoridectomy, which is the partial or total removal of the clitoris and/or the clitoral hood (prepuce).

Type 2: This type is known as excision and involves the partial or total removal of the clitoris and the labia minora, with or without excision of the labia majora.

Type 3: This type is known as infibulation and involves removal of the external genitalia and the narrowing of the vaginal opening through the creation of a covering seal. The seal is created by cutting and repositioning the inner, or outer, labia, with or without removal of the clitoris. A small opening is left for menstruation and the passage of urine. Women who undergo this procedure must be later cut open for intercourse and childbirth.

Type 4: This type involves other harmful procedures to the female genitalia for non-medical purposes, such as pricking, piercing, incising, scraping, and cauterizing the genital area.

Female genital mutilation is practiced to reinforce traditional views of femininity, such as the enhancement of female docility and obedience, and to initiate girls into womanhood. It is also done as a cleansing or purification ritual to rid girls or women of past actions considered socially unacceptable to their communities (Sanctuary for Families, 2013). Some communities believe that female genital mutilation physically differentiates women from men in that the removal of the "male-like" clitoris and labia is viewed as marking a girl's identity as female. A woman who does not undergo the procedure is often considered not fully female and can be ostracized by her community. The female genitals may be viewed as ugly and bulky, whereas removal brings about smoothness which is considered beautiful, particularly in communities that perform infibulations (Sanctuary for Families, 2013).

Female genital mutilation is commonly practiced as a strict requirement for marriage because it ensures premarital virginity and marital fidelity, both highly valued and carefully policed in many communities. The clitoridectomy is believed to control a woman's sexuality through removal of her site of sexual desire. Whereas infibulations prevent premarital intercourse and maintain virginity until marriage, a clitoridectomy is believed to control sexual desire. Some cultures believe that female genital mutilation enhances sexual pleasure for men. Women with infibulations may be frequently cut open for intercourse and then reinfibulated after childbirth to tighten the vagina to increase the husband's sexual pleasure (Sanctuary for Families, 2013).

Another cultural belief associated with female genital mutilation is the view of women as gatekeepers of family honor. Thus, the practice of female genital mutilation is believed to bring greater social value, status, respectability and honor to both the girl undergoing the procedure and her family members (Sanctuary for Families, 2013). Because of its association with gender identity, family honor, social status, and being marriageable, women who do not undergo the procedure face stigmatization, isolation, and will be unmarriageable. In some communities, women who refuse to have the procedure may be considered unclean and thus forbidden from handling food and water. Consequently, many women face immense social pressure for themselves and their daughters to undergo the procedure in order to avoid rejection by the community and to preserve marriageable status and social status (Sanctuary for Families, 2013).

Although female genital mutilation is against the law in the United States, the practice continues to be performed. The procedure is typically performed on girls who are part of a community originally from a country where female genital mutilation is prevalent, by traditional practitioners who operate covertly and illegally. Certain healthcare providers in this country who come from countries where the practice is prevalent perform the procedure on girls from their own communities at parental request (Sanctuary for Families, 2013).

Many girls who are young immigrant, permanent U.S. residents, and U.S. citizens are sent abroad to be subjected to female genital mutilation, typically during their school vacation, as part of a trip organized by their parents to expose their daughters to the customs of their homelands. This practice has been termed "vacation cutting." Sometimes parents use vacation cutting as a way to temper the influence of American culture on their daughters, especially if the daughters demonstrate too much assimilation to American social mores (Sanctuary for Families, 2013). Some girls are unaware that they are being sent to their homeland to be cut until they are actually forced to have the procedure. Girls are often sent overseas to have the procedure without their own knowledge and consent, as well as without the knowledge or consent of one or both parents. Controlling spouses, elder relatives, and community members often have overriding authority over a dissenting parent's wishes. In some cases the daughter may be kidnapped and sent abroad to have the procedure against the parents' express will (Sanctuary for Families, 2013).

Elder Abuse

According to the 2010 census, the proportion of the total U.S. population 65 years of age or older is 13%, or 40.3 million people. By 2050, people aged 65 or older will likely comprise 20% of the population. In 2010, 5.8 million people were 85 years of age or older. In 2050, that number is expected to reach 19 million (NCEA, 2014b). As the number of elderly people increases, so does the number of elder abuse cases. Elder abuse is a critical problem for women because women tend to live longer than men. Although both men and women can be subjected to elder abuse, women make up a larger share of the aging population and account for two-thirds of all reports of elder abuse (OWL-The Voice of Women 40+, 2009).

Elder abuse constitutes intentional actions by a caregiver or other person that cause harm or a serious risk of harm (whether or not harm is intended) to a vulnerable elderly person. These actions include failure to satisfy the basic needs of the elder or failure to protect the elder from harm. The caregiver or other person stands in a trust relationship with the elderly person (OWL, 2009). Two major situations characterize elder abuse:

Domestic abuse. Domestic abuse is mistreatment that is committed by someone with whom the elder has a special relationship, such as a spouse, sibling, child, friend, or caregiver (NCEA, 2014a).

Institutional abuse. Institutional abuse is mistreatment that occurs in a residential facility such as a nursing home, assisted living facility, group home, board and care facility, foster home, etc., and is commonly perpetrated by someone with a legal or contractual obligation to provide some element of care or protection (NCEA, 2014a).

According to the National Center on Elder Abuse (NCEA, 2014a), the following types of elder abuse can occur:

Physical abuse. The threat to inflict, or inflicting physical pain or injury on a vulnerable elder, or depriving an elder of a basic need.

Emotional or psychological abuse. The act of causing mental pain, anguish, or distress in an elderly person through verbal or nonverbal acts.

Sexual abuse. Nonconsensual sexual contact of any kind, or coercing an elder to witness sexual behaviors.

Exploitation or financial abuse. The illegal taking, misuse, or concealment of funds, property, or assets of a vulnerable elder.

Neglect. The refusal or failure by those responsible to provide food, shelter, health care, or protection for a vulnerable elder. Neglect can be active, when the refusal or failure is intentional, or passive, when the refusal or failure is unintentional.

Abandonment. The desertion of a vulnerable elder by anyone who has assumed the responsibility for care or custody of that person.

It is common for elders to be subjected to more than one type of mistreatment at the same or different times. For example, a person neglecting to provide an elder with appropriate care, food, or medication may also be financially exploiting that elder (NCEA, 2014a). Indicators of elder abuse are presented in **Box 9–4**.

Sometimes elders may neglect their own care, which can result in illness or injury. Self-neglect can be manifested by behaviors that include the hoarding of objects, newspapers, magazines, mail/paperwork, etc., and/or animal hoarding to the extent that the safety of the individual (and/or other household or community members) is threatened or compromised (NCEA, 2014a). The elder may fail to adequately provide food and nutrition for oneself or become dehydrated. They may neglect to take essential medications or refuse to seek medical treatment for serious illness. They may leave a burning stove unattended or be unable to attend to housekeeping. They may be confused and be unable to dress appropriately for the weather, or be unable to maintain appropriate hygiene. The problem of self-neglect is frequently paired with declining health, isolation, Alzheimer's disease, dementia, or substance dependency. Self-neglect is one of the most commonly reported concerns brought to the attention of adult protective services. In some of these cases, connecting the elders

---

Box 9–4: Indicators of Elder Abuse

Common indicators that elder abuse might be taking place:

- Bruises, pressure marks, broken bones, abrasions, and burns may be signs of physical abuse, neglect, or mistreatment.

- Unexplained withdrawal from normal activities, a sudden change in alertness, and unusual depression may be signs of emotional abuse.

- Bruises around the breasts or genital area may be signs of sexual abuse.

- Sudden changes in financial situations may be signs of exploitation.

- Bedsores, unattended medical needs, poor hygiene, and unusual weight loss are signs of possible neglect.

- Belittling, threats and other uses of power and control by spouses are signs of verbal or emotional abuse.

- Strained or tense relationships and frequent arguments between the caregiver and elderly person may also be signs of an abusive relationship.

Modified from National Center on Elder Abuse. (2014a). Frequently asked questions. Retrieved from http://www.ncea.aoa.gov/faq/index.aspx

to supportive services in the community can allow such individuals to continue living on their own. Conditions such as depression and malnutrition could be treated successfully with medical intervention. If the problems of the elder are severe enough, a guardian may be appointed (NCEA, 2014a).

As with other types of domestic violence, elder abuse is a complex problem. A combination of psychological, social, and economic factors, along with the mental and physical conditions of the victim and the perpetrator, contribute to the occurrence of elder abuse. The majority of elder abuse cases is perpetrated by known and trusted others, especially family members, including adult children, spouses, and others. Abusers can be women or men and be of any age, race, or socio-economic status. Elder abuse can be committed by family members, friends, service providers, peers, and strangers (NCEA, 2014a).

The following factors do not explain all types of elder abuse, since a variety of causal factors are involved with different types of abuse, as well as with each single incident. Evidence suggests, however, that there are some risk factors that are commonly associated with elder abuse. Elders who have dementia or Alzheimer's disease are at higher risk for abuse or neglect than the general population of elderly. Caregivers of the elderly with dementia often have a heightened perception of burden and develop depressive symptoms. Caregivers can be exposed to the psychological aggression and physical assault behaviors of elders with dementia (NCEA, 2014a). Other factors that contribute to elder abuse are caregiver stress, impairment of the dependent elder, and resentment of the dependency, especially as the level of dependency increases. In many cases of abuse, caregivers are unprepared, unwilling, or unable to provide the necessary care.

Elders who have remained in an abusive marital/partner relationship are also at risk for abuse. Spouses/intimate partners make up a large proportion of elder abusers, and thus have continued their abusive behavior into old age. If one partner has traditionally tried to exert power and control over the other through psychological aggression, physical violence, threats, isolation, and other tactics, then elder abuse becomes a continuation of the couples' history of domestic violence (NCEA, 2014a).

Abusers are often adult children who are dependent on their victims for financial assistance, housing, and other forms of support. Such adult children may need this support because they suffer from personal problems, such as mental illness, alcohol or drug abuse, or other dysfunctional personality characteristics, and lack of community support. The risk of elder abuse may be especially high when these adult children reside with the elder (NCEA, 2014a). It has been posited that an abuser may be repeating a cycle of violence similar to the cycle identified in cases of child abuse or neglect. The abuser of an elderly parent may have been abused by that parent in childhood, or the abuser may have witnessed the same type of elder abuse by the parent against the abuser's grandparent.

Higher rates of elder abuse are also associated with living with someone else, as well as being socially isolated. Although incongruous, these findings are related in that abusers residing with elders have a greater opportunity to abuse. The abuser may be isolated from the rest of the community themselves or endeavor to isolate the elder from others in order to hide the abuse. Further research is needed to clarify the association between these factors (NCEA, 2014a).

Quality of Life Issues Associated With Violence Against Women

Women bear a disproportionate burden as victims of violence. Violence impacts women as the actual victims of crimes, as well as the wives, daughters, mothers, and girlfriends of male victims or male perpetrators, and as perpetrators themselves. These women, and the women who are victims of violence, are all at risk for traumatic consequences of violence. Not only are there physical and psychological consequences, but violence leads to high societal costs and an overall decrease in quality of life for victims, families, and communities (Alexander, LaRosa, Bader, Garfield, & Alexander, 2010, p. 416).

Quality of life issues and concerns associated with violence against women are complex, multidimensional, and commonly involve the domains of health and physical functioning, psychological and spiritual well-being, socioeconomic integrity, and family well-being.

Health and Physical Functioning

Although the prevalence and forms of violence against women may differ across the globe, the health consequences seem to be similar across all settings. The characteristics or the severity of the consequences of violence can be impacted by context-specific factors such as poverty, gender inequality, cultural or religious practices, access to health, legal and other supportive services, conflict or natural disaster, HIV/AIDS prevalence, and legal and policy environments (WHO, 2012).

The effects of violence on health and physical functioning can be acute and immediate, chronic and long-lasting, and, in worst cases, fatal. Evidence has consistently indicated that the more severe the abuse, the greater its impact on the physical and mental health of women. The negative health consequences can continue long after the abuse has ended. The consequences of violence are likely to be more critical when women are subjected to more than one type of violence, such as physical and sexual, and/or multiple incidents of violence over time (WHO, 2012).

Women who are subjected to physical violence by intimate partners are more likely than men to experience acute or immediate physical injury. In addition, women who have been subjected to physical or sexual violence by a partner after the age of 15 are more likely to experience poor overall health, chronic pain, memory loss, difficulty walking, and problems carrying out activities of daily living, as compared to other women. Women with a history of abuse are more likely than other women to experience a variety of health problems such as headaches, chronic pelvic pain, back pain, abdominal pain, irritable bowel syndrome, and gastrointestinal disorders. In addition, worldwide, women are more likely to be killed by male intimate partners (WHO, 2012).

Women who are subjected to female genital mutilation experience no health benefits and have serious health implications. The procedure involves removal of normal healthy female genital tissue and interferes with the natural function of the female body. Immediate complications of the procedure include severe pain, shock, hemorrhage, tetanus, sepsis, urine retention, open sores in the genital area, and trauma to nearby genital tissue (WHO, 2014a). Women can also experience long-term complications, such as recurrent bladder and urinary tract infections, cysts, infertility, increased risk of childbirth complications and newborn fatalities, and the need for additional surgeries later, such as required to be cut open for intercourse and childbirth. Women may need repeated stitching and opening procedures to allow for childbirth, which further increases the risk and occurrence of immediate and long-term complications (WHO, 2014a). Sexual problems are also common to women who have undergone these procedures. They are likely to experience pain during sexual intercourse, less sexual satisfaction, and a lack of sexual desire (WHO, 2012).

Women who are subjected to sexual violence are more likely to experience higher rates of gynecological problems. These problems include vaginal infection, pain during intercourse, chronic pelvic pain, and urinary tract infections. Women who experience intimate partner violence without sexual violence have a higher risk of gynecological problems, though it is unclear why this is so. Women subjected to sexual violence have a greater incidence of gynecological trauma, especially in situations involving rape with objects, or when a girl is forced to have sexual intercourse and give birth before her pelvis is fully developed. Gynecological trauma may entail vaginal tearing, fistula formation between the vagina and bladder or rectum, or both, hemorrhage, infection, ulceration, other genital injuries, or complications during childbirth (WHO, 2012).

Women who are subjected to physical violence or forced sexual intercourse by any perpetrator are likely at higher risk of having an unintended pregnancy or unwanted pregnancy as compared to women with no history of abuse, both in the short-term and over the course of their reproductive lives. Unwanted pregnancy risk can be directly related to forced sexual intercourse or difficulty negotiating contraceptive use in an abusive relationship. It can also be indirectly related to high-risk sexual behaviors associated with a history of sexual abuse in childhood or adolescence. Girls and women faced with an unwanted pregnancy resulting from forced sexual intercourse will often terminate the pregnancy, whether or not safe abortion is available. Higher rates of pregnancy termination are associated with intimate partner violence, rape by non-partners, and transactional sex. Moreover, women subjected to physical or sexual violence by intimate partners also experienced higher rates of induced abortion (WHO, 2012).

Women who are HIV positive are more likely than other women to have been subjected to physical and sexual violence. Women subjected to physical and sexual violence are more vulnerable to contracting HIV and other sexually transmitted diseases through direct and indirect means (WHO, 2012). Women who are in violent relationships may have more difficulty refusing sexual intercourse or negotiating condom use. Vaginal trauma from forced sexual intercourse can increase the risk of contracting HIV. Women who were exposed to childhood sexual abuse often engage in risky sexual behaviors later in life, such as having multiple sex partners, lack of condom use, and

experiencing subsequent violence. Furthermore, fear of violence may stop women from seeking HIV testing, counseling, health services, as well as services for prevention of HIV transmission to infants. Thus, not only is violence associated with increased risk of HIV transmission, but it can be a consequence of disclosure of HIV positive status (WHO, 2012).

Physical and sexual violence during pregnancy is associated with numerous complications, including low maternal weight gain, miscarriage, stillbirth, and low-birth-weight babies. A frequently overlooked outcome of violence during pregnancy is maternal death. Evidence suggests that partner violence is associated with a substantial number of deaths among pregnant women (WHO, 2012).

Issues Affecting Psychological and Spiritual Functioning

Psychological Functioning

Women subjected to violence are at great risk for adverse mental health outcomes that substantially impact quality of life. The adverse mental health sequelae of violence tend to be chronic, and often persist well after a woman has achieved safety (Mechanic, 2004). The effects of violence on women are wide ranged and vary according to the type of assault experienced as well as sociocultural and trauma-related factors specific to each victim (Briere & Jordan, 2004). It is widely documented that women subjected to violence often experience anxiety and stress disorders, depression, helplessness, low self-esteem, dissociation, psychosomatic disorders, sexual problems, substance abuse, sleeping and eating disorders, and suicidality.

The sexual and physical abuse of girls can be similarly injurious, and produces a wide range of symptoms that can last well into adulthood (Briere & Jordan, 2004; WHO, 2012). Childhood sexual and physical abuse increases the risk of victims engaging in subsequent risky behaviors such as early sexual activity, substance abuse, multiple sexual partners, choosing abusive partners later in life, and lower rates of contraceptive and condom use. Women who have been subjected to childhood sexual abuse may suffer from feelings of worthlessness and have difficulty distinguishing sexual from affectionate behavior. They may have difficulty maintaining appropriate personal boundaries and refusing unwanted sexual advances. Women with a history of childhood sexual abuse have been shown to have a higher risk of experiencing sexual violence later in life (WHO, 2012).

A common psychological reaction to violent encounters such as intimate partner violence or rape is PTSD. PTSD can be extremely debilitating, and women may experience symptoms such as hypervigilance, emotional numbness and avoidance, and hyperarousal. Women with PTSD often turn to alcohol and drugs to help them cope with the symptoms. Substance abuse may also begin during an abusive relationship as a way to escape from the reality of the abusive situation.

Women who have been raped often experience rape trauma syndrome. This condition may occur in two phases. The first phase (the acute phase) includes the immediate emotional reactions following the event. These responses may vary and include but are not limited to shock, anger, numbness, guilt, disbelief, embarrassment, shame, feelings of being unclean, anxiety, fear, denial, self-blame, or restlessness. Women often experience significant disruption of their lives in the acute phase. The second phase of rape trauma syndrome involves women's attempts at reorganizing their lives and lifestyle, and learning to cope again. Women may decide to change schools, jobs, or routes to school or work in an effort to remove reminders of the rape from their daily lives. Overwhelming feelings frequently emerge that women may not directly link to the rape. Frequently, the rape may be repressed and not acknowledged, sometimes for years, but the feelings persist. Depression, guilt, and poor self-esteem are

common reactions during this phase. Suicidality, substance abuse, social phobias, and eating disorders may occur. The experience of rape can affect women's capacity for sexual health and intimacy. How a woman reacts to a rape experience may be mediated by individual coping and reaction patterns, demographic variables, characteristics of the assault, historical variables, and social support.

Spirituality

Spirituality and religiosity can influence the lives of victimized women in a number of ways. In the realm of domestic violence, spirituality and religious beliefs can strongly define women's conceptualization of marriage, love, gender roles, and expectations of marriage, hence influencing whether victims stay in or leave abusive relationships. The occurrence of domestic violence can either strengthen or weaken the spiritual or religious orientation of the victim. Victims may experience a spiritual vacuum in which they lose spiritual connection with God, themselves, and other people. On the other hand, victims of domestic violence may turn to religious and spiritual resources to cope and find meaning (Yick, 2008).

Religious ideology often reinforces commitment to marriage vows, the traditional nuclear family household, and the concept of being a dutiful wife and nurturing mother. This influence may compel a woman to stay in an abusive marriage. Religion may also serve as a cultural barrier to seeking help in domestic violence situations. Some religious belief systems emphasize the notions of forgiveness or perseverance, which may make women in abusive relationships reluctant to obtain help. Religion and spirituality can openly as well as covertly encourage abuse through emphasis of gender role expectations associated with husband leadership and wifely submissiveness (Yick, 2008).

In some instances, religion can decrease the risk of domestic violence. Many religious communities seem to adhere to values emphasizing commitment, personal growth, and family orientation, all of which might serve as buffer to domestic violence. Evidence suggests religious attendance is influential in decreasing the likelihood of perpetrating violence against one's partner. Thus, when both men and women engage in increased church attendance, the likelihood of perpetrating violence is decreased (Yick, 2008).

Spirituality and religion can be important coping mechanisms for women in violent relationships. The world is often viewed as unsafe, unjust, and unpredictable by victims of abuse, violence, and trauma. Religion and spirituality can provide victims with a meaning to life, a sense of mastery out of what appears futile, and support by connecting them to a larger community (Yick, 2008). As such, religion and spirituality can provide a system that creates meaning for individuals trying to reevaluate adversity. Some victims may view adversity as an opportunity for growth. Some may attribute adversity to the will of God or a superior being, and some use religious and spiritual strategies, such as prayer and meditation, to find solace and strength. Women in abusive relationships may rely on God or a superior being as a source of strength, and abused women with higher levels of spiritual involvement may experience better psychological well-being (Yick, 2008).

Issues Affecting Socioeconomic Integrity

The costs of violence against women in this country are estimated to exceed $5.8 billion. The largest component of this estimate is the nearly $4.1 billion dollars, more than two-thirds of the total costs, attributed to direct costs associated with medical care and mental health care. Of these costs, 89.7% are attributable to intimate partner physical assaults. Approximately $1.8 billion dollars is attributed to indirect costs of lost productivity from employment, household chores, and the value of lost lifetime earnings of homicide victims had they been able to live out

their full life expectancies (National Center for Injury Prevention and Control [NCIPC], 2003).

Healthcare needs that are associated with violence against women place a disproportionate burden on the healthcare system. Women subjected to violence have greater need for health care and seek healthcare services more frequently than women in the general population. Furthermore, as the frequency and severity of the violence increases, women's use of healthcare services increases accordingly. Evidence suggests that the use of healthcare services is highest among women in ongoing abusive relationships (WHO, 2012). On the other hand, women subjected to violence are less likely to seek preventive care, such as cancer screenings, mammograms, and cholesterol and blood pressure screening. Preventive care is commonly more cost-effective than treatment. The implications to lack of preventive care among women subjected to violence are poorer overall health and higher healthcare costs. In the United States, annual healthcare costs are significantly higher among women experiencing physical intimate partner violence and those who had experienced it within the past 5 years (WHO, 2012).

A key issue that emerges in the domain of violence against women is victim blame. Women may be made to feel at fault for having triggered violence by their behavior, or that the violence was deserved so they may not report the abuse or rape. Certain societal attitudes about the victim's style of dress, her relationship with the abuser or assailant, evidence of resistance, the presence of alcohol or drugs, and location of the incident can shift the onus of blame onto the victim. Such societal attitudes frequently influence victims to avoid reporting violence due to fear, shame, stigma, or perceived lack of support from family or community. These attitudes can be a significant factor toward the perpetuation of the cycle of violence in intimate relationships and in communities.

Social isolation is frequently a part of violent intimate relationships. Abusive partners will often act to separate women from their networks of support. Women's social activities may be restricted, and contact with relatives and friends may be forbidden or severely limited by abusive partners. Abusive partners may also separate women from the means to be self-sufficient by forbidding them to work outside the home or by prohibiting access to money or severely limiting the use of money. These acts are perpetrated by abusive partners in order to maintain power and control over women in their relationships.

Issues Affecting Family Well-Being

Violence against women produces numerous issues and concerns that affect family well-being and quality of life. Women as well as their children are severely affected by domestic violence. Children in violent households commonly witness the violence in their homes as well as being abused themselves. Violence in the home has severe short- and long-term implications for children (UNICEF, 2006). Children in families experiencing domestic violence may develop behavioral, social, and emotional problems. They may exhibit aggressive and antisocial behavior, depression, and anxiety. In addition, these children may have higher levels of anger, hostility, oppositional behavior, and disobedience (UNICEF, 2006). Children in violent households often experience low self-esteem, fear and withdrawal, poor relationships with siblings and peers, poor social relationships, and are more likely to suffer from cognitive and attitudinal problems. They may experience difficulties in school and have poor academic performance, and may exhibit slower cognitive development, lack of skills in conflict resolution, and limited problem-solving capabilities. They may also exhibit pro-violence attitudes and belief in rigid gender stereotypes and male privilege (UNICEF, 2006).

Children exposed to domestic violence often suffer from long-term complications. Evidence suggests that males exposed to domestic violence as children are more likely to engage in domestic violence as adults. Similarly, females exposed to domestic violence as children are more likely to become victims as adults. Children exposed to domestic violence are also more likely to suffer from depression and trauma symptoms as adults. They are also at higher risk for premature death and for developing risk factors for many common causes of death in the United States (UNICEF, 2006).

Family and friends are an important source of support for women in abusive relationships. Support from family and friends helps abused women to emotionally cope with the abuse and provide a safe haven and source of protection for women and their children. When able, women frequently turn to family and friends for advice, inspiration, encouragement, a place to stay, help with children, and financial assistance. Having a larger network of supportive and empathic family and friends can be helpful in maintaining better psychological well-being. Moreover, receipt of tangible support from family and friends is very important for women seeking to leave an abusive relationship. Lack of tangible and emotional support contributes to the distress of women in abusive relationships. Thus, the role of social support networks in mitigating the adverse impact of violence that battered women experience is substantial (Goodkind, Gillum, Bybee, & Sullivan, 2003).

On the other hand, not all abused women are surrounded by loving, supportive families who have the financial means to help them. Many women have family and friends who do not believe them, who blame them for provoking the abuse, and/or may be too fearful themselves to intervene. If some abused women repeatedly leave and return to the abusive relationship, family and friends may become less supportive over time. Some may provide tangible support but in an emotionally unsupportive, blaming manner that may ultimately turn out to be more harmful than helpful to the woman's overall well-being (Goodkind et al., 2003).

Implications for Healthcare Providers

Women subjected to violence—in particular, intimate partner violence—have a greater need for, and use of, healthcare services. Healthcare providers are well positioned to provide support to victims of violence; however, healthcare settings predominantly focus on screening and referral of women to domestic violence services. More inclusive services, especially those aimed at improving women's health and quality of life over time, have still to be widely integrated into health care (Ford-Gilbe, Merritt-Gray, Varcoe, & Wuest, 2011).

Primary healthcare providers need to take the lead in screening all women for self-reports of actual or possible experiences of relationship violence in order to prevent the actual, potential, or possible adverse outcomes of violence. Early identification of victims and survivors of violence is essential in order to promote healing and restoration. Healthcare providers must also screen adults and adolescents for online or technology-based stalking, harassment, bullying, or unsolicited sexual encounters. Such forms of interpersonal violence can cause psychological, social, emotional, and physical distress in adult and adolescent victims, as well as increase the risk of suicide ideation, suicide, and depression (Shavers, 2013).

In the primary care setting, women should be screened during their periodic examinations, especially gynecological visits. Women who present with gynecological problems, particularly multiple problems, chronic stress-related symptoms, and central nervous system symptoms, should be routinely considered for exposure to violence. The effects of stress and mental distress commonly accompany physical health problems in victims of relationship violence.

Many women who have been subjected to relationship violence do not come to healthcare facilities with apparent trauma or injuries. On the other hand, women who are battered and go to an emergency department frequently present with more injuries to the head, face, neck, thorax, breasts, and abdomen than women who have not been physically abused (Campbell, 2002). When there is a question of violence, either past or present, it is essential that healthcare providers obtain a focused history and perform a systematic physical examination to assess the severity and timing of trauma, injuries, gynecological conditions, central nervous system disorders, and chronic stress-related conditions.

It is essential that healthcare providers gain a general understanding of the relationships and patterns associated with relationship violence in order to understand the development of stress-related illnesses and mental disorders in women who have been subjected to violence. It is common for women to exhibit generalized and vague symptoms when they present for health care, including generalized concerns such as unexplained pain or malaise. Sometimes healthcare providers have preconceived ideas that such women have some other psychological disorder or might be exhibiting drug-seeking behavior, when in reality this behavior may be a woman's cry for help, or an attempt on her part to prove to her abusive partner that she is afflicted with some medical disorder as a way to preclude further violence or receive sympathy. Moreover, fear of further abuse, embarrassment, or some other reason may prevent an abused woman from revealing that she has been abused. Thus it is essential that healthcare providers understand how to identify signs of interpersonal violence.

Violence against women is a complicated problem that is best addressed through collaboration across health, domestic violence, social service, and legal sectors, as well as with community stakeholders, including women themselves. The development of supportive interventions for women who have been subjected to violence is a research priority. More evidence-based interventions need to be developed, especially those that center on women's lives beyond the crisis of leaving abusive relationships (Ford-Gilboe et al., 2011). Of interventions that have been tested, evidence suggests that domestic violence advocacy consisting of information and support to deal with abuse and to access needed services is associated with improvements in quality of life, safety actions, social support, access to services, and a reduction in violence when provided to women who sought assistance, particularly through shelters. In a similar vein, brief interventions aimed at providing women with information and support to assist with problem solving and decision making related to intimate partner violence is associated with decreased violence and increased use of safety behaviors. Such brief interventions may also be associated with decreased depressive symptoms and improved physical function (Ford-Gilboe et al., 2011). On the other hand, advocacy interventions provided by paraprofessionals that focus on system navigation or support and problem-solving interventions provided by social workers may not be effective in improving women's health. While interventions centered on support, safety, and system navigation are important for women who have left abusive relationships, they may not adequately deal with the health consequences of violence (Ford-Gilboe et al., 2011).

Although evidence suggests that cognitive behavioral therapy is helpful in mitigating the psychological effects of violence, complex interventions that concurrently attend to women's safety, the physical and mental health consequences of intimate partner violence, as well as social and economic challenges that create barriers to change have yet to be developed and methodically tested. Interventions that are trauma-informed and specifically focus on the impact of interpersonal violence and victimization on the life, health, and development of women are needed (Ford-Gilboe et al., 2011).

Special Concerns of Age and Ethnicity

During routine health encounters, all young women should be questioned about experiencing violence. The incidence of violence among adolescents is high, usually involving dating violence. Physical or sexual dating violence can result in serious and adverse health outcomes that carry lifelong implications. Healthcare providers should ask adolescents in a safe and private location about dating violence victimization and perpetration; this may be an important initial step toward effective intervention and prevention approaches. Questioning teenagers about jealous or possessive partners could provide clues to the existence of dating violence. Teenagers often feel uncomfortable about revealing they are experiencing relationship violence, and may present with vague physical complaints that may be indicative of distress. Many adolescents accept physical and sexual aggression as normal in dating and partner relationships. Healthcare providers can be a valuable resource in providing an alternative view regarding types of behavior that are appropriate in an intimate relationship.

Violence affects women of all ages; however, the literature often addresses violence experienced by women during the childbearing years. The unique problems of aging women who are subjected to violence are frequently overlooked. Elder abuse and mistreatment are often addressed from the perspective of inadequate care, which obscures important issues. As previously discussed, some forms of elder abuse and mistreatment are derived from a perspective of inadequate care and are rooted in the dynamics of caregiving. This may obscure the fact that other forms of elder abuse and mistreatment, particularly physical assaults, are interpersonal violence (Philips, 2000). Also, the notion that elder abuse is a product of inadequate care masks the gender issues and power dynamics inherent in intimate partner violence as they apply to older women. A wife or partner subjected to abuse at any age can experience serious physical and emotional harm, and even death. Because their physical vulnerability increases with age, older women can suffer serious injury or death even from low severity violence (Phillips, 2000).

Although injury may be the reason older women seek health care, the physical and mental consequences of violence may be more subtle, including depression, sleeplessness, chronic pain, atypical chest pain, and other types of somatic symptoms (Phillips, 2000). Healthcare providers who interact with cognitively impaired or unresponsive women need to assess for nonverbal cues and focus the assessment on the caregiver. Perpetrators of abuse may trigger suspicion by exhibiting behavior that includes showing possessiveness or jealousy toward the victim, denying or minimizing the seriousness of the violence, refusing to take responsibility for the violence, and holding a rigid view of gender roles or negative attitudes toward women.

The scrutiny of violence against women requires the consideration of cultural differences in values, attitudes, and behavioral norms across racial and ethnic groups. Data is scarce in this area, and on the whole, it is difficult to assess attitudes toward rape and other violent crimes. Some societal attitudes tend to place the burden of blame on rape victims rather than on those who commit the violent act. In some cases, the belief that the violence was justified may persist.

Societal acceptance of male dominance can strongly impact cultural attitudes about violence against women. It is a prevailing belief in many cultures by both men and women that a man has the right to control the behavior of his wife and daughters, and disobedient women should be punished. The legitimization of these acts of violence perpetuates violence against women in these cultures. Societal practices and beliefs that make women especially vulnerable to abuse by their intimate partners include marked inequalities between men and women, rigid gender roles, weak sanctions against violent behavior, and cultural norms that espouse man's right to sex regardless of a woman's feelings (Krug et al., 2002). Findings from a wide range of studies conducted in both industrialized and developing countries suggest that violence in intimate relationships can be triggered by a remarkably consistent list of factors that include a woman disobeying her husband, arguing back, not having food ready on time, not caring adequately for the children or home, questioning the man about money or girlfriends, going somewhere without the man's permission, refusing the man sex, and the man suspecting the woman of infidelity (Krug et al., 2002).

Research Review

Do prevalence, frequency, and severity of intimate partner violence differ by rurality?

Peek-Asa, C., Wallis, A., Harland, K., & Beyer, K. (2011). Rural disparity in domestic violence prevalence and access to resources. *Journal of Women's Health, 20*(11), 1743–1749.

Disparity exists in this country regarding access to health, prevention, and protection services based on population density. Specifically, women who live in rural areas have less access to domestic violence shelters, physical and mental health professionals, law enforcement, and judicial personnel than urban-dwelling women. Rural-dwelling women face barriers to accessing services because of lack of service availability in their communities, geographic distance, and isolation. The purpose of this study was to determine if prevalence, frequency, and severity of intimate partner violence differ by rurality, and to identify variance in geographic access to intimate partner violence resources.

This study used a cross-sectional clinic-based survey design to measure the 1-year prevalence of physical, sexual, and psychological intimate partner violence in 1,478 women living in a rural section of an upper midwestern state in the United States. Women were asked to provide their zip codes, which identified their location of residence in this otherwise anonymous survey. Physical and sexual abuse was measured using a modified version of the Abuse Assessment Screen. Psychological abuse was assessed using the Women's Experience with Battering scale. Rural Urban Commuting Area Codes, which examine rurality on a continuum of population density considering influence of population density in neighboring zip codes were used to identify whether women were living in an urban, suburban, large rural, or small rural town, or an isolated rural area. Intimate partner violence intervention programs in the state were inventoried and mapped, and the distance to the closest program was estimated for each participant based on an algorithm developed for use when only zip code location is available. Demographic data also collected from participants.

The findings of this study indicated that the prevalence, frequency, and severity of physical and sexual intimate partner violence was higher among women living in small or isolated rural areas than in urban or large rural towns. Psychological abuse prevalence did not vary by rurality. These findings were consistent with previous research. Findings also revealed that domestic violence intervention programs in rural or remote rural counties covered considerably more counties per program, had fewer on-site shelter services, and had far fewer total shelter beds available per county. The results also indicated that in addition to the lack of health and domestic violence intervention program resources in many rural counties, the distance to these services for rural women represents a barrier to access. Women in urban, suburban, or large rural towns had an average drive of less than 10 miles to the closest domestic violence intervention program resources, whereas women in small or isolated rural areas faced distances averaging greater than 25 miles. This distance represented a significant hardship for rural women to access resources, which is especially important considering they are victims of more frequent and severe intimate partner violence. The findings revealed that rural women were more likely to experience abuse and more likely to suffer frequent and severe abuse, yet they have less access to domestic violence intervention program services and must travel a much greater distance to reach existing services. The results of this study documented the health disparities present among rural populations of women experiencing intimate partner violence. In addition, this study underscored the critical need for increased preventive services and domestic violence intervention programs in rural areas.

Chapter Summary Points

- Violence against women is any act of gender-based violence of which the outcome or likely outcome is physical, sexual, or mental harm or suffering to women. This includes threats of such acts, coercion or arbitrary deprivation of liberty, occurring in public or in private life.
- Violence against women impedes the attainment of equality, development, and peace, and weakens or nullifies the enjoyment by women of their human rights and basic freedoms.
- Women and girls in all societies, to a greater or lesser extent, experience physical, psychological, and sexual abuse that cuts across the boundaries of income, class, and culture.
- Violence against women is a worldwide pandemic that occurs throughout the life cycle, is an indication of the historically disparate power relations between men and women, and is perpetuated by traditional and customary practices that give women subordinate status in family, workplace, community, and society.
- In the United States, violence against women is a major public health problem that affects women and girls of all ages, in all types of personal and family relationships, and in all economic, educational, cultural, racial, age, and religious levels.
- These acts of violence encompass intimate partner violence (also known as domestic violence), sexual violence, stalking, psychological aggression, as well as bullying, teen violence, human trafficking, and other forms of trauma and abuse.
- Women across all racial and ethnic groups are subjected to violence. Hence, a woman's experience of violence is shaped by her racial and ethnic background and is understood or experienced differently between women of different racial or ethnic groups.
- A combination of individual, relational, community, and societal factors contributes to the risk of becoming a victim or perpetrator of intimate partner violence, yet these may or may not be direct causes.
- The most effective way to stop violence against women and girls is by preventing its occurrence through addressing its root and structural causes.
- Preventive efforts should be directed towards the promotion of gender equality and women's empowerment and their enjoyment of human rights in communities.
- Primary interventions are needed to make the home and public spaces safer for women and girls, to ensure women's economic autonomy and security, and increase women's participation and decision-making powers in the home and relationships, as well as in public life and politics.
- Gender differences in prevalence of intimate partner violence remain disputed because research in this area has produced mixed results.
- Violence against women has serious physical and psychological consequences, high societal costs, and leads to an overall decrease in quality of life for victims, families, and communities.
- Women subjected to violence have a greater need for, and use of, healthcare services. Healthcare providers are well positioned to provide support to victims of violence.

- Healthcare settings predominantly focus on screening and referral of women to domestic violence services. More inclusive services, especially those aimed at improving women's health and quality of life over time have still to be widely integrated into health care.
- Violence against women is best addressed through collaboration across health, domestic violence, social service, and legal sectors, as well as with community stakeholders, including women themselves.
- The literature often focuses on violence experienced by women during the childbearing years. The unique problems of aging women who are subjected to violence are often overlooked.
- The notion that elder abuse is a product of inadequate care masks the gender issues and power dynamics inherent in intimate partner violence as they apply to older women. A wife or partner subjected to abuse at any age can experience serious physical and emotional harm, and even death.
- The scrutiny of violence against women requires the consideration of cultural differences in values, attitudes, and behavioral norms across racial and ethnic groups. Societal acceptance of male dominance strongly impacts cultural attitudes about violence against women.
- A prevailing belief of men and women in many cultures is that a man has the right to control the behavior of his wife and daughters, and disobedient women should be punished. The legitimization of such acts of violence perpetuates violence against women in these cultures.

Critical Thinking Exercise

Case Study

Karen C. is a 24-year-old woman with a history of having been physically abused by her father up until the age of 13. The abuse stopped when her parents divorced and she went to live with her grandmother. Karen graduated from high school and went to work as a cashier at the local Walmart. About a year ago, Karen met Larry, a 30-year-old construction worker, at a neighborhood tavern, and they started seeing each other. They dated steadily for 3 months, during which time Larry was an ideal boyfriend. He was handsome and attentive, took Karen out on enjoyable dates, and made her feel special and loved. He swept her off her feet and wanted them to spend every minute together. Karen fell in love with Larry and was delighted when he proposed marriage. They married 6 weeks later.

At first, the marriage was great. However, as time went on, the honeymoon ended and reality settled in. Karen started to feel inconsequential, as if her opinion did not matter. Larry was often judgmental and cruel. If she mentioned this he would laugh it off and say she was imagining it. However, it seemed that Larry's opinion was the only one that mattered. Karen became very insecure and tried hard to get his approval. Whenever Larry wanted to have sex, Karen did so no matter how tired or poorly she felt. She did her best to keep a tidy house and have dinner ready when Larry came home from work. Often she felt that no matter how hard she tried, her efforts just were not good enough.

Larry would become angry when Karen would talk on the phone to her girlfriends. He would demand to know to whom she was talking and what they were talking about. Larry complained that Karen was not paying enough attention to him and she seemed to enjoy paying attention to her friends more than to him. Karen stopped talking to her friends on the phone while Larry was home. Larry would also become moody if Karen wanted to get together with a female friend after work, so she stopped meeting up with her friends. Larry would text message Karen very frequently while she was at work, asking what she was doing, to whom she had been talking and what was said. After being reprimanded by her supervisor for excessive cell phone usage during working hours, Karen texted that she could not answer any more text messages and turned off her phone. That evening Larry began shouting at her, and accused her of ignoring him, of thinking only of herself and of not caring about him.

Larry was critical and demanding. He complained that Karen was spending too much money and placed her on a strict allowance that barely covered household necessities. Larry would look for any reason to punish Karen. He repeatedly criticized her about her appearance or behavior during social engagements, and accused her of being interested in other men. He would slap or shove her during arguments. After hitting her, Larry would blame her for driving him to violence, and make Karen apologize for doing so. Karen admitted to herself that Larry was difficult to live with but believed that if only she could improve herself and be the kind of wife Larry wanted then things would be better.

The intensity and frequency of Larry's anger had increased as well as the persistence and efforts of Karen to appease him. Karen grew more anxious, depressed, and worn down by humiliation. Recently Karen discovered that she was pregnant and felt overwhelmingly fearful and uncertain. Karen dreaded telling Larry because he was constantly complaining about money. Having a baby was expensive and might mean that eventually she would have to stay home to take care of the baby. When Karen told Larry about the pregnancy, he slapped her and accused her of getting pregnant on purpose so she would not have to take care of him. Due to the severity of the shouting in this argument, neighbors called the police. However, when the police arrived, Larry denied any violence and explained they just had a normal disagreement between couples. Karen, fearful of saying otherwise, quietly agreed with her husband.

Karen went to her first prenatal visit at the obstetrical clinic and after the initial examination and tests were taken, Karen was asked routine screening questions for domestic violence. At first she denied there was anything wrong with her marriage, but upon further questioning Karen admitted that she and her husband fought a lot and she was not happy in her marriage. She had nowhere else to go and had to make her marriage work for the sake of her baby. Karen's physician provided her with information regarding the different types of domestic abuse and asked Karen if she was experiencing any of those. Karen felt too humiliated to answer and started to sob. Her physician explained the potential danger of Karen's situation and assisted her in safety planning, including a referral to a shelter for battered women. Karen promised she would consider her options.

Questions for Seminar Discussion

1. What factors make Karen vulnerable to intimate partner violence?
2. Explain the different types of intimate partner violence that are present in Karen's relationship.
3. What are the risk factors involved for Karen and her unborn child?
4. Why can't Karen just leave the relationship?
5. If Karen left the relationship, what factors would make her return to it?
6. Describe the physical, psychological/spiritual, socioeconomic, and family quality of life issues that are readily manifested in this relationship as a result of intimate partner violence.
7. What community referrals and resources are available that would assist Karen in leaving her abusive relationship and in improving her quality of life?

Internet Resources

Advocates for Human Rights: Stop Violence Against Women Project: provides information, advocacy, and change in the promotion of women's human rights around the world. http://www.stopvaw.org/

AHA Foundation: provides advocacy to protect and defend the rights of women in the United States from religiously and culturally instigated oppression. http://theahafoundation.org/

National Center on Elder Abuse: provides information regarding research, training, best practices, news and resources on elder abuse, neglect and exploitation. http://www.ncea.aoa.gov/

National Network to End Domestic Violence: a membership and advocacy organization of state domestic violence coalitions, allied organizations, and supportive individuals who work closely with its members to understand the ongoing and emerging needs of domestic violence victims and advocacy programs. This organization ensures that those needs are heard and understood by policymakers at the national level. http://nnedv.org/

Polaris Project: provides information, advocacy, support, training, technical assistance, and client services that will combat human trafficking. http://www.polarisproject.org/

Rape, Abuse, and Incest National Network: Provides information, services, advocacy, and programs to prevent sexual violence, assist victims and ensure that rapists are brought to justice. https://rainn.org

Sanctuary for Families: provides service and advocacy for survivors of domestic violence, sex trafficking, and related forms of gender violence. http://www.sanctuaryforfamilies.org/

UN Women: the United Nations organization dedicated to elimination of discrimination against women and girls, the empowerment of women, and achievement of equality between women and men as partners and beneficiaries of development, human rights, humanitarian action, and peace and security. http://www.unwomen.org/

WomenWatch: provides information and resources on the promotion of gender equality and the empowerment of women throughout the United Nations system. http://www.un.org/womenwatch

References

Advocates for Human Rights. (2010). Prevalence of sexual harassment. Retrieved from http://www.stopvaw.org/prevalence_of_sexual_harassment

Alexander, L. L., LaRosa, J. H., Bader, H., Garfield, S., & Alexander, W. J. (2010). *New dimensions in women's health* (5th ed.). Sudbury, MA: Jones and Bartlett Publishers.

Black, M., Basile, K., Breiding, M., Smith, S., Walters, M., Merrick, M., ... Stevens, M. (2011). *The National Intimate Partner and Sexual Violence Survey (NISVS): 2010 summary report.* Atlanta, GA: National Center for Injury Prevention and Control, Centers for Disease Control and Prevention.

Brandle, B., & Dawson, L. (2011). Responding to victims of abuse in later life. *The Journal of Adult Protection, 13*(6), 315–322.

Breiding, M., Basile, K., Smith, S., Black, M., & Mahendra, R. (2015). *Intimate partner violence surveillance: Uniform definitions and recommended data elements, Version 2.0.* Atlanta, GA: National Center for Injury Prevention and Control, Centers for Disease Control and Prevention.

Briere, J., & Jordan, C. (2004). Violence against women: Outcome complexity and implications for assessment and treatment. *Journal of Interpersonal Violence, 19*(11), 1252–1276.

Bureau of Justice Statistics. (2014). Rape and sexual assault. Retrieved from http://www.bjs.gov/index.cfm?ty=tp&tid=317

Campbell, J. (2002). Health consequences of intimate partner violence. *Lancet 359*(9314), 1331–1336.

Center for American Progress. (2011). Domestic violence in the LGBT community: A fact sheet. Retrieved from http://www.americanprogress.org/issues/lgbt/news/2011/06/14/9850/domestic-violence-in-the-lgbt-community/

Centers for Disease Control and Prevention. (2013). Intimate partner violence: Risk and protective factors. Retrieved from http://www.cdc.gov/violenceprevention/intimatepartnerviolence/riskprotectivefactors.html

Chan, K. (2012). Gender differences in self-reports of intimate partner violence: A review. *Aggression and Violent Behavior, 16*(2), 167–175.

Chapleau, K., Oswald, D., & Russell, B. (2008). Male rape myths: The role of gender, violence, and sexism. *Journal of Interpersonal Violence, 23*(5), 600–615.

Cho, H. (2012a). Examining gender differences in the nature and context of intimate partner violence. *Journal of Interpersonal Violence, 27*(2), 2665–2684.

Cho, H. (2012b). Racial differences in the prevalence of intimate partner violence against women and associated factors. *Journal of Interpersonal Violence, 27*(13), 344–363.

Cho, H., & Wilke, D. (2010). Gender differences in the nature of the intimate partner violence and effects of perpetrator arrest on revictimization. *Journal of Family Violence, 25,* 393–400.

Commission on the Status of Women. (2013). Elimination and prevention of all forms of violence against women and girls: Focus on prevention of violence against women and girls. Retrieved from http://www.un.org/womenwatch/daw/csw/csw57/panels/panel1_moderators_summary.pdf

Department of Defense Sexual Assault Prevention and Response. (2014). Department of defense annual report on sexual assault in the military: Fiscal year 2013. Retrieved from http://www.sapr.mil/public/docs/reports/FY13_DoD_SAPRO_Annual_Report_on_Sexual_Assault.pdf

Department of State, United States of America. (2010). Trafficking in persons report (10th ed.). Retrieved from http://www.state.gov/documents/organization/142979.pdf

Department of State, United States of America. (2015). Trafficking in persons report July 2015. Retrieved from http://www.state.gov/j/tip/rls/tiprpt/2015/index.htm

El-Bassel, N., Gilbert, L., Wu, E., Go, H., & Hill, J. (2005). Relationship between drug abuse and intimate partner violence: A longitudinal study among women receiving methadone. *American Journal of Public Health*, 95(3), 465–470.

Ford-Gilboe, M., Merritt-Gray, M., Varcoe, C., & Wuest, J. (2011). A theory-based primary health care intervention for women who have left abusive partners. *Advances in Nursing Science*, 34(3), 198–214.

Goodkind, J., Gillum, T., Bybee, D., & Sullivan, C. (2003). The impact of family and friends reactions on the well-being of women with abusive partners. *Violence Against Women*, 9(3), 347–373.

Johnson, M., & Ferraro, K. (2000). Research on domestic violence in the 1990s: Making distinctions. *Journal of Marriage and Family*, 62, 948–963.

Krug, E., Dahlberg, L., Mercy, J., Zwi, A., & Lozano, R. (Eds). (2002). *World report on violence and health*. Geneva: World Health Organization.

Mechanic, M. (2004). Beyond PTSD: Mental health consequences of violence against women: A response to Briere and Jordan. *Journal of Interpersonal Violence*, 19(11), 1283–1289.

National Center for Injury Prevention and Control. (2003). *Costs of intimate partner violence against women in the United States*. Atlanta, GA: Centers for Disease Control and Prevention. Retrieved from http://www.cdc.gov/violenceprevention/pdf/ipvbook-a.pdf

National Center on Elder Abuse. (2014a). Frequently asked questions. Retrieved from http://www.ncea.aoa.gov/faq/index.aspx

National Center on Elder Abuse. (2014b). NCEA statistics/data. Retrieved from http://www.ncea.aoa.gov/Library/Data/index.aspx

National Human Trafficking Resource Center. (2015). Hotline statistics. Retrieved from http://www.traffickingresourcecenter.org/states

National Institute of Justice. (2007). Stalking. Retrieved from http://www.nij.gov/topics/crime/stalking/Pages/welcome.aspx

National Network to End Domestic Violence. (2014a). About financial abuse. Retrieved from http://nnedv.org/resources/ejresources/about-financial-abuse.html

National Network to End Domestic Violence (2014b). Forms of abuse. Retrieved from http://nnedv.org/resources/stats/gethelp/formsofabuse.html

OWL-The Voice of Women 40+. (2009). Elder abuse: A women's issue. Mothers day report, 2009. Retrieved from http://www.owl-national.org/Mothers_Day_Reports_files/OWL_MothersDay_Report_09_Final_2.pdf

Peek-Asa, C., Wallis, A., Harland, K., & Beyer, K. (2011). Rural disparity in domestic violence prevalence and access to resources. *Journal of Women's Health*, 20(11), 1743–1749.

Philips, L. (2000). Domestic violence and aging women. *Geriatric Nursing*, 21(4), 188–193.

Planty, M., Langton, L., Krebs, C., Berzofsky, M., & Smiley-McDonald, H. (2013). Female victims of sexual violence, 1994-2010. U.S. Department of Justice, Office of Justice Programs: Special Report. Retrieved from http://www.bjs.gov/content/pub/pdf/fvsv9410.pdf

Polaris Project. (2012). Human trafficking cheat sheet. Retrieved from file:///C:/Documents%20and%20Settings/Admin/My%20Documents/Downloads/Human%20Trafficking%20Cheat%20Sheet.pdf

Rape, Abuse, and Incest National Network. (2014). Intimate partner sexual violence. Retrieved from https://www.rainn.org/public-policy/sexual-assault-issues/marital-rape

Regional Offices on Women's Health. (2010). The prevention of violence against women and girls, 2009-2010. Retrieved from http://womenshealth.gov/publications/federal-report/prevention-of-violence-against-women-and-girls.pdf

Sanctuary for Families. (2013). Female genital mutilation in the United States. Retrieved from file:///C:/Documents%20and%20Settings/Admin/My%20Documents/My%20PDF/Violence%20Against%20Women/fgm%20report%20sanctuaryforfamilies.pdf

Shavers, C. (2013). Intimate partner violence: A guide for primary care providers. *The Nurse Practitioner*, 38(12), 39–46.

Tjaden, P., & Thoennes, N. (2000). Extent, nature, and consequences of intimate partner violence. Washington, DC: U.S. Department of Justice, National Institute of Justice. Retrieved from https://www.ncjrs.gov/pdffiles1/nij/181867.pdf

UK Center for Research on Violence Against Women. (2011). How do women from different racial/ethnic backgrounds experience intimate partner violence or sexual assault? Does race and ethnicity matter? Retrieved from https://opsvaw.as.uky.edu/sites/default/files/10_Race.pdf

UNICEF. (2006). Behind closed doors: The impact of domestic violence on children. Retrieved from http://www.unicef.org/protection/files/BehindClosedDoors.pdf

United Nations. (2010). The world's women 2010: Trends and statistics. Retrieved from http://unstats.un.org/unsd/demographic/products/Worldswomen/WW_full%20report_color.pdf

United Nations. (2014). Background information on sexual violence used as a tool of war. Retrieved from http://www.un.org/en/preventgenocide/rwanda/about/bgsexualviolence.shtml

United Nations Children's Fund. (2013). Female genital mutilation/cutting: A statistical overview and exploration of the dynamics of change. New York, NY: UNICEF. Retrieved from http://www.unicef.org/publications/index_69875.html

United Nations Office on Drugs and Crime. (2012). Global report on trafficking in persons 2012 (United Nations publication, Sales No. E.13.IV.1). Retrieved from http://www.unodc.org/documents/data-and-analysis/glotip/Trafficking_in_Persons_2012_web.pdf

UN Women. (2014a). Facts and figures: Ending violence against women. Retrieved from http://www.unwomen.org/en/what-we-do/ending-violence-against-women/facts-and-figures

UN Women. (2014b). Focusing on prevention to stop the violence. Retrieved from http://www.unwomen.org/en/what-we-do/ending-violence-against-women/prevention

World Health Organization. (2008). Eliminating female genital mutilation: An interagency statement. Retrieved from http://whqlibdoc.who.int/publications/2008/9789241596442_eng.pdf?ua=1

World Health Organization. (2012). Understanding and addressing violence against women: Health consequences. Retrieved from http://apps.who.int/iris/bitstream/10665/77431/1/WHO_RHR_12.43_eng.pdf?ua=1

World Health Organization. (2014a). Female genital mutilation. Fact sheet No. 241. Retrieved from http://www.who.int/mediacentre/factsheets/fs241/en/

World Health Organization. (2014b). Sexual and reproductive health: Female genital mutilation and other harmful practices. Retrieved from http://www.who.int/reproductivehealth/topics/fgm/prevalence/en/

World Health Organization. (2014c). Violence against women: Fact sheet No. 239. Retrieved from http://www.who.int/mediacentre/factsheets/fs239/en/

Yick, A. (2008). A metasynthesis of qualitative findings on the role of spirituality and religiosity among culturally diverse domestic violence survivors. *Qualitative Health Research*, *18*(9), 1289–1306.

Breast Cancer

Introduction

Breast cancer occurs across a wide spectrum of ages in women, with incidence and mortality generally increasing with age. Since the majority of breast cancer incidence is found in older women, it would appear to be suitable that the discussion of the health and quality of life issues of women with breast cancer takes place within the context of this age group. Still, age is a significant factor that defines various dimensions of prognosis, treatment, and influences on quality of life. Nevertheless, this chapter will endeavor to address the needs and issues of women with breast cancer and indicate differences that may exist specific to younger or older women.

Incidence

Breast cancer is a major public health problem in the United States. It was estimated that 232,670 new cases of breast cancer were diagnosed among women in this country in 2014 (Siegel, Ma, Zou, & Jemal, 2014). It was estimated that 48,910, or 21%, of the invasive breast cancer cases and 15,650, or 24%, of the breast cancer in situ cases occurred in women younger than 50 years of age. It was also estimated that 40,430 women would die from the disease (Siegel et al., 2014). A woman living in the United States has a 12.3%, or 1 in 8, lifetime risk of being diagnosed with breast cancer (American Cancer Society [ACS], 2013a).

Non-Hispanic white women have a higher incidence of breast cancer than African-American women across all age groups; however, African-American women have a higher incidence of the disease under the age of 40. In addition, African-American women are more likely to die from breast cancer across the age spectrum (ACS, 2013a). Among Latina women, breast cancer is the most commonly diagnosed cancer as well as the leading cause of death (ACS, 2012). Overall, the incidence and death rates of breast cancer in Latinas, Asian/Pacific Islanders, and Native American/Alaskan Natives are lower in comparison to white and African-American women. The lowest breast cancer incidence and death rates are among Asian/Pacific Islander women (ACS, 2013a).

Ethnic Considerations

The higher incidence of breast cancer among white women is likely attributed to changes in their reproductive patterns, which have shifted to first childbirth at an older age and having fewer children. The greater utilization of mammography screening that detects tumors too small to be felt, as well as obesity and use of hormone replacement therapy (HRT), may also contribute to the higher incidence rate (ACS, 2013a).

Among African-American women, breast cancer is the second highest cause of death behind lung cancer. African-American women often lack access to timely, high-quality treatment, and therefore breast cancer is likely to be diagnosed at a later stage, with tumors that evince more aggressive characteristics. These aspects contribute to African-American women having the highest death rates and lowest 5-year survival rates as compared to white women (ACS, 2013b). Furthermore, socioeconomic factors and racial discrimination are apt to influence the death and survival rates in African-American women with breast cancer (Field et al., 2005). Disparities in employment, wealth, income, education, housing, and overall standard of living have been found to create socio-economic barriers to high-quality breast cancer prevention, early detection, and treatment services for African Americans (ACS, 2013b).

The lower incidence of breast cancer among Latinas as compared to non-Latina white women may be attributed in part to the protective reproductive patterns found more often among Latinas. These patterns include younger age at first childbirth, having a larger number of children, and less use of HRT. However, lower incidence may also reflect decreased use of mammography screening and underdiagnosis of breast cancer (ACS, 2012). Similar to African-American women, Latinas are likely to evince disease at more advanced stages and experience lower 5-year survival rates than white women. Socioeconomic factors such as poverty, lack of health insurance, linguistic isolation, inadequate health information, lack of ethnically sensitive and culturally competent health facilities, and lack of understanding of the American healthcare system create barriers to access of high quality breast cancer prevention, detection, and treatment services (Huerta, 2003).

Etiology and Risk Factors

Instead of one disease, breast cancer is increasingly regarded as a group of diseases distinguished by different molecular subtypes, risk factors, clinical behaviors, and responses to treatment (ACS, 2013a). There is no single known causative agent for breast cancer. Breast cancer is believed to be caused by an interaction of multiple hormonal, environmental, hereditary, and lifestyle factors (Pruthi, et al., 2007). Two major predisposing factors associated with breast cancer are age and female gender. Advancing age increases the risk of breast cancer in women. Other commonly accepted factors that increase the risk of developing breast cancer include early onset of menarche, late menopause, nulliparity, and older age (over 30) at first childbirth. Such reproductive patterns may increase the exposure of breast tissue to spikes in the ovarian hormones of estrogen and progesterone from longer duration of active menstrual cycles over the lifetime.

Women with a family history of breast cancer are at higher risk for developing the disease. Factors such as having a first-degree female relative (i.e., mother, daughter, or sister) who has had breast cancer, having more than one relative affected, and if that relative was diagnosed at an early age or had bilateral disease, significantly raise the risk of breast cancer. Hereditary breast cancer is a subset of familial breast cancer that is associated with the inherited genetic mutations of BRCA1 and BRCA2 genes that predispose a woman to breast cancer. Although hereditary breast cancer accounts for 5% to 10% of total breast cancer cases, carriers of BRCA1 and BRCA2 gene mutation are considered to be at very high risk for developing breast cancer (Pruthi et al., 2007).

The presence of epithelial proliferative changes to breast tissue is another factor that increases the risk of breast cancer. Atypical hyperplasia has been noted to increase breast cancer risk 4- to 5-fold, and as much as 11-fold when combined with family history of an affected first-degree relative (Sakorafas, 2003). Likewise, premalignant lesions such as lobular carcinoma in situ (LCIS) are highly associated with the subsequent development of invasive breast cancer (Pruthi et al., 2007). Women who have had a past history of breast cancer are at increased risk of developing breast cancer in the other breast. It is estimated that women with a previous breast cancer diagnosis are five times more likely than the general population to develop breast cancer, especially when other factors such as hereditary, familial, young age at primary diagnosis, proliferative atypical changes, radiation exposure, or multifocal cancer are also present (Sakorafas, 2003).

Environmental and lifestyle factors also increase the risk of developing breast cancer. Combination (estrogen and medroxyprogesterone) HRT has been shown to substantially increase breast cancer risk (Pruthi et al., 2007). Moderate to high radiation exposure on breast tissue, especially before the age of 20, has been associated with higher risk for breast cancer. Lifestyle factors such as increased alcohol consumption, increased dietary fat intake, and postmenopausal obesity have also been associated with increased risk of developing breast cancer (Osuch, 2002; Pruthi et al., 2007). Although most hormonal, reproductive, and hereditary factors are not modifiable, environmental and lifestyle factors are potentially modifiable and offer prospects for reducing breast cancer risk for many women (Pruthi et al., 2007).

Degree of Breast Cancer Risk

Defining women's degree of risk for developing breast cancer has prospective implications for medical decision making, especially for determining preventive management interventions. Risk assessment is achieved through taking an accurate history, using validated tools that will estimate a woman's risk of developing breast cancer, and timely application of risk management strategies based on the degree of risk (Pruthi et al., 2007). Risk assessment is a complex, ongoing, informed decision-making process that requires open dialogue between the healthcare provider and woman, and periodic reassessment during the woman's lifetime (Pruthi et al., 2007). Various breast cancer risk prediction models exist. Among those available, the most common prediction model used is the Gail model, developed by the National Cancer Institute. The Gail model calculates the 5-year and lifetime risk for developing breast cancer for women over 35 years of age who have not been previously diagnosed with breast cancer and takes into account age, age at menarche, number of biopsies, number of first-degree relatives with breast cancer, age at first live birth, and race (National Cancer Institute [NCI], 2015b). Women may be designated as having low to average risk, high risk, and very high risk for developing breast cancer.

Women with a low to average risk have risk factors that confer a 1.5% or less relative risk of developing breast cancer. Women with a Gail model score of 1.7% or higher are considered at high risk for developing breast cancer and may demonstrate a prior history of atypical hyperplasia or family history of at least one affected first-degree relative. Women with very high risk include BRCA1 or BRCA2 gene mutation carriers and women who have had LCIS, ductal carcinoma in situ (DCIS), or significant thoracic radiation exposure before age 20 (Pruthi et al., 2007). Limitations of the Gail model include risk prediction for women as a group rather than individual risk prediction and underestimation of risk for those with extensive family history of breast cancer, paternal family history of breast cancer, or family history of ovarian cancer (NCI, 2015b). The model has been shown to estimate risk in African-American women but may underestimate risk in African-American women with previous biopsies. Further research is needed to validate use of the Gail model in other minority populations (NCI, 2015b).

Other statistical models have been developed for risk assessment in women with certain groupings of risk factors, such as the Claus model, BRCAPRO model, Myriad model, and Couch model, and each offers specific benefits and limitations to its use. The Claus model, for example, may be particularly useful in estimating breast cancer risk in women with a strong family history of breast or ovarian cancer (NCI, 2015b). Nevertheless, more research is needed to improve the discriminatory functions of the risk assessment models. Currently, use of the Gail model in modified form is approved for identifying women eligible for risk reduction strategies (NCI, 2015b).

Risk Reduction

Women who demonstrate an increased risk for breast cancer with a >1.7% 5-year risk according to the modified Gail model for risk assessment can be offered risk reduction strategies by their healthcare provider. Risk reduction strategies consist of chemoprevention, risk-reducing surgical procedures, specific lifestyle modifications, and surveillance. Surveillance strategies include clinical breast examinations and breast imaging procedures that detect breast cancer at an earlier stage of progression. (National Comprehensive Cancer Network [NCCN], 2015b).

Chemoprevention

Tamoxifen is a first-generation selective estrogen receptor modulator (SERM) that blocks the action of estrogen on breast tissue, thereby blocking the growth of estrogen receptive breast cancers or preventing the development of new breast cancers. In 1998, after extensive clinical trials, the Food and Drug Administration approved the use of tamoxifen to reduce the risk of breast cancer in high-risk women. It is currently recommended that tamoxifen be given to healthy pre- and postmenopausal women 35 years of age or older who have a 1.7% or greater 5-year risk for breast cancer as determined by the modified Gail model (NCCN, 2015b). Tamoxifen has been noted to increase the risk of developing adverse effects such as endometrial cancer, thromboembolic disease, hot flashes, and vaginal discharge. The risk of developing adverse effects of tamoxifen seems to be more pronounced in postmenopausal women and in those with other medical comorbidities (Pruthi et al., 2007).

Raloxifene is a second-generation SERM that is chemically different from tamoxifen but has similar antiestrogenic action on breast tissue with considerably less stimulation of endometrial tissue (NCCN, 2015b). Raloxifene is used primarily in postmenopausal women for risk reduction. Adverse effects associated with raloxifene include hot flashes, influenza-like symptoms, peripheral edema, leg cramps, endometrial cavity fluid, and increased risk of deep vein thrombosis and pulmonary embolus. Current practice recommends that raloxifene can be given to healthy postmenopausal women who are 35 years of age or older, who have demonstrated 1.7% or greater 5-year risk for breast cancer as determined by the modified Gail model. Raloxifene has also been approved for risk reduction in women who have a history of LCIS (NCCN, 2015b).

Aromatase inhibitors block the conversion of androgens to estrogen by inactivating the aromatase enzyme. This will result in estrogen suppression and significantly lower the levels of estrogen in breast and other tissues in postmenopausal women. Anastrozole and exemestane have been studied in clinical trials as adjunctive therapy in postmenopausal women with invasive breast cancer and these drugs have shown notable reduction in the incidence of breast cancer recurrence. Presently, use of aromatase inhibitors for risk reduction in healthy postmenopausal women is restricted to ongoing clinical trials only (NCCN, 2015b).

The use of risk reduction agents incurs risks and benefits that should be discussed with individual women as part of a shared decision making process. Women undergoing risk reduction therapy must be closely monitored for potential adverse side effects that may develop as a result of using these agents (NCCN, 2015b).

Risk-Reduction Surgery

Women who are at very high risk for developing breast cancer may be offered the option of risk reduction surgical procedures. Prophylactic bilateral mastectomy has been shown to reduce the incidence of breast cancer by 90%, and prophylactic bilateral salpingo-oophorectomy has been found to decrease breast cancer risk in BRCA1/2 carriers by 50% (NCCN, 2015b). The prophylactic salpingo-oophorectomy, performed after completion of childbearing, is frequently chosen as the initial procedure because it may be seen as less threatening to body image and self-esteem than prophylactic mastectomy (Pruthi et al., 2007). Women who undergo bilateral mastectomy for risk reduction must have all breast tissue removed but

do not require axillary node dissection. Women may also select breast reconstruction to be performed immediately following the bilateral mastectomy (NCCN, 2015b).

All women who are eligible for risk reduction interventions should receive counseling that thoroughly explains all available options to reduce risk of breast cancer, including lifestyle modifications, risks and benefits, and possible adverse effects, individualized according to one's specific overall health status (NCCN, 2015b). Risk reduction interventions pose a significant impact on the quality of life of healthy women at high risk for breast cancer, and adequate preparation and support services will be needed.

Surveillance

Comprehensive breast cancer surveillance involves clinical breast examination, mammography, and breast self-exam, also known as breast awareness. The degree of risk for developing breast cancer determines the age at which surveillance begins and the frequency with which the screening modalities are performed. For women with low to average risk for developing breast cancer, clinical breast exam as part of periodic health exam should be conducted every 1–3 years in the 25- and 30 but less than 40-year-old age groups (NCCN, 2015c). Periodic self-breast exam is encouraged, as it is important for women to become familiar with the landscape of their breasts in order to detect any changes. For women 40 years of age and older, annual clinical breast examination with mammography and periodic self-breast exam should be done (NCCN, 2015c). For women who have high and very high risk of developing breast cancer, enhanced surveillance is recommended. The age at which screening begins and frequency of screening modalities are determined by the presence of specific high risk factors.

Lifestyle Modification

Although evidence supports the link between HRT, postmenopausal obesity, alcohol consumption, high-fat diet and increased risk of breast cancer, definitive association between modification of these factors and risk reduction has not been clearly established (NCCN, 2014b). Nonetheless, in clinical trials of predominantly postmenopausal women, evidence trends toward risk reduction in changes and modifications that are congruent with a healthy lifestyle. Such modifications include weight reduction and maintenance of healthy weight, participation in regular exercise, following a low-fat diet, and avoidance of HRT. Research findings suggest an association between moderate intake of alcohol (1 to 2 drinks per day) and an increased risk of developing breast cancer. However, the effect of reduced alcohol consumption on the reduction of breast cancer incidence has not been established. One drink per day may elevate breast cancer risk modestly. Therefore, women should limit intake of alcohol to less than one drink per day. One drink is defined as 1 ounce of liquor, 6 ounces of wine, or 8 ounces of beer (NCCN, 2015b).

Gender Similarities and Differences

Male breast cancer is a rare disease and accounts for 1% of all breast cancer cases in the United States. It was estimated that 2,360 new cases of breast cancer were diagnosed among men in 2014, and 430 men would die from the disease (Siegel et al., 2014). Men generally tend to have risk factors that are similar to women, such as advancing age, increased exposure to estrogen (from Klinefelter syndrome or exogenous administration of estrogen or estrogen-related drugs), obesity, heavy alcohol intake, familial history, inherited mutations of BRCA1 or BRCA2 genes, and radiation exposure to the chest. In addition, testicular damage, occupational risks of high temperature environments (that can affect the testicles), and exposure to gasoline exhaust fumes have been noted

to increase breast cancer risk in men (Fentiman, Fourquet, & Hortobagyi, 2006; Ouzounakis, Tsiligiri, & Kourkouta, 2014). The rarity of the disease in men also explains the paucity of research on the subject and small sample sizes in existing research collected from long-range retrospective reviews (Schaub et al., 2008).

The prognosis of breast cancer, however, tends to be poorer in men than in women. The 5- and 10-year survival for stage I breast cancer in men is about 58% and 38%, respectively. For stage II, 5- and 10-year survival is approximately 38% and 10%. The overall 5- and 10-year survival for all stages is approximately 36% and 17%, respectively (Ouzounakis et al., 2014). Men may be reluctant to seek medical attention because of lack of awareness, embarrassment, or denial. Because of this, the diagnosis of breast cancer in men tends to occur when the disease is at a later stage, which can subsequently decrease treatment success and chances of survival.

Diagnosing Breast Cancer

Mammography is the primary imaging modality used to detect breast cancer. Mammography allows breast cancer to be detected at earlier stages, and is associated with significant reductions in breast cancer mortality and better cure rates (NCCN, 2015c). Screening mammography entails two views of each breast, one from the top (craniocaudal) and one from the side (mediolateral oblique). When abnormalities are detected, additional views are taken with specific magnification or compression. Increased breast density limits the sensitivity of mammography and other screening methods for women with dense breasts are preferred. Digital mammography produces an electronic image of the breast and permits computer storage and manipulation. Both types of mammography are similar in accuracy but digital mammography tends to be more accurate in younger women with increased breast density. Digital mammography is not as widely available and is more expensive than traditional film mammography (NCCN, 2015c).

Ultrasonography is an important diagnostic test and is used adjunctively to mammography in high-risk screening. Ultrasonography is effective in identifying tumors that may be missed by mammography in women with dense breasts. It can differentiate cysts from solid lesions; however, it does not detect most calcifications. Although painless and inexpensive, accuracy is dependent on the skill of the operator and there is risk of false-positive in detection. Lack of standardization, unknown sensitivity and specificity, and inability to detect microcalcifications make ultrasonography problematic as a screening modality for the general population at this time (NCCN, 2015c; Pruthi et al., 2007).

Breast MRI is another important imaging modality that is used adjunctively to mammography and as a screening tool in certain women at high risk for developing breast cancer. The MRI is highly sensitive for invasive cancers, and breast density does not reduce effectiveness. The MRI is limited in specificity, since the appearance of malignant and benign disease may overlap. A higher rate of false-positive findings can result. This may incur additional workups, biopsies, costs, and anxiety for women with MRI-detected benign disease (NCCN, 2015c; Pruthi et al., 2007).

When suspicious lesions are detected on imaging, needle localization excisional biopsy or core needle biopsy with ultrasound, stereotactic (mammographic) or MRI guidance is done to obtain a definitive diagnosis. Benign results do not require further surgery. Biopsy results that are positive for cancer require further treatment.

Adherence to breast cancer screening modalities varies among different groups of women. Women over 60 years of age, those from lower socioeconomic groups, and women of ethnic minorities tend to have poor compliance. Three domains have been identified that appear to be most influential in predicting screening adherence: demographic factors, cognitive factors, and socio-emotional factors (Magai, Consedine, Neugut, & Hershman, 2007). Demographic factors that contribute to poor compliance to breast cancer screening include financial barriers, lack of access to services, and lack of health insurance (Kerans, 2004). Cognitive factors include misinformation and lack of accurate knowledge about breast cancer risk, treatments, and outcomes, and fatalistic attitudes about cancer. Socio-emotional factors include lack of social support, cultural beliefs, fear of social consequences of cancer, fear of the medical consequences of cancer, embarrassment, denial, and inaccurate risk perception (Magai et al., 2007). Healthcare providers need to be aware of the influence that these factors may have on women's adherence to screening and incorporate this awareness into further efforts to improve adherence to breast cancer screening. Many of these factors are modifiable and eminently suited to intervention directed toward improving survival and quality of life (Magai et al., 2007).

Treatment

The treatment of breast cancer encompasses treating local disease, axillary disease, and systemic disease. Local disease and axillary disease are managed by surgery, radiation therapy, or both. Systemic disease is managed by cytotoxic chemotherapy, hormonal therapy, biologic therapy, or a combination of these options. The selection of appropriate therapeutic options for women diagnosed with breast cancer is based on a number of prognostic and predictive factors. These factors include specific histological and pathological characteristics of the tumor, tumor staging, tumor hormone receptor status, tumor HER2 status, the presence or absence of metastatic disease, presence of additional diseases, patient age, menopausal status, and patient preference. All of these factors must be taken into consideration in order to determine the most suitable treatment plan for an individual woman. Patient preference is considered a major component of the decision-making process, especially regarding treatment options that offer equivalent survival rates (NCCN, 2015a).

The staging of breast cancer is the process of establishing the extent of the cancer in the body when it is diagnosed, and it is an essential factor for determining prognosis and treatment options. The stage of cancer is based on whether the cancer is invasive or noninvasive, the size of the tumor, lymph node involvement, and whether the cancer has spread to other parts of the body (ACS, 2013a). A staging system is a standardized method used to communicate information about the extent of a cancer in the body. Stage is indicated by Roman numerals from stage I (the least advanced stage) to stage IV (the most advanced stage). Stage 0 designates noninvasive cancer (ACS, 2015). The staging system for breast cancer is presented in **Box 10–1**.

The clinical stage of breast cancer is based on the results of the physical exam, biopsy, and imaging tests. The pathologic stage of breast cancer is based on the results of these tests plus the results of surgery. Pathologic staging is likely to be more accurate than clinical staging as it determines the extent of the cancer based on tissue analysis of tumor, lymph nodes, and areas of possible metastasis. After the staging categories have been determined, the information is then pooled into stage groupings. Similar stages of breast cancer will have a comparable outlook and are frequently treated in a similar way. The pathologic stages of breast cancer are presented in **Table 10–1**.

Surgery

SURGICAL TREATMENT

The primary goals of surgical treatment are to remove the cancer from the breast and to establish the stage of disease. A simple or total mastectomy entails removal of the entire breast, including the nipple and areola. Modified radical mastectomy involves removal of the entire breast and axillary lymph nodes. Radical mastectomy, which involves removal of the breast, axillary lymph nodes and underlying chest muscles is rarely used because in most cases removal of the chest muscles is not needed to remove all of the cancer. Breast conservation surgery involves removal of the tumor with cancer-free

---

Box 10–1: The Stages of Breast Cancer

- Stage 0 (carcinoma in situ)
- Stage I
- Stage II
- Stage IIIA
- Stage IIIB
- Stage IIIC
- Stage IV

Reproduced from National Cancer Institute. (2015a). Breast cancer treatment (PDQ®). Retrieved from http://www.cancer.gov/types/breast/patient/breast-treatment-pdq#link/stoc_h2_1

Table 10–1 PATHOLOGIC STAGING OF BREAST CANCER

Stage	Description
0	Carcinoma in situ: includes three types: Ductal carcinoma in situ (DCIS) Lobular carcinoma in situ (LCIS) Pagets disease of the nipple
I	
IA	Tumor is 2 centimeters (cm) or smaller. Cancer has not spread beyond the breast.
IB	Small clusters of cancer cells (bigger than 0.2 millimeters (mm) but smaller than 2 mm) are found in the lymph nodes and either: • no tumor is found in the breast; OR • tumor is 2 cm or smaller
II	
IIA	• No tumor is found in the breast or the tumor is <u>less than or equal to </u>2 cm. Cancer larger than 2 mm is found in 1-3 axillary lymph nodes or in the lymph nodes near the breastbone, OR • Tumor is larger than 2 cm but not larger than 5 cm. Cancer has not spread to the lymph nodes.
IIB	• Tumor is larger than 2 cm but not larger than 5 cm. Small clusters of breast cancer cells (larger than 0.2 mm but not larger than 2 mm) are found in the lymph nodes; OR • Tumor is larger than 2 cm but not larger than 5 cm. Cancer has spread to 1-3 axillary lymph nodes or to the lymph nodes near the breastbone; OR • Tumor is larger than 5 cm. Cancer has not spread to the lymph nodes.
III	
IIIA	• No tumor is found in the breast or tumor may be any size. Cancer is found in 4-9 axillary lymph nodes or in the lymph nodes near the breastbone; OR • Tumor is larger than 5 cm. Small clusters of breast cancer cells (larger than 0.2 mm but not larger than 2 mm) are found in the lymph nodes; OR • Tumor is larger than 5 cm. Cancer has spread to 1-3 axillary lymph nodes or to the lymph nodes near the breastbone.
IIIB	Tumor may be any size and cancer has spread to the chest wall and/or to the skin of the breast and caused swelling or an ulcer. Also, cancer may have spread to: • Up to 9 axillary lymph nodes; OR • To the lymph nodes near the breastbone.
IIIC	No tumor is found in the breast or tumor may be any size. Cancer may have spread to the skin of the breast and caused swelling or an ulcer and/or has spread to the chest wall. Cancer also has spread to: • 10 or more axillary lymph nodes; OR • Lymph nodes above or below the collarbone; OR • Axillary lymph nodes and lymph nodes near the breastbone.
IV	Cancer has spread to other organs of the body, most often the lungs, liver, or brain.

Modified from National Cancer Institute. (2015a). Breast cancer treatment (PDQ®). Retrieved from http://www.cancer.gov/types/breast/patient/breast-treatment-pdq#link/stoc_h2_1

margins of breast tissue. The rest of the breast, nipple, and areola remain intact (ACS, 2013a).

Analysis of axillary lymph nodes is an essential part of breast cancer management because the absence or presence of metastases in the axillary lymph nodes is a crucial prognostic indicator. Clinical examination and imaging alone cannot definitively determine the presence of cancer cells. Therefore, further assessment will necessitate sentinel node biopsy or axillary node dissection. Sentinel node biopsy involves injecting tracers that are picked up by the lymphatic channel and converge in the sentinel lymph node that drains from the locus of the breast cancer site. The sentinel node is removed through a small incision and evaluated for the presence of cancer cells (ACS, 2013a). Axillary dissection is a safe, yet more complex, procedure, involving removal of level 1 and level 2 axillary lymph nodes for evaluation of the presence of cancer cells. Axillary node dissection is associated with increased risk of developing decreased range of motion, parasthesia, pain, and lymphedema as postoperative complications (NCCN, 2015a). Sentinel node mapping does not differ significantly from axillary dissection in detecting the presence or absence of metastasized cells in the axillary lymph nodes, and is the preferred method. Studies have shown decreased incidence of arm and shoulder pain, lymphedema, and sensory loss resulting from sentinel node biopsy as compared to axillary node dissection (NCCN, 2015a).

BREAST RECONSTRUCTION

The cosmetic defect that often accompanies surgical treatment of breast cancer can have a powerful influence on quality of life. Women who undergo a mastectomy or a lumpectomy that leaves a significant defect in the appearance of the breast may choose to have breast reconstruction. Breast reconstruction may be performed directly following the initial surgical treatment (immediate reconstruction) or at a future date (delayed reconstruction). A variety of simple or complex reconstruction procedures are available that range from the insertion of subpectoral implants to use of the woman's skin, muscle, and fat tissue from a different part of her body to construct a breast (autologous reconstruction), or a combination of both. Breast reconstruction does not influence the probability rates of disease recurrence or length of survival in breast cancer survivors; however, it is associated with better quality of life (NCCN, 2015a).

Radiation Therapy

Women who undergo a lumpectomy for primary breast cancer may also need to receive adjuvant whole breast radiation therapy to kill any cancer cells that may remain in the breast tissue and reduce the chance of disease recurrence. Radiation therapy may also be necessary in women who have had a mastectomy for large tumors or tumors that have spread to the axillary lymph nodes (NCCN, 2015a). Radiation therapy is performed by using external beam or by brachytherapy, which is localized radiation through the use of indwelling catheters. External radiation therapy is delivered in a dose of 45 to 50Gy over a period of 5 to 6 weeks. Brachytherapy delivers the maximum therapeutic dose of radiation over a shorter period of time. Women may experience local side effects to radiation therapy that include dermatitis, moist desquamation, and mild edema. Women who have axillary lymph node dissection with axillary radiation may develop lymphedema of the involved arm. A systemic side effect of radiation therapy that commonly occurs is fatigue. Side effects may last for weeks or months following completion of treatment.

Systemic Therapy

After surgical treatment, systemic therapy may be initiated. In certain cases that meet specific criteria, chemotherapy may be given prior to surgical treatment. When considering systemic therapy, the risk of disease recurrence with local treatment alone must be weighed against the magnitude of benefits possible with adjuvant therapy, toxic effects of the therapy, and the presence of additional illnesses and chronic conditions. The selection of a specific systemic therapeutic regimen is based on the risk of disease recurrence, prognostic factors of age, menopausal status, comorbidities, tumor histology, clinical and pathologic characteristics of the tumor, tumor estrogen receptor status, number of involved axillary lymph nodes, absence or presence of metastasis, multi-gene testing, and HER2 status of the tumor (NCCN, 2015a). Systemic therapy for breast cancer includes cytotoxic chemotherapy and endocrine therapy. Chemotherapeutic drugs commonly used in the systemic treatment of breast cancer include anthracyclines, cyclophosphamide, methotrexate, antimetabolites, trastuzumab, taxanes, and 5-fluorouracil (NCCN, 2015a).

Research has indicated that for the most part, combinations of drugs are more effective than one drug alone for breast cancer treatment. Numerous drug combinations are employed, yet it is unclear that any single combination is the best. Certain drug combinations seem to be more effective than others, based on previously listed characteristics of the patient and tumor. The length of treatment with chemotherapy is usually 3 to 6 months, depending on the combination of drugs used. The full efficacy of chemotherapy is achieved when the complete dose and cycle of drugs are finished in a timely manner (ACS, 2013a).

The adverse effects of cytotoxic chemotherapy include alopecia, fatigue, nausea and vomiting, oral mucositis, increased susceptibility to infection, and premature menopause. Some adverse effects often last for weeks or months following completion of treatment and can exert a dramatic influence on quality of life. Moreover, research has suggested that women who enter systemic chemotherapy with an initially poor quality of life may be at risk for prematurely discontinuing treatment, which can further threaten quality of life and ultimately survival (Richardson, Wang, Hartzema, & Wagner, 2007).

Endocrine Therapy

All primary invasive breast cancers are evaluated regarding estrogen (ER) and progesterone (PR) receptor status. With few exceptions, most women with hormone-receptor positive status should be given adjuvant endocrine therapy for a period of 5 years. Endocrine therapy can significantly reduce the rate of breast cancer recurrence and significantly increase rate of survival, regardless of age, menopausal status, axillary lymph node involvement, or use of chemotherapy (ACS, 2013a; NCCN, 2015a). Endocrine therapy decreases estrogen levels or blocks the effects of estrogen on the growth of breast cancer cells. Tamoxifen and toremifene are drugs that inhibit estrogen from binding to breast cancer cells and are effective in both postmenopausal and premenopausal women (ACS, 2013a).

Aromatase inhibitors are another class of drugs that are effective in treating both early and advanced hormone receptor positive breast cancer in postmenopausal women. Aromatase inhibitors include anastrozole, letrozole, and exemestane. These drugs have been effective in reducing recurrence and extending survival in postmenopausal women, either as initial therapy, sequential therapy with tamoxifen, or extended therapy following tamoxifen therapy completion (ACS, 2013a; NCCN, 2015a). Fulvestrant is a recent drug that is administered by injection once a month. Fulvestrant blocks estrogen binding and decreases the number of estrogen receptors on breast tumors. Fulvestrant is frequently effective in postmenopausal women even if the breast cancer no longer responds to tamoxifen (ACS, 2013a).

Side effects of tamoxifen and aromatase inhibitors have similarities and specific differences.

Both tamoxifen and aromatase inhibitors cause hot flashes, vaginal dryness, and night sweats. However, tamoxifen causes increased risk of uterine cancer and deep vein thrombosis, while aromatase inhibitors are associated with increased risk of osteoporosis, musculoskeletal symptoms, and bone fracture (NCCN, 2015a).

Quality of Life Issues Associated With Breast Cancer

While much attention focuses on active disease and the immediate effects of therapies, it is essential to consider that breast cancer continues to influence women's lives for years after diagnosis and treatment. Women who have had breast cancer generally move forward with their lives and many thrive, but many women continue to be troubled by breast cancer-related problems long into survivorship (Ferrell, Grant, Funk, Otis-Green, & Garcia, 1997, 1998a; Janz et al., 2007; Rustøen & Begnum, 2000; Sammarco, 2001a, 2003). Immediate and long-term quality of life issues and concerns associated with breast cancer are frequently multidimensional and extend across the various domains of life. The diagnosis of breast cancer, the chosen treatment modalities, the after-effects of those modalities, and the demands of survivorship are key factors that will challenge women's ability to maintain an acceptable quality of life.

Breast cancer and the effects of treatment can disturb quality of life by influencing health and physical functioning, psychological and spiritual well-being, socioeconomic integrity, and family well-being. Surgical treatment and adjunctive therapies such as radiation therapy and systemic chemotherapy frequently produce disruptive and distressing short- and long-term symptoms that can cause physical discomfort and psychosocial distress. Symptoms frequently interrelate, appear in clusters, contribute to the development and exacerbation of other symptoms, and concurrently impact across various domains of quality of life (Hunter et al., 2004).

Issues Affecting Health and Physical Functioning

The most common and persistent symptoms affecting health and physical functioning include fatigue, pain, lymphedema, menopausal symptoms, sexual dysfunction, and sleep disturbance.

Fatigue

Fatigue is a broad feeling of lack of energy that is associated with difficulty concentrating, reduced motivation, and decreased physical activity (Gélinas & Fillion, 2004). Breast cancer survivors have reported some of the highest rates of fatigue as compared to other types of cancer, with incidence ranging from 99% during adjuvant treatment to 38% after conclusion of treatment (Dirksen & Epstein, 2008). Fatigue is often triggered by hematologic changes during chemotherapy or radiation therapy, and may appear in relation to the presence of menopausal symptoms or pain, as well as emotional distress, sleep disturbance, and depression. Fatigue may also accompany stressors such as future concerns, functional disabilities, social problems, self-image concerns, and medical and treatment problems that may be experienced by women during and after cancer treatment (Gélinas & Fillion, 2004). Fatigue is a pervasive and disturbing symptom in breast cancer survivors that exerts dramatic impact across a number of dimensions of quality of life (Janz et al., 2007). Fatigue in women with breast cancer may have numerous etiologies but persistent, severe fatigue should prompt evaluation for anemia and depression and determination of appropriate treatment. For example, treatment of anemia-related fatigue with erythropoeisis-stimulating drugs has shown significant effectiveness in reducing fatigue and improving quality of life (Cella, 2006). Furthermore, aggressive application of strategies such as psychological counseling, cognitive behavioral interventions for insomnia, and social support can be effective in reducing fatigue and improving physical and emotional well-being (Dirksen & Epstein, 2008).

Pain

The presence of postsurgical pain is another post-treatment symptom experienced by breast cancer survivors. Postsurgical pain is a chronic neuropathic pain syndrome. Women with neuropathic pain experience a burning, shooting, or electric shock-like pain and altered skin sensation in the lateral chest wall, medial upper arm, and axilla, which is prevalent after mastectomy, lumpectomy, and axillary dissection (Blunt & Schmeidel, 2004; Eversley et al., 2005). The cause of neuropathic pain syndrome is unclear, though it is thought to be attributed to damaged nerve pathways acquired during the surgical procedures, and, in some cases, pressure exerted by axillary hematoma (Blunt & Schmeidel, 2004). The pain syndrome is estimated to appear in approximately 40% of women who have had a mastectomy, with a significantly higher incidence in younger women, Latinas, and African-American women (Eversley et al., 2005). Pain intensity may range from mild discomfort that does not require treatment to continuous severe pain that interrupts sleep and considerably restricts quality of life (Blunt & Schmeidel, 2004). The persistence of pain in breast cancer survivors can lead to fatigue, disability, and psychological distress, and contributes to poor physical and emotional well-being (Janz et al., 2007). Treatment of neuropathic pain syndrome entails drug therapy. Neuropathic pain is poorly responsive to opioids and nonsteroidal anti-inflammatory agents. Relief has been obtained with venlafaxine, a selective serotonin reuptake inhibitor (SSRI) antidepressant,

which is better tolerated with less adverse effects (Reuben, Makari-Judson, & Lurie, 2004). Topical administration of capsaicin has shown promise in clinical trials for relieving symptoms of cancer related neuropathic pain syndrome (England & Bhaskar, 2012; England & Hand, 2012). Acupuncture may also be offered as an additional treatment option (Eustachi, 2007).

Lymphedema

Lymphedema occurs as both an acute and chronic condition and is characterized by an abnormal accumulation of protein-rich lymph fluid in the interstitial space of the arm, breast, and chest of persons treated for breast cancer. Lymphedema most commonly affects the arm on the same side of the treated breast (Armer et al., 2008). In women with breast cancer lymphedema can develop from tumor compression or lymphatic vessel obstruction but is most often an after-effect of therapies such as axillary lymph node dissection and radiation. Removal of axillary lymph nodes increases the risk of impaired lymph drainage. Radiation can cause inflammation and constriction of the lymph channels, which can induce abnormal accumulation of lymph in the interstitial spaces of the affected arm (Acebedo, 2015).

The incidence of lymphedema among breast cancer survivors has been estimated at 20% to 40% (Acebedo, 2015). It is believed that lymphedema symptoms are often underreported, unsolicited, and underdiagnosed in clinical practice due to the fact that to date, no single, valid and reliable method for regularly assessing limb volume is routinely applied in practice (Acebedo, 2015; Lawrance, & Stammers, 2008). Although increased use of sentinel lymph node biopsy, in which only three or less lymph nodes are removed as compared to ten or more lymph nodes with axillary dissection, has lessened relative lymphedema incidence, the condition nevertheless remains prevalent in susceptible women.

Conditions that may prompt the development of lymphedema in at-risk women include infections, injuries, burns, muscle strain, restriction, excessive heat, and air travel (Fu, Axelrod, & Haber, 2008). Symptoms of lymphedema may begin as a sensation of arm fullness and mild discomfort. As lymphedema further develops, joint immobility, limb enlargement, pain, and skin changes occur in the later stages of the condition (Acebedo, 2015). Cellulitis and lymphangitis can predispose afflicted women to repeated infections. Lymphedema can adversely impact quality of life by impairing functional abilities, self-image, self-esteem, interpersonal and family relationships, and occupational roles.

Treatment of lymphedema comprises multifaceted interventions known as complex decongestive physiotherapy. This therapy consists of a set of interventions that includes manual lymphatic drainage, external compression devices, and specific exercises administered by trained therapists. Manual lymphatic drainage performed by a trained physiotherapist involves light massage that stimulates functioning lymph vessels in the trunk and contralateral arm and pushes stagnant lymph fluid from the edematous arm. Compression therapy involves application of compression bandages, compression garments, gradient compression devices, or pneumatic compression devices to the affected limb. Compression therapy is aimed at mobilization of lymph fluid. Therapeutic exercises are individualized exercises that assist lymph flow in the course of repeated contraction and relaxation of muscles. Evidence suggests that empirical patient education based on women's awareness levels and potential vulnerability may substantially improve patient outcomes in the prevention and management of lymphedema (Acebedo, 2015).

MENOPAUSAL SYMPTOMS

Symptoms of menopause are a common and distressing occurrence for women who have breast cancer. A large number of postmenopausal women may experience symptoms of their natural menopause at the time breast cancer is first discovered. Menopausal symptoms can develop in postmenopausal women who have had to discontinue HRT when diagnosed with breast cancer. Premenopausal women will develop menopausal symptoms as a result of undergoing treatment-induced premature menopause, which is the abrupt cessation of ovarian function from the effects of chemotherapy, estrogen-blocking drugs, or oophorectomy (Daniel, Mitchell, Higham, Timpson, & Foy, 2014). The abrupt cessation of ovarian function and subsequent reduction of hormone levels can bring about a rapid onset of severe menopausal symptoms, which pose a major problem in younger women (Daniel et al., 2014). Although cessation of ovarian function is permanent with ovarian ablation and oophorectomy, factors such as a woman's age and the type and dosage of drugs received may influence a temporary or permanent cessation of ovarian function with chemotherapy or endocrine therapy (MacDonald, 2007). Menopausal symptoms in women taking tamoxifen, as well as in younger women who have experienced premature menopause, tend to be more severe and disruptive than symptoms experienced in healthy women undergoing natural menopause (Daniel et al., 2014). Menopausal symptoms include hot flashes, night sweats, fatigue, joint pain, palpitations, loss of libido, vaginal dryness and atrophy, amenorrhea, anxiety, depression, irritability, weight gain, insomnia, mood swings, loss of energy, thinning hair, and dry skin (Archibald, Lemieux, Byers, Tamlyn, & Worth, 2006; MacDonald, 2007).

Numerous quality of life issues emerge in relation to menopausal symptoms, especially when treatment-induced premature menopause has occurred. Women experience physical and emotional distress associated with menopausal symptoms. Hot flashes and night sweats are the most prevalent symptoms and are frequently associated with poor emotional function, poor body image, anxiety, sleep disturbance, embarrassment, and emotional distress (Daniel et al., 2014). Young women rendered suddenly menopausal are particularly vulnerable to emotional distress. The transition to lost or impaired fertility, a permanently changed body image, and uncertainty of personal, social, and sexual worth can be devastating (Hunter et al., 2004). The physical and emotional effects of menopausal symptoms can diminish quality of life.

Safe and effective treatment for menopausal symptoms is challenging. HRT for breast cancer survivors is not recommended. Specific symptoms such as depression can respond well to antidepressant therapy and counseling. Dietary modification may be considered in managing body weight. A variety of treatment options are available to treat menopausal symptoms (see Chapter 12). Relaxation therapy combined with cognitive behavioral therapy that includes stress management, counseling, and patient education have also been helpful in assisting breast cancer survivors to reduce menopausal symptoms (Hunter et al., 2004). Lifestyle modifications that incorporate avoiding alcohol, smoking, hot spicy foods, and hot environments can help to moderate hot flashes. Wearing layered clothing made of cotton, and avoiding silk, wool, and synthetic fibers can be helpful. At night, fans, air conditioning, cotton sheets, and lightweight cotton nightwear can help promote a more comfortable sleeping environment (MacDonald, 2007).

SEXUAL DYSFUNCTION

Breast cancer and its treatment modalities affect women in a variety of physical and psychosocial ways that can lead to sexual dysfunction. In Western society, female breasts are considered an integral part of female sexual identity. Total or partial loss of a breast can greatly influence the sexuality of breast cancer survivors (Dean, 2008). Breast cancer surgery, whether it entails lumpectomy or mastectomy with or without breast reconstruction, results in reduced or lost tactile stimulation and disfigurement that can substantially affect body image and sexual response (Dean, 2008). Radiation therapy can create temporary skin changes such as radiation tattoos, erythema, and burns that may resolve within months, or chronic changes that may be sustained over a number of years. Chronic changes include altered skin pigment, retraction, telangiectasias, erythema, fibrosis, and diminished arm mobility (Dean, 2008). Chemotherapy produces numerous acute and chronic changes that can have persistent impact on body image and sexual function. Acute side effects such as alopecia, stomatitis, nausea, vomiting, pallor, weight gain, and fatigue may resolve soon after treatment is completed. Chronic changes related to chemotherapy-induced menopause may include vaginal dryness, vaginal atrophy, fatigue, loss of libido, hot flashes, and dyspareunia that can be long lasting or permanent in many cases, and can cause diminished sexual satisfaction and sexual dysfunction (Dean, 2008). The side effects of endocrine therapy can cause hot flashes, vaginal dryness, vaginal discharge, mood changes, weight gain, abnormal uterine bleeding, and bone pain that can contribute to diminished sexual health and sexual dysfunction (Dean, 2008).

Sexual dysfunction can substantially affect the quality of life of breast cancer survivors. Treatment effects can cause physical and emotional distress, impairment of sexual satisfaction, diminished self-esteem, and altered body image. Women's perceptions of femininity, sexual identity, childbearing capabilities, and intimacy can be adversely affected. Sexual dysfunction can negatively influence depression and aggravate anxiety, family maladjustment, and relational discord (Dizon, 2009).

The management of sexual dysfunction in breast cancer survivors is challenging because the issues involved are often overlooked by nurses and other healthcare providers, even though the problem is widespread (Dean 2008). Without adequate assessment and discussion of sexual dysfunction with their patients, healthcare providers are limited in being able to offer effective treatment. When sexual issues are not addressed by healthcare providers, women may be uncomfortable raising the issues, or believe them unimportant (Dean, 2008; Dizon, 2009). If women do not recognize or report the development of sexual problems in their lives, their healthcare providers may assume that none exist or that adequate resolution has been achieved. Such ineffective or non-communication about these sensitive issues may create a major barrier to providing helpful treatment (Dean, 2008).

The first step toward effective treatment of sexual dysfunction is for healthcare providers to routinely assess the sexual health of breast cancer survivors. This assessment can help diminish women's fears, improve their comfort level, and provide an open forum for further discussion. An invitation for further discussion of sexual issues can validate women's concerns as well as underscore their importance. Providing adequate information prior to breast cancer treatment is important to help prepare women for eventual physical changes and their impact on sexual function. Women who develop sexual dysfunction need to be informed about various treatment options that are available to help them manage their sexual difficulties (Dean, 2008).

Many of the problems that define sexual dysfunction are amenable to treatment. Interventions may include drug therapy to relieve hot flashes and other menopausal symptoms, the application of vaginal lubricant for relief of vaginal dryness and dyspareunia, the use of clothing and breast prostheses to disguise surgical defects, and recommending sexual positions that may be more comfortable and satisfying (Dean, 2008; Dizon, 2009). Counseling is a significant part of the treatment plan for sexual dysfunction and is strongly recommended to help women manage the psychosocial aspects of sexual dysfunction and improve quality of life. Counseling can help women adjust to the changes brought about by diagnosis and treatment, improve body image and self-esteem, manage distressful life changes, and improve communication with their partner. Some women and their partners may need only suggestions and recommendations about ways to resume sex comfortably, while others may require more intensive therapy (Dizon, 2009).

Sleep Disturbance

Sleep disturbance is a widespread problem among long-term breast cancer survivors. It is estimated that sleep disturbance occurs in 30–70% of cancer patients. Breast cancer survivors are particularly susceptible to sleep difficulties because of the adverse effects of treatment such as pain and hot flashes (Dirksen & Epstein, 2008). Restful, undisturbed sleep is essential in enabling women to manage the demands of breast cancer and related posttreatment symptoms. Sleep disturbance can be physiologically disruptive to the system by diminishing women's resiliency to the stress response, resulting in greater vulnerability to the effects of stress. Sleep disturbance in breast cancer survivors is often accompanied by fatigue, depression, and anxiety, with interrelationships that seem to contribute to severity among the symptom cluster (Janz et al., 2007).

Treatment for sleep disturbance commonly includes pharmacologic intervention with benzodiazepine receptor agonists or melatonin agonists. Nonpharmacologic methods for treating sleep disturbance have resulted in reliable and durable sleep improvement. Individuals with sleep disturbance who have been treated with nonpharmacologic methods tend to find these treatments more acceptable and suitable (Epstein & Dirksen, 2007). Cognitive behavioral therapy is an effective nonpharmacologic therapy that consists of stimulus control instructions, sleep restriction therapy, and sleep education and hygiene. Stimulus control instructions teach individuals to associate the bed and bedroom with sleep and avoid associations with non-sleep activities. Sleep restriction therapy aims to restrict the amount of time that an individual spends in bed to that spent sleeping. Sleep education and hygiene entails imparting information regarding sleep processes and functions, circadian rhythms, specific sleep needs, sleep deprivation, and supportive information. Cognitive behavioral therapy has shown effectiveness in reducing sleep disturbance and improving fatigue, anxiety, depression, and quality of life in breast cancer survivors (Dirksen & Epstein, 2008, Epstein & Dirksen, 2007).

Issues Affecting Psychological and Spiritual Functioning

PSYCHOLOGICAL FUNCTION

Countless women experience distress in the course of diagnosis and treatment of breast cancer, and a considerable subgroup of distressed women experience clinically significant depression. It is estimated that the incidence of depression among breast cancer survivors could be as high as 25%. (Fann et al., 2008). Women appear to be most vulnerable to depression for the first year following diagnosis, with a greater incidence of depression taking place among women younger than 50 and older than 70, women who live alone, women with comorbidities, women with lower levels of education, women who undergo chemotherapy, and women who have a previous history of depression (Fann et al., 2008; Suppli et al., 2014). Anxiety that often accompanies depression may be substantially increased when primary treatment for breast cancer is completed and women must face fear of disease recurrence and feelings of loss subsequent to reduced contact with their healthcare providers (Fann et al., 2008). Perceptions of impaired body image, altered femininity, impaired sexuality and attractiveness can also increase the risk of developing depression (Reich, Lesur, & Perdrizet-Chevallier, 2008).

Although depression is a prevalent condition among breast cancer survivors, it is frequently unrecognized and untreated. This could be explained by the likelihood that women may be reluctant to reveal their emotional distress to their oncologists and, in turn, oncologists may be unfamiliar with screening measures for depressive symptoms (Reich et al., 2008). The level of depression in patients is often underestimated by healthcare providers. Depression can exert a serious influence on the lives of breast cancer survivors. It is strongly associated with pain, fatigue, and cognitive dysfunction in women with breast cancer. Depression can also hamper social and occupational role performance, affect stress, and impair discernment of health and physical symptoms. It can seriously hinder quality of life, reduce compliance with treatment modalities, and decrease survival (Fann et al., 2008; Reich et al., 2008).

Treatment options for depression in breast cancer survivors consists of pharmacologic therapy and psychotherapeutic interventions (Wu, Brothers, Farrar, & Andersen, 2014). Pharmacologic therapies consisting of tricyclic antidepressants and SSRI antidepressants have been effective in treating depression and improving quality of life. Psychotherapeutic interventions address women's needs for information, social support, emotional expression, and improvement of coping abilities. Strategies such as supportive-expressive group therapy, individual psychosocial support, adjuvant psychotherapy, cancer support group, online support for adjuvant psychological treatment, and cognitive behavioral stress management intervention have been efficacious for breast cancer survivors with depression (Reich et al, 2008). Evidence suggests that breast cancer survivors show a greater preference for psychotherapeutic modalities of treatment over pharmacologic modalities. Healthcare providers should tailor treatment recommendations to patient preference and concerns regarding both pharmacologic and psychotherapeutic therapies (Wu et al., 2014).

SPIRITUALITY

Evidence suggests that spirituality, religion, and prayer are very important to quality of life for some people who have been diagnosed with cancer and may be a helpful addition to conventional medical care. Prayer may help to reduce stress and anxiety, promote a more positive outlook and a stronger will to live (Breastcancer.org, 2013). Interest has been growing in spirituality and how it can help cancer survivors cope. Although most studies of spirituality are small, findings indicate that spiritual coping may be one of the most powerful ways that individuals draw on their own resources to deal with serious illness. Evidence suggests that a high level of spirituality in seriously ill individuals may be associated with lower anxiety about death (Breastcancer.org, 2013). Individuals with advanced cancer who reported spiritual well-being were able to cope more effectively with their illnesses and find meaning in their experience. In women with breast cancer, spirituality and prayer have been associated with less depression and a more positive sense of well-being. Moreover, women with breast cancer who have high levels of religiosity tend to have significantly lower levels of depression. Evidence also suggests that in women with breast cancer, prayer is associated with psychological well-being (Breastcancer. org, 2013).

Issues Affecting Socioeconomic Integrity

Numerous socioeconomic issues can adversely affect the quality of life of breast cancer survivors. Even though the majority of women with breast cancer return to work following completion of treatment, a considerable portion of women are not successful in resuming employment. It is estimated that approximately 35% of breast cancer survivors do not return to work after diagnosis and treatment. Although some of these women age 60 and older may have developed breast cancer around the time they were anticipating retirement, and carry through with their plans, a noteworthy segment of women experience disruption in vocational functioning (Reid-Arndt, 2006). Various employment concerns emerge. Women may delay reentry into the workplace, feel unable to fulfill their career capability, or they may switch jobs or retire earlier than planned because of breast cancer. Women may be reluctant to change jobs in the event breast cancer returns, and annual income may decline commensurate with a reduction in hours worked. Physical factors such as disease severity, physical dysfunction, and fatigue could deter returning to work. Furthermore, women may encounter employment-related discrimination related to having had cancer that could result in job demotion or denial of promotion (Reid-Arndt, 2006). Strategies that address disruptions in vocational functioning should include aggressive treatment of lingering physical symptoms that may interfere with physical stamina and functional ability to perform job-related duties. Career counseling can be helpful for women who want to switch jobs. Employment education programs that focus on specific needs of breast cancer survivors and dispel myths and misinformation can help improve employer-employee relations (Sammarco, 2004).

In addition to employment-related difficulties, women frequently experience financial constraints, concerns about insurability and coverage, problems with disclosure and confidentiality issues, and concerns regarding stigmatization from breast cancer. The economic burden of treatment for breast cancer can be especially problematic, especially for those women with limited income and who lack health insurance (Lalani, 2011). Women of lower socioeconomic status face significant financial and/or knowledge barriers that influence receipt of treatment. Structural barriers such as access to transportation, distance of residence to treatment facilities, type of hospital performing breast cancer surgery, and patient preferences are factors that contribute to disparities in receipt of treatment among women of differing socioeconomic strata (White, Richardson, Kronitras, & Pisu, 2014). Treatment availability, cost, and quality can influence initial treatment selection as well as continuance with follow-up care (Sammarco, 2004). The presence of barriers to care must be assessed and women should be given timely referrals to available resources to help them navigate through financial difficulties (Lalani, 2011). Targeted interventions are needed to address these barriers.

Breast cancer survivors often encounter disruption in social and role functioning within the community. Friends may distance themselves out of fear or misinformation. Women may experience communication difficulties with family, friends, and healthcare providers including uneasiness in expressing thoughts and feelings, intimidation, or reluctance to being perceived as burdensome (Sammarco, 2004). Breast cancer survivors may reduce participation in leisure activities, social integration, and community involvement, often associated with the presence of physical and emotional distress caused by the disease (Reid-Arndt, 2006). The aggressive management of physical symptoms, provision of counseling, and participation in individual or group support activities is important in helping breast cancer survivors regain social and community integration (Reid-Arndt, 2006; Sammarco, 2004).

Issues Affecting Family Well-Being

The diagnosis and treatment of breast cancer can negatively impact family well-being and quality of life (Costa-Requena, Rodriguez, & Fernández-Ortega, 2013). Breast cancer survivors frequently experience disruption in family and spousal relationships that produces distress, anxiety, and role disturbance. Sexual dysfunction and communication difficulties may adversely affect the marital/partner relationship (Dean, 2008). Spouses and partners may develop distress, anxiety, and

depression, which can impair the ability of family members to carry out domestic roles. The presence of poor psychosocial adjustment, advanced disease, and physical debilitation in breast cancer survivors often influences profound distress, anxiety, helplessness, and fear of maternal death in their children (Sammarco, 2003). Fear and anxiety regarding the possibility of breast cancer developing in daughters, especially in the presence of positive familial history, may be present. Family dynamics may change, with women shifting from the role of care provider to care recipient, and spouse/partner or adult children assuming the role of caregiver, and consequently women may experience distress associated with feeling burdensome to their families (Sammarco, 2003). Marital and family counseling, family education, and participation in support and advocacy groups should be encouraged to help reduce the burden of distress on family quality of life (Sammarco, 2004).

Implications for Healthcare Providers

Healthcare providers need to be mindful of the fact that symptoms frequently persist beyond completion of treatment. All too often, attention is strongly focused on treatment and supportive care of women undergoing initial breast cancer therapies, but after treatment ends, less attention may be given to improving recovery and quality of life. In the posttreatment period, women have reduced contact with healthcare providers and the emphasis of follow-up visits is frequently on detection of disease recurrence. Thus, various physical symptoms may be overlooked or underreported. Women may be uncomfortable, reluctant, or embarrassed to discuss sensitive issues such as vaginal dryness or sexual dissatisfaction. Symptom assessment as well as quality of life assessment should be a routine part of follow-up visits with breast cancer survivors. The assessment of symptoms should continue with attention to whether symptoms are worsening, stable, improved, or resolved (Janz et al., 2007), with particular emphasis on monitoring the state of women's quality of life. Many symptoms are amenable to treatment strategies that can reduce symptom burden and improve quality of life. Prior to breast cancer treatment, women should be thoroughly prepared about what to expect in the course of surgery, radiation therapy, and systemic therapy, with periodic reassessments of understanding and expectations. Aggressive symptom management should be implemented during treatment and continued for as long as needed to alleviate distress and maintain women's well-being.

In addition to physical symptom burden, healthcare providers need to be aware of the prevalence of psychological burdens that affect quality of life. Altered body image, fear of recurrence and metastasis, uncertainty, spiritual distress, grief, loneliness, and depression are commonly experienced by breast cancer survivors and may also be unseen, underdiagnosed, or minimized by healthcare providers. Women may be reluctant to express the true depth of their concerns and distress due to embarrassment, anxiety, or perceived lack of support and concern on the part of healthcare providers (Sammarco, 2004). Healthcare providers should encourage individual and family counseling with therapists who specialize in breast cancer issues to reduce distress and relieve unmanageable psychological burdens of affected women. Social support is a valuable resource in assisting women to adjust to the emotional demands of breast cancer. Healthcare providers should assist women to identify supportive resources and utilize those resources to enhance their quality of life. Participation in support groups can provide information, training in coping abilities, relaxation and emotional support, and practice in expressing thoughts and feelings. Interaction with other women who have undergone similar experiences can be particularly helpful to women who experience loneliness or have minimal social networks.

Spirituality is another valuable source of support and comfort for breast cancer survivors. Spiritual care can augment quality of life regardless of religious affiliation or practice. Healthcare providers should encourage women to express their spiritual concerns and spiritual experiences as part of their efforts to come to terms with breast cancer as a life-threatening illness (Sammarco, 2004).

Work resumption is a significant indicator of recovery from breast cancer and a valuable resource of support and positive reinforcement (Reid-Arndt, 2006). Timely referrals to social workers and community agencies that can provide vocational guidance and assistance are key strategies that can address socioeconomic needs. Women should be encouraged to confer with their human resources representatives at their workplace concerning their legal rights regarding disability, disclosure, and workplace discrimination. A thorough follow-up of long-term breast cancer survivors is indicated, with particular emphasis on the economic circumstances of women and their families and the cumulative effect on the functional abilities of women with comorbidities (Chirikos, Jacobs, & Jacobsen, 2002).

Healthcare providers need to be mindful of the effects of breast cancer on family roles and dynamics. The needs of families can be overlooked, since attention is mainly directed toward diagnosis, treatment, and follow-up care of women with breast cancer. Family vulnerabilities should be assessed as part of routine quality of life assessment, with particular emphasis on coping abilities and social support resources of women and their families.

Special Concerns of Age and Ethnicity

Although adult women across the life cycle share common experiences, concerns, and anxieties associated with diagnosis, treatment, and survivorship of breast cancer, certain quality of life issues prevail among specific age cohorts and ethnic minorities. Evidence suggests that younger, premenopausal women with breast cancer encounter more distress, more life disruption, poorer psychosocial adjustment, and poorer well-being than their older counterparts (Ferrell, Grant, Funk, Otis-Green, & Garcia, 1998b; Ganz, Greendale, Petersen, Kahn, & Bower, 2003; Kroenke et al., 2004; Sammarco, 2001b; Wenzel et al., 1999). Younger women are more susceptible to the distressing effects of breast cancer because a life-threatening disease at this stage of life is unforeseen and disruptive. The impact of treatment on reproductive health, fertility, and premature menopause is especially troublesome to younger women (Ganz et al., 2003). Older women tend to sustain better psychosocial adjustment and emotional functioning than younger women. Women who are older at time of diagnosis may have greater emotional flexibility honed from prior life experience and are better able to manage the psychosocial demands of breast cancer. However, older women may have less physical resiliency when faced with the demands of breast cancer and treatment. They are likely to experience decreased physical functioning from the presence of comorbid conditions and physical limitations associated with aging, which can adversely affect quality of life (Ganz et al., 2003).

Poverty, lack of education, and unemployment, factors common to the lower socioeconomic strata of society, can hinder access to health care and negatively influence health outcomes. The lowest socioeconomic level is known to have an overrepresentation of ethnic minorities (Ashing-Giwa & Lim, 2009). Multiethnic breast cancer survivors who live in depressed economic and socioecologic conditions can be vulnerable to poor quality of health care, family and functional distress, and economic hardship. Evidence suggests that African-American and Latina breast cancer survivors who have lower socioeconomic means are likely to experience more episodes of psychosocial and socioecologic instability. Lower socioeconomic means and higher socioecologic stress can adversely affect physical health, emotional well-being, and influence poor quality of life (Ashing-Giwa & Lim, 2009).

Healthcare providers need to consider the challenges that age and ethnicity can render in women's ability to sustain an acceptable quality of life throughout breast cancer survivorship. Ongoing assessment of quality of life is fundamental to identify the specific needs of vulnerable women. Proactive intervention that integrates supportive resources and services is essential in assisting vulnerable younger, older, and multiethnic women in maintaining acceptable quality of life.

Research Review

How Do Latina and Caucasian Breast Cancer Survivors Differ in Quality of Life?
Sammarco, A., & Konecny, L. (2010). Quality of life, social support, and uncertainty among Latina and Caucasian breast cancer survivors: A comparative study. *Oncology Nursing Forum*, *37*(1), 93–99.

The purpose of this study was to examine the differences between Latina and Caucasian breast cancer survivors in perceived social support, uncertainty, and quality of life, and on various demographic variables. A descriptive comparative research design was employed. A sample of 182 Caucasian and 98 Latina breast cancer survivors was recruited from various sites in the New York metropolitan area, and study participants completed the Northouse Social Support Questionnaire, Mishel Uncertainty in Illness Scale Community Form, and the Ferrans and Powers Quality of Life Index-Cancer Version III. Data were analyzed using descriptive, parametric, and nonparametric statistical analyses.

The findings revealed differences between Caucasian and Latina breast cancer survivors in perceived social support, uncertainty, and quality of life. The results suggest that ethnicity had an influence on the variables of the study. Caucasian breast cancer survivors perceived significantly more total social support than the Latina cohort. Significantly more Caucasian breast cancer survivors were married, and the Latina cohort reported higher rates of divorce and separation, which possibly explained this finding. Latina breast cancer survivors reported significantly higher levels of uncertainty than the Caucasian cohort. This finding was likely influenced by the Latina cohort having reported lower levels of education, greater presence of psychiatric illness, and having undergone more aggressive breast cancer treatments than the Caucasian cohort. These findings may have contributed to the higher levels of uncertainty among the Latina cohort. Uncertainty can be triggered by factors such as presence of comorbidities, treatment side effects, fear of death and suffering, and financial concerns for health-related costs. The Latina breast cancer survivors reported significantly poorer total quality of life than the Caucasian cohort, especially in the health and functioning and socioeconomic domains. The disparity in quality of life scores was likely influenced by lower socioeconomic status, psychiatric illness comorbidity, and lower levels of education, all of which are factors that have been shown to diminish quality of life. Latina cultural values such as *paternalismo*, *fatalismo*, and *familialism* may contribute to the disparities noted between cohorts. In the overall comparison of total quality of life, the pattern of less perceived social support in the presence of increased uncertainty together influenced a poorer quality of life in the Latina cohort. This pattern of prediction has been supported by findings from previous studies.

Nurses and other healthcare providers need to be cognizant of the essential association between perceived social support, uncertainty, and quality of life in Latina breast cancer survivors and how Latinas are likely to differ from Caucasian breast cancer survivors. Factors such as cultural values, comorbidities, and education level may influence perceived social support, uncertainty, and quality of life. Nurses and other healthcare providers need to be aware of Latina cultural values and address these values through culturally meaningful interventions that will augment perceived social support, reduce uncertainty, and enhance quality of life of Latina breast cancer survivors.

Chapter Summary Points

- Breast cancer is believed to be caused by an interaction of multiple hormonal, environmental, hereditary, and lifestyle factors.
- Advancing age increases the risk of breast cancer in women, as does early onset of menarche, late menopause, nulliparity, and older age (over 30) at first childbirth.
- Women with a family history of breast cancer, genetic mutations of BRCA1 and BRCA2 genes, epithelial proliferative changes to breast tissue, and a past history of breast cancer are at higher risk for developing the disease.
- Women who demonstrate a significant risk for breast cancer may be offered risk reduction strategies by their healthcare provider.
- African-Americans and Latinas are likely to be diagnosed with breast cancer at more advanced stages and experience lower 5-year survival rates than white women.
- Diagnosis of breast cancer in men is often made at a later stage, with a poorer prognosis, which is associated with a lack of awareness, screening, or timely response of men to changes in their breasts.
- Healthcare providers need to be alert to the demographic, cognitive, and socio-emotional factors that contribute to poor compliance to breast cancer screening, and incorporate this awareness into further efforts to improve adherence to breast cancer screening.
- Local and axillary disease is treated with surgery, radiation therapy, or both, and systemic disease is treated with cytotoxic chemotherapy, hormonal therapy, biologic therapy, or a combination of these options.
- Quality of life issues and concerns associated with breast cancer are multidimensional, distributed across various domains of life, and may be persistent for years into survivorship.
- Breast cancer diagnosis and treatment adversely affects quality of life by influencing health and physical functioning, psychological and spiritual well-being, socioeconomic integrity, and family well-being.
- Routine assessment for the presence of physical, psychological, socioeconomical, and family burdens that affect quality of life is essential to ascertain if worsening, stabilization, improvement, or resolution has occurred.
- Unique demands associated with age and ethnicity can further challenge women's ability to sustain an acceptable quality of life, and vulnerable women should be identified.
- Proactive intervention with integration of supportive resources and services is essential to assist women in maintaining acceptable quality of life.

Critical Thinking Exercise

Case Study

Mrs. C. is a 55-year-old breast cancer survivor. She is divorced and lives with her two children, a 19-year-old daughter who has started college and a 17-year-old son who is a junior in high school. Mrs. C. was employed as a secretary for a small business firm and supplemented her salary with a part-time job a few evenings a week as a billing clerk for a dental practice prior to being diagnosed with breast cancer. Mrs. C.'s ex-husband lives in another city and does not contribute financial support. Mrs. C. has a small circle of friends and an elderly widowed mother. Mrs. C. had a left modified radical mastectomy with axillary lymph node dissection. Her pathology report indicated that 4 out of 19 lymph nodes were positive for cancer cells, and the tumor was estrogen receptor and progesterone receptor positive. Further workup revealed that Mrs. C. was negative for distant metastasis. Mrs. C. received six cycles of CAF systemic chemotherapy (cyclophosphamide, anthracyclines, and 5-fluorouracil) and has been taking tamoxifen since completion of chemotherapy.

Mrs. C. experienced alopecia, fatigue, and nausea during her chemotherapy treatments and was unable to work. When chemotherapy was completed, her hair grew back, the nausea resolved, and fatigue improved enough for her to return to her day job. However, by the end of the day Mrs. C. feels totally drained. She does not sleep well and awakens frequently from hot flashes and night sweats. She experienced natural menopause at age 52, accompanied by various mild to moderate menopausal symptoms, which seem to have become more severe since she began taking tamoxifen. She is saddened and distressed by having had cancer and a mastectomy. She feels unattractive and hides her sadness from her children since she doesn't want to upset them. Although she assumes an upbeat attitude in front of others, she is terrified for the future. She fears disease recurrence and dying, fears losing her job, being unable to pay for her medical care, and being unable to provide for her family. She drags herself through her days and wonders if her life will ever improve.

Questions for Seminar Discussion

1. What overt physical, psychological/spiritual, socioeconomic, and family issues threaten Mrs. C.'s quality of life?
2. What issues and concerns are not readily apparent but could become problematic to Mrs. C. and her family?
3. What further information would be needed from Mrs. C. in order to obtain a thorough assessment of her quality of life?
4. What strengths and weaknesses are present that factor into Mrs. C.'s ability to manage her illness and quality of life demands?
5. What treatment options and interventions are available to help Mrs. C. resolve breast cancer related problems that continue to plague her?
6. What community referrals could be made that would help Mrs. C. improve her quality of life?

Internet Resources

American Cancer Society: breast cancer information and resources for patients, family, survivors, and professionals. http://www.cancer.org

BreastCancer.Org: a breast cancer community-based forum for online support. http://www.breastcancer.org/

National Breast Cancer Foundation: a breast cancer community-based forum for online support. http://community.nationalbreastcancer.org/

National Cancer Institute: breast cancer information and resources for patients, family, survivors, and professionals. http://www.cancer.gov/cancertopics/types/breast

Susan G. Komen Breast Cancer Foundation: a grassroots network for breast cancer survivors and activists, which focuses on information, support, and advocacy. http://ww5.komen.org/

References

Acebedo, J. (2015). Minimizing breast cancer-related lymphoedema. *Practice Nursing, 26*(2), 79–83.

American Cancer Society. (2012). *Cancer facts and figures for Hispanics/Latinos 2012–2014.* Atlanta, GA: American Cancer Society, Inc.

American Cancer Society. (2013a). *Breast cancer facts and figures 2013–2014.* Atlanta, GA: American Cancer Society, Inc.

American Cancer Society. (2013b). *Cancer facts and figures for African Americans 2013–2014.* Atlanta: American Cancer Society, Inc.

American Cancer Society. (2015). How is breast cancer staged? Retrieved from http://www.cancer.org/cancer/breastcancer/detailedguide/breast-cancer-staging

Archibald, S., Lemieux, S., Byers, E., Tamlyn, K., & Worth, J. (2006). Chemically-induced menopause and the sexual functioning of breast cancer survivors. *Women & Therapy, 29*(1/2), 83–106.

Armer, J., Henggeler, M., Brooks, C., Zagar, E., Homan, S., & Stewart, R. (2008). The health deviation of post-breast cancer lymphedema: Symptom assessment and impact on self-care agency. *Self Care, Dependent Care & Nursing, 16*(1), 14–21.

Ashing-Giwa, K., & Lim, J. (2009). Examining the impact of socioeconomic status and socioecologic stress on physical and mental health quality of life among breast cancer survivors. *Oncology Nursing Forum, 36*(1), 79–88.

Blunt, C., & Schmiedel, A. (2004). Some cases of severe post-mastectomy pain syndrome may be caused by an axillary haematoma. *Pain, 108*(3), 294–296.

Breastcancer.org. (2013). Spirituality and prayer. Retrieved from ww.breastcancer.org/treatment/comp_med/types/spirituality

Cella, D. (2006). Quality of life in clinical decisions in chemotherapy-induced anemia. *Oncology, 20*(8 Suppl 6), 25–28.

Chirikos, T., Russell-Jacobs, A., & Jacobsen, P. (2002). Functional impairment and the economic consequences of female breast cancer. *Women & Health, 36*(1), 1–20.

Costa-Requena, G., Rodriguez, A., & Fernández-Ortega, P. (2013). Longitudinal assessment of distress and quality of life in the early stages of breast cancer treatment. *Scandinavian Journal of Caring Sciences, 27*, 77–83.

Daniel, B., Mitchell, H., Higham, P., Timpson, J., & Foy, S. (2014). Management of menopausal symptoms for breast cancer patients. *British Journal of Nursing, 23*(8), 427–432.

Dean, A. (2008). Supporting women experiencing sexual problems after treatment for breast cancer. *Cancer Nursing Practice, 7*(8), 29–33.

Dirksen, S., & Epstein, D. (2008). Efficacy of an insomnia intervention on fatigue, mood, and quality of life in breast cancer survivors. *Journal of Advanced Nursing, 61*(6), 664–675.

Dizon, D. (2009). Quality of life after breast cancer: Survivorship and sexuality. *The Breast Journal, 15*(5), 500–504.

England, J., & Bhaskar, A. (2012). 68 Management of cancer-related neuropathic pain using the Capsaicin 8% patch. *European Journal of Oncology Nursing, 16*, S25.

England, J., & Hand, J. (2012). 69 The Capsaicin 8% patch for the treatment of cancer-related neuropathic pain – the importance of appropriate patient management and clinic set up. *European Journal of Oncology Nursing, 16*, S25.

Epstein, D., & Dirksen, S. (2007). Randomized trial of a cognitive-behavioral intervention for insomnia in breast cancer survivors. *Oncology Nursing Forum, 34*(5), E51–59.

Eustachi, A. (2007). Complementary therapies in breast cancer patients. *Breast Care, 2*, 209–216.

Eversley, R., Estrin, D., Dibble, S., Wardlaw, L., Pedrosa, M., & Favilla-Penney, W. (2005). Post-treatment symptoms among ethnic minority breast cancer survivors. *Oncology Nursing Forum, 32*(2), 250–256.

Fann, J., Thomas-Rich, A., Katon, W., Cowley, D., Pepping, M., McGregor, B., & Gralow, J. (2008). Major depression after breast cancer: A review of epidemiology and treatment. *General Hospital Psychiatry, 30*, 112–126.

Fentiman, I., Fourquet, A., & Hortobagyi, G. (2008). Male breast cancer. *Lancet, 367*, 595–604.

Ferrell, B., Grant, M., Funk, B., Otis-Green, S., & Garcia, N. (1997). Quality of life in breast cancer. Part I: Physical and social well-being. *Cancer Nursing, 20*(6), 398–498.

Ferrell, B., Grant, M., Funk, B., Otis-Green, S., & Garcia, N. (1998a). Quality of life in breast cancer. Part II: Psychological and spiritual well-being. *Cancer Nursing, 21*(1), 1–9.

Ferrell, B., Grant, M., Funk, B., Otis-Green, S., & Garcia, N. (1998b). Quality of life in breast cancer survivors: implications for developing support services. *Oncology Nursing Forum, 25*, 887–895.

Field, T.A., Buist, D.S., Doubeni, C., Enger, S., Fouayzi, H., Hart, G., ... Yao, J. (2005). Disparities and survival among breast cancer patients. *Journal of the National Cancer Institute Monograph, 35*, 88–95.

Fu, M., Axelrod, D., & Haber, J. (2008). Breast-cancer-related lymphedema: Information, symptoms, and risk-reduction behaviors. *Journal of Nursing Scholarship, 40*(4), 341–348.

Ganz, P., Greendale, G., Petersen, L., Kahn, B., & Bower, J. (2003). Breast cancer in younger women: Reproductive and late health effects of treatment. *Journal of Clinical Oncology, 21*(22), 4184–4193.

Gélinas, C., & Fillion, L. (2004). Factors related to persistent fatigue following completion of breast cancer treatment. *Oncology Nursing Forum, 31*(2), 269–278.

Huerta, E. (2003). Cancer statistics for Hispanics, 2003: Good news, bad news, and the need for a health system paradigm change. *CA Cancer Journal for Clinicians, 53*(4), 205–207.

Hunter, M., Grunfeld, E., Mittal, S., Sikka, P., Ramirez, A., Fentiman, I., & Hamad, H. (2004). Menopausal symptoms in women with breast cancer: Prevalence and treatment preferences. *Psycho-Oncology, 13*, 769–778.

Janz, N., Mujahid, M., Chung, L., Lantz, P., Hawley, S., Morrow, M., ... Katz, S. (2007). Symptom experience and quality of life of women following breast cancer treatment. *Journal of Women's Health, 16*(9), 1348–1361.

Kerans, M. (2004). Breast cancer screening behavior among low-income and minority women. *Clinical Excellence for Nurse Practitioners, 8*(1), 14–21.

Kroenke, C., Rosner, B., Chen, W., Kawachi, I., Colditz, G., & Holmes, M. (2004). Functional impact of breast cancer by age at diagnosis. *Journal of Clinical Oncology, 22*, 1849–1856.

Lalani, N. (2011). The impact of socioeconomic status on the breast cancer journey. *Journal of Cancer Education, 26*(1), 200–201.

Lawrance, S., & Stammers, T. (2007). A model of care optimizing recovery after breast cancer surgery. *Cancer Nursing Practice, 7*(6), 35–39.

MacDonald, P. (2007). Support in early menopause. *Practice Nurse, 33*(3), 39–40.

Magai, C., Consedine, N., Neugut, A., & Hershman, D. (2007). Common psychosocial factors underlying breast cancer screening and breast cancer treatment adherence: A conceptual review and synthesis. *Journal of Women's Health, 16*(1), 11–23.

National Cancer Institute. (2015a). Breast cancer treatment (PDQ®). Retrieved from http://www.cancer.gov/types/breast/patient/breast-treatment-pdq#link/stoc_h2_1

National Cancer Institute. (2015b). Genetics of breast and gynecologic cancers–for health professionals (PDQ®). Retrieved from http://www.cancer.gov/cancertopics/pdq/genetics/breast-and-ovarian/HealthProfessional/page2#Section_66

National Comprehensive Cancer Network. (2015a). *National clinical practice guidelines in oncology v 3.2015: Breast cancer.* Retrieved from http://www.nccn.org/professionals/physician_gls/pdf/breast.pdf

National Comprehensive Cancer Network. (2015b). *National clinical practice guidelines in oncology v.2.2015: Breast cancer risk reduction.* Retrieved from http://www.nccn.org/professionals/physician_gls/pdf/breast_risk.pdf

National Comprehensive Cancer Network. (2015c). *National clinical practice guidelines in oncology v 1.2015: Breast cancer screening and diagnosis guidelines.* Retrieved from http://www.nccn.org/professionals/physician_gls/pdf/breast-screening.pdf

Osuch, J. (2002). Breast health and disease over a lifetime. *Clinical Obstetrics and Gynecology, 45*(4), 1140–1161.

Ouzounakis, P., Tsiligiri, M., & Kourkouta, L. (2014). Prevention of male breast cancer. *International Journal of Caring Sciences, 7*(2), 375–378.

Pruthi, S., Brandt, K., Degnim, A., Goetz, M., Perez, E., Reynolds, C., ... Ingle, J. (2007). A multidisciplinary approach to the management of breast cancer, part 1: Prevention and diagnosis. *Mayo Clinic Proceedings, 82*(8), 999–1012.

Reich, M., Lesur, A., & Perdrizet-Chevallier, C. (2008). Depression, quality of life, and breast cancer: a review of the literature. *Breast Cancer Research and Treatment, 110*, 9–17.

Reid-Arndt, S. (2006). The potential for neuropsychology to inform functional outcomes research with breast cancer survivors. *Neurorehabilitation, 21*, 51–64.

Reuben, S., Makari-Judson, G., & Lurie, S. (2004). Evaluation of efficacy of the perioperative administration of venlafaxine XR in the prevention of postmastectomy pain syndrome. *Journal of Pain and Symptom Management, 27*(2), 133–139.

Richardson, L., Wang, W., Hartzema, A., & Wagner, W. (2007). The role of health related quality of life in early discontinuation of chemotherapy for breast cancer. *The Breast Journal, 13*(6), 581–587.

Rustøen, T., & Begnum, S. (2000). Quality of life in women with breast cancer: A review of the literature and implications for nursing practice. *Cancer Nursing, 23*(6), 416–421.

Sakorafas, G. (2003). The management of women at high risk for the development of breast cancer: Risk estimation and prevention. *Cancer Treatment Reviews, 29*, 79–89.

Sammarco, A. (2004). Enhancing the quality of life of survivors of breast cancer. *Annals of Long-Term Care, 12*(3), 40–45.

Sammarco, A. (2001a). Perceived social support, uncertainty, and quality of life among younger women with breast cancer. *Cancer Nursing, 24*(3), 212–219.

Sammarco, A. (2001b). Psychosocial stages and quality of life of women with breast cancer. *Cancer Nursing, 24*(4), 272–277.

Sammarco, A. (2003). Quality of life among older survivors of breast cancer. *Cancer Nursing, 26*(5), 408–415.

Sammarco, A., & Konecny, L. (2010). Quality of life, social support, and uncertainty among Latina and Caucasian Breast Cancer Survivors: A comparative study. *Oncology Nursing Forum, 37*(1), 93–99.

Schaub, N., Maloney, N., Schneider, H., Feliberti, E., & Perry, R. (2006). Changes in male breast cancer over a 30-year period. *The American Surgeon, 74*, 707–712.

Siegel, R., Ma, J., Zou, Z., & Jemal, A. (2014). Cancer statistics, 2014. *CA: A Cancer Journal for Clinicians, 64*, 9–29.

Suppli, N., Johansen, C., Christensen, J., Kessing, L., Kromen, N., & Dalton, S. (2014). Increased risk for depression after breast cancer: A nationwide population-based cohort study of associated factors in Denmark, 1998-2011. *Journal of Clinical Oncology, 32*(34), 3831–3839.

Wenzel, L., Fairclough, D., Brady, M., Cella, D., Garrett, K., Kluhsman, B., et al. (1999). Age related differences in the quality of life of breast carcinoma patients after treatment. *Cancer, 86*(9), 1768–1774.

White, A., Richardson, L., Kronitras, H., & Pisu, M. (2014). Socioeconomic disparities in breast cancer treatment among older women. *Journal of Women's Health, 23*(4), 335–341.

Wu, S., Brothers, B., Farrar, W., & Andersen, B. (2014). Individual counseling is the preferred treatment for depression in breast cancer survivors. *Journal of Psychosocial Oncology, 32*, 637–646.

Gynecologic Cancers

Introduction

Gynecologic cancers are serious and life-threatening conditions. As women age, their risk for developing gynecologic cancers increases considerably. Gynecologic cancers are challenging because the vague and subtle symptoms that are often presented by these cancers tend to make early diagnosis, treatment, and successful recovery difficult. Gynecologic cancers cause substantial impact on the quality of life of adult women. This chapter explores three gynecologic cancers that commonly occur in women during midlife and beyond: endometrial cancer, ovarian cancer, and cervical cancer. The various issues of gynecologic cancers that impact on the quality of life of adult women will also be examined.

Incidence

The American Cancer Society estimated that in 2015 approximately 98,280 women would be diagnosed with gynecologic cancers and 30,440 women would die from the diseases (American Cancer Society [ACS], 2015a). The most prevalent gynecologic malignancy is carcinoma of the endometrium—it is the fourth most common malignant neoplasm in women after breast, lung, and colon cancers. In 2015, approximately 54,870 new cases of endometrial cancer were expected to occur, which accounts for approximately 7% of overall annual cancer occurrences in women. Furthermore, 10,170 cancer deaths from endometrial cancer were estimated to occur in the United States, which accounts for approximately 4% of the overall deaths from cancer in women (ACS, 2015a). Approximately 2.7% of women will be diagnosed with endometrial cancer at some point during their lifetime (National Cancer Institute [NCI], 2013). The overall survival rate of endometrial cancer is 81.5%. The survival rates based on staging of the disease include 95.3% for localized disease that is confined to the primary site, 67.5% for regional disease that has spread to the lymph nodes, 16.9% for distant disease that has metastasized, and 47.8% for unknown (unstaged) disease (NCI, 2013).

Following endometrial cancer, ovarian cancer is the next most common gynecologic cancer. In 2015, 21,290 new cases of ovarian cancer were estimated to occur in the United States. The incidence of ovarian cancer has been declining since the mid 1980s. An annual decline of 0.9% per year has been observed between 2007 and 2011. Deaths from ovarian cancer in 2015 were estimated to be 10,170, which accounts for 5% of annual cancer deaths in women. Ovarian cancer causes more deaths in women than any other cancer of the reproductive system (ACS, 2015a). Women have a 1.4% lifetime risk of being diagnosed with ovarian cancer. The overall survival rate of ovarian cancer is 44.2%. The survival rates based on staging of the disease include 91.9% for localized disease, 72% for regional disease, 27.3% for distant disease, and 21.5% for unstaged disease (NCI, 2013).

After cancers of the endometrium and ovary, cancer of the cervix is the third most common gynecologic cancer in women in this country. In 2015, 12,900 new cases of cervical cancer were estimated to occur. The incidence rates of cervical cancer have substantially declined over most of the past several decades, particularly among younger women. These declines have begun to taper off (ACS, 2015a). In 2015, 4,100 deaths were estimated to occur. The death rates have declined rapidly in past decades as a result of prevention and early detection from screening with the Pap test, but rates in recent years have begun to level off, particularly among younger women. From 2007 to 2011 rates stabilized among women younger but decreased 1.1% annually among women older than 50 years (ACS, 2015a). Women have a 0.7% lifetime risk of being diagnosed with cervical cancer. The overall survival rate of cervical cancer is 67.9%. The survival rates based on staging of the disease include 90.9% for localized disease, 57.1% for regional disease, 26.1% for distant disease, and 54.3% for unstaged disease (NCI, 2013).

Ethnic Considerations

The incidence of endometrial cancer is higher in white women than in African-American women. However, the mortality rate from endometrial cancer in African-American women is nearly twice as high as that in white women. Along with barriers to early detection and effective treatment, a major factor explaining the increased mortality rate in African-American women is the significant occurrence of higher grade and more aggressive histologies in this population (Allard & Maxwell, 2009).

On the other hand, the incidence of ovarian cancer is lower in African-American women than in white women. Similarly, the mortality rate of ovarian cancer is lower in African-American women. Disparity is noted with respect to 5-year survival rates for ovarian cancer. The 5-year survival rate for ovarian cancer is 39.5% for African-American women, compared to 44.2% for white women (Schoenstadt, 2013).

Significant differences exist in the incidence of cervical cancer in white women and

African-American women. From 2007 to 2011, incidence rates stabilized in white women younger than 50 years yet decreased annually by 3.4% per year in African-American women. In women 50 years and older, incidence rates declined annually by 2.5% in white women and 3.8% in African-American women (ACS, 2015a). Moreover, even though mortality rates for all U.S. women are decreasing, the risk of death from cervical cancer for African-American women remains twice that of white women. Between 2003 and 2007, the estimated mortality rate from cervical cancer was 4.4 per 100,000 for African-American women and 2.2 per 100,000 for white women (Collins, Holcomb, Chapman-Davis, Khabele, & Farley, 2014).

Etiology and Risk Factors

Endometrial Cancer

Endometrial cancer is classified into three types. The most common type is estrogen-dependent endometrial cancer (type I), which accounts for 80% of cases. Type I is caused by an excess of endogenous or exogenous estrogen, unopposed by progesterone. Long-term unopposed estrogen exposure allows for continued endometrial growth and the development of hyperplasia with or without atypia. The resulting tumors are usually low grade and have a favorable prognosis. Type I cancers usually occur in younger women who are obese and perimenopausal (American College of Obstetricians and Gynecologists [ACOG], 2005, reaffirmed 2011; Chiang, 2013; Sorosky 2008).

Type II endometrial cancer is unrelated to endometrial hyperplaysia or estrogen. It accounts for 10% of cases. The endometrium is generally atrophic or has polyps. Type II endometrial cancer occurs spontaneously and tends to present with higher-grade tumors or poor prognostic cell types, such as papillary serous or clear cell tumors. Patients with type II endometrial cancer are often

multiparous and normal weight. Type II cancer often occurs in women who are older and postmenopausal, and is more common in African-American women (ACOG, 2005, reaffirmed 2011; Chiang, 2013; Sorosky, 2008).

The third type of endometrial cancer is familial endometrial carcinoma, which is a hereditary form of the disease. Familial endometrial carcinoma accounts for as many as 10% of cases, of which 5% are associated with Lynch II syndrome, also known as hereditary nonpolyposis colorectal cancer (HNPCC). While endometrial cancer is the most common cancer associated with HNPCC (40% to 60% lifetime risk), other malignancies, such as ovarian cancer, may occur. HNPCC is an autosomal-dominant condition characterized by germline mutations in any one of six genes located on chromosomes 2, 3, and 7. Although as many as 35% of endometrial cancers in this syndrome are associated with high-grade tumors, Lynch II syndrome may produce a neoplasm of any grade or histology, (ACOG, 2005, reaffirmed 2011; Chiang, 2013; Sorosky 2008).

Endometrioid adenocarcinoma is the most common endometrial cancer cell type. This constitutes 75% to 80% of endometrial carcinoma cases. Adenocarcinomas arise from glandular epithelial cells of the endometrium. Less common types include papillary serous (5% to 10%), clear cell (less than 5%), adenosquamous (2%) and mucinous (2%). Papillary serous and clear cell carcinomas are considered to be high grade and tend to be more aggressive than endometrial adenocarcinomas. They tend to be detected at advanced stages and have poor prognosis (Chaing, 2013).

RISK FACTORS FOR ENDOMETRIAL CANCER

While the exact cause of endometrial cancer is not known, the current understanding of risk factors helps to identify women at risk for type I endometrial cancer due to estrogen excess. Risk factors associated with exogenous sources of estrogen include the following:

ESTROGEN THERAPY (ET) For women with a uterus, the risk of endometrial cancer associated with unopposed estrogen use for 5 or more years is more than tenfold higher compared with women not taking ET. However, adding progesterone therapy to estrogen eliminates the risk of endometrial cancer (ACS, 2015c).

TAMOXIFEN Tamoxifen, when used for chemoprevention of breast cancer, increases the risk of endometrial cancer nearly threefold (Sorosky, 2008). A selective estrogen receptor modulator, (SERM), tamoxifen has site-specific activity in different tissues. It suppresses growth in breast tissue but stimulates the growth of the endometrial lining (ACS, 2015c; Sorosky, 2008).

Risk factors associated with endogenous sources of estrogen include the following:

EARLY MENARCHE Menstruation that begins before the age of 12 years increases the number of years that the endometrium is exposed to estrogen (ACS, 2015c).

LATE MENOPAUSE Menopause occurring after the age of 52 increases the duration of estrogen exposure (ACS, 2015c).

HISTORY OF INFERTILITY OR NULLIPARITY During pregnancy, the hormonal balance shifts toward more progesterone, which protects the uterus. As a consequence, women who have had many pregnancies have a reduced risk of developing endometrial cancer, and women who are infertile or who have never been pregnant have an increased risk (ACS, 2015c).

OBESITY The majority of women who develop endometrial cancer tend to be obese. Women who are 30 pounds over ideal weight have a threefold increased risk of developing endometrial cancer, whereas women who are 50 pounds or more over

ideal weight have a tenfold increased risk (Chiang, 2013). Women who are obese have higher levels of endogenous estrogen as a result of the conversion of androstenedione to estrone and the aromatization of androgens to estradiol, both of which occur in peripheral adipose tissue (Chiang, 2013).

CHRONIC ANNOVULATION Annovulation is a common cause of infertility and may be caused by several factors. One of the leading causes of chronic annovulation is polycystic ovary syndrome (PCOS). Women with PCOS have excess androgens and elevated luteinizing hormone (LH) and normal or low follicle-stimulating hormone (FSH) levels. Patients may also have elevated levels of free estrogen, owing to the peripheral conversion of androgens to estrogens and the decreased production of sex hormone binding globulin (SHBG) in the liver, which serves to increase the unopposed effects of estrogen over time (ACS, 2015c; Lucidi, 2013).

DIABETES There may be as much as a fourfold increased risk of endometrial cancer in women with diabetes. Diabetes is more common in individuals who are overweight, but even women with diabetes who are not overweight have a higher risk of developing endometrial cancer (ACS, 2015c).

HIGH-FAT DIET Consumption of a high-fat diet may lead to obesity, which is a documented risk factor for endometrial cancer. Some researchers believe that fatty foods may also have a direct effect on estrogen metabolism, thereby increasing the risk of endometrial cancer (ACS, 2015c).

OVARIAN CANCER Certain ovarian tumors, such as granulose theca cell tumors, produce estrogen, thereby increasing a woman's risk of developing endometrial cancer (ACS, 2015c).

Ovarian Cancer

Epithelial ovarian carcinomas are the most common type of ovarian cancer and account for approximately 90% of diagnoses. Most of these occurrences develop in postmenopausal women (Green, 2013b). Epithelial ovarian cancers arise from the epithelial lining of the ovary. As the ovary enlarges with tumor growth, cells from the surface of the ovary are shed into the peritoneal cavity, where they are implanted on the peritoneal surface and omentum and become small tumor sites. Invasive spread to the regional para-aortic and pelvic lymph nodes, bowel, and bladder, accompanied by ascites with peritoneal seeding of the liver surface, diaphragm, bladder, and intestines is common (Green, 2013b).

Epithelial ovarian cancer can be further subdivided into serous or mucinous, (the two most common cell types), and endometroid, clear cell, and Brenner carcinomas. Epithelial tumors of low malignancy potential (borderline ovarian carcinoma) are usually found in younger women and are often confined to the ovary at diagnosis. Germ cell and sex cord-stromal tumors account for 5% of all ovarian cancers (Green, 2013a; 2013b).

Risk Factors for Ovarian Cancer

Family History   Family history is a very important risk factor in developing ovarian cancer. The lifetime risk in the general population for developing ovarian cancer is 1.6%. When one first-degree family member is affected, the risk elevates 4% to 5%. When two first-degree family members are affected, the lifetime risk increases to 7%. Approximately 5% to 10% of ovarian cancer cases occur in women with family history of the disease (Green, 2013b).

When a woman carries the *BRCA1* or *BRCA2* genetic mutation, her hereditary risk for ovarian cancer is significantly increased. Women who carry the *BRCA1* gene mutation have a 50% to 85% lifetime risk for developing breast cancer and a 15% to 45% risk for developing epithelial ovarian cancer. Women who carry the *BRCA2* gene mutation have a 50% to 85% lifetime risk for developing breast

cancer and a 10% to 20% risk for developing epithelial ovarian cancer. Furthermore, families that carry the *BRCA2* gene mutation are also at risk for developing cancers of the prostate, larynx, pancreas, and male breast (Green, 2013b).

Age   Age is a significant risk factor for developing ovarian cancer, as the risk of developing ovarian cancer increases as women age. Women younger than 40 years of age rarely develop ovarian cancer. Most ovarian cancers tend to develop after menopause. Half of all ovarian cancers are found in women older than 63 years of age (ACS, 2015d).

Parity   Parity is a significant risk factor for ovarian cancer. Women who have not had children have increased risk of developing epithelial ovarian cancer, as possibly women with early menarche or late menopause. Women who have experienced full term pregnancy have a 50% decreased risk for developing ovarian cancer compared to women who have never been pregnant. The risk continues to decline with subsequent pregnancies (Green, 2013b).

Hormonal Contraceptives   Use of oral contraceptives lowers the risk of ovarian cancer since conditions that suppress the ovulatory cycle may play a protective role (Green, 2013b). The risk decreases only after 3 to 6 months of using oral contraceptives, and the risk decreases the longer oral contraceptives are used. The benefits of lower risk continue for many years after discontinuation of oral contraceptives (ACS, 2015d). Evidence suggests that the women who used depot medroxyprogesterone acetate (DMPA or Depo-Provera CI˚), an injectable hormonal contraceptive, had decreased risk of ovarian cancer. The risk was further decreased if the women had used it for 3 or more years (ACS, 2015d).

Obesity   Evidence suggests that obesity is associated with risk for ovarian cancer. Overall, research findings suggest that obese women (those with a body mass index of at least 30) have a higher risk of developing ovarian cancer (ACS, 2015d).

Previous Hormonal Therapy   Prolonged hormonal estrogen therapy in postmenopausal women may be associated with increased risk for developing ovarian cancer. Risk may also decline as years since hormonal therapy increase (Green, 2013b).

Fertility Drugs   The fertility drug clomiphene citrate may increase the risk for developing ovarian tumors when used for longer than 1 year. Women who did not become pregnant while taking this drug appeared to have highest risk. Fertility drugs may increase the risk for developing the type of ovarian tumors known as "low malignant potential." However, women who are infertile may be at higher risk (compared to fertile women) even if they do not use fertility drugs. This might be related in part to not having had the protective effects of carrying a pregnancy to term or having used oral contraceptives (ACS, 2015d).

Cervical Cancer

With rare exceptions, cervical cancer can develop from genital infection with human papillomavirus (HPV), which is a known human carcinogen. Although HPV infections can be transmitted via nonsexual routes, the majority of infections are sexually transmitted (Boardman, 2013). HPV is the most common sexually transmitted infection worldwide. It is estimated that approximately 79 million Americans are currently infected with HPV, and approximately 14 million people become newly infected each year. HPV is so widespread that nearly all sexually active men and women will acquire at least one type of HPV at some point in their lives (Centers for Disease Control and Prevention [CDC], 2013).

In order for cervical cancer to occur, HPV infection must be present. Although HPV infection occurs in a high percentage of sexually active women, approximately 90% of HPV infections clear on their own within months to a few years and with no sequelae. However, cytology reports in the 2 years following HPV infection might reveal a low-grade squamous intraepithelial lesion (SIL). On average, the outcome of only 5% of HPV infections will be the development of cervical intraepithelial neoplasia (CIN) grade 2 or 3 lesions (which is the recognized cervical cancer precursor) within 3 years of infection. Only 20% of CIN 3 lesions lead to invasive cervical cancer within 5 years, and only 40% of CIN 3 lesions lead to invasive cervical cancer within 30 years (Boardman, 2013).

Cervical cancer is characterized by a well-defined premalignant phase that can be identified through cytological examination of exfoliated cells (Pap test) and confirmed on histological examination. These premalignant changes can represent a spectrum of cervical abnormalities inclusive of SIL or CIN lesions. Such early lesions form a continuum that is divided into low-grade or high-grade SIL or CIN 1, 2, 3 and reflects the increasingly abnormal changes of the cervical epithelium. Over time, the premalignant lesions can persist, regress, or progress to invasive malignancy. CIN1 often regresses spontaneously, whereas CIN 2 and 3 are more likely to persist and progress. The premalignant changes almost always occur in metaplastic epithelium at the squamocolumnar junction. This is the region of the cervix where the squamous lining of the vagina transitions into the columnar epithelium of the uterus. Unfortunately, cytological and histological examinations cannot reliably distinguish the few women with abnormal cytology who will progress to invasive cancer from the vast majority of those whose abnormalities will spontaneously regress (ACS, 2015b; Boardman, 2013).

Cervical cancers and cervical pre-cancers are classified by cytologic and histologic characteristics. Cervical cancers are categorized into two main types: squamous cell carcinoma and adenocarcinoma. Squamous cell carcinomas account for approximately 80% to 90% of cervical cancers. These cancers arise from the squamous cells that cover the surface of the exocervix. Squamous cell carcinomas most frequently start at the juncture of the exocervix and the endocervix. Adenocarcinomas make up most of the other cervical cancers, which have become more common in the past 20 to 30 years. This type of cervical cancer develops from the mucus-producing gland cells of the endocervix. Adenosquamous carcinomas, or mixed carcinomas, are cervical cancers that occur less commonly and have features of both squamous cell carcinomas and adenocarcinomas (ACS, 2015b).

Since only a small fraction of HPV infections develop into cancer, other factors must be involved in the course of carcinogenesis. Factors that influence the progression of CIN 3 lesions include type and duration of infection (i.e., high-risk HPV type and persistent infection), compromised immunity, environmental factors, and lack of access to routine cytology screening (Boardman, 2013).

Currently, more than 115 different genotypes of HPV have been identified and cloned, and approximately 40% infect the genital area. More than 90% of all cervical cancers worldwide are caused by eight HPV types: 16, 18, 31, 33, 35, 45, 52, and 58 (Boardman, 2013). These types are known to cause persistent infections leading to high-grade cervical changes such as moderate or severe dysplasia and neoplasia. HPV types 16, 18, and 45 are known to cause 94% of cervical adenocarcinomas. The cervical cancer risk of HPV type 16 is likely an order of magnitude higher than that posed by other high-risk HPV types (Boardman, 2013).

RISK FACTORS FOR CERVICAL CANCER

The risk factors for cervical cancer include those that increase risk for acquiring HPV infection. These include the following:

AGE   Early age at first intercourse (age 18 or younger) is a risk factor for HPV, because it is believed that the younger-developing cervix is more likely to be infected due to the normal physiologic process of squamous metaplasia. This process occurs at the squamocolumnar junction, or transformation zone, in which the more fragile columnar epithelial cells are replaced with hardier squamous epithelial cells. Squamous metaplasia is initiated by the eversion of the columnar epithelium onto the ectocervix under the influence of estrogen and its ensuing exposure to the acidic vaginal pH. Although metaplasia occurs throughout the reproductive years, it is most active during adolescence and first pregnancy. Cells undergoing metaplasia are more vulnerable to carcinogenic agents such as HPV (ACS, 2015b; Sellors & Sankaranarayanan, 2014).

SEXUAL BEHAVIOR   Having multiple sex partners or having a partner with multiple sex partners increases the risk of multiple exposures to HPV. However, only a small proportion of women infected with HPV go on to develop cervical cancer (Boardman, 2013).

Factors thought to play a contributing role in the evolution of cervical cancer from HPV infection include the following:

SMOKING   Current and former smokers have approximately two to three times the incidence of high-grade cervical intraepithelial lesions or invasive cancer among women infected with HPV. Increased risk is also associated with passive smoking, although to a lesser extent. Cervical cancer is twice as likely to develop in women who smoke cigarettes as opposed to nonsmokers. The carcinogens that the body is exposed to from smoking affect more than just the lungs, since carcinogens absorbed by the lungs are carried in the bloodstream throughout the body. Tobacco by-products have been discovered in the cervical mucus of women who smoke, and it is believed that these tobacco by-products damage DNA in cervical cells. Smoking may also impair the immune response, thereby interfering with the ability of the immune system to fight HPV infection (ACS, 2015b).

IMMUNOSUPPRESSION   Women who are immunocompromised from HIV infection or other causes, such as medications, have increased prevalence and persistence of HPV infections. This may explain why women with HIV/AIDS have a five-fold increase in risk of cervical cancer. An impaired immune system decreases the ability of the immune system for destroying cancer cells and slowing their growth and spread (ACS, 2015b; Boardman, 2013).

ORAL CONTRACEPTIVES   Evidence suggests that taking oral contraceptives for an extended period of time increases the risk of cervical cancer. Evidence also suggests that the longer a woman takes oral contraceptives, the risk of cervical cancer increases, but the risk decreases after a woman ceases taking oral contraceptives. Research findings conclude that the risk of cervical cancer was doubled in women who took oral contraceptives longer than 5 years; however, the risk normalized 10 years after they were discontinued (ACS, 2015b).

HIGH PARITY   Evidence suggests that the risk of developing cervical cancer is increased in women who have had 3 or more full-term pregnancies. The reason for this remains unclear; however, it is posited that women who have higher parity may likely have had unprotected intercourse to get pregnant, resulting in higher exposure to HPV. Also, hormonal changes during pregnancy may make women more susceptible to HPV infection or cancer growth. Another theory is that pregnant women might have weakened immune response, allowing for HPV infection and cancer growth (ACS, 2015b).

AGE AT FIRST FULL-TERM PREGNANCY   Women who are younger than 17 years of age when they have their first full-term pregnancy likely have twice the risk of developing cervical cancer later in life than women who become pregnant at 25 years of age or older (ACS, 2015b).

POVERTY   Another risk factor for cervical cancer is poverty. Many low-income women lack ready access to adequate healthcare services, including Pap tests. Poor access to healthcare services prevents low income women from receiving adequate screening and treatment for cervical pre-cancers (ACS, 2015b).

DIETHYLSTILBESTEROL   Diethylstilbesterol (DES) is a hormonal drug that was prescribed between 1940 and 1971 to prevent miscarriage in some women. Daughters of women who took DES (while in utero) later develop clear-cell adenocarcinoma of the vagina or cervix more frequently than would usually be expected. Clear-cell carcinoma is extremely rare in women who have not been exposed to DES. Approximately 1 case of clear cell carcinoma develops in every 1,000 women whose mothers took DES during pregnancy. The risk is likely greatest in women whose mothers took the drug during their first 16 weeks of pregnancy. Women with DES-related clear-cell adenocarcinoma tend to be diagnosed at about 19 years of age. Since the use of DES during pregnancy was discontinued in 1971 by the FDA, the youngest DES daughters are older than 35, which places them beyond the age of highest risk. However, it is unknown if these women are safe from DES-related cancer. Furthermore, it is unknown how long DES-exposed women will remain at risk. DES daughters might also have increased risk of developing squamous cell cancers and precancers of the cervix linked to HPV (ACS, 2015b).

GENETIC PREDISPOSITION   Women whose mother or sisters have had cervical cancer are 2 to 3 times more likely to develop the disease than if no one in the family had it. It is suspected that familial tendency toward cervical cancer is caused by an inherited condition that makes some women more susceptible to HPV infection than others (ACS, 2015b).

Chlamydia Infection   Chlamydia is a common sexually transmitted infection that can cause pelvic inflammation, leading to infertility. Evidence suggests that there is a higher risk of cervical cancer in women whose blood test results show evidence of past or current chlamydia infection, as compared with women who have normal test results (ACS, 2015b).

Nutritional Status   Diets low in fruits and vegetables may be potential contributing factors in the development of cervical cancer. Low levels of retinol and vitamin A, low levels of antioxidants such as vitamins C and E, and low levels of folate and carotenoids are likely associated with higher risk of persistent HPV infection and cervical cancer (ACS, 2015b; Chih, Lee, Colville, Binns, & Xu, 2013). Obese women are at higher risk for developing cervical cancer. Evidence suggests that obese women are more likely to avoid cervical cancer screening (López-de-Andrés et al., 2010).

Risk Reduction

Endometrial Cancer

Although most cases of endometrial cancer cannot be prevented, there are some strategies that may lower the risk of developing this disease. Modifying risk factors whenever possible will help to reduce the risk of endometrial cancer. Obesity or being overweight more than triples the risk of developing endometrial cancer as compared to women with a healthy weight. Thus, attaining and maintaining a healthy weight can reduce the risk of this cancer.

Higher levels of physical activity are associated with lower risk of endometrial cancer. Thus, engaging in regular physical activity (exercise) may help decrease the risk of endometrial cancer. Engaging in an active lifestyle and low-fat diet can help in maintaining a healthy weight and lower the risk of high blood pressure and diabetes, which are other risk factors for endometrial cancer (ACS, 2015c).

Women who have their uterus and take estrogen therapy for menopausal symptoms need to be informed about the associated risk of endometrial cancer. Progestins (progesterone-like drugs) can reduce the risk of endometrial cancer in women taking estrogen therapy; however, this combination may increase the risk of breast cancer (ACS, 2015c).

Another risk reduction strategy is to get precancerous disorders of the endometrium properly treated. Many endometrial cancers develop over a period of years. Endometrial hyperplasia, a less serious endometrial abnormality, may be a precursor to endometrial cancer. Some cases of hyperplasia will resolve without treatment; however, sometimes hyperplasia needs to be treated with hormones or surgery. Treatment with progestins as well as dilation and curettage (D&C) or hysterectomy can prevent hyperplasia from becoming cancerous. Abnormal vaginal bleeding, the most common symptom of endometrial pre-cancers and cancers, must be investigated and treated in a timely manner (ACS, 2015c).

Women with hereditary nonpolyposis colorectal cancer (HNPCC, Lynch syndrome) are at very high risk for developing endometrial cancer. Thus, options for risk reduction to prevent endometrial cancer in women with HNPCC may include hysterectomy after finishing having children. In a study of 61 women with HNPCC, none who had prophylactic hysterectomies later developed endometrial cancer, while 1/3 of the women who did not have a hysterectomy went on to be diagnosed with endometrial cancer within the next 7 years (ACS, 2015c).

Ovarian Cancer

Although nearly all women have one or more risk factors for ovarian cancer, most of the common factors only slightly increase risk and subsequently only partly explain the frequency of the disease. Consequently, knowledge thus far about risk factors has not translated into practical ways to prevent most cases of ovarian cancer.

Although little is known about ways to reduce the risk of developing germ cell and stromal tumors of the ovaries, several options for reducing the risk of developing epithelial ovarian cancer exist. Some strategies may reduce the risk only minimally, and some to a greater extent. Some strategies are easily followed, and some require surgery. Women at risk for developing ovarian cancer should consult with their healthcare professionals who can help them consider strategies applicable to their personal situations (ACS, 2015d).

Oral Contraceptives

The use of oral contraceptives decreases the risk of developing ovarian cancer, especially among women who use them for several years. Evidence suggests that women who used oral contraceptives for 5 or more years have about a 50% lower risk of developing ovarian cancer as compared with women who never used oral contraceptives. Nonetheless, oral contraceptives have some serious risks and side effects. Women who are considering taking these drugs for any reason should discuss the possible risks and benefits with their physicians. (ACS, 2015d).

Gynecologic Surgery

Both tubal ligation and hysterectomy may reduce the risk of developing ovarian cancer. However, experts recommend that these surgeries should only be done for valid medical reasons, and not for their effect on ovarian cancer risk (ACS, 2015d). Women who have a strong family history of ovarian or breast cancer and need to undergo a hysterectomy for a valid medical reason should consider removal of both ovaries and fallopian tubes as part of that procedure. Women who have already gone through menopause or are close to menopause and do not have an increased risk of ovarian cancer are often advised by their physicians to have the ovaries removed in conjunction with a hysterectomy. Women over the age of 40 who plan to undergo a hysterectomy should be advised by their physicians to have their ovaries removed (ACS, 2015d).

Prevention Strategies for Women With a Family History of Ovarian Cancer, Including Cancer Due to *BRCA* Mutation

Genetic counseling can predict whether women are likely to have one of the gene mutations associated with an increased ovarian cancer risk. Women who have a family history that indicates the likelihood of gene mutation should consider genetic testing.

Genetic testing can help determine if women or their family members carry certain gene mutations that cause a high risk of ovarian cancer. The results of genetic testing are not always clear cut, and a genetic counselor can assist women in determining what the results mean to them. Some women who have a strong family history of ovarian cancer can be greatly relieved knowing they do not have a mutation that increases their ovarian cancer risk and that of their children. Although discovering that they have such a mutation can be stressful for women, many find this information very helpful in making important decisions about prevention strategies for themselves and their children.

Many women use oral contraceptives to reduce their risk of developing ovarian cancer. Oral contraceptives seem to reduce the risk for women with *BRCA1* and *BRCA2* mutations. However, women without these mutations may experience increased breast cancer risk while taking oral contraceptives, and the increased risk continues for some time after oral contraceptives are discontinued. Research that has investigated the use of oral contraceptives in women with *BRCA* mutations has produced mixed results regarding breast cancer risk. Research investigating the risks and benefits of oral contraceptives for women at high ovarian and breast cancer risk is ongoing (ACS, 2015d).

Whether tubal ligation effectively reduces the risk of ovarian cancer in women who have *BRCA1* or *BRCA2* mutations remains unclear. Findings of studies that have investigated this issue have been inconsistent. However, researchers are in agreement that removal of both ovaries and fallopian tubes (salpingo-oophorectomy) protects women with *BRCA1* or *BRCA2* mutations against cancer of the ovaries and fallopian tubes (ACS, 2015d). Some women may opt to have risk-reducing or prophylactic surgery to decrease the risk of ovarian cancer before cancer is even suspected. Generally, salpingo-oophorectomy is recommended for women who are very high-risk patients and have finished having children. Although this surgery substantially lowers risk of ovarian cancer, risk is not entirely eliminated because some women who have a high risk of ovarian cancer already have a cancer at the time of surgery. These cancers can be microscopic and only found when the ovaries and fallopian tubes are examined after removal. Moreover, an increased risk of primary peritoneal carcinoma (PPC) is noted in women with *BRCA1* or *BRCA2* gene mutations. Although the risk is low, PPC can still develop after the ovaries are removed (ACS, 2015d).

Women with mutations in *BRCA1* or *BRCA2* have increased risk of cancer of the fallopian tubes. Early fallopian tube cancers are often found unexpectedly when the fallopian tubes are removed as a part of a risk-reducing surgery. Thus it is recommended that women at high risk of ovarian cancer who are having their ovaries removed should have their fallopian tubes completely removed as well.

Evidence suggests that premenopausal women who have *BRCA* gene mutations and have had their ovaries removed reduce their risk of breast cancer as well as their risk of ovarian cancer. The risk of breast cancer is reduced by 85% to 95%, and the risk of ovarian cancer is reduced by 50% to 60% (ACS, 2015d).

Cervical Cancer

CERVICAL CANCER SCREENING

The Pap smear is a highly effective means of reducing the risk of cervical cancer in many women. The Pap smear can detect changes in cervical tissue early before turning into cancer. The U.S. Preventive Services Task Force [USPSTF] recommends that screening cytology (Pap smear) for cervical cancer should occur every 3 years in women aged 21 to 65. Evidence indicates cervical cancer incidence and mortality is substantially reduced when screening occurs every 3 years in this age group. For women aged 30 to 65 years who want to lengthen the screening interval, screening with a combination of Pap smear and human papillomavirus (HPV) testing should be done every 5 years to provide benefits similar to those seen with cytology screening alone every 3 years. Adequate evidence indicates that screening with HPV testing (alone or in combination with cytology) in women younger than 30 years of age bestows little or no benefit (USPSTF, 2012).

According to the USPSTF (2012), potential harms of screening can include more frequent testing and invasive diagnostic procedures, as well as mild psychological anxiety, distress, and concerns about health. Overdiagnosis confers risk of unnecessary surveillance, diagnostic tests, and treatments with associated adverse effects. Potential harms of screening likely outweigh potential benefits in the following instances. Screening for cervical cancer in women younger than age 21 is not recommended because evidence indicates that screening in this age group, regardless of sexual history, does not reduce cervical cancer incidence and mortality as compared to screening beginning at age 21. Screening is not recommended in women older than age 65 who have had sufficient prior screening and are not otherwise at high risk for cervical cancer. Screening would have little or no benefit to this population. Furthermore, the USPSTF does not recommend screening for cervical cancer in women who have had a hysterectomy with removal of the cervix and who do not have a history of a high-grade precancerous lesion (i.e., CIN grade 2 or 3) or cervical cancer. Convincing evidence indicates that continuing screening in this population provides no benefits. In addition, cervical cancer screening with HPV testing, alone or in combination with cytology, in women younger than 30 years of age is not recommended (USPSTF, 2012).

Follow-Up on Abnormal Pap Smears

Women who have abnormal Pap smear results need to follow up with regular Pap smears or colposcopies. Women who have been treated for cervical dysplasia still need to follow up with Pap smears or colposcopies. Dysplasia can return, and when undetected can turn into cervical cancer (ACS, 2015b). The identification and treatment of early precancerous lesions is essential to the prevention of cervical cancer. Scheduling and keeping regular gynecological exams and Pap tests reduces the incidence and mortality of cervical cancer (NCI, 2015a). Abnormal changes in the cervix are readily detected by the Pap test and are easily cured before cancer develops.

Limiting Sexual Partners

Evidence suggests that women who have multiple sexual partners increase their risk for cervical cancer. Women who have multiple sexual partners, have sex with a partner who has multiple sexual partners, or begin having sex at an early age increase their risk of developing HPV, which can

lead to cervical cancer. Thus, limiting the number of sexual partners, avoiding sex with a partner who has had many sex partners, and waiting until being older to have sex are measures that can reduce risk of developing HPV, and subsequently decreases the risk of cervical cancer (ACS, 2015b).

Smoking Cessation and Avoiding Secondhand Smoke

Smoking cigarettes and exposure to secondhand smoke increases the risk of developing many cancers, including cervical cancer. Smoking combined with an HPV infection may accelerate cervical dysplasia. Smoking cessation may reduce the risk of developing cervical cancer (ACS, 2015b).

Condom Use

Women who have unprotected sex are at increased risk for contracting sexually transmitted infections that can increase the risk for developing cervical cancer. Use of condoms during sex will decrease the risk of sexually transmitted infections and subsequent cervical cancer risk. Evidence suggests that when condoms are used correctly, the rate of HPV infection in women is lowered by 70% when used each time women have sex. Although condoms do not offer complete protection against every possible HPV-infected area of the body, such as skin of the genital and anal area, they do provide some protection against HPV as well as HIV and some other sexually transmitted infections (ACS, 2015b).

HPV Vaccines

Vaccines are available to protect women from HPV infections. Gardasil® is given to protect against HPV types 6, 11, 16, and 18. Cervarix® protects against types 16 and 18. Gardasil is approved to prevent anal and genital warts, as well as anal, vaginal, and vulvar cancers and precancers. Both Cervarix and Gardasil are given in a series of three injections over a 6-month period. The side effects are usually mild, with the most common being short-term redness, swelling, and soreness at the injection site. Cervarix is given to girls and young women ages 10 to 25 years, and Gardasil is approved for use in both males and females aged 9 to 26 years old (ACS, 2015b).

Diagnosis and Treatment of Gynecologic Cancers

Endometrial Cancer

Few symptoms are indicative of endometrial cancer; however, as this cancer becomes advanced, certain symptoms are more common.

Abnormal Uterine Bleeding, Spotting, or Other Discharge

The most common symptom in about 90% of women diagnosed with endometrial cancer is abnormal uterine bleeding. In women who are menstruating, this symptom can appear as bleeding between menstrual periods or excessive, prolonged menstrual flow. In postmenopausal women, any bleeding is abnormal and should be evaluated. Another symptom of endometrial cancer is non-bloody vaginal discharge, which can occur in about 10% of cases (ACS, 2015c).

Pelvic Pain and/or Mass and Weight Loss

Symptoms that are more common in later stages of endometrial cancer include pelvic pain, pelvic mass, and weight loss. Although any of these symptoms can be associated with conditions other than endometrial cancer, it is important that women not delay in seeking medical evaluation. Delay in diagnosing endometrial cancer can lower the odds for successful treatment (ACS, 2015c).

There is no screening test currently available to detect endometrial cancer. In particular, a Pap smear is not effective in detecting endometrial

cancer, although the finding of atypical glandular cells is strongly suggestive of uterine malignancy in postmenopausal women. If endometrial cancer is suspected or if a woman is at high risk for its development, a gynecologist or gynecologic oncologist should be consulted immediately (ACS, 2015c).

A history and physical exam is essential in diagnosing endometrial cancer. The physical exam should include a thorough abdominal, inguinal lymph node, pelvic, vaginal, and rectal examination. Abnormal bleeding from the genital tract can occur from the vagina, cervix, uterus, or fallopian tubes. Metastatic spread of endometrial cancer occurs in a characteristic pattern, which is commonly to the pelvic and para-aortic lymph nodes. Distant metastasis usually appears in the lungs, inguinal and supraclavicular lymph nodes, liver, bones, brain, and vagina.

The first step in diagnosing endometrial cancer in women with postmenopausal bleeding is obtaining an endometrial biopsy. The biopsy is performed through the use of an endometrial suction catheter that is inserted through the cervix into the uterine cavity. An endometrial biopsy can detect 80% to 90% of endometrial cancers if an adequate tissue sample is obtained. However, if the biopsy result fails to provide sufficient diagnostic information or if abnormal bleeding persists, dilatation and curettage (D&C) with or without hysteroscopy is recommended. D&C is a very effective method for assessing uterine bleeding and diagnosing endometrial cancer. D&C under anesthesia is recommended to exclude malignancy when endometrial biopsy results are negative or inadequate, if the endometrial thickness by transvaginal ultrasound is greater than 5 mm, or if a high degree of suspicion exists. A hysteroscopy is used to directly visualize the uterine cavity. In conjunction with a D&C, hysteroscopy is a helpful tool that provides a diagnosis for abnormal bleeding and guides directed biopsies of suspicious areas. There is risk however, that hysteroscopy may enable transtubal intraperitoneal expulsion of cancer cells. (ACS, 2015c; NCI, 2015c).

Endometrial tissue samples removed by biopsy or D&C are microscopically examined to determine whether cancer is present. If cancer is present, the cytology report will indicate the type of endometrial cancer that is present, such as endometroid or clear cell, as well as the grade of cancer. Endometrial cancer is graded on a scale of 1 to 3 according to how closely the cancer cells resemble normal endometrial cells. Women who have lower grade cancers are less likely to have advanced disease or recurrences. If HNPCC is suspected as the underlying cause of endometrial cancer, the tumor tissue can be tested for protein changes (such as having fewer mismatch repair proteins) or DNA changes such as microsatellite instability (MSI). MSI can occur when one of the genes associated with HNPCC becomes faulty. If these protein or DNA changes are present, genetic counseling and genetic testing is recommended to test for the genes that cause HNPCC. Testing for low mismatch repair protein levels or for MSI is most frequently done in women who develop endometrial cancer at an earlier than usual age or who have a family history of endometrial or colon cancer (ACS, 2015c; National Comprehensive Cancer Network [NCCN], 2016).

The staging of endometrial cancer is an essential factor in determining a treatment plan. Endometrial cancer is staged based on examination of tissue removed during surgery (surgical staging). The American Joint Committee on Cancer [AJCC] and the International Federation of Gynecology and Obstetrics (FIGO) have designated staging to classify the staging of endometrial cancer. Most commonly, the FIGO system is used (NCI, 2015d), and it is presented in **Table 11–1**.

Table 11–1 FIGO STAGES OF ENDOMETRIAL CANCER

Stage I	The cancer is confined to the corpus uteri (body of the uterus).
Stage IA	The tumor is less than halfway through the myometrium. No lymph node or distant site involvement.
Stage IB	The cancer has grown more than halfway through the myometrium yet still contained within the body of the uterus.
Stage II	The tumor has spread into the cervical stroma (supporting tissue of the uterus) but has not spread outside of the uterus.
Stage III	The tumor has spread locally outside of the uterus and/or has spread regionally.
Stage III A	The tumor invades the serosa (outer surface of the uterus) and/or the fallopian tubes or adnexae (ovaries).
Stage III B	The tumor invades the vagina and/or the parametrium (tissues around the uterus).
Stage III C	The tumor has spread to pelvic and /or para-aortic lymph nodes.
Stage III C1	The pelvic lymph nodes are positive for tumor cells.
Stage III C2	The para-aortic lymph nodes are positive for tumor cells with or without positive pelvic lymph nodes.
Stage IV	The tumor invades bladder and/or bowel and/or distant metastases.
Stage IV A	The tumor invades bladder and/or bowel mucosa.
Stage IV B	Metastases to distant organs including intra-abdominal organs and/or inguinal lymph nodes.

Modified from National Cancer Institute. (2015d). Endometrial cancer treatment for health professionals (PDQ®). Retrieved from http://www.cancer.gov/types/uterine/hp/endometrial-treatment-pdq

The 5-year survival rate for endometrial cancer (the percentage of patients who live at least 5 years after their cancer is diagnosed) is a standard way of discussing an individual's prognosis. Five-year relative survival rates estimate the percentage of patients who would be expected to survive the effects of their cancer (NCI, 2015d). Relative survival rates give a more accurate reflection of the impact of the cancer on survival (ACS, 2015c). Survival rates are frequently based on previous outcomes of large numbers of women who had endometrial cancer; however, these rates cannot predict what will happen in any particular woman's case. Many other factors, such as a woman's general health and how well the cancer responds to treatment influence individual prognosis (ACS, 2015c). The overall 5-year relative survival rate for endometrial cancer is 81.5% (NCI, 2015g). The 5-year relative survival rate for endometrial adenocarcinoma by stage at diagnosis is presented in **Table 11–2**.

The choice of treatment for endometrial cancer depends mainly on the type and stage of the disease, the level of differentiation, the woman's overall health, age, and her personal preferences and considerations. The treatment options are hysterectomy, radiation therapy, and hormonal therapy. Radiation therapy may be given by external beam radiation or intracavitary (vaginal) brachytherapy. Chemotherapy may be used in recurrent or advanced cases of endometrial cancer. Women with endometrial cancer who qualify should participate in clinical trials as a way to access state-of-the-art cancer treatment (ACS, 2015c; NCCN, 2016).

The surgical procedure recommended is a total abdominal hysterectomy with bilateral salpingo-oophorectomy. Women with localized disease may just require surgery alone to be cured. On the other hand, women with myometrial invasion are usually treated with a combination of surgery and adjuvant radiation therapy. Lymph node sampling or dissection, as well as peritoneal lavage, may also be done at the same time as surgery. Depending on the extent of cancer, an omentectomy, peritoneal biopsies, and tumor debulking procedures may also be performed during the surgery. Recovery from surgery usually takes approximately 4 to 6 weeks (ACS, 2015c; NCCN, 2016).

Women who are not candidates for surgery or radiation, or who have advanced disease, are treated with hormonal therapy. The hormonal agents commonly administered for this purpose include progestin agents such as medroxyprogesterone acetate and megestrol acetate, luteinizing hormone-releasing hormone agonists such as goserelin and leuprolide, tamoxifen, and aromatase inhibitors such as letrozole, anastrozole, and exemestane (ACS, 2015c; NCCN, 2016).

In instances where a high-grade endometrial cancer such as papillary serous carcinoma or clear cell carcinoma is present, or endometrial cancer is

Table 11–2 ENDOMETRIAL ADENOCARCINOMA 5-YEAR RELATIVE SURVIVAL RATE BY STAGE AT DIAGNOSIS

Stage	5-Year Relative Survival Rate
Localized	95.3%
Regional	68.2%
Distant	16.9%
Unstaged	48.5%

Modified from National Cancer Institute. (2015g). SEER Stat fact sheets: Endometrial cancer. Retrieved from http://seer.cancer.gov/statfacts/html/corp.html

in advanced stages, women will have surgery followed by chemotherapy, radiation therapy, or both. Chemotherapy drugs that may be used include cisplatin, carboplatin, paclitaxel, doxorubicin, and ifosfamide. Multi-agent chemotherapy regimens are preferred if tolerated by the patient. Chemotherapy drugs are administered in cycles, which are schedules of regular doses followed by a period of time without drugs to allow the body to rest and recover from side effects. Cycles of chemotherapy drugs are administered every 3 to 4 weeks for approximately four to six cycles. When chemotherapy and radiation therapy are given together, chemotherapy will be administered for a few cycles, followed by radiation therapy. Then chemotherapy is administered again; this pattern is known as "sandwich therapy." Sandwich therapy may be used for endometrial papillary serous cancer and uterine carcinosarcoma (ACS, 2015c; NCCN, 2016).

An essential part of the treatment plan is a specific schedule of follow-up visits after completion of treatment. Endometrial cancer is most likely to return within the first few years after treatment. Frequency of surveillance depends on the stage and grade of cancer. Women who had stage IA low-grade endometrioid cancers (grades 1 and 2) should be seen every 6 months for the first year after treatment, and then yearly after that. Women who had stage IB or II low-grade endometrioid cancers (grades 1 and 2), should be evaluated every 3 months for the first year, then every 6 months for the next 4 years, and then once a year. Women with higher stage or grade cancers (stages III or IV, or cancers that were grade III, including papillary serous, clear cell, or carcinosarcomas) require more frequent follow-up visits. Recommended frequency of follow-up visits for high-grade or advanced stages is every 3 months for the first 2 years, every 6 months for the next 3 years, and then yearly after that (ACS, 2015c). At each visit, an examination of the abdomen and inguinal lymph nodes along with speculum and rectovaginal examinations should be done. Questioning about symptoms that might indicate cancer recurrence

should be made since most recurrences are discovered during evaluation of symptomatic patients. If symptoms or physical examination results suggest recurrent cancer, tests such as CT scan, ultrasound, CA-125 blood test, or biopsies should be performed. Evidence suggests that routine blood tests and imaging are not needed unless symptoms or physical exam abnormalities are present (ACS, 2015c).

Ovarian Cancer

The majority of cases of ovarian cancer are diagnosed when the disease has already reached an advanced stage. Symptoms of ovarian cancer are vague and offer only subtle signs of its presence, such as abdominal bloating and discomfort, dyspepsia, and fatigue or weakness, all of which can be attributed to many factors. Additional symptoms that may or may not be attributed to ovarian cancer include pelvic pressure or abdominal pain, difficulty eating or feeling full quickly, unexplained weight gain or loss, back pain, pain during sex, menstrual changes, changes in bowel patterns (diarrhea or constipation), urinary incontinence, and/or urinary urgency, fullness, and frequency. Thus, by the time ovarian cancer is considered as a possible cause of these symptoms, the cancer frequently has advanced beyond the ovaries. In addition, certain types of ovarian cancer can rapidly spread to the surface of nearby organs. Symptoms associated with advanced disease include anorexia, nausea, vomiting, ascites, abdominal or back pain, pleural effusion, and palpable abdominal or pelvic mass. Effective screening is difficult since women may be asymptomatic in the premalignant or very early stages of the disease. Nevertheless, prompt attention to symptoms can improve the odds of early diagnosis and successful treatment (ACS, 2015d).

Research directed toward developing an effective screening test for ovarian cancer has yet to be successful. Transvaginal ultrasound and tumor-associated antigen CA-125 tests are useful for detecting and monitoring the presence of advanced disease but are not sufficiently sensitive or specific enough to be recommended for screening asymptomatic women for ovarian cancer (ACS, 2015d).

Diagnosing ovarian cancer begins with a history and physical examination to detect the presence of a pelvic mass and signs of ascites. Transvaginal and abdominal ultrasound, color-flow Doppler ultrasound, computed tomography (CT scan), positron emission tomography (PET scan), and magnetic resonance imaging (MRI) will likely be performed to confirm the presence of a mass. If test results suggest ovarian cancer, a referral to a gynecologic oncologist is appropriate at this point to make sure proper staging and debulking (removal) of the tumor is done. Evidence suggests that treatment of ovarian cancer by a gynecologic oncologist ensures increased adherence to guideline-based procedures that produce better clinical outcomes as well as a 6-to 9-month median survival benefit for women with this disease (ACS, 2015d; Stewart, Rim, & Richards, 2011).

In order to make a definitive diagnosis of cancer, stage the extent of disease, and debulk all visible tumor in the abdomen and pelvis, surgical exploration must be performed. Surgical staging of ovarian cancer and the accuracy of staging is essential since ovarian cancers have different prognoses and treatment guidelines at different stages. The accuracy of staging may influence whether or not a cure will be achieved. Cancer that is inaccurately staged may lead to underestimation of the extent of the cancer, which then may not be adequately treated. Once the cancer has been staged, the stage does not change even in the event of disease recurrence or subsequent metastasis to new locations in the body. Therefore, treatment by a gynecologic oncologist is indispensable for increasing the likelihood of accurate staging of ovarian cancer.

The staging system most commonly used in staging ovarian cancer is the FIGO system (NCI, 2015e). The FIGO staging system relies on the results of surgery for the determination of the actual stage of disease. The staging of ovarian cancer is presented in **Table 11–3**.

Table 11–3 Staging of Ovarian Cancer

Stage	
I	The tumor is confined to ovaries or fallopian tube(s).
Ia	The tumor is confined to one ovary or one fallopian tube, and is not on the outer surface of the ovary or fallopian tube. No cancer cells are present in ascites or peritoneal washings.
Ib	The tumor is confined to both ovaries or fallopian tubes but is not present on outer surfaces of ovaries or fallopian tubes. No cancer cells are present in ascites or peritoneal washings.
Ic	The tumor is present in one or both ovaries or fallopian tubes with any of the following: (Ic1) Intraoperative surgical spill, (Ic2) The capsule (outer wall of the tumor) has ruptured before surgery or tumor is present on ovarian or fallopian tube surface, (Ic3) Cancer cells are present in ascites or peritoneal washings.
II	The tumor is present in one or both ovaries or fallopian tubes with pelvic extension (below pelvic brim) or peritoneal cancer (Tp).
IIa	The tumor has extended to and/or invaded the uterus and/or fallopian tubes, and/or ovaries.
IIb	The tumor has invaded other pelvic intraperitoneal tissues.

(continues)

Table 11–3 STAGING OF OVARIAN CANCER (*continued*)

Stage	
III	The tumor has spread to one or both ovaries, or fallopian tubes, or there is primary peritoneal cancer, and: • Cytologically or histologically confirmed spread to the peritoneum outside of the pelvis and/or • Metastasis to the retroperitoneal lymph nodes.
IIIa	Tumor has metastasized to the retroperitoneal lymph nodes with or without microscopic peritoneal involvement beyond the pelvis.
IIIa(i)	Positive (cytologically or histologically proven) retroperitoneal lymph nodes.
IIIa(ii)	Metastases present, greater than 10 millimeters (mm) in largest dimension.
IIIa2	Microscopic involvement above the pelvic brim, with or without positive retropritoneal lymph nodes.
IIIb	Macroscopic (i.e. large enough to be visible to the naked eye) peritoneal metastases beyond the pelvic brim, less than 2 centimeters (cm) in largest dimension with or without metastases to retroperitoneal lymph nodes.
IIIc	Macroscopic peritoneal metastases beyond the pelvic brim, greater than or equal to 2 cm in largest dimension with or without metastases to retroperitoneal lymph nodes.
IV	Distant metastases without peritoneal metastases.
IVA	Pleural effusion positive for presence of cancer cells.
IVB	Metastases to extra-abdominal organs, with cancer cells present in inguinal lymph nodes and lymph nodes outside of the abdominal cavity.

Modified from National Cancer Institute. (2015e). Ovarian epithelial, fallopian tube, and primary peritoneal cancer treatment for health professionals (PDQ®). Retrieved from http://www.cancer.gov/types/ovarian/hp/ovarian-epithelial-treatment-pdq

The survival rates for ovarian cancer are substantially less than other cancers that affect women. The overall 5-year relative survival rate for all types of ovarian cancer is 44.5% (NCI, 2015h). Women who are diagnosed with an early stage of ovarian cancer have a much higher 5-year survival rate than those diagnosed at a later stage. Nonetheless, approximately 15% of women with ovarian cancer are diagnosed early (ACS, 2015d). The 5-year relative survival rate for invasive epithelial ovarian cancer by stage at diagnosis is presented in **Table 11–4**.

Treatment options for ovarian cancer include surgery, chemotherapy, hormone therapy, targeted therapy, and radiation therapy. All women diagnosed with ovarian cancer are potential candidates for clinical trials and should be offered participation in them if they meet the selection criteria. Choice of treatment options depends on numerous factors such as stage and grade of cancer, age, state of health, whether childbearing is a concern, and other personal considerations.

The main treatment option for most ovarian cancers is surgery. The extent of surgery depends on the woman's general state of health and how far the cancer has spread. For epithelial ovarian cancer, two main goals of surgery are staging and debulking. Debulking surgery should be done by a gynecologic oncologist who is trained in staging and debulking procedures. Cancers that are debulked correctly are described as *optimally debulked*. Women with optimally debulked cancers have a better survival outlook than those with cancers

Table 11–4 Invasive Epithelial Ovarian Cancer 5-Year Relative Survival Rate by Stage at Diagnosis

Stage	5-Year Relative Survival Rate
Localized	92.1%
Regional	73.2%
Distant	28.3%
Unstaged	22.9%

Modified from National Cancer Institute. (2015h). SEER Stat fact sheets: Ovary cancer. Retrieved from http://seer.cancer.gov/statfacts/html/ovary.html

that are not debulked properly (*sub-optimally debulked*). Women with suboptimally debulked ovarian cancer may need to have additional surgery later (ACS, 2015d).

Surgery for epithelial ovarian cancer involves performing a total abdominal hysterectomy with bilateral salpingo-oophorectomy. In addition, the omentum is removed along with removal of some pelvic and abdominal lymph nodes, removal of ascitis fluid for analysis, visualization and biopsy of the undersurface of the diaphragm, pelvic and peritoneal biopsies, and peritoneal washings. Surgery also involves tumor debulking, which removes as much of the tumor as possible, especially if the tumor is found to be widely spread throughout the abdomen at the time of surgery. The goal of debulking surgery is to leave behind no tumors larger than 1 cm, at which point the tumor would then be considered optimally debulked. In the course of debulking the tumor, sections of bowel, urinary bladder, stomach, liver, and/or pancreas, as well as the appendix, spleen and/or gallbladder may be removed. Premenopausal women will experience surgical menopause from removal of the ovaries (ACS, 2015d).

If eligible for chemotherapy, patients may receive a regimen of drugs intravenously, intraperitoneally, or in some cases by a combination of both routes. Chemotherapy drugs that are administered via intravenous regimens include paclitaxel and carboplatin, docetaxel and carboplatin, or bevacizumab, paclitaxel and carboplatin. Chemotherapy drugs that may be administered in combined intravenous and intraperitoneal regimens include paclitaxel (given intravenously) and cisplatin (given intraperitoneally). Chemotherapy candidates must be assessed for adequate organ function prior to beginning treatment, especially intraperitoneal chemotherapy, and must be monitored carefully following each cycle for signs of toxicities. The common course of chemotherapy for ovarian cancer involves three to six cycles for earlier stage disease and six to eight cycles for advanced stage disease, with 3 to 4 weeks between each cycle (ACS, 2015d; NCCN, 2015b).

The side effects of chemotherapy can be unpleasant and distressing, and certain chemotherapy drugs place women at risk for dangerous toxicities. Intraperitoneal chemotherapy requires concentrated dosages of chemotherapy drugs to be instilled into the peritoneal cavity. Evidence suggests that intraperitoneal chemotherapy improves survival from ovarian cancer; however, side effects tend to be more severe than those experienced from intravenous chemotherapy. Women who receive combined intravenous and intraperitoneal chemotherapy are at risk for increased toxicities such as myelosuppression, renal toxicities, abdominal pain, neuropathy, gastrointestinal toxicities, hepatic toxicities, and metabolic toxicities (ACS, 2015d).

Factors that can favorably influence the prognosis of ovarian cancer include diagnosis at a younger age, a lower stage of disease at diagnosis, a well-differentiated tumor, absence of ascitis, good performance status, cell type other than mucinous or clear cell, smaller volume of disease prior to any debulking surgery, and smaller residual volume of tumor following debulking surgery (NCI, 2015e).

The annual mortality in ovarian cancer is approximately 65% of the incidence rate, since most patients have widespread disease at presentation. As more effective treatments have become available, increasing numbers of women with advanced disease at diagnosis are surviving, and they are having remissions of 2 years or longer. Overall, the rate of relapse in patients after completion of first-line platinum-based and taxane-based treatment is 80% (NCI, 2015e). The median time to recurrence in high-risk early ovarian cancer patients is 24 months following initial treatment and 17 months in patients with advanced ovarian cancer (Chua, Liauw, Robertson, & Morris, 2010).

The main goal of follow-up care is the early detection of recurrence so that additional treatment will offer the possibility of disease control. A therapeutic alliance and partnership between clinician and patient improves the possibility that early, subtle signs of recurrence will be promptly reported and evaluated. Lifelong follow-up will be required at regularly scheduled intervals. Follow-up visits should be scheduled every 2 to 4 months for the first 2 years, then every 3 to 6 months for 3 years, then annually after 5 years. A physical exam including pelvic exam should be done, and routine blood work as well as CA-125 and other tumor markers should be drawn. Chest, abdomen, and pelvic imaging should be done as clinically indicated. If results suggest recurrent disease, treatment options will include clinical trials, recurrence therapy, or supportive/palliative care, as warranted (NCCN, 2015b).

Cervical Cancer

Women with early cervical cancers and pre-cancers are usually asymptomatic. Symptoms often do not develop until the cancer becomes invasive and spreads into nearby tissue. The most common symptoms of cervical cancer include abnormal vaginal bleeding such as postcoital bleeding, postmenopausal bleeding, bleeding and spotting between periods, and heavy menstrual flow or irregular menses. Bleeding after douching or following a pelvic exam may also take place. Abnormal vaginal discharge may occur, which can be watery, purulent, mucoid, or contain some blood. Dyspareunia may also be present. These signs and symptoms can be attributed to conditions other than cervical cancer. Nonetheless, prompt attention to suspicious signs and symptoms should be sought. Ignoring symptoms can increase the probability of cancer being diagnosed at a more advanced stage, which decreases the likelihood for effective treatment (ACS, 2015b).

Diagnosing cervical cancer begins with a thorough history that focuses on key areas of information related to risk factors and symptoms of cervical cancer. A complete physical examination that includes a thorough pelvic, abdominal, inguinal lymph node, and rectal examination should be performed. A Pap smear is done to detect the presence of pre-cancer or cancer. If abnormal cells are found, then a colposcopy is performed, and biopsies of cervical tissue are taken for diagnostic purposes. Biopsies may include colposcopic biopsy, endocervical curettage, and cone biopsies. If a diagnosis of invasive cervical cancer is determined, referral to a gynecologic oncologist is an appropriate course of action (ACS, 2015b).

If the biopsy confirms the presence of cervical cancer, diagnostic tests must be done to evaluate the spread of cancer. In addition to local invasion, cervical cancer can spread via the bloodstream or regional lymphatics. Dissemination of the tumor is commonly a function of the extent of invasiveness of the local tumor. Although cervical cancer usually progresses in an orderly sequence, a small tumor may present distant metastases. Thus, patients must be carefully assessed for metastatic disease (NCI, 2015b). Cystoscopy, proctoscopy, pelvic exam under anesthesia, as well as MRI, PET, and CT imaging studies may be done. Intravenous urography and chest x-ray may also be performed (ACS, 2015b).

The most accurate method by which to determine the extent of cervical cancer is pretreatment surgical staging. However, because there is little evidence that shows overall improved survival with routine surgical staging, surgical staging should be performed only as part of a clinical trial (NCI, 2015b). Thus staging of cervical cancer is, for the most part, based on clinical rather than surgical findings. This means that the extent of disease is usually evaluated by the doctor's physical examination and a few other tests that are done in some cases, such as cystoscopy and proctoscopy—it is not based on the findings at surgery (ACS, 2015b). Pretreatment surgical staging in bulky but locally curable disease may be performed in certain cases when a nonsurgical search for metastatic disease is negative. If abnormal lymph nodes should be detected by CT scan or lymphangiography, a negative fine-needle aspiration should be obtained before a surgical staging procedure is done (NCI, 2015b).

The staging that defines cervical cancer has been designated by AJCC and FIGO, with the FIGO system most commonly used. The stages of cervical cancer are presented in **Table 11–5**. The

---

Table 11–5 STAGING OF CERVICAL CANCER

Stage	
I	The tumor is contained to the cervix. It has not spread outside the cervix. The cancer has not spread to nearby lymph nodes or distant sites. There is a very small amount of cancer, visible only under a microscope. The deepest invasion is ≤5 mm and largest extension is ≥7 mm.
IA1	The cancer is ≤3 mm (about 1/8-inch) deep and ≤7 mm (about 1/4-inch) wide. The cancer has not spread to nearby lymph nodes or distant sites.
IA2	The cancer is between 3 mm and 5 mm (about 1/5-inch) deep and <7 mm (about 1/4-inch) wide. The cancer has not spread to nearby lymph nodes or distant sites.
IB	Includes stage I cancers that can be seen without a microscope as well as cancers that can only be seen with a microscope if they have spread deeper than 5 mm (about 1/5 inch) into connective tissue of the cervix or are wider than 7 mm. These lesions have not spread to nearby lymph nodes or distant sites.
IB1	The cancer is clinically visible and is ≤4 cm (about 1 3/5 inches). Lesion has not spread to nearby lymph nodes or distant sites.
IB2	The cancer is clinically visible and is >4 cm in greatest dimension. Lesion has not spread to nearby lymph nodes or distant sites.
II	The cancer has invaded beyond the uterus but not to the pelvic wall or lower third of the vagina.

(continues)

Table 11–5 STAGING OF CERVICAL CANCER (*continued*)

Stage	
IIA	The cancer has not spread into the parametria. The cancer may have grown into the upper part of the vagina. Lesion has not spread to nearby lymph nodes or distant sites.
IIA1	The cancer is clinically visible and is ≤4 cm. Lesion has not spread to nearby lymph nodes or distant sites.
IIA2	The cancer is clinically visible and is >4 cm in greatest dimension. Lesion has not spread to nearby lymph nodes or distant sites.
IIB	The cancer has spread into the parametria. It has not spread to nearby lymph nodes or distant sites.
III	The cancer has spread to the lower part of the vagina or the walls of the pelvis. The cancer may be blocking the ureters causing hydronephrosis or nonfunctioning kidney. Lesion has not spread to nearby lymph nodes or distant sites.
IIIA	The cancer has spread to the lower third of the vagina but not to the walls of the pelvis. Lesion has not spread to nearby lymph nodes or distant sites.
IIIB	The cancer has grown into the walls of the pelvis and/or has blocked one or both ureters causing hydronephrosis, but has not spread to lymph nodes or distant sites. The cancer has spread to lymph nodes in the pelvis but not to distant sites. The tumor can be any size and may have spread to the lower part of the vagina or walls of the pelvis.
IV	The cancer has extended beyond the true pelvis or has invaded the mucosa of the bladder or rectum.
IVA	The cancer has spread to adjacent organs such as the bladder or rectum. Lesion has not spread to nearby lymph nodes or distant sites.
IVB	The cancer has spread to distant organs beyond the pelvic area, such as the lungs or liver.

Modified from National Cancer Institute. (2015b). Cervical cancer treatment—for health professionals (PDQ®). Retrieved from http://www.cancer.gov/cancertopics/pdq/treatment/cervical/HealthProfessional/allpages

stage of cervical cancer at diagnosis is indicative of the extent of cancer in the body and determines treatment options as well as strongly influences length of survival. The earlier cervical cancer is found, the better the chances of survival five years after being diagnosed (NCI, 2015f). The overall 5-year relative survival rate for cervical cancer is 69.9%. The relative 5-year survival rate for cervical cancer by stage at diagnosis is presented in **Table 11–6**.

Treatment of cervical cancer is determined by the stage of disease at the time of diagnosis. Other factors such as the woman's age, general health, and individual preferences may also influence treatment options. Treatment of precancerous lesions and carcinoma in situ lesions may include removal of lesions by cryosurgery, laser ablation, loop electrosurgical excision procedure (LEEP), or conization. After treatment, women require lifelong surveillance at regular intervals. Timing and frequency of follow-up is based on Pap test results and colposcopy examinations (ACS, 2015b; NCCN, 2015a).

Treatment of advanced cervical cancer encompasses surgery, radiation therapy, and chemotherapy. A gynecologic oncologist, radiation oncologist, and medical oncologist will likely be involved in managing treatment since two or

Table 11–6 CERVICAL CANCER 5-YEAR RELATIVE SURVIVAL RATE BY STAGE AT DIAGNOSIS

Stage	5-Year Relative Survival Rate
Localized	91.5%
Regional	57.4%
Distant	16.5%
Unstaged	53.2%

Modified from National Cancer Institute. (2015f). SEER Stat fact sheets: Cervix uteri cancer. Retrieved from http://seer.cancer.gov/statfacts/html/cervix.html

more treatment approaches are commonly used. Depending on the stage of cancer, surgical options may include simple hysterectomy, modified radical hysterectomy, or extend to radical hysterectomy with pelvic exenteration, which is the removal of all pelvic organs including the bladder, rectum, vulva, and vagina. Pelvic lymph node dissection is also performed. For young women who wish to preserve their fertility, a radical trachelectomy may be done, which removes the cervix and upper part of the vagina but retains the body of the uterus (ACS, 2015b; NCCN, 2015a).

Options for radiation therapy include external beam or intracavitary (brachytherapy) irradiation. Radiation is frequently combined with chemotherapy. Clinical trial findings suggest combining radiation therapy with chemotherapy with cisplatin is more effective than radiation alone (NCI, 2015b).

Systemic chemotherapy may be given as part of the main treatment for some stages of cervical cancer. Chemotherapy may be given together with radiation as concurrent chemoradiation. In this option, cisplatin is administered every week during radiation, about 4 to 5 hours before the radiation appointment. Cisplatin may also be given with 5-fluorouracil (5-FU) every 4 weeks during radiation. Other drug combinations can also be used. Chemotherapy may be given (without radiation) before and/or after concurrent chemoradiation. Chemotherapy is also given if cancer has relapsed or spread. The drugs that are frequently used to treat relapse or disease spread include cisplatin, carboplatin, paclitaxel, topotecan, and gemcitabine. Docetaxel, ifosfamide, 5-FU, irinotecan, and mitomycin may also be used. Combination therapy is recommended (ACS, 2015b; NCCN, 2015a).

A specific schedule of follow-up care is essential to detect disease recurrence. Follow-up visits should be scheduled every 3 to 6 months for the first 2 years following completion of treatment, then every 6 to 12 months for the next 3 to 5 years. Thereafter, follow-up visits should be scheduled annually based on the woman's risk of disease recurrence. Women at high risk for recurrence will be assessed more frequently than women at low risk. Follow-up visits should entail detailed history and physical examination with annual, as indicated, cervical/vaginal cytology performed for the detection of lower genital tract neoplasia. Imaging, such as MRI, PET, CT scans, and chest x-ray, as well as laboratory assessment will be indicated based on the presence of symptoms or examination findings suspicious for recurrence (NCCN, 2015a).

Quality of Life Issues Associated With Gynecologic Cancer

Gynecologic cancer can significantly influence the quality of life of women. The diagnosis of cancer, its treatment and aftermath, and the demands of survivorship are crucial factors that often defy the capability of women to maintain an acceptable quality of life. Quality of life issues associated with gynecologic cancers and their treatment can be multidimensional and have a widespread impact across the various domains of quality of life.

Gynecologic cancer and the effects of treatment can influence health and physical functioning, psychological and spiritual well-being, socioeconomic integrity, and family well-being. Surgical treatment and adjuvant therapies, such as hormonal therapy, chemotherapy, and radiation therapy often engender short- and long-term consequences that can produce physical discomfort, psychological distress, familial role disruption, and economic burden. These issues can profoundly affect the quality of life of women and their families.

Issues Affecting Health and Physical Functioning

As previously noted, symptoms of gynecologic cancers may be vague or absent in early stages of disease, and may later manifest as persistent symptoms in advanced stages, such as pain, bleeding, and organ dysfunction. The vagueness and variability of symptoms as well as lack of screening adherence may contribute to diagnosis of gynecologic cancers in more advanced stages. Disease that is diagnosed at an advanced stage is ultimately more challenging to treat effectively and will likely require more extensive and complex treatment modalities.

Total abdominal hysterectomy and bilateral salpingo-oophorectomy are surgical procedures that are commonly performed to stage and treat gynecologic cancers. Women with localized disease may be cured with surgery alone, whereas women with more extensive disease may be treated with a combination of surgery and adjuvant therapies. Sexual dysfunction may occur, depending on the extent of surgery performed as well as result from adjuvant therapies. Younger women who are premenopausal will experience induced premature menopause and loss of fertility. Symptoms of induced menopause tend to be more severe than symptoms of natural menopause.

Chemotherapy is a common adjunctive therapy given in treatment of gynecologic cancer and acts to systemically destroy cancer cells. However, in the course of killing cancer cells, chemotherapeutic drugs can damage normal cells of the body, particularly cells that rapidly regenerate such as hair, gastrointestinal mucosa, and blood-producing cells in the bone marrow. Common side effects of chemotherapy include nausea and vomiting, loss of appetite, mouth and vaginal sores, peripheral neuropathy, tinnitus, and hair loss. Younger women who have retained their ovaries may experience induced menopause as a result of chemotherapy. Women receiving chemotherapy may also develop low blood cell counts that can lead to anemia, leukopenia, and thrombocytopenia. Consequently, women receiving chemotherapy often experience fatigue, shortness of breath, bruising and bleeding after minor cuts or injuries, and increased risk for infection. It is important to note that over time, some chemotherapy drugs can have lasting toxic effects on the function of certain organs, such as the heart and kidneys (**Table 11–7**). Dosages and treatment schedules must be adjusted and monitored closely to decrease the risk of drug toxicity.

Radiation therapy may be given by external beam radiation or intracavitary (vaginal) brachytherapy. In some cases, women with gynecologic cancer may receive both methods of radiation therapy, or concurrent chemotherapy and radiation therapy. Evidence suggests that women treated with radiation therapy tend to have more impairment from

Table 11–7 TOXIC EFFECTS OF CHEMOTHERAPY DRUGS

Chemotherapy Drug	Toxic Effect
Doxorubicin	Cardiomyopathy
Cisplatin	Kidney damage, neuropathy, ototoxicity
Paclitaxel	Neuropathy
Ifosfamide	Hemorrhagic cystitis

Data from American Cancer Society (2015d). Ovarian cancer. Retrieved from http://www.cancer.org/acs/groups/cid/documents/webcontent/003130-pdf.pdf

adverse effects than those treated with other modalities (Gonçalves, 2010). Common short-term side effects of radiation therapy include diarrhea, fatigue, skin irritation, radiation cystitis, radiation proctitis, radiation vaginitis, vaginal stenosis, anemia, and leukopenia. Long-term side effects of radiation therapy include premature menopause in younger women who retained their ovaries, defecation urgency with fecal leakage, vaginal stenosis, and lymphedema of the lower extremities. Pelvic radiation may also weaken bones, which may lead to pathologic fractures of the hips and pelvic bones (ACS, 2015c; Dunberger et al., 2010; NCCN, 2016).

Adverse side effects of treatment frequently challenge the health and physical functioning of women with gynecologic cancer. Treatment side effects can be uncomfortable, distressing, painful, and may be temporary or permanent. The severity of side effect symptoms is associated with the types of chemotherapy drugs used and the combination of modalities and delivery routes. Symptom severity can also vary during the trajectory of cancer treatment (Trudel-Fitzgerald, Savall, & Ivers, 2013). While many side effects are temporary and will disappear at the completion of treatment, there are numerous symptoms that may persist long after completion of treatment and/or become permanent conditions, such as vaginal stenosis and induced menopause. Supportive therapies such as antiemetics, acupuncture, and cannabinoids, as well as complementary therapies, may be prescribed as needed to relieve adverse side effects, increase comfort, and improve quality of life (Cotter, 2009; Lu, 2005).

Lymphedema of the lower extremity may develop from tumor involvement of the lymphatics or as an adverse result of surgery or radiation therapy. Lymphedema might develop several months after completion of treatment. Women with lymphedema experience a swollen, uncomfortable limb that is restricted in range of motion and may become aggravated by fibrosis and joint contracture. The affected limb may also have altered sensitivity, and can be prone to repeated episodes of infections. Evidence suggests that complex decongestive physiotherapy is an effective modality for the management of lymphedema and will likely improve the quality of life of affected women (Kim & Park, 2008).

Sexual dysfunction may develop as a result of surgery or adjuvant treatment. Pre- and postmenopausal women may experience decreased libido upon removal of the ovaries. Menopausal symptoms of vaginal dryness and atrophy can contribute to discomfort during sexual intercourse. Vaginal dryness and atrophy can be treated with water-based lubricants, and some women may be able to use low-dose estrogen treatment in the vagina. Pain, inability to reach orgasm, loss of sensation, reduced libido, shortening of the vagina, and incomplete penis penetration are also common sexual problems, especially associated with surgery and radiotherapy (Barros & Labate, 2008; Reis, Beji, & Coskun, 2010). Radiation treatments, particularly intravaginal treatment (brachytherapy), can create vaginal scarring, and the vagina can scar closed. This condition can seriously impact a woman's ability to engage in penetrative intercourse and can affect her genital, pelvic, and perhaps clitoral sensitivity. Sexual sensation or orgasms may be less intense and a longer time may be required to reach the level of excitement and arousal that was experienced prior to cancer treatment. The use of vaginal dilators is frequently prescribed to maintain the length and integrity of the vagina. Continued use of dilators with consistent sexual health follow-up can help to maintain vaginal health and the capacity for vaginal intercourse.

Issues Affecting Psychological and Spiritual Functioning

PSYCHOLOGICAL FUNCTIONING

Gynecologic cancer and its treatment can have an adverse effect on women's psychological functioning. Evidence suggests that women most commonly experience fatigue and symptoms of anxiety and depression. Fatigue is one of the most common and distressing concerns, and most women will develop fatigue across the trajectory of survivorship. Fatigue is present well past the completion of treatment and can substantially affect quality of life (Harrington, Hanson, Moskowitz, Todd, & Feuerstein, 2010).

Symptoms of anxiety and depression also impact the quality of life of women with gynecologic cancer (Harrington et al., 2010). Depression hinders the ability of women to have meaningful relationships, maintain social connections, meet business obligations, and manage an acceptable quality of life. Women with depression may exhibit overwhelming sadness, anxiety, feelings of guilt, inability to concentrate, loss of appetite, loss of interest in

usual activities and hobbies, sleeplessness, and suicidality. Adverse treatment side effects frequently contribute to distress and feelings of depression. Evidence suggests that stressors experienced over the long-term differ from the stressors experienced during treatment or immediately following diagnosis, and therefore the cause of depression and anxiety may change throughout the trajectory of treatment and recovery (Harrington et al., 2010).

Uncertainty and fear of recurrence commonly persist for years following completion of treatment (Seske, Gjengedal, & Råheim, 2013). Women may experience interludes of remission followed by episodes of recurrence that necessitate further treatment. These events can keep women in an ongoing state of uncertainty and anxiety (Ferrell, Smith, Ervin, Itano, & Melancon, 2003). Women who are at risk for poor long-term coping and poor quality of life following a life-threatening illness tend to be young in age, have previous stressful life events, have a history of depression, are in pain, have a hopeless/helpless outlook, have low perceived control, and have little social support (Matthews et al., 2000).

Body image is a major area of concern among women with gynecologic cancer. The extent of disrupted body image depends on the disease and its treatment. Evidence suggests that for women with gynecologic cancer, the loss of parts of the body, loss of reproductive organs, and development of sexual dysfunction causes great sadness and pain (Reis et al., 2010). Loss of reproductive function in women of childbearing age can be very distressing. Gynecologic cancer surgery tends to be one of the most significant factors that damage a woman's body image. Surgical treatment frequently necessitates removal of some or all of the reproductive organs, which can damage women's self-esteem, self-confidence, and how they view themselves as women. Women may mourn the loss of a youthful body and femininity. Radical surgeries and those requiring extensive resection may result in functional changes such as ileostomies, colostomies, and ileoconduits that are perceived as embarrassing or ugly. Such surgeries impair the bodily completeness of a woman and damage body image (Reis et al., 2010).

Sexual dysfunction is a complex area of concern for women with gynecologic cancer. In addition to the physical factors that impair sexual function, many women experience psychosexual issues such as lack of interest, fear of sexual intercourse, and inorgasmia that impede sexual function. Sexual dysfunction can interfere with women's role identity, engendering feelings of inadequacy and inability to function as a complete woman in a sexual relationship with their husbands/partners. Consequently, the marital/partner relationship can be disrupted (Reis et al., 2010). Chronic sexual dysfunction is a legitimate singular concern; however, evidence suggests that sexual difficulties are associated with various problems in the areas of mood, quality of life, and adjustment. Women with sexual difficulties are more likely to perceive poorer physical health, have moderate to severe levels of depressive symptoms, and use nonprescription or recreational drugs as a coping strategy (Matthews et al., 2000).

SPIRITUALITY

Spirituality is an important aspect of quality of life for women with gynecologic cancer. Spirituality is comprised of dimensions that include not only religiosity but hopefulness, transcendence, and purpose. Since spirituality is linked to life meaning, it is an important component of deriving meaning from cancer. Spiritual beliefs and affirming relationships are important to women's sense of hope. Finding meaning through spirituality and spiritual practices facilitates positive reappraisal during stressful situations. Deriving meaning from cancer through spirituality helps women and their families to cope, maintain a sense of hopefulness, and recognize positive changes in their lives that may result from having cancer. The process of finding meaning involves reflection, reevaluation, and creation of new short-term goals. This process occurs over time and entails assessment of personal resources

and preferences within the context of women's social environments (Ferrell, Smith, Juarez, & Melancon, 2003; Reb, 2007; Wenzel et al., 2002).

Issues Affecting Socioeconomic Integrity

Numerous socioeconomic concerns can impact the quality of life of gynecologic cancer survivors. The direct and indirect financial costs of gynecologic cancer care produces considerable economic burden on women, especially women over the age of 45, on their families, and on society as a whole. Direct costs are those associated with medical care, such as screening, treatment, hospitalization, outpatient care, follow-up care, home health care, medications, and nursing home care. Indirect costs are those costs other than direct medical costs and are more difficult to quantify, such as lost productivity from being unable to work, increased caregiver burden, and the effects on quality of life of women and their families.

In the United States, the national expenditures for cancer care have been increasing. In 2010, the estimated medical care expenditures for cancer care in this country were $124.6 billion. Of this total, the estimated national medical care expenditures for gynecologic cancer were $5.1 billion for ovarian cancer, $2.6 billion for uterine cancer, and $1.6 billion for cervical cancer (NCI, 2012). In the near future, it is likely that cancer costs may increase at a faster rate than overall medical expenditures. As the population ages, it is likely that the number of women treated for gynecologic cancer will increase faster than the overall population of women, and the prevalence of gynecologic cancers will likely increase. Furthermore, medical costs are also likely to increase as new, more advanced, and more expensive treatments are adopted as standards of care (NCI, 2012).

Since direct medical expenditures account for only one component of the total economic burden of gynecologic cancer, it is important to also consider indirect costs. The indirect costs consist of losses in time and economic productivity consequential to cancer-related illness and death.

Overall lost productivity based on lost earnings related to premature cancer deaths in the United States (mortality costs associated with an approximately 600,000 cancer deaths in 2005) was estimated to be $134.8 billion. Of this total, lost productivity was approximately $2.8 billion for ovarian cancer, $1.8 billion for cervical cancer, and $1 billion for uterine cancer. Considering the projected growth and aging of the U.S. population, productivity costs are likely to increase if cancer mortality rates remain constant in the future (NCI, 2012).

Barriers that prevent many women from receiving optimal health care include lack of health insurance, financial constraints, and lack of accessibility. Uninsured women and women from ethnic minorities are considerably more likely to be diagnosed with gynecologic cancer at a more advanced stage, when treatment can be more extensive and more costly. The Affordable Care Act is expected to reduce the number of women who are uninsured and improve the healthcare system for cancer patients (ACS, 2015a).

Numerous women of working age who have gynecologic cancer were in the workforce when diagnosed and many may choose to continue working during treatment or return to work after completion of treatment. The rate that women eventually return to work will vary by a number of factors such as type of cancer and type of occupation, However, evidence suggests that women with gynecologic cancer are more likely to be unemployed than healthy women, and being unemployed may be a long-lasting effect. Furthermore, it is likely that women with gynecologic cancer will have lower employment rates and work fewer hours than similarly aged adults for as long as 2 to 6 years following diagnosis (Nachreiner, Shanley, & Ghebre, 2013).

Various factors may influence a woman's decision to return to work, such as physical and psychological effects of cancer and its treatment, supervisor and coworker support, job flexibility, and ignorance about cancer from supervisor and coworkers. The effects of cancer and its treatment can impact women's job performance by challenging their ability to perform physical as well as cognitive tasks. The effects of radiation therapy, for example, may influence the capacity to perform physical activities, and the effects of chemotherapy may affect concentration. In addition, whether the workplace has employer-based policies that assist in the return to work process may influence women's decision or capability to return to work (Nachreiner et al., 2013).

Women with gynecologic cancer frequently experience disruption of social relationships. At first, they may feel isolated and wish to avoid others who have the disease, particularly those women with advanced disease. After a time, women recently diagnosed will seek relationships with other women who have gynecologic cancer in an effort to share the lived experience and find emotional support (Ferrell, Smith, Ervin et al., 2003). Women with gynecologic cancer frequently live through feelings of devastation and fluctuation of hope during the course of their illness. They commonly experience uncertainty, loss of control, losses associated with social and work roles, and losses related to a limited future (Reb, 2007). It has long been known that social support is an important situational resource that can improve the health and quality of life of cancer survivors. Social support plays an essential role in reducing uncertainty in illness and in enhancing hope. Women often use social comparisons, that is, comparing themselves to other women with cancer, to inspire hope and motivation. Although some women avoid support groups, those who participate in these groups can connect with others living through similar experiences, providing hope and optimism about the future. Participation in a support group enables women to validate their experiences and helps them realize they are not alone (Ferrell, Smith, Ervin et al., 2003; Reb, 2007).

The presence of a system of support in women's lives and the positive perception of support can enhance adjustment (Lim & Zebrack, 2008). On the other hand, unsupportive interactions with family or friends may contribute to emotional distress (Reb, 2007). Sometimes the support of husbands or partners may not be perceived as an effective source of support. The supportiveness of the intimate partner could be affected by problems that women may have with sexual functioning, emotional adjustment, and possibly satisfaction with the relationship. Evidence suggests that supportiveness of the intimate partner may be inversely associated with women's self-rated health, total number of gynecological problems, and reliance on psychotherapy or counseling to cope with gynecologic cancer (Matthews et al., 2008).

Issues Affecting Family Well-Being

Gynecologic cancer produces numerous issues and concerns that affect family well-being and quality of life. Women are not the only persons affected by the diagnosis and treatment of cancer. Their families also experience the crisis and fallout surrounding the cancer diagnosis. The household roles and lifestyles of family members can be adversely affected by the cancer experience. Some roles are relinquished, assumed by other family members, or performed inadequately. These changes frequently impact on the ability of the family to cope with the illness and function as a unit. Roles and responsibilities of the ill woman must be redistributed to other family members to bridge the gap created by the demands of illness, resulting in the shifting and transformation of the roles of other family members. Women shift from the role of caregiver to that of receiver of care. This can be distressful and engender feelings of loss of control (Giovanetti de Jesus & Bergamasco, 1998).

Family members often assume the role of caregiver, particularly if treatment side effects are debilitating or the cancer is advanced and the woman requires extensive physical care. Family members must bear the financial burden of cancer, which can be especially stressful when financial resources and health insurance coverage are limited or absent. Family members who are caregivers commonly experience fatigue and stress associated with the burden. Family members may also experience psychological distress associated with feelings of helplessness and lack of control, often exacerbated by fear of recurrence and stress of the initial diagnosis of cancer (Ferrell, Ervin, Smith, Marek, & Melancon, 2001). Family caregivers may experience distress associated with cancer treatments received by their loved one, especially since the treatments can be intensive, prolonged, and produce substantial side effects. Social isolation is frequently encountered because family caregivers often relinquish outside social activities in order to devote their time and attention to the physical care of their ill family member. Furthermore, fear and uncertainty may develop when the cancer has strong genetic susceptibility, such as with ovarian cancer. Women may fear the development of cancer in daughters, sisters, or other female relatives (Ferrell, Ervin, Smith et al., 2001).

Implications for Healthcare Providers

A major area of consideration in the care of women who have gynecologic cancer is symptom management. Symptoms of various types accompany treatment and frequently linger long past completion of primary treatment, or may become permanent. It is essential that healthcare providers responsible for the long-term care of gynecologic cancer survivors realize the many challenges of symptom burden that women continue to face once cancer treatment has ended (Harrington, et al., 2010). During followup visits symptoms must be carefully evaluated. Whether related to tumor pathology, recurrence, or after-effects of treatment, symptoms must be considered as targets for management. This is especially true for symptoms that hamper either the physical and psychosocial dimensions of function. Healthcare providers must be alert for the development of symptoms and offer appropriate options for aggressive management. Quality care for survivors of gynecologic cancer encompasses surveillance of cancer over time, as well as enhanced preventive health and management of long-term and late effects from cancer and its aggressive and often toxic treatments (Harrington et al., 2010).

Patient education must be an essential focus of follow-up visits. Healthcare providers should teach women to recognize symptoms that might be suggestive of disease recurrence, such as vaginal discharge, weight loss, pain in the pelvis, hips, back, or legs, and persistent coughing. Women who smoke should be encouraged to cease and abstain from smoking. Patients who received radiation therapy may develop vaginal stenosis, which can interfere with sexual function and make physical examination uncomfortable or painful. Encouraging the use of vaginal dilators may be effective in preventing or treating vaginal stenosis. Use of a vaginal dilator should start 2 to 4 weeks following completion of radiation therapy and may be performed indefinitely (NCCN, 2015a).

Women are often not prepared for the bodily changes that result from gynecologic cancer and may find it difficult to ask questions related to these changes during follow-up visits. Having had cancer engenders feelings of loss, uncertainty, vulnerability, and loss of control over bodily processes. Women have a need for information and guidance about the physical as well as emotional repercussions of cancer throughout the treatment process and survivorship. Healthcare providers need to be active in addressing physical, psychological, emotional, and sexual issues in their conversations with their patients (Matzo, Graham, Troup, & Ferrell, 2014; Seske et al., 2013).

Special Concerns of Age and Ethnicity

The majority of gynecologic cancers tend to be diseases of older women in their postmenopausal years. A uniform definition of old or elderly does not exist, and it is important to acknowledge that the concept of being old or elderly spans a wide range of years inclusive of varied personal and social perspectives. Aging is exhibited in different persons in diverse ways and at different times. For practical purposes, elderly individuals have been referred to as younger-old (65 to 74 years of age), older-old (75 to 84 years of age), and oldest-old (85 years of age and older). However, biological age becomes more important than chronological age when considering implications of gynecologic cancer and its treatment (McGowan, 1995; Van Rijswijk & Vermorken, 2000).

In Western societies, the incidence of endometrial and ovarian cancers is more common in older women age 65 and above, whereas cervical cancer is more likely to develop in younger women 35 to 39 years of age, with another peak incidence between 70 and 74 years of age. In the United States, 55% of women with uterine cancer and 46% of women with ovarian cancer are over the age of 65 (Van Rijswijk & Vermorken, 2000). Elderly women have the highest risk of developing gynecologic cancers. Women over the age of 65 have a twofold risk of developing uterine cancer, a threefold risk of developing ovarian cancer, and a 10% higher risk of developing cervical cancer as compared to women 40 to 65 years of age (Mirhashemi, Nieves-Neira, & Averette, 2001).

The risk of cancer-related death is also higher in elderly women, and this risk appears to be independent of the increased incidence (Mirhashemi et al., 2001). The mortality rates of older patients with gynecologic cancer are significantly higher in comparison with younger patients. The poorer prognosis of elderly women with gynecologic cancer is likely influenced by the fact that older women tend to be diagnosed with tumors of a more advanced stage as compared to younger women. Elderly women are inclined to avoid routine gynecologic examination and screening procedures. Medical office visits tend to decrease by half after the age of 65. Barriers to compliance with cancer screening procedures encompass socioeconomical, educational, cultural, and physician attitudes. Other factors contributing to poorer prognosis among elderly patients include a preference of elderly women to delay diagnosis or avoid active treatment, general poor health, or the presence of comorbid medical conditions (Mirhashemi et al., 2001; Van Rijswijk & Vermorken, 2000).

Older women exhibit different patterns of care and extent of surgery as compared to younger women. They are likely to have surgery less often, or if they have surgical treatment it is likely to be less extensive as compared to younger women. Chemotherapy may also be used less frequently in older women. The degrees of comorbid conditions, organ dysfunction, and social support resources vary in elderly women and these factors are influential when cancer treatment, particularly chemotherapy, is considered. Furthermore, chronic diseases, decreased functional capacity, and dementia can adversely affect the survival rates of elderly women with gynecologic cancer. Having numerous comorbid conditions substantially increases the risk of dying from gynecologic malignancy. Cognitive impairment and disability are particularly prevalent in women over the age of 85 and can negatively impact survival. In addition, lack of social support is a considerable risk factor for poor survival among elderly patients (Van Rijswijk & Vermorken, 2000).

It is important for healthcare providers to be cognizant of the biology of aging as well as the physiological changes that occur in elderly women in order to develop better care strategies for women with gynecologic cancer. Age should not be the only consideration that directs diagnostic and treatment decisions for elderly patients. Many elderly women can undergo radical surgery and receive multiagent chemotherapy and radiation therapy safely. Evidence indicates that elderly patients can tolerate standard treatment modalities safely without increased morbidity or mortality (Mirhashemi et al., 2001). Elderly women with good functional status can tolerate surgery and adjuvant treatment with similar effectiveness as younger patients. Adjustments in chemotherapy dosage will be needed for elderly patients with compromised function, and attention to comorbid factors is essential for anticipating particular care needs. Nonetheless, certain treatments may only make marginal differences in survival but impose side effects that can significantly impact quality of life, especially for elderly women who are in advanced stages of disease. Thus, treatment goals and decisions need to incorporate quality of life considerations as an integral part of the treatment plan. The effects of treatment should never be worse than the disease itself (McGowan, 1995).

Elderly women should be encouraged to maintain routine gynecological examinations and screening. Healthcare providers should use every healthcare visit as an opportunity to educate patients about the benefits of regular pelvic examinations and Pap smears, and recommend appropriate screening. Physician recommendation has been found to be a major predictor of patient compliance with screening tests (Mirhashemi et al., 2001).

Women from medically underserved populations have a greater likelihood for being diagnosed with late-stage diseases that could have been treated more effectively or cured if diagnosed earlier. Obstacles that prevent individuals or groups from obtaining effective health care include physical barriers, financial barriers, and cultural beliefs (Collins et al., 2014). African-Americans have the highest mortality rate and shortest survival of any racial and ethnic group in the United States for most cancers. The origins of these disparities are complex and are considered to reflect social and economic inequalities more than biological differences connected with race. Socioeconomic disparities encompass disproportion in work, wealth, income, education, housing, and overall standard of living in addition to barriers to high-quality cancer prevention, early detection, and treatment services (ACS, 2013).

In the United States, cervical cancer in particular remains a disease of socioeconomic disparity.

African-American and Hispanic women are more likely to be diagnosed with cervical cancer and more likely to die from it than white women. The disproportionate burden of cervical cancer in ethnic minority women is primarily due to lack of compliance with preventive vaccination measures, lack of screening and follow-up, and lack of aggressive treatment (Collins et al., 2014). The high incidence and mortality rates of cervical cancer are indicative of barriers and lack of access to health care among poor and minority women (ACS, 2013; Freeman & Wingrove, 2005).

Healthcare providers need to develop and implement strategies that will serve to diminish disparities and facilitate earlier diagnosis and optimal treatment of ethnic minority women. Of major importance is improving access to quality health care. Healthcare providers should strive to improve outreach to ethnic minority women. Rural or inner-city healthcare providers should enhance partnerships with regional referral centers as well as increase referrals of minority women to specialized regional centers for treatment. Increased efforts should be made to refer ethnic minority women to the care of gynecologic oncologists. Policies are needed that further increase the inclusion of ethnic minority women in clinical trials, as well as expand access to prevention, screening, and treatment. Higher priority should be given to research that investigates disparities in gynecologic cancer. Healthcare providers need to increase awareness and incorporate health disparities and equity topics into national meetings. Moreover, healthcare providers need to further enhance individual patient participation in care, which is a vital step in eliminating disparities in gynecologic cancer. Ethnic minority women need more outreach, education, and awareness about gynecologic cancer, as well as increased awareness and interventions for healthy behavior and lifestyle (Collins et al., 2014).

Research Review

What are the quality of life levels of survivors of gynecologic cancer and the problems that affect their quality of life, sexual health, and sexual functioning?

Reis, N., Beji, N., & Coskun, A. (2010). Quality of life and sexual functioning in gynecological cancer patients: Results from quantitative and qualitative data. *European Journal of Oncology Nursing, 14*(2), 137–146.

The purpose of this study was to determine the quality of life levels of survivors of gynecologic cancer and to find out the problems that affect their quality of life, sexual health, and sexual functioning. This study used a cross-sectional design to elicit information about quality of life and sexual functioning through both quantitative data and qualitative interviews. A sample of 100 gynecologic cancer survivors who had completed treatment at least 6 months previously were recruited from the gynecological oncology clinics of Istanbul University and constituted the sample of this study. Study participants completed a demographic questionnaire, the Quality of Life Cancer Survivors Instrument, and a subsample of 30 participants were randomly selected and interviewed in depth about issues related to their sexual functioning and health. Quantitative data were analyzed using descriptive statistics, independent t-test, and analysis of variance. Qualitative data were analyzed based on methods of descriptive and content analysis.

The findings of this study indicated that the sample had a moderately low quality of life. The diagnosis and treatment of gynecologic cancer produced substantial problems that impacted adversely on the physical, psychological, social, and spiritual aspects of quality of life. Study participants reported that fatigue and problems such as menstrual changes and loss of fertility were key issues that affected their physical well-being. Anxiety and depression caused by the probability of developing a second cancer, recurrence, or spread of the cancer, as well as anticipating future diagnostic tests were reported to be among the most crucial issues that impacted on the psychological well-being of the participants. A moderate level of social well-being was reported by the participants, and the results pointed to a high level of social support from parents, family, and friends that likely contributed to an improvement in social well-being. However, familial stress and sexual problems were reported to be the most important issues affecting social aspects of quality of life. Study participants also reported a moderate level of spiritual well-being, and those who had strong religious and moral activity had a more positive spiritual well-being. However, spiritual well-being was likely affected adversely with negative thoughts about their disease and the persistence of uncertainty about the future.

The results of the qualitative arm of the study suggest that four important components of sexual health—body image, gender role, sexual functioning, and reproductive ability—were affected by gynecologic cancer and its treatment, likely contributing to a number of problems related to women's sexual health and functioning. Many women have to cope with these problems alone. Thus, preparation, education, and support of women with gynecologic cancer by healthcare professionals in relation to quality of life aspects and sexual functioning/health are a high priority and should be an integral part of follow-up care.

Chapter Summary Points

- It was estimated that in 2015, approximately 98,280 women would be diagnosed with gynecologic cancers and 30,440 women would die from the diseases.
- Cancers of the endometrium, ovary, and cervix are the most common gynecologic cancers in women in this country.
- Risk factors for endometrial cancer include exposure to exogenous sources of estrogen, early menarche, late menopause, obesity, infertility or nulliparity, annovulation, diabetes, high-fat diet, and ovarian cancer.
- Risk factors for ovarian cancer include family history, *BRCA1* or *BRCA2* genetic mutation, increasing age, nulliparity, obesity, prolonged estrogen therapy, and fertility drugs.
- Risk factors for cervical cancer include behaviors that increase the risk of acquiring HPV infection, smoking, immunosuppression, oral contraceptives, high parity, young age at first pregnancy, poverty, diethylstilbesterol use, chlamydia, and genetic predisposition.
- Women who demonstrate a significant risk for gynecologic cancer should be offered risk reduction strategies by their healthcare provider.
- African-American women are likely to be diagnosed with gynecologic cancer at more advanced stages and experience higher mortality rates than white women.

- Healthcare providers need to be alert to the demographic, cognitive, and socio-emotional factors that contribute to poor compliance to cervical cancer screening, and incorporate this awareness into further efforts to improve adherence to cervical cancer screening.
- Surgical staging of gynecologic cancer and the accuracy of staging is essential since gynecologic cancers have different prognoses and treatment guidelines at different stages. Cancer that is inaccurately staged may lead to underestimation of the extent of the cancer, inadequate treatment, and poorer survival.
- Treatment by a gynecologic oncologist is an indispensable factor for increasing the likelihood of accurate staging of gynecologic cancer.
- The main treatment options for gynecologic cancers include surgery, chemotherapy, radiation therapy; and hormonal therapy. Other factors such as the woman's age, general health, and individual preferences may also influence treatment options.
- The diagnosis of cancer, its treatment and aftermath, and the demands of survivorship are crucial factors that often defy the capability of women to maintain an acceptable quality of life.
- Surgical treatment and adjuvant therapies, such as hormonal therapy, chemotherapy and radiation therapy often engender troublesome and distressing short- and long-term consequences that can produce physical discomfort, psychological distress, familial role disruption, and economic burden. These issues can profoundly affect the quality of life of women and their families.
- Healthcare providers responsible for the long-term care of gynecologic cancer survivors need to realize the many challenges of symptom burden that women continue to face once cancer treatment cancer has ended.
- It is essential for healthcare providers to be cognizant of the biology of aging as well as the physiological changes that occur in elderly women in order to develop better care strategies for women with gynecologic cancer.
- Women from medically underserved populations have a greater likelihood for being diagnosed with late-stage diseases that could have been treated more effectively or cured if diagnosed earlier. Obstacles that prevent individuals or groups from obtaining effective healthcare include physical barriers, financial barriers, and cultural beliefs.
- Healthcare providers need to develop and implement strategies that will serve to diminish disparities and facilitate earlier diagnosis and optimal treatment of ethnic minority women. Of major importance is improving access to quality health care.

Critical Thinking Exercise

Case Study

Mrs. G. is a 75-year-old African-American woman who was diagnosed with stage IIIB cervical cancer. Mrs. G. has long-standing hypertension for which she takes antihypertensive medication. She is a widow who lives with her adult daughter and 3-year-old granddaughter in a one-bedroom apartment in an urban housing project. Mrs. G. is retired and receives a fixed income of social security and a small pension. Her daughter works as a waitress in a local diner and also has a part-time job as a bartender in a neighborhood bar to help make ends meet. Up until she became sick, Mrs. G. babysat her granddaughter. Since her illness, her granddaughter has had to go into day care. Mrs. G. has a small circle of friends, and attended the Baptist church in her neighborhood.

Mrs. G. was treated at the oncology clinic of her local community hospital. Her treatment plan consisted of a radical hysterectomy with bilateral salpingo-oopherectomy and radiation therapy. She experienced skin irritation, fatigue, and radiation proctitis from radiation therapy that has persisted since completion of her treatment. She needs to wear adult incontinence protection because the proctitis has caused stool leakage. Mrs. G. is distressed from having had cancer and fears cancer recurrence and dying. She is upset and embarrassed by her incontinence problem and avoids leaving her apartment for fear of becoming incontinent at church or in the presence of her friends. Mrs. G. tries to help take care of her granddaughter but is limited by fatigue and weakness.

Questions for Seminar Discussion

1. What physical, psychological/spiritual, socioeconomic, and family quality of life issues does Mrs. G. readily manifest as a result of having had gynecologic cancer?
2. What issues and concerns are not readily apparent but could become problematic for Mrs. G. and her family?
3. What further information will the healthcare provider need to obtain in order to create a thorough assessment of Mrs. G.'s quality of life?
4. What type of coping strengths and weaknesses does Mrs. G. exhibit?
5. What treatment options and interventions might help Mrs. G. resolve the quality of life issues that continue to plague her in her recovery?
6. What community referrals and resources are available that would assist Mrs. G. in adjusting to having had cervical cancer and improve her quality of life?

Internet Resources

American Cancer Society: provides gynecologic cancer information and resources for patients, family, survivors, and professionals. http://www.cancer.org

CDC: Cancer Prevention and Control: provides gynecologic cancer information and resources for patients, family, survivors, and professionals. http://www.cdc.gov/cancer/

Foundation for Women's Cancer: provides comprehensive information and resources about gynecologic cancer risk, prevention, early detection, and optimal treatment for patients, family, survivors, and professionals. http://www.wcn.org or http://www.foundationforwomenscancer.org

National Cancer Institute: as part of the National Institutes of Health, provides gynecologic cancer information and resources for patients, family, survivors, and professionals. http://www.cancer.gov

National Cervical Cancer Coalition: provides women, family members, and caregivers with advocacy, information, and resources related to cervical cancer and HPV, and promotes prevention through education about early vaccination, Pap testing and HPV testing. http://www.nccc-online.org

National Ovarian Cancer Coalition: provides information and resources related to ovarian cancer for patients, family, and survivors. http://www.ovarian.org

Ovarian Cancer National Alliance: Provides advocacy, support, information and resources to survivors, caregivers, and health care providers. http://www.ovariancancer.org

References

Allard, J., & Maxwell, G. (2009). Race disparities between black and white women in the incidence, treatment, and prognosis of endometrial cancer. *Cancer Control, 16*(1), 53–56.

American Cancer Society. (2013). *Cancer facts & figures for African Americans 2013-2014.* Atlanta, GA: American Cancer Society.

American Cancer Society. (2015a). *Cancer facts & figures 2015.* Atlanta, GA: American Cancer Society.

American Cancer Society (2015b). Cervical cancer. Retrieved from http://www.cancer.org/cancer/cervicalcancer/detailedguide/index

American Cancer Society (2015c). Endometrial cancer. Retrieved from http://www.cancer.org/cancer/endometrialcancer/index

American Cancer Society (2015d). Ovarian cancer. Retrieved from http://www.cancer.org/acs/groups/cid/documents/webcontent/003130-pdf.pdf

American College of Obstetricians and Gynecologists. (2005, reaffirmed 2011). Management of endometrial cancer (ACOG Practice Bulletin No. 65). *Obstetrics and Gynecology, 106,* 413–425.

Barros, G., & Labate, R. (2008). Psychological repercussions related to brachytherapy treatment in women with gynecological cancer: Analysis of production from 1987 to 2007. *Revista Latino-Americana de Enfermagem (RLAE), 16*(6), 1049–1053.

Boardman, C. (2013). Cervical cancer. Retrieved from http://emedicine.medscape.com/article/253513-overview#aw2aab6b2b3

Centers for Disease Control and Prevention. (2013). Genital HPV infection—Fact sheet. Retrieved from http://www.cdc.gov/std/HPV/STDFact-HPV.htm

Chiang, J.W. (2013). Uterine cancer. Retrieved from http://emedicine.medscape.com/article/258148-overview#aw2aab6b2b1aa

Chih, H., Lee, A., Colville, L., Binns, C., & Xu, D. (2013). A review of dietary prevention of human papillomavirus-related infection of the cervix and cervical intraepithelial neoplasia. *Nutrition and Cancer, 65*(3), 317–328.

Chua, T., Liauw, W., Robertson, G., & Morris, D. (2010). Second line treatment of first relapse recurrent ovarian cancer. *Australian & New Zealand Journal of Obstetrics & Gynaecology, 50*(5), 465–471.

Collins, Y., Holcomb, K., Chapman-Davis, E., Khabele, D., & Farley, J. (2014). Gynecologic cancer disparities: A report from the Health Disparities Taskforce of the Society of Gynecologic Oncology. *Gynecologic Oncology, 133*(2), 353–361.

Cotter, J. (2009). Efficacy of crude marijuana and synthetic Delta-9-Tetrahydrocannabinol as treatment for chemotherapy-induced nausea and vomiting: A systematic literature review. *Oncology Nursing Forum, 36*(3), 345–352.

Dunberger, G., Lind, H., Steineck, G., Waldenstrom, A., Nyberg, T., Al-Abany, M., … Åvall-Lundqvist, E. (2010). Self-reported symptoms of faecal incontinence among long-term gynaecological cancer survivors and population-based controls. *European Journal of Cancer, 46*(3), 606–615.

Ferrell, B., Ervin, K., Smith, S., Marek, T., & Melancon, C. (2003). Family perspectives of ovarian cancer. *Cancer Practice, 10*(6), 269–276.

Ferrell, B., Smith, S., Ervin, K., Itano, J., & Melancon, C. (2003). A qualitative analysis of social concerns of women with ovarian cancer. *Psycho-Oncology, 12,* 647–663.

Ferrell, B., Smith, S., Juarez, G., & Melancon, C. (2003). Meaning of illness and spirituality in ovarian cancer survivors. *Oncology Nursing Forum, 30*(2), 249–257.

Freeman, H., & Wingrove, B. (2005). *Excess cervical cancer mortality: A marker for low access to health care in poor communities.* Rockville, MD: National Cancer Institute, Center to Reduce Cancer Health Disparities. NIH Pub. No. 05–5282. Retrieved from http://www.cancer.gov /about-nci/organization/crchd/about-health-disparities /resources/excess-cervical-cancer-mortality.pdf

Giovanetti de Jesus, J., Bergamasco, R. (1998). When the housewife is missing. *Journal of Family Nursing, 4*(4), 387–393.

Gonçalves, V. (2010). Long term quality of life in gynecological cancer survivors. *Current Opinion in Obstetrics and Gynecology, 22*, 30–35.

Green, A. (2013a). Borderline ovarian cancer borderline tumor overview. Retrieved from http://emedicine .medscape.com/article/1950573-overview#aw2aab6b2

Green, A. (2013b). Ovarian cancer. Retrieved from http://emedicine.medscape.com/article/255771 -overview#aw2aab6b2b4

Harrington, C., Hanson, J., Moskowitz, M., Todd, B., & Feuerstein, M. (2010). It's not over when it's over: Long-term symptoms in cancer survivors—A systematic review. *International Journal of Psychiatry in Medicine, 40*(2), 163–181.

Kim, S., & Park, Y. (2008). Effects of complex decongestive physiotherapy on the oedema and the quality of life of lower unilateral lymphoedema following treatment for gynecological cancer. *European Journal of Cancer Care, 17*, 463–468.

López-de-Andrés, A., Martin-López, R., Hernández-Barrera, V., Carrasco-Garrido, P., Gil-de-Miguel, A., Esteban y Peña, M., Jiménez-García, R. (2010). Predictors of breast and cervical cancer screening in a Spanish metropolitan area. *Journal of Women's Health, 19*(9), 1675–1681.

Lim, J., & Zebrack, B. (2008). Different pathways in social support and quality of life between Korean American and Korean breast and gynecological cancer survivors. *Quality of Life Research, 17*, 679–689.

Lu, W. (2005). Accupuncture for side effects of chemoradiation therapy in cancer patients. *Seminars in Oncology Nursing, 21*(3), 190–195.

Lucidi, R. (2013). Polycystic ovarian syndrome. Retrieved from http://emedicine.medscape.com/article/256806 -overview#a0101

Matthews, A., Aikens, J., Helmrich, S., Anderson, D., Herbst, A., & Waggoner, S. (2000) Sexual functioning and mood among long-term survivors of clear-cell adenocarcinoma of the vagina or cervix. *Journal of Psychosocial Oncology, 17*(3-4), 27–45.

Matzo, M., Graham, C., Troup, C., & Ferrell, B. (2014). Development of a patient education resource for women with gynecologic cancers: Cancer treatment

and sexual health. *Clinical Journal of Oncology Nursing, 18*(3), 343–348.

McGowan, L. (1995). The management of elderly patients with gynecologic cancer. *Current Opinion in Obstetrics and Gynecology, 7*, 53–56.

Mirhashemi, R., Nieves-Neira, W., & Averette, H. (2001). Gynecologic malignancies in older women. *Oncology, 15*(5), 580–586.

Nachreiner, N., Shanley, R., & Ghebre, R. (2013). Cancer and treatment effects on job task performance for gynecological cancer survivors. *Work, 46*, 433–438.

National Cancer Institute. (2012). Cancer trends progress report: 2011/2012 update. Retrieved from http://www .progressreport.cancer.gov/

National Cancer Institute. (2013). SEER Stat fact sheets: Endometrial cancer. Retrieved from http://seer.cancer .gov/statfacts/html/corp.html

National Cancer Institute. (2015a). Cervical cancer prevention—for health professionals (PDQ®). Retrieved from http://www.cancer.gov/cancertopics/pdq/prevention /cervical/HealthProfessional

National Cancer Institute. (2015b). Cervical cancer treatment—for health professionals (PDQ®). Retrieved from http://www.cancer.gov/cancertopics/pdq /treatment/cervical/HealthProfessional/allpages

National Cancer Institute. (2015c). Endometrial cancer screening-for health professionals (PDQ®). Retrieved from http://www.cancer.gov/cancertopics/pdq/screening /endometrial/healthprofessional/allpages

National Cancer Institute. (2015d). Endometrial cancer treatment for health professionals (PDQ®). Retrieved from http://www.cancer.gov/types/uterine/hp /endometrial-treatment-pdq

National Cancer Institute. (2015e). Ovarian epithelial, fallopian tube, and primary peritoneal cancer treatment for health professionals (PDQ®). Retrieved from http://www .cancer.gov/types/ovarian/hp/ovarian-epithelial -treatment-pdq/

National Cancer Institute. (2015f). SEER Stat fact sheets: Cervix uteri cancer. Retrieved from http://seer.cancer .gov/statfacts/html/cervix.html

National Cancer Institute. (2015g). SEER Stat fact sheets: Endometrial cancer. Retrieved from http://seer.cancer .gov/statfacts/html/corp.html

National Cancer Institute. (2015h). SEER Stat fact sheets: Ovary cancer. Retrieved from http://seer.cancer.gov /statfacts/html/ovary.html

National Comprehensive Cancer Network. (2015a). NCCN clinical practice guidelines in oncology: Cervical cancer. Version 2.2015. Retrieved from http://www .nccn.org/professionals/physician_gls/pdf/cervical .pdf

National Comprehensive Cancer Network. (2015b). NCCN clinical practice guidelines in oncology: Ovarian cancer including fallopian tube cancer and primary peritoneal cancer. Version 2.2015. Retrieved from http://www.nccn.org/professionals/physician_gls/pdf/ovarian.pdf

National Comprehensive Cancer Network. (2016). NCCN clinical practice guidelines in oncology: Uterine neoplasms. Version 1.2016. Retrieved from http://www.nccn.org/professionals/physician_gls/pdf/uterine.pdf

Reb, A. (2007). Transforming the death sentence: Elements of hope in women with advanced ovarian cancer. *Oncology Nursing Forum, 34*(6), E70–E81.

Reis, N., Beji, N., & Coskun, A. (2010). Quality of life and sexual functioning in gynecological cancer patients: Results from quantitative and qualitative data. *European Journal of Oncology Nursing, 14*(2), 137–146.

Schoenstadt, A. (2013). Ovarian cancer survival rate. Retrieved from http://ovarian-cancer.emedtv.com/ovarian-cancer/ovarian-cancer-survival-rate.html

Sellors, J., & Sankaranarayanan, R. (Eds.). (2014). Colposcopy and treatment of cervical intraepithelial neoplasia: A beginner's manual. Retrieved from http://screening.iarc.fr/colpo.php

Seske, R., Gjengedal, E., & Råheim, M. (2013). Living in a changed female body after gynecological cancer. *Health Care for Women International, 34*, 14–33.

Sorosky, J. (2008). Clinical expert series: Endometrial cancer. *American College of Obstetricians and Gynecologists, 111*, 436–447.

Stewart, S., Rim, S., & Richards, T. (2011). Gynecologic oncologists and ovarian cancer treatment: Avenues for improved survival. *Journal of Women's Health, 20*(9), 1257–1260.

Trudel-Fitzgerald, C., Savall, J., & Ivers, H. (2013). Evolution of cancer-related symptoms over an 18-month period. *Journal of Pain and Symptom Management, 45*(6), 1007–1018.

U.S. Preventive Services Task Force. (2012). Cervical cancer: Screening. Retrieved from http://www.uspreventiveservicestaskforce.org/uspstf11/cervcancer/cervcancerrs.htm

van Rijswijk, R., & Vermorken, J. (2000). Drug therapy for gynaecological cancer in older women. *Drugs and Aging, 17*(1), 13–32.

Wenzel, L., Donnelly, J., Fowler, J., Habbal, R., Taylor, T., Aziz, N., & Cella, D. (2002). Resilience, reflection, and residual stress in ovarian cancer survivorship: A gynecologic oncology group study. *Psycho-Oncology, 11*, 142–153.

The Climacteric and Menopause

Introduction

Over the last century, the life expectancy of women in the United States has risen dramatically. As of 2014, the life expectancy for women from birth is 81 years. By race, the life expectancy is 81.3 years for white women, 78 years for African-American women, and 83.8 years for Hispanic women (Arias, 2014). Not only are women living longer but many are living one-third to one-half of their lives beyond the menopause. Subsequently, health issues associated with aging women have come to the forefront of society and health care.

All aging women, regardless of color, socioeconomic status, education level, or religion, are united by menopause. Menopause is a milestone experience that is unique and individual among women (Brockie, 2008). The menopause produces physical, psychological, social, and emotional changes in women's lives. For some, menopause can be a tumultuous event in their lives, and for others it can occur with hardly any difficulty. Overall, the changes brought about by menopause can greatly influence quality of life. This chapter will focus on the multidimensional process of menopause and the impact of menopause on the quality of life of women.

Conceptualizations of Menopause

Specific assumptions about menopause and the current state of knowledge of menopause have led to the emergence of distinct conceptualizations of this natural occurrence in the reproductive cycle of women. These diverse conceptualizations have shaped current attitudes and therapeutic approaches. The conceptualizations of menopause found in North American culture include biomedical, psychological/psychosocial, sociocultural, and feminist perspectives. Although no individual conceptualization is comprehensive enough to explain all of the complexities of menopause, examining each perspective and its underlying assumptions will enhance understanding of the multidimensional nature of menopause.

Biomedical Conceptualization

The biomedical conceptualization defines menopause as an estrogen deficiency condition. The symptoms of menopause, both physical and psychological, are the result of cessation of ovarian function and subsequent estrogen withdrawal. The treatment approach is therefore hormonal replacement (Barile, 1997). The basis of the biomedical perspective attributes the event of menopause to biology with medical treatment as the appropriate response and eliminates the assignment of blame or punishment to women for their symptoms (Barile, 1997). However, this perspective "medicalizes" menopause and in essence, transfers control of menopause from women to physicians. This view promotes dependency of women on physicians for treatment. In addition, it is posited that the medicalization of menopause reinforces the gender bias that has shaped medical treatment and research, and fosters the stereotypical view of women as biologically inferior to men (Barile, 1997; Meyer, 2001, 2003).

Psychological/Psychosocial Conceptualization

The psychological/psychosocial conceptualization of menopause views menopausal symptoms—in particular, depression—as being associated with social factors such as multiple roles, marital stress, social circumstances, and losses, specifically the loss of femininity and youth (Barile, 1997). Changes and losses related to menopause and aging are numerous and encompass physical aspects such as altered appearance, changes in mental and sensory acuity, decreased mobility, and altered health, as well as psychosocial losses such as retirement, children leaving the nest, and loss of spouse and friends to illness and death. Within this framework, depression, stress, or premorbid personality patterns help explain the underlying cause of menopausal symptoms. Treatment strategies are aimed at alleviating depression or anxiety with psychotherapy or pharmacologic therapy, particularly for the psychological symptoms (Barile, 1997). The basis of this perspective attributes the event of menopause to psychological rather than biological cause, and the burden of blame and responsibility for menopause symptoms is placed on the woman. This perspective emphasizes a need for medical treatment, social supports, and coping skills (Barile, 1997). It eliminates consideration of biological factors and reduces women to a set of roles and functions or to a composite of reactions to society and environment (Li, Carlson, Snyder, & Holm, 1995).

Sociocultural Conceptualization

The sociocultural conceptualization views menopause within the context of social or cultural-symbolic events, with role changes or cultural attitudes toward menopause and aging identified as primary factors related to menopausal symptoms (Li et al., 1995). Within the sociocultural perspective, women's social and cultural history determines their reactions to menopause, and thus women from diverse cultures will cope differently with the event (Barile, 1997). In cultures where age is respected and women's status and prestige increase with age, menopause is viewed positively as transition to higher status. Furthermore, in cultures where menopause is viewed as an unavoidable and normal stage of the life cycle, the event brings freedom from anxiety over pregnancy and menstruation. Women from these cultures tend to experience fewer problems with menopause (Barile, 1997). In cultures where age is devalued and youth and sex highly valued, menopause and aging are generally viewed negatively and perceived with apprehension (Li et al., 1995). Treatment strategies are aimed at cognitive restructuring, encouraging women to assume an active, advocate role in changing their environment, and to learn effective coping responses to the attitudes and values of their culture toward women and aging. The sociocultural perspective expands the view of menopause to explain cultural differences; however, it can foster self-blame and feelings of inadequacy in women who compare themselves to women of other cultures (Barile, 1997).

Feminist Conceptualization

The feminist conceptualization views menopause as a normal physiological and developmental process that is health-enhancing rather than health-compromising, and is an inevitable life transition or passage associated with challenges and freedoms (Barile, 1997; Meyer, 2003). From this perspective, treatment strategies highlight the normality of life transitions and cognitive restructuring that enhance the view of menopause as a challenge within women's control. Also, coping strategies for managing the challenges of life transition are emphasized, as well as alternative natural and homeopathic treatments (Barile, 1997). The feminist perspective places women in control of their experiences and empowers them to learn about their bodies and be active participants in their own health. While this view assimilates well with the other perspectives, there may be a tendency to underestimate the biological, psychological, and sociocultural facets of menopause when attitude alone is considered an adequate approach to the process (Barile, 1997).

Menopause is a multidimensional process and the conceptualizations discussed here reflect that multidimensionality. These perspectives are not mutually exclusive, and contain several overlapping facets. This chapter discusses menopause from an integrative perspective that incorporates the biomedical, psychological/psychosocial, sociocultural, and feminist views of the process and its symptoms, treatment strategies, and impact on quality of life.

Incidence

Menopause marks the end of ovarian endocrine function in women, and subsequently the end of menstruation. The median age at which final menses occurs in American women is approximately 51.4 years. Preceding the end of menses is the climacteric, or perimenopause, a period of physiologic changes that marks the transition from fertility to infertility. The median age for the onset of the climacteric is 47 years (Santoro & Chervenak, 2004). Menopause that occurs before age 30 is likely associated with chromosomal abnormalities or autoimmune disorders. Early or premature menopause occurs between the ages of 31 to 40 years and accounts for about 1% of women who experience natural menopause. This number does not include women who have surgically or medically induced menopause. Menopause after the age of 40 is considered normal, and is considered late after the age of 55. Late menopause occurs in approximately 2% of the women undergoing natural menopause (Santoro, 2007).

The characteristic perimenopause, or transition to menopause, starts with menstrual irregularity at the approximate age of 47, followed by intermittent cycling that continues for about 4 years. Then complete amenorrhea is achieved at approximately 51 to 52 years of age (Santoro, 2007). Transition ends 12 months after the final menses.

Various lifestyle and social factors play a role in influencing the age at which menopause occurs. Cigarette smoking has been associated with advancing the onset of menopause by approximately 2 years (Santoro & Chervenak, 2004). Findings from the Study of Women's Health Across the Nation (SWAN) suggest that higher body mass index, smoking, non-contraceptive hormone use, and a history of osteoporosis were also associated with premature menopause (Santoro, 2004).

Ethnic Considerations

Ethnic differences associated with the age at final menses have been noted. Findings from the SWAN study indicate that African-American and Latina women tend to experience menopause slightly earlier than the median age while Japanese-American and Chinese-American women tend to complete menopausal transition slightly later than the median age (Santoro & Chervenak, 2004). Latina women experience menopause approximately 6 months earlier than women of other ethnic groups (SWAN: Study of Women's Health Across the Nation [SWAN], 2003).

African-American and Latina women are more likely to experience premature menopause while Chinese and Japanese women are least likely to have an early menopause (Green & Santoro, 2009). In addition, ethnic variation exists in the prevalence of hysterectomy at an earlier age that can induce premature menopause. Hysterectomy that is indicated for benign conditions such as uterine fibroids, abnormal bleeding, endometriosis, and pelvic organ prolapse is more prevalent in African-American and Latina women (Green & Santoro, 2009).

Some menopausal symptoms seem to be more common among various ethnic groups. In the SWAN study, approximately 46.5% of African-American women and 49.4% of Latina women experience hot flashes and night sweats as opposed to 36.6% Chinese, 34.3% Japanese, and 28.9% Caucasian women (Green & Santoro, 2009). Latina and African-American women are more likely to be vulnerable to depressive symptoms and sleep disturbances than Chinese and Japanese women. In addition, Latina women are more likely to suffer from vaginal symptoms than other ethnic groups (Green & Santoro, 2009). It is important to note that ethnicity alone may not explain the disparities in menopausal symptoms that appear among the various ethnic groups. Acculturation, or lack of it, may be a confounding factor in influencing ethnic disparity in menopausal symptoms (Green & Santoro, 2009). Lower socioeconomic status is associated with increased symptom burden, greater functional limitations, higher prevalence of disease at baseline, greater perceived stress, and earlier age at menopause (Santoro, 2004; Santoro & Sutton-Tyrell, 2011).

Etiology and Risk Factors

Natural menopause occurs in response to changes in the functioning of the hypothalamic-pituitary-ovarian axis. The perimenopausal period starts approximately 2 to 8 years preceding the cessation of menses and includes the 12 months of amenorrhea following the final menses. During perimenopause, women experience a change in the length and character of the menstrual cycle. Elevated levels of follicle stimulating hormone (FSH) and luteinizing hormone (LH), as well as decreased levels of estradiol and inhibin, occur. Aging ovaries produce follicles that are less responsive to FSH. The negative feedback effect of elevated estrogen and progesterone on hypothalamic production of gonadotropin releasing-hormone is no longer functional, and anterior pituitary production of FSH and LH persists.

As a result, women commonly experience irregular menstrual cycles characterized by longer or shorter cycles, heavier or lighter flow, periods of amenorrhea, and worsening or newly developing premenstrual syndrome. In due course, fewer ovarian follicles develop, until the follicle supply is completely depleted. Estrogen and progesterone levels are low and FSH and LH levels continue to be elevated. Complete cessation of menstruation will occur. However, until menstruation ceases, unpredictable ovarian function can lead to ovulation. If contraception is not used, an unexpected pregnancy is possible.

Menopause may be surgically or medically induced. Surgical menopause occurs when the ovaries are surgically removed in a bilateral oophorectomy. Medically induced menopause can be caused by medications, chemotherapy, or radiation that destroys ovarian function. Women who undergo medical or surgical menopause experience untimely loss of fertility as well as symptoms that tend to be more severe than those experienced with natural menopause. In addition, women who experience induced menopause are likely younger than the women who undergo natural menopause, and thus lack the protective influence of estrogen for a longer period of time. Consequently, women who experience induced menopause may face a greater risk of developing cardiovascular disease and osteoporosis as well as congestive heart failure, stroke, fractures, parkinsonism, dementia, cognitive impairment, depression, and anxiety (Gallagher, 2007; Lobo, 2007; Santoro & Sutton-Tyrell, 2011).

Following menopause, women are at a higher risk for developing chronic disorders. Hormonal and physiologic changes that occur at midlife and are associated with menopause may significantly increase women's risk for the development of, most notably, cardiovascular disease, osteoarthritis, osteoporosis, and Alzheimer's disease. Strategies for the reduction of risk for the following diseases will be discussed in other chapters of this unit.

Cardiovascular Disease

Many risk factors for cardiovascular disease are unfavorably modified as a result of menopausal changes. Women experience alterations in lipid metabolism and fat distribution in the body. Levels of low density lipoprotein (LDL) cholesterol, very low density lipoprotein (VLDL) cholesterol, and levels of triglycerides tend to increase during menopause, while levels of high density lipoprotein (HDL) cholesterol tend to decrease (Abernethy, 2008). These changes in lipoproteins significantly increase women's risk of developing cardiovascular disease. Additionally, estrogen and progestin reduction that results from menopause may be associated with reduced vascular elasticity, which contributes to increased risk of hypertension.

Body fat redistribution and weight gain frequently occur at midlife. Adipose tissue that was more likely to accumulate at the thighs of younger women, which contributed to a "pear"-shaped silhouette, is redistributed to the waist and contributes to an "apple"-shaped silhouette. A waist circumference larger than 35 cm along with a body mass index (BMI) greater than 30 kg/m^2 are associated with an increased risk of developing insulin resistance and can lead to cardiovascular disease and diabetes. Moreover, a higher incidence of hot flashes, night sweats, and soreness or stiffness in the back, shoulders, and neck is associated with having a BMI greater than 27 kg/m^2 (Abernethy, 2008).

Osteoarthritis

Estrogen deficiency increases the risk of developing osteoarthritis in postmenopausal women (National Institute of Arthritis, and Musculoskeletal and Skin Diseases [NIAMS], 2013). The incidence of osteoarthritis and related joint symptoms has been noted to increase at menopause (Cimmino & Parodi, 2005). Joint cartilage has estrogen receptors and its metabolism is hormonally sensitive. The estrogen deficiency associated with menopause likely contributes to the pathogenesis of the disease (Cimmino & Parodi, 2005; Von Mühlen, Morton, Von Mühlen, & Barrett-Connor, 2002).

Osteoporosis

Postmenopausal women have an escalated risk of developing osteoporosis. Bone remodeling is an ongoing process in which bone resorption activity is equal to that of bone formation activity. Peak bone mass is achieved in women in their late 20s to mid 30s, after which bone resorption and formation become relatively stable. At menopause, estrogen decline influences increased bone turnover and excessive bone resorption that results in decreased bone mass throughout the entire skeleton. The rate of bone loss in the first year after menopause is rapid, between 1% and 5%, and slows to approximately 1% per year thereafter.

Alzheimer's Disease

The risk of developing Alzheimer's disease is significantly higher in women than in men. This statistic contributes to the premise that deficiency of estrogen at menopause may play a role in the cascade of pathological processes that leads to Alzheimer's disease (Craig & Murphy, 2009). However, research that has investigated the influence of estrogen therapy on the prevention and treatment of Alzheimer's disease has produced equivocal results. Findings have indicated that estrogen therapy given to women at the time of menopause may delay or reduce the risk of developing Alzheimer's disease but does not have clinical benefits as a treatment for it (Craig & Murphy, 2009).

Gender Similarities and Differences

While menopause occurs in women, a similar condition of hormonal decline is thought to occur in men. This natural decline in testosterone in middle-aged men is referred to as andropause, male menopause, male climacteric, androgen deficiency, or partial androgen deficiency in the aging male (PADAM). Women experience estrogen decline rather abruptly over a period of several months, or continuing for a number of years. Men, on the other hand, experience a natural decline in testosterone production gradually, beginning any time after age 30, and the decline progresses over decades. More frequently than not, symptoms appear in men in their fifties (Varner, 2013).

Andropause is thought to produce physiological and psychological symptoms similar to those experienced by women during menopause. The symptoms that men commonly report include mood swings, anger, fatigue, loss of cognitive skills, depression, insomnia, irritability, loss of body hair, erectile dysfunction, decreased libido, weakness, loss of lean body and bone mass, skin changes, loss of muscle strength, increased abdominal and visceral body fat, and hot flashes (Varner, 2013). Decreased testosterone levels are thought to contribute to an increased risk of hyperlipidemia, heart disease, diabetes, and osteoporosis in men (Varner, 2013).

The insidious onset and nonspecific nature of the symptoms makes andropause difficult to diagnose for a number of reasons. Men are often reluctant to seek help or advice because of embarrassment or because they perceive their symptoms as part of aging and thus rarely seek medical help (Peate, 2003). If men do seek medical help for their symptoms, the physician often confirms that the symptoms are a normal part of aging and further investigation is infrequent (Gould, 2005). Testosterone levels decline with advancing age, and they vary during the day. There is also considerable variability in the range of normal laboratory values of testosterone, which implies that a substantial decline in hormone levels can occur but still be considered within a normal range. Hormone levels can greatly differ among healthy older men and can be influenced by health and lifestyle, including such factors as smoking, obesity, alcohol use, and various disease states (Leonard, 2004; McKinlay, Travison, Araujo, & Kupelian, 2007; Peate, 2003; Tunuguntla, 2005).

Once the diagnosis of andropause is made, treatment is clear-cut. Hormone replacement therapy (HRT) is prescribed in order to gain relief of symptoms related to the androgenic deficiency. Delivery methods of hormone replacement include oral androgens, transdermal adhesives and gels, subcutaneous implants, and injectable androgens. However, HRT is not without risk. Testosterone therapy can increase the risk of prostate cancer, lipid abnormalities, sleep apnea, polycythemia, liver toxicity, heart disease, gynecomastia, water retention, irritability, acne, hair loss, and testicular atrophy (de Melo, Soares, & Baragatti, 2013; Ginsberg & Cavalieri, 2008).

Although research in the area of female menopause has been abundant, comparable investigation related to andropause tends to be scarce, especially concerning safety and efficacy of testosterone replacement therapy. Moreover, similar to the varied perceptions of female menopause, the healthcare community also debates whether andropause is a normal part of aging, a psychosocial construct, or a disease of hormone deficiency that should be treated with hormone replacement (Vainiopää & Topo, 2006).

Diagnosing Menopause

The occurrence of menopause is most evident by a woman's age, changes in the menstrual cycle, and presence of menopausal symptoms. Menopause is definitively diagnosed when menses have ceased for a period of twelve months. Resumption of the menses after the 12-month absence is extremely rare and might be seen in circumstances where menopause was temporarily induced by a medical condition or chemotherapy. Testing serum FSH levels is not considered a reliable method for diagnosing menopause. FSH levels may be used to indicate decline in ovarian function but results can be misleading. FSH levels are unpredictable based on whether the ovary secretes estrogen. Consequently, consistently elevated FSH greater than 40 IU/ml suggests menopause but does not predict *when* final ovarian failure has occurred.

As women transition through menopause, symptoms occur mainly due to the diminished effect of estrogen on target organs in the body as well as aging. The prevalence and severity of symptoms vary among women and may be influenced by environmental and lifestyle factors such as climate, culture, diet, women's roles, attitudes towards cessation of reproductive abilities, and aging (Brockie, 2008). The classic symptoms of menopause include vasomotor reactivity, urogenital atrophy, and psychological distress. Each of these problems can greatly influence the quality of life of menopausal women (Van der Mooren & Kenemans, 2004).

Vasomotor Reactivity

Vasomotor symptoms are the most common symptoms experienced by nearly all women undergoing menopausal transition, although severity and frequency can vary widely. Vasomotor symptoms include hot flashes, sweating, and palpitations. The hot flash is caused by unexpected vasodilation of the superficial blood vessels in the skin, and is characterized by a feeling of intense heat that rushes through the body, neck, and head. The skin may redden to a blush and perspiration can develop. Hot flashes may last from a few seconds to several minutes and occur frequently at night, often severely.

Urogenital Atrophy

The reduction of estrogen in menopause affects the collagen content in the skin and urogenital structures as well as contractile response of smooth muscle, leading to atrophy. Atrophy consequently leads to urinary, vaginal, and vulvar symptoms, which are presented in **Table 12–1**. Urinary

Table 12–1 UROGENITAL SYMPTOMS ASSOCIATED WITH MENOPAUSE

Urinary Symptoms	Vaginal Symptoms	Vulvar Symptoms
Frequency	Vaginal dryness	Pruritus
Urgency	Atrophic vaginitis	Vulvar atrophy
Incontinence	Dyspareunia	Progressive loss of pubic hair
Urethritis	Postcoital bleeding	
Cystitis	Uterine prolapse	

incontinence is not unusual with aging but is never normal. Lower estrogen levels are associated with urethral atrophy, which can further increase the likelihood of developing incontinence. Women commonly experience stress incontinence, urge incontinence, or a combination of both. Incontinence conditions that are less common include overflow incontinence (leakage related to urinary retention) and extraurethral incontinence, in which urine leaks through a bladder fistula, which could develop as a complication caused by bladder injury during a hysterectomy. In addition to the physical changes of the vagina, women may experience lowered libido, decreased arousal, and decline in sexual function.

Psychosomatic Symptoms

Women often experience psychosomatic symptoms that include mood swings, irritability, forgetfulness, nervous tension, dizzy spells, poor concentration, sleep disruption, insomnia, tiredness, and depression. Symptoms may be interrelated as well as occur independently of each other, a complex phenomenon that is not well understood (Avis, Brockwell, & Colvin, 2005). In some women, psychosomatic symptoms may develop as a domino effect of vasomotor symptoms. For example, women experiencing hot flashes that repeatedly interrupt sleep are likely to experience tiredness, irritability, and poor concentration. Psychosomatic symptoms may occur in the absence of vasomotor symptoms or

may be attributed to aging or other physical or psychosocial factors. Midlife women often face considerable stress and pressures from responsibilities and worries involving family, finances, health, bereavement, and employment issues, which can influence psychosomatic symptoms (Brockie, 2008).

Research evidence suggests that negative attitudes and views of menopause and aging may adversely influence symptom presentation and severity (Deeks, 2004). Results of several cross-racial and multiethnic studies indicate that race, ethnicity, and differing cultural beliefs and values can be influential factors in symptom experience (Avis, Brockwell, & Colvin, 2005).

Treatment of Symptoms

Whether menopause is viewed as a normal transition in life, sociocultural phenomenon, or hormonal deficiency, the experience is unique to each woman and several options are available to reduce the impact associated with menopausal symptoms. Treatment approaches include lifestyle modification, nonprescription therapies, and prescription therapies. No treatment is needed unless menopausal symptoms become bothersome. Women with mild vasomotor symptoms are treated with lifestyle modification and nonprescription options. Women with moderate to severe vasomotor symptoms can be offered prescription systemic hormone and nonhormonal products.

Lifestyle Modification

Lifestyle modification consists of strategies that help to reduce discomfort and improve well-being. These strategies include dietary modification, exercise, improvement of personal comfort and well-being, sleep hygiene therapies, and cognitive engagement.

DIETARY MODIFICATION

A balanced diet low in saturated fat, containing adequate fiber, and rich in calcium and vitamin D is recommended (Murkies, 2004). Recommended calcium intake should be approximately 1,000 mg per day for women 50 years and younger; and 1,200 mg per day for women over 50 years of age. Recommended vitamin D intake is 600 IU per day for adult women 70 years of age and younger and 800 IU per day for women older than 70. (Shifren & Gass, 2014). Foods such as sugar (especially refined sugar), caffeinated beverages and foods containing caffeine, spicy foods, and alcohol can contribute to more frequent or severe hot flashes. Avoidance or decreased intake of these foods is suggested (Holloway, 2008; Loprinzi, Wolf, Barton, & Laack, 2008).

Women may experience increased loss of body fluids through excessive perspiration. Increasing water intake (especially cold water) to at least six to eight glasses per day will maintain adequate hydration and can help reduce discomfort associated with hot flashes and sweating. Women who experience nocturia or urinary incontinence will need to coordinate water consumption according to time of day, needs for social occasions, or availability of bathroom facilities.

EXERCISE

It is well known that exercise is beneficial for enhancing well-being. Exercise increases the release of endorphins, which can improve mood and chronic pain. Regular exercise can also reduce the risk of developing heart disease, osteoporosis, diabetes, and obesity. Evidence suggests that increased physical activity is associated with lower prevalence of certain of menopausal symptoms, such as forgetfulness, depressive mood, sleep disturbance, stiffness/soreness, and heart palpitations (McAndrew et al., 2009; Wilbur, Miller, McDevitt, Wang, & Miller, 2005); however, findings have been inconsistent regarding the effects of exercise in preventing or reducing vasomotor symptoms (Aiello et al., 2004; Daley, Stokes-Lampard, Mutrie, & MacArthur, 2007; Whitcomb, Whiteman, Lagenberg, Flaws, & Romani, 2007). Daily weight bearing exercise, such as walking briskly for at least 30 minutes, combined with a resistance training program twice a week is an ideal regimen for obtaining beneficial effects on bone density, muscle strength, and cardiac fitness (Asikainen, Kukkonen-Harjula, & Miilunpalo, 2004). Women should be advised to consult with their healthcare provider prior to beginning an exercise regimen.

IMPROVEMENT OF PERSONAL COMFORT AND WELL-BEING

Relief of vaginal dryness and dyspareunia may be optimized by the use of nonhormonal vaginal lubricants that are available without prescription. Products on the market include water-based lubricants and polycarbophil moisturizers. Water-based lubricants (such as Astroglide, Intimate Options, K-Y Personal Lubricant, Lubrin, Moist Again, and Silk E), contain water-soluble substances that coat the vagina and provide surface lubrication that eases penetration during intercourse. Polycarbophil moisturizers contain a bioadhesive polymer that is water swellable, not water soluble, and binds directly to vaginal tissue, providing more than surface lubrication. The hydrating characteristic of the polycarbophil moisturizer tends to restore vaginal pH to premenopausal levels and decreases vaginal dryness, itching, and irritation (North American Menopause Society [NAMS], 2015; Wiggins & Dizon, 2008). Women who experience vaginal dryness should be advised to use products designed solely for vaginal use and to avoid products that contain perfumes or alcohol, such as hand creams, which can increase burning and itching. Furthermore, women should avoid using oil-based products such as baby oil or petroleum jelly, which can cause irritation, damage to condoms and diaphragms, and can harbor abnormal vaginal and bladder bacteria, leading to increased infections.

Women who experience incontinence may be encouraged to use incontinence pads to protect clothing and reduce embarrassment. Incontinence pads are more absorbent than menstrual pads and offer better skin protection. Women may also be fitted with incontinence pessaries to be worn continuously or just during activities that induce incontinence, such as running or aerobics. Women should try drinking adequate water to keep urine diluted (clear and pale yellow), and avoid foods or beverages with a high acid or caffeine content, which may irritate the bladder lining (NAMS, 2015). Foods to avoid include grapefruit, oranges, tomatoes, coffee, and caffeine-containing soft drinks. Voiding at regular intervals rather than waiting for the physical sensation of the urge to urinate can reduce the amount of urine in the bladder and decrease incontinence episodes. Practicing Kegel exercises to strengthen the pelvic floor muscle can also be effective in improving incontinence episodes (NAMS, 2015). Also, women who cough due to smoking, allergies, or asthma should quit smoking or seek treatment to control coughing, which would help reduce stress incontinence episodes. If conservative measures are unsuccessful, anticholinergic medication or surgical options may be considered.

Women who experience hot flashes can increase their personal comfort by wearing fabrics that absorb perspiration and allow air to circulate, such as cotton or linen. Women should wear layers of clothing that can be removed during a hot flash. Ambient temperatures are thought to influence frequency and severity of hot flashes; thus maintaining a cool environment with use of air conditioning, fans, or open windows is recommended. Reducing core body temperature by ingesting cold foods and beverages can also be helpful (Loprinzi et al., 2008; Ravnikar, Santoro, & Utian, 2005).

Because smoking is associated with higher prevalence and severity of vasomotor symptoms as well as increased morbidity and mortality associated with diseases such as cardiovascular disease, cancer, and osteoporosis, smoking cessation is strongly recommended. Numerous options are available that can assist individuals to stop smoking, such as medication, counseling, hypnosis, and support programs. Motivation and a desire to quit are essential factors for success in smoking cessation.

Stress has been associated with increased prevalence of menopausal symptoms (Balk, 2003). Research suggests that stress management and relaxation may improve symptoms such as hot flashes, night sweats, sleep disturbance, depressed mood, and anxiety (Hunter, 2003; Hunter, Coventry, Hamed, Fentiman, & Grunfeld, 2009). Techniques such as regular exercise, relaxation therapy, deep breathing, cognitive behavioral therapy, yoga, tai chi, massage therapy, and spiritual practices have been efficacious in reducing stress and moderating a variety of menopausal symptoms (Balk, 2003; Hunter, 2003; Hunter et al., 2009; Alexander & Andrist, 2013). Since the menopausal experience is unique to each woman and symptom prevalence and intensity varies from woman to woman, stress management should be individualized to each woman and her lifestyle.

Sleep Hygiene

Sleep disturbances in midlife women are often attributed to menopausal symptoms such as hot flashes and night sweats, but may also be associated with sleep disorders, stress, social and family factors, depressive symptoms, and other comorbid health conditions (Minarik, 2009). A vicious cycle often develops in which the various physical or psychosocial symptoms or conditions disrupt sleep, which in turn further influences the presence, frequency, or severity of symptoms or conditions. The complexity of sleep disturbance necessitates that women receive a thorough clinical assessment that contains both subjective and objective descriptions of sleep habits, sleep patterns, sleep environment, health problems, cognitive and behavioral status, menopausal vasomotor symptoms, lifestyle behaviors, and depression. Appropriate referrals for care of underlying physical and mental conditions that affect sleep, such as obesity, diabetes, nocturia, and depression should be made. Women who are identified with primary sleep disorders should be referred to an accredited sleep clinic for care (Minarik, 2009).

Various strategies can be helpful in improving quality of sleep in menopausal women. Vasomotor symptom control is an important step in restoring healthy sleep patterns. Maintaining a cool and comfortable sleep environment, wearing lightweight cotton sleepwear, use of lightweight cotton bedding, and utilizing previously discussed strategies to reduce frequency and intensity of vasomotor symptoms will be helpful.

Midlife psychosocial factors also influence sleep disruption, so additional strategies to enhance sleep should be considered. Stress reduction techniques, relaxation, and cognitive behavioral therapy are effective options. In addition, stimulus control therapy can be used to form a positive association between the individual's bed and sleep to establish a stable sleep–wake pattern. Another behavioral therapy, sleep restriction, limits time in bed to total sleep time, which helps to improve sleep continuity. Biofeedback techniques are helpful in reducing somatic arousal, as is cognitive therapy, which confronts an individual's fear of staying awake and its potential effects in order to eliminate anxiety about sleep performance (Schutte-Rodin, Broch, Buysse, Dorsey & Sateia, 2008).

Sleep hygiene therapy involves engaging in healthy lifestyle practices to improve quality of sleep. Women should be taught to keep to a regular sleeping schedule in a quiet sleeping environment. They should consume a healthy diet and avoid alcohol and stimulants such as caffeine and nicotine. Excessive fluids should not be taken before bedtime. Regular exercise is recommended, but stimulating activities should be avoided before bedtime. The bedroom should be used only for sleep or sexual activities. Daytime napping should also be avoided. Engaging in relaxation behaviors at bedtime can also be helpful (Schutte-Rodin et al., 2008).

COGNITIVE ENGAGEMENT

Cognitive difficulties such as forgetfulness and lack of concentration are thought to be associated with estrogen deficiency in relation to estrogen receptors in the brain, and can also be a result of aging. In addition, fatigue, moodiness, sleep disturbance, stress, or an underlying medical condition can negatively influence cognitive function. Research findings suggest that among menopausal women, forgetfulness is a frequently perceived symptom and is ranked high in severity (Berg, Larson, & Pasvogel, 2008).

The initial approach should be a thorough assessment to rule out physical or psychological conditions that may be producing cognitive symptoms. Once the potential for organic conditions has been eliminated, women should be advised that forgetfulness is likely due to menopause, and is aging related, and strategies that increase cognitive engagement may be helpful in managing cognitive symptoms. Use of calendars, visual reminders, and lists for task completion can help reduce the stress of forgetfulness. Participation in intellectually energizing pursuits, puzzles, hobbies, and other activities can help to maintain cognitive engagement and improve function. Obtaining adequate sleep and rest are also important strategies for improving cognitive function.

Nonprescription Therapies

Nonprescription therapies are mainly complementary and alternative remedies, which comprise a broad range of healing strategies that women may use to find relief from menopausal symptoms. The use of complementary and alternative therapies by perimenopausal and postmenopausal women in this regard has increased significantly. Therapies frequently used for symptom relief include alternative medical systems, such as traditional Chinese medicine, mind-body medicine, and biologically based treatment. Research findings as to the effectiveness of these strategies for symptom reduction are generally scarce or equivocal.

Traditional Chinese Medicine

As noted in Chapter 4, traditional Chinese medicine (TCM) is a system of healing that emphasizes proper balance of two opposing and inseparable forces: yin and yang. An imbalance of yin and yang is thought to lead to the blockage of blood and vital energy of the body, known as *qi*, along pathways known as meridians. In TCM, menopause is considered to be part of an occurrence that involves an imbalance of vital energy. The TCM practitioner may use an individualized combination of herbs, meditation, breathing exercises, diet, or acupuncture to bring the body back into harmony and reduce menopausal symptoms.

Mind-Body Medicine

This system focuses on the interaction of brain, mind, body, and behavior and the powerful ways in which emotional, mental, social, spiritual, and behavioral factors can directly influence health. Strategies such as hypnosis, dance, music, prayer, mental healing, relaxation and visual imagery, meditation, and yoga appear to be helpful when used in conjunction with conventional medicine to reduce anxiety and pain, and improve quality of life. Biofeedback techniques have been effective in reducing episodes of hot flashes and stress incontinence. Major advantages to using mind-body techniques are the lack of adverse side effects and minimal health risks.

Biologically Based Treatment

The biologically based treatments used most often by perimenopausal and postmenopausal women include botanical therapies derived from herbs and phytoestrogens. Botanical therapies are complex mixtures of preparations made from the whole plant or plant part, such as root, leaves, gum, resin, or essential oil. Most botanical therapies are medicinal herbs, which produce and contain chemical substances that act on the body. Although herbal therapies are natural and thought to be safer than prescription drugs, herbs can have pharmacological effects and adverse side effects. It is imperative that women who use herbs be advised that herbal therapies can interact with prescription drugs and result in enhanced or diminished effects of the herb, the drug, or both, or an entirely new effect that is not seen when either substance is taken alone. Caution must be exercised by women who use herbal therapies, and their healthcare providers should be consulted regarding herbal use. Common botanical therapies and adverse effects are presented in **Table 12–2**.

Phytoestrogens are complex plant compounds that are metabolized from plant foods high in fiber, such as legumes, soybeans, vegetables, and cereals. Soy isoflavones, a subgroup of phytoestrogens thought to possess estrogenic properties, are most commonly associated with menopausal symptom management. Although research results pointing to soy and soy isoflavone effectiveness in relief of vasomotor symptoms has been equivocal, there may be small benefit in symptom reduction (Shifren & Gass, 2014). The most promising results of soy and soy isoflavone effectiveness appear to be in maintaining cognitive function of postmenopausal women—in particular, in

Table 12–2 Common Botanical Therapies Used by Perimenopausal and Postmenopausal Women

Botanical	Use	Adverse Effects
Black Cohosh (*Cimicifuga racemosa* or *Actaea racemosa*)	Relief of hot flushes. Efficacy of treatment is inconclusive in clinical trials.	Occasional gastrointestinal discomfort, nausea, vomiting, frontal headache, bradycardia, rare possibility of liver failure.
Chastetree Berry (*Vitex agnus-castus*)	Irregular menstruation, heavy irregular uterine bleeding premenstrual syndrome, cyclical mastalgia. Significant improvement of symptoms demonstrated in clinical trials.	Nausea, headache, gastrointestinal disturbances, menstrual disorders, acne, pruritis, erythematous rash, decreased libido. Not recommended for women with low libido.
Dong Quai (*Angelica sinensis*)	Used with other herbs in TCM to treat gynecological conditions. Efficacy for relief of hot flushes has not been confirmed by clinical trials.	Photosensitivity, hypotension, and anticoagulation. May trigger heavy uterine bleeding. Contraindicated in women with fibroids, blood clotting problems. Contraindicated for use with anticoagulants.
Evening Primrose Oil (*Oenothera biennis*)	Relief of hot flushes. Efficacy of treatment is inconclusive in clinical trials.	Inflammation, thrombosis, immunosuppression, nausea, diarrhea. Increased risk of seizures in seizure disorders, those taking antipsychotic drugs and drugs that lower seizure threshhold. Contraindicated for use with phenothiazines.
Ginkgo (*Ginkgo biloba*)	Improve memory and cognitive function. Efficacy of treatment is promising in clinical trials.	Gastrointestinal distress and headache. Large doses may cause restlessness, anxiety, allergic skin reactions, sleep disturbance, diarrhea, nausea, vomiting. Chronic use may increase risk of bleeding, subdural hematoma, and subarachnoid hemorrhage.
Ginseng: Chinese, Korean, Asian (*Panax ginseng*); American (*Panax quinquefolius*)	Relief of hot flushes. Efficacy of treatment is inconclusive in clinical trials.	Nervousness, insomnia, dizziness, hypertension, mastalgia with diffuse breast nodularity, reduction in blood glucose levels. Contraindicated for those with breast cancer, and for use with antihypertensives, stimulants, MAO inhibitors, digoxin, anticoagulants. Has multiple drug interactions.

(continues)

Table 12–2 Common Botanical Therapies Used by Perimenopausal and Postmenopausal Women (*continued*)

Botanical	Use	Adverse Effects
Kava (*Piper methysticum*)	Anxiety, irritability, insomnia hot flushes. Significant improvement of symptoms demonstrated in clinical trials.	Minor gastrointestinal upset, headache, sedation, restlessness. Heavy chronic use causes yellowing and scaling of skin, and eye irritation. Product is associated with liver toxicity. Contraindicated for use with depression, alcohol, psychotropics, antihistamine, or substances that cause sleepiness or confusion.
Licorice Root (*Glycyrrhiza glabra*)	Used with other herbs in TCM formulations for menopause-related symptoms. Efficacy of treatment is inconclusive in clinical trials.	Large chronic doses may cause pseudoprimary aldosteronism with symptoms of edema, hypertension, and hypokalemia. Contraindicated in heart failure, arrhythmias, hypertension, hypokalemia, hypertonis, kidney failure, liver disease, diabetes, cirrhosis, or diuretic use.
Passion Flower (*Passiflora incarnata)*	Relief of insomnia. Efficacy of treatment is inconclusive in clinical trials.	Contraindicated for use with MAO inhibitors.
Red Clover (*Trifolium pretense*)	Relief of hot flushes. Isoflavones are often isolated from the herb. Efficacy of treatment is inconclusive in clinical trials.	High doses may cause rash. Contraindicated in use with estrogen, progesterone, blood thinners, pregnancy, or in breast cancer.
Sage (*Salvia officinalis*)	Relief of hot flushes, night sweats. Safe for use as a tea. Ethanolic extracts containing thujone are not recommended.	Prolonged or excessive use of ethanolic extract can cause vomiting, vertigo, kidney damage, convulsions.
St. John's Wort (*Hypericum perforatum*)	Relief of depression. Significant improvement of symptoms demonstrated in clinical trials. Also used in combination with black cohosh for relief of hot flushes.	Photosensitivity and cataract formation, gastrointestinal distress, fatigue. Users should avoid sunbathing and protect themselves from sun exposure. Contraindicated for concomitant use with psychotropic drugs, SSRIs, warfarin, digoxin, theophylline, idinavir, cyclosporine, and phenprocoumon. Breakthrough vaginal bleeding may occur when used with oral contraceptives containing ethinyl estradiol and desogestrel.
Valerian (*Valeriana officinalis*)	Nervousness and insomnia. Significant improvement of symptoms demonstrated in clinical trials.	Long-term administration may be associated with headache, restlessness, sleeplessness, cardiac disorders.

improving category fluency, verbal memory, mental flexibility, and planning ability. Accordingly, the inclusion of soy in the diet of nonallergic perimenopausal and postmenopausal women may be beneficial (Geller & Studee, 2005).

Prescription Therapies

When lifestyle modification and nonprescription therapies do not provide desired relief from menopausal symptoms, women may be offered prescription therapies. These include systemic hormone therapy, nonhormonal prescription options, and vaginal preparations.

SYSTEMIC HORMONE THERAPY

Hormone therapy should be considered for treatment of moderate to severe vasomotor symptoms only when an indication for therapy has been clearly identified. Before prescribing hormone therapy it is imperative that healthcare providers and their patients review any cautions or contraindications to hormone use, and discuss potential individual risks and benefits so that an informed decision can be made (NAMS, 2010). A comprehensive history and physical examination are essential, as well as an assessment of risk factors for stroke, coronary heart disease, venous thromboembolism, osteoporosis,

and breast cancer (NAMS, 2010). There is no FDA-approved hormonal therapy for treating hot flashes in women at high risk for or who have been diagnosed with breast cancer. Nonhormonal agents may provide relief of hot flashes for women who have had breast cancer. Women with breast cancer risk or history who consider herbal alternatives to hormone therapy should be advised to use caution since some botanicals can have estrogen-like activity. A summary of contraindications for hormone therapy is presented in **Table 12–3**.

It is essential that women considering hormone therapy be informed of known risks, but it cannot be assumed that benefits and risks of therapy apply to all age ranges and durations of therapy. Numerous individual factors may influence a woman's willingness to accept the risks of hormone therapy, particularly if hormone therapy is being considered for menopausal symptom relief or to lower risk of osteoporotic fractures that may or may not occur. Furthermore, since disease incidence increases with age and time since menopause, the risk-benefit ratio of short-term use of hormone therapy is more acceptable for symptom reduction in younger women, whereas long-term use or hormone therapy initiation in older women will have a less acceptable risk-benefit ratio (NAMS, 2010). Women who have undergone premature

Table 12–3 CONTRAINDICATIONS FOR HORMONE THERAPY

Contraindications for Estrogen Use	Contraindications for Progestogen Use
Known or suspected cancer of the breast	Known or suspected cancer of the breast
Known or suspected estrogen-dependent neoplasia	Active thrombophlebitis or thromboembolic disorders
History of uterine or ovarian cancer	Liver dysfunction or disease
History of coronary heart disease or stroke	Undiagnosed abnormal vaginal bleeding
History of biliary tract disorder	Pregnancy
Undiagnosed abnormal genital bleeding	
History of or active thrombophlebitis or thromboembolic disorder	

menopause, whether natural or induced, will have different circumstances because they have increased risk of cardiovascular disease and osteoporosis as well as increased severity of symptoms as compared to women who experience menopause at the median age. Treatment recommendations for women who are beginning use of hormones will differ from women who have previously used hormone therapy for several years. Each woman who considers hormone therapy is unique and has her own risk profile. Individualization of therapy is vital to providing health benefits with minimal risks, thereby enhancing quality of life (NAMS, 2010).

Estrogen Therapy/Estrogen-Progestogen Therapy For women without contraindications, systemic estrogen therapy (ET) and estrogen-progestogen therapy (EPT) are the therapeutic standard for treating moderate to severe menopause-related hot flashes and are government approved in the United States and Canada for this indication as well as for osteoporosis prevention (NAMS, 2015). Systemic ET is prescribed for women who have had a hysterectomy, as the use of unopposed estrogen increases the risk of endometrial hyperplasia and cancer. Systemic EPT is prescribed for women who have a uterus, as progestogen reduces the risk of uterine cancer to the level of using no hormones. For most healthy, symptomatic women under the age of 60 or within 10 years of their final menstrual period, the benefits of ET/EPT outweigh the risks (Shifren & Gass, 2014).

Progestogen Therapy Progestogens are a wide range of hormones with properties of the naturally occurring hormone progesterone, which is produced by the ovary after ovulation and by the placenta during pregnancy. The most common types of progestogen products used in prescription preparations are progesterone, progestins, pregnane and nonpregnane derivatives, and compounds resembling testosterone. Progestogen therapy is an option for treating vasomotor symptoms and other conditions at menopause and after. As previously noted, the primary use in menopausal treatment is to oppose the action of estrogen in women with a uterus to reduce the risk of endometrial hyperplasia and risk from unopposed estrogen. Progestogen-only therapy may also be prescribed for women without contraindications who do not wish to take estrogens but are not opposed to trying another hormone. Evidence suggests that there is an increased risk of breast cancer with estrogen-progestogen use for 3 to 5 years, as noted in the Women's Health Initiative study. However, there was no increased risk of breast cancer noted with 7 years of ET use, allowing for more flexibility in duration of ET use in women without a uterus. (Shifren & Gass, 2014).

Evidence from observational studies suggests that both transdermal ET and low-dose oral ET have been associated with a lower risk of venous thromboembolism and stroke compared with standard-dose oral ET. However, evidence from randomized, controlled trials is lacking (Shifren & Gass, 2014). In women with a uterus, a combination of the selective estrogen receptor modulator bazedoxifene with conjugated estrogen has been approved for the treatment of vasomotor symptoms and prevention of osteoporosis (Shifren & Gass, 2014). Systemic hormone therapy and low-dose vaginal ET are effective treatments for moderate to severe symptoms of vulvar and vaginal atrophy. Additionally, the estrogen agonist/antagonist ospemifene is now approved for this indication (Shifren & Gass, 2014). A summary of hormone therapy options along with advantages and disadvantages of use is presented in **Table 12–4**.

It is recommended that the lowest dose of hormone therapy should be used for the shortest duration needed to manage menopausal symptoms. The decision to use hormone therapy must be a shared decision between a woman and her healthcare provider. Treatment should be individualized and must incorporate women's personal risk factors as well as their quality of life priorities

Table 12–4 HORMONE THERAPY OPTIONS

Type	Product Name	Active Ingredient	Advantages/Disadvantages
Estrogens, oral	Cenestin	Conjugated estrogens	Rapidly metabolized in the gut and liver before reaching circulation (first-pass effect). Stimulates greater increase in high-density lipoprotein cholesterol (HDL-C), triglycerides, hepatic globulins, coagulation factors, and C-reactive than other routes of administration.
	Estrace	Micronized estradiol	
	Estratab	Esterified estrogens	
	Menest	Esterified estrogens	
	Ogen	Estropipate	
	Ortho-est	Estropipate	
	Premarin	Conjugated equine estrogens(CEE)	
Estrogens, transdermal	Climara	Estradiol	Avoids first-pass effect and does not increase triglycerides. Does not increase HDL-C. Has less adverse effects on gallbladder disease and coagulation factors.
	Esclim	Estradiol	
	Vivelle,	Estradiol	
	Vivelle-Dot	Estradiol	
	Alora	Estradiol	
	Estrogel	Estradiol	
	Estraderm	Estradiol	
	Estrasorb Cream	Estradiol	
Progestogens, oral	Provera	Medroxyprogesterone acetate (MPA)	Has first-pass effect, provides endometrial protection at adequate dose and duration. Prometrium is contraindicated in women with peanut allergy.
	Prometrium	Micronized progesterone	
	Aygestin	Norethindrone acetate	
	Amen	MPA	
	Cycrin	MPA	
	Megace	Megestrol acetate	
	Micronor	Norethidrone	
	Nor-QD	Norethidrone	
	Orvette	Norgestrel	
Combination estrogen + progestogen, oral preparation	Prempro	CEE+ MPA	Has first-pass effect, provides protection against endometrial hyperplasia and cancer.
	Premphase	CEE (14 tabs), then CEE + MPA (14 tabs)	
	Femhrt		
	Prefest	Norethindrone acetate + ethinyl estradiol	
	Activella	Estradiol 3 tabs then estradiol + norgestimate 3 tabs	
		Estradiol + norethindrone acetate	
Combination estrogen + progestogen transdermals	Climara Pro	Estradiol + levonorgestrel	Low doses of transdermal progestogens have metabolic advantage over high doses of oral therapy by avoiding first-pass hepatic effects.
	Combipatch	Estradiol + norethindrone acetate	

(continues)

Table 12–4 Hormone Therapy Options (*continued*)

Type	Product Name	Active Ingredient	Advantages/Disadvantages
Combination estrogen + androgens, oral	Estratest HS Estratest	Esterified estrogens + methytestosterone Esterified estrogens + methytestosterone	Used for moderate to severe vasomotor symptoms unresponsive to estrogen.
Estrogen, vaginal creams	Estrace Premarin	Micronized 17β–estradiol CEE	Systemic absorption of estrogen is uncommon but possible.
Estrogen, vaginal tablets	Vagifem	Estradiol hemihydrate	Systemic estrogen absorption can occur. Tablets are less messy than vaginal cream.
Estrogen, vaginal ring	Estring Femring	Micronized 17β–estradiol Estradiol acetate	Systemic absorption of estrogen can occur. Estring is used to treat atrophic vaginitis. Femring may be used to treat hot flashes.
Progestogen, gel	Prochieve 4%	Progesterone	Provides sustained and controlled delivery of progesterone to vaginal tissue.
Progestogen, IUS	Mirena	Levonorgestrel	Systemic absorption can occur. Delivers highest concentration of levonorgestrel to the endometrium.

(Shifren & Gass, 2014). When hormone therapy is used in symptomatic women or for the prevention of osteoporosis, extended duration of treatment may be appropriate if alternative therapies are not tolerated. A careful assessment of individual risks and benefits should be performed in these cases. When treatment is considered solely for moderate to severe symptoms of vulvar and vaginal atrophy, the use of low-dose vaginal ET is preferred over systemic ET due to the greater safety profile of low-dose vaginal ET (Shifren & Gass, 2014).

Custom-compounded hormones refers to hormones that are mixed by a pharmacy based on a prescription supposedly customized for an individual woman based on blood or salivary hormone levels. Such hormone therapy products are made into a cream, lozenge, gel, tablet, spray, or skin pellet that typically contains one or more hormone in differing amounts in addition to other ingredients. Custom-compounded hormones are often described as "bioidentical," and purported to contain only hormones structurally identical to the hormones manufactured by a woman's ovaries during the reproductive years. However, *bioidentical* is a term invented by marketers and has no clear scientific meaning (Shifren & Gass, 2014). The use of custom-compounded hormone therapy has increased significantly among women seeking alternative therapies. Although compounding pharmacies are regulated by state pharmacy boards, very little oversight is provided by the Food and Drug Administration (FDA). Moreover, compounded hormones are not tested for safety or efficacy, as opposed to commercially manufactured FDA-approved hormone therapy products, and they frequently do not come with product information sheets which are otherwise required by FDA-approved commercially manufactured hormone therapy products. Consumers are generally unaware that the FDA has limited control over the marketing and safety monitoring of compounded hormones, and the advertising and promotional claims of safety and efficacy of compounded hormones are unsupported by medical evidence (Shifren & Gass, 2014).

Custom-compounded bioidentical hormone therapy should not be used. The lack of product quality control and regulatory oversight as well as lack of evidence regarding safety or effectiveness makes this therapy ill-advised (Shifren & Gass, 2014). Women who request custom-compounded hormone therapy should be advised to use hormone therapy products that are FDA-approved and biochemically identical to the hormones naturally produced by the ovaries during reproductive life, such as estradiol and progesterone. FDA-approved hormone therapy products are available in a wide range of doses that may be tailored to meet the individual needs of each woman (Shifren & Gass, 2014).

Women who have primary ovarian insufficiency or early menopause may be candidates for combined estrogen-progestogen contraceptives until they reach the average age of natural menopause at 52 years. Symptomatic women may require longer duration. The prescription of hormone therapy for the prevention of chronic disease is not recommended (Shifren & Gass, 2014).

After initiation of hormone therapy, vasomotor symptom relief is usually obtained in 2 to 6 weeks. Women should be offered anticipatory guidance about management of side effects of treatment, should they occur. Possible side effects are presented in **Box 12–1**. Women should return to their healthcare provider for a follow-up visit 6 to 8 weeks after initiation of therapy for evaluation of progress. If the initial dosage of ET/EPT is not adequate, it can be increased or dosage schedule modified as necessary. Ongoing evaluation for potential adverse effects should also be done. Annual return visits are recommended at which time the decision to continue or discontinue treatment should be revisited. Duration of use is a challenging issue and will vary according to the individual woman and her particular circumstances for treatment. The shortest duration of hormone therapy that is consistent with treatment goals, benefits, and risks for the individual woman is essential. If the lowest effective dose of hormones is used and the woman has been

---

Box 12–1: Adverse Effects of Hormone Therapy

Adverse effects of estrogen therapy/estrogen-progestogen therapy include:

- Uterine bleeding
- Breast tenderness
- Nausea
- Abdominal bloating
- Fluid retention in extremities
- Headache
- Dizziness
- Hair loss
- Mood changes with EPT
- Changes in the shape of the cornea

well advised of the potential risks and benefits, and there is clinical supervision and consultation, extension of therapy for the woman's treatment goals is acceptable under certain circumstances. A woman may perceive that the benefits of symptom relief outweigh risks, especially after failing an attempt to discontinue hormone therapy. In addition, a woman with established loss of bone mass may find that alternate therapies are inappropriate or cause unacceptable adverse effects, or the benefit-risk ratio of extended use is unknown (NAMS, 2010).

ANDROGEN THERAPY Androgens in women function as the immediate precursors for estrogen biosynthesis, and affect sexual desire, muscle mass, distribution of adipose tissue, bone mineral density, energy, and psychological well-being. Androgen levels decline with age and with other conditions such as adrenal insufficiency, corticosteroid use, and hypopituitarism. There is no abrupt decline of androgens at menopause, as seen with ovarian estrogen, except in cases of surgical menopause (NAMS, 2015).

Testosterone therapy may be used in trials to treat female sexual interest/arousal disorder (previously known as hypoactive sexual desire disorder) in carefully selected postmenopausal women when no other etiology is identified for this disorder. The long-term risks of testosterone therapy for women are unknown, including possible effects on the risk of cardiovascular disease or breast cancer. Women who are prescribed testosterone therapy need to be advised of both possible risks and adverse effects. Adverse effects of testosterone therapy include acne, weight gain, hirsutism, permanent lowering of the voice, clitoral enlargement, changes in emotion, such as increased anger, and adverse changes in lipids and liver function tests. Women receiving testosterone therapy should have blood testosterone levels checked intermittently to ensure that levels remain in the normal range for reproductive-aged women (Shifren & Gass, 2014).

SELECTIVE ESTROGEN RECEPTOR MODULATORS

Selective estrogen receptor modulators (SERMs) act as estrogen agonists in some tissues and as estrogen antagonists in others. Selective tissue-specific actions may be obtained by different SERMs, which allows for individualization of therapy, depending on the medical needs of the postmenopausal woman. Women at high risk for thrombosis should not be given SERMs since SERMs increase the risk of venous thromboembolytic events similar to oral estrogen therapy (Shifren & Gass, 2014).

In the United States and Canada, tamoxifen has been approved for prevention and treatment of breast cancer, toremifene has been approved for treatment of breast cancer, raloxifene has been approved for prevention and treatment of osteoporosis and prevention of breast cancer, and ospemifene has been approved for treatment of dyspareunia due to postmenopausal vaginal atrophy (Shifren & Gass, 2014). In addition, the first tissue-selective estrogen complex (TSEC), which consists of the pairing of conjugated estrogens with the SERM bazedoxifene, has been approved for the treatment of vasomotor symptoms and the prevention of osteoporosis in women with a uterus. Bazedoxifene provides endometrial protection, which eliminates the need for a progestogen (Shifren & Gass, 2014).

Tamoxifen is well known for its benefits in the prevention and treatment of breast cancer. It is also an estrogen agonist in bone, and decreases bone loss in the spine and hip of postmenopausal women. However, women who use tamoxifen experience an increased risk for uterine cancer, venous thromboembolytic events, and cataracts (Shifren & Gass, 2014). Raloxifene increases bone mineral density and decreases the risk of osteoporotic vertebral fractures. It does not decrease the risk of hip or nonvertebral fractures. In postmenopausal women with increased risk for breast cancer, raloxifene also reduces the risk of invasive breast cancer. Like tamoxifen, raloxifene increases the risk of venous thromboembolytic events, however unlike tamoxifen, raloxifene does not increase the risk of uterine cancer (Shifren & Gass, 2014). In postmenopausal women, ospemifene improves vaginal pH and vaginal maturation, and reduces dyspareunia due to vulvovaginal atrophy. However, no studies have yet investigated whether ospemifene is effective in the prevention or treatment of breast cancer or osteoporosis (Shifren & Gass, 2014).

Nonhormonal Prescription Options

Nonhormonal prescription options are available for women who are not candidates for hormonal therapy. Some nonhormonal prescription drugs have shown efficacy in relieving hot flashes, but none is as effective as systemic estrogen therapy (NAMS, 2015). Treatment options include antidepressants (namely fluoxetine, paroxetine, sertraline, or venlafaxine), the anticonvulsive drug, gabapentin; and the anthypertensive, clonidine. The nonhormonal prescription options along with dosage, adverse effects, and contraindications are presented in **Table 12–5**.

Ongoing Treatment

Any treatment for vasomotor symptoms may need to be adjusted from time to time since estrogen production will gradually lessen over the period of menopause transition. Furthermore, women may develop medical conditions unrelated to menopause or menopause treatment. Changing from one therapy to another may require a washout period. Regardless of the therapy chosen, the treatment option should be periodically evaluated to determine if it is still needed because menopausal vasomotor symptoms will eventually subside in nearly all women.

Table 12–5 Nonhormonal Prescription Options for Vasomotor Symptoms

Category	Drug	Side Effects	Contraindications	Comments
Antidepressants	Venlafaxine (Effexor)	Nausea, vomiting, mouth dryness, decreased appetite	Concomitant use of MAO inhibitors; taper when discontinuing	Response is immediate, antidepressants can be used by women with breast cancer
	Fluoxetine (Prozac)	Asthenia, sweating, nausea, somnolence, anorgasmia, decreased libido	Concomitant use of MAO inhibitors or thioridazine; caution with warfarin	Taper when discontinuing
	Paroxetine (Paxil)	Same as fluoxetine	Same as fluoxetine	
	Sertraline (Zoloft)	Weight gain, blurred vision	May interfere with tamoxifen metabolism	
Anticonvulsants	Gabapentin (Neurontin)	Somnolence, dizziness, ataxia, weight gain	Avoid antacids within 2 hours of use	Taper when discontinuing

(continues)

Table 12–5 Nonhormonal Prescription Options for Vasomotor Symptoms (*continued*)

Category	Drug	Side Effects	Contraindications	Comments
Antihypertensives	Clonidine (Catapres)	Dry mouth, drowsiness, dizziness, weakness, constipation, rash, myalgia, urticaria, insomnia, nausea, agitation, orthostatic hypotension, impotence, arrhythmias		Taper when discontinuing to avoid nervousness, headache, agitation, confusion, and rapid rise of blood pressure
Others	Methyldopa (Aldomet) Combined belladonna, phenobarbital, ergotamine (Bellergal)		Use for vasomotor symptoms is not recommended due to limited efficacy and potential for adverse effects	

Quality of Life Issues Associated With Menopause

Menopause marks an important milestone in women's lives. Not only does it signal the end of the menstrual cycle, it also indicates the end of a woman's capability to bear children. For some, this may be welcome, but for some it may be difficult if the goal of bearing children has not come to fruition even after years of unsuccessful intervention (van der Mooren & Kenemans, 2004).

Women who experience the menopausal transition are vulnerable to one or more physical or psychological symptoms or conditions that are related, either directly or indirectly, to hormonal changes associated with ovarian insufficiency.

These symptoms and conditions can greatly impact on quality of life. Estrogen decline also increases women's risk of numerous chronic diseases such as cardiovascular disease, osteoporosis, osteoarthritis, and Alzheimer's disease. These diseases can significantly reduce life expectancy and well-being (van der Mooren & Kenemans, 2004).

Menopause encompasses more than a hormonal phenomenon. For many women, menopause coincides with other major life events that signal transition toward aging. These life events may include illnesses, death of spouse or friends, children reaching adulthood and leaving the family home, retirement, caring for elderly parents, marital problems, and divorce (van der Mooren & Kenemans, 2004). The added stress of menopausal symptoms to the demands of these life events can impair women's ability to adequately cope, and subsequently may threaten quality of life.

The quality of life issues that emerge in women transitioning through menopause are multidimensional and encompass health and physical functioning, psychological and spiritual well-being, socioeconomic integrity, and family well-being. Menopausal symptoms, side effects of treatment therapies, the likelihood of comorbid conditions, all occurring against the backdrop of major life events, present a formidable challenge to women's ability to maintain an acceptable quality of life across these domains.

Issues Affecting Health and Physical Functioning

For women, the menopause experience is unique and personal. Some women have severe symptoms that disrupt all aspects of their lives, while others find it almost a "non-event" and report no bothersome symptoms. The type and severity of menopausal symptoms varies. Symptoms usually begin in the perimenopausal period and may gradually increase in frequency and severity. Postmenopausal women generally experience more symptoms with greater severity than perimenopausal women. The symptoms most frequently reported are hot flashes, and these reach highest occurrence during the first 2 years postmenopause and then decline over time. Most women generally experience hot flashes for 6 months to 2 years, although some women have them for 10 years or longer. Hot flashes can be disruptive to daily activities as well as quality of sleep. They diminish quality of life by causing acute physical discomfort and sleep disturbances that can lead to fatigue, irritability, and forgetfulness.

Symptoms associated with urogenital atrophy often interfere with women's personal and relational satisfaction, self-esteem, and well-being. Vaginal dryness and irritation may cause painful sexual intercourse (dyspareunia), which can hinder intimate relationships. Problems with their partner's sexual performance or with the relationship can make some women less interested in sex. In addition, urinary problems such as frequency and incontinence can cause embarrassment and social isolation.

The various treatment options for menopausal symptoms that were discussed earlier can be effective in obtaining relief of discomfort, management of symptoms, and improvement of quality of life. Treatment should be individualized according to the specific needs of the woman, with particular awareness of the risks and benefits of each modality. Women who are prescribed hormone therapy may experience bothersome side effects that can impact quality of life. Fluid retention may be managed by decreasing salt intake, exercise, or use of a mild diuretic. Bloating may require modification of type or dosage of hormones. Breast tenderness may be relieved by modification of type or dosage of hormones, and a decrease in salt, caffeine, and chocolate intake. Headache may be related to type and dosage of hormones, therefore modification may be warranted along with reduction of salt, caffeine, and alcohol intake. Mood changes may respond to modification in type or dosage of hormones as well as ensuring adequate water intake and restricting salt, caffeine, and alcohol. Nausea may be relieved by taking hormones with meals and modification of type or dosage of hormone.

Women may be less inclined to discuss sexual issues with their healthcare providers due to embarrassment or unawareness that sexual dysfunction may be related to menopause, or that treatments are available to help mitigate sexual problems. Counseling and sex therapy can be effective for many women and couples who have sexual issues. Continuation of sexual activity is a realistic and expected part of aging, and thus referrals for counseling should be considered even when pharmacological interventions are indicated.

Women should be thoroughly evaluated with history, physical examination, and selective laboratory testing in order to rule out other health problems that can mimic the symptoms of menopause. Women may have several diagnoses to contend with at once, such as hypertension, diabetes, and menopause. Often, a significant improvement in quality of life may be obtained by bringing comorbid conditions under control, which can lessen menopausal symptoms enough so that they are no longer bothersome.

Issues Affecting Psychological and Spiritual Functioning

Psychological Functioning

The psychological impact of menopause can vary from woman to woman. Some women may take the transition in stride while others may feel anxiety, stress, depressed mood, and decreased sense of well-being. Although most women do not experience a major depressive disorder, some women may be vulnerable to a first episode of major depression during menopause, especially if they have a history of an anxiety disorder or recent stressful life event (Bromberger et al., 2009).

Women may experience mood changes that range from depression to anxiety to irritability, which can negatively impact on quality of life. They may feel depressed, exhausted and weak, or unable to cope. They may experience odd memory problems, especially with retrieving words, or sleep disturbance, that further add to distress (Derry, 2004). It remains unclear whether these psychological responses are primary or secondary to physical symptoms such as hot flashes and consequent sleep disturbance, or, if directly associated with menopause status, what the source may be. Adverse psychological symptoms may resolve for some women when physical symptoms are relieved, as with hormone therapy. For others, psychological symptoms may not improve with

hormone therapy, or medication side effects such as depression, headache, or odd bodily sensations may develop (Derry, 2004).

Women are more likely to experience confusion, uncertainty, or pessimism about menopause early on but over time may gradually readjust their self-image regarding midlife, menopause, and the meaning of symptoms. From a developmental point of view, women at midlife may experience an inner reorganization that produces a redefinition of self, other, and a greater sense of autonomy and congruence. For some women, menopause may become entwined in this reorganization process and represent positive or negative aspects of psychological changes. Menopause may also represent wider apprehensions about aging (Derry, 2004).

The complex nature of menopausal distress presents a challenge for determining interventions that would mitigate psychological symptoms. Effective coping begins with obtaining a comprehensive individualized psychosocial assessment. This assessment should reveal the woman's psychosocial history, perception of symptoms, and how symptoms, both physical and psychological, impact on her life. Coping with menopausal distress can be facilitated by engendering a positive self-image and sense of mastery, a positive consideration for and comfort with one's body, a positive perspective of one's life stage, and accurate information about health problems and health-promoting strategies (Derry, 2004). Healthcare providers should be attentive to these basic components and provide assistance in strengthening women's coping mechanisms in response to menopausal distress.

Numerous treatment options are available that will help relieve distress, treat more serious mood disturbances, and improve quality of life. As discussed earlier, these interventions include prescription hormones and antidepressants, nonprescription herbal remedies, lifestyle approaches, stress reduction therapies, and counseling. Because different options appear to work for some women but not others, women need to work closely with their healthcare providers to determine which strategies are most effective for them. Women who take an active, informed role in managing their menopause regain a sense of control that helps strengthen their ability to cope and ultimately enhances their quality of life.

SPIRITUALITY

It is well known that religious and spiritual factors have a positive influence on health status and psychological well-being. The reason for this may be that religious involvement is associated with positive health behaviors and having a more optimistic worldview. In addition, religion is known to be a positive source of support and coping, especially for aging women. For many women, religion becomes an important coping mechanism as they age (Steffen, 2011). In midlife spirituality may help women meet losses, deepen their spiritual roots, and find new meaning in life. For midlife women faith may continue to develop and flourish when children leave home, leading to new life goals and identity. Evidence suggests that having faith is a frequently used self-care strategy during menopause. Well-being in midlife is associated with early religious socialization and church attendance (Steffen, 2011).

Research findings suggest that spirituality may contribute to increased severity in menopausal symptoms if women perceive a significant loss of identity and purpose during menopausal transition. On the other hand, spirituality may contribute to decreased severity in menopausal symptoms if women perceive that they are strengthened by their spirituality during menopausal transition. In addition, research has shown that spiritual strength is related to decreased levels of menopausal symptoms (Steffen, 2011).

Issues Affecting Socioeconomic Integrity

Menopause can have a significant socioeconomic effect on the quality of life of women. Menopausal symptoms often interfere with social functioning. Symptoms such as hot flashes and urinary incontinence can cause physical discomfort, embarrassment, and distress. Women may be reluctant to participate in social activities, which can increase social isolation. Sleep disruption can increase fatigue and exhaustion, making it difficult to participate in household or community activities. Women may find that exhaustion as well as cognitive symptoms such as inability to concentrate and forgetfulness hinder their work productivity and job performance.

Vaginal atrophy, reduced libido, and decreased sexual arousal, as well as psychological distress and depression can impede sexual function and satisfaction. As a result, women may have difficulty with social and marital relationships. Distress and depression can contribute to higher rates of marital dissatisfaction and divorce (Hash, Rubinow, & Schmidt, 2008).

Increased healthcare expenditures may be incurred from treatment of menopausal symptoms or concurrent health conditions that become more prevalent in association with menopause. Changes in health insurance status and ability to pay for health care as a result of retirement or unemployment can influence the quality of care that women receive as well as their ability to comply with treatments recommendations.

The aggressive management of physical symptoms, provision of counseling, and participation in individual or group support activities are essential considerations that can help women regain social and community integration.

Issues Affecting Family Well-Being

Menopause coincides with many significant midlife issues that can impact family well-being and quality of life, including children reaching adulthood and leaving home (or returning home after college or economic downturns), retirement of women or spouse/partners, physical and emotional changes that occur in spousal/partner relationships, development of chronic diseases in both women and spouse/part-ners, and becoming caregivers of elderly parents or grandchildren. These issues can bring about changes in family roles and responsibilities, changes in pri-vacy and independence, uncertainty, and changes in identity and self-concept. How successfully women manage the challenges of menopause within the context of these life events will depend on the effi-cacy of their coping mechanisms, attitudes about menopause and aging, expectations of treatment and lifestyle modalities, and sources of social and family support. Marital and family counseling, family education, and participation in support and advocacy groups can play a significant part in help-ing women and families through menopause transi-tion and changing life events, and subsequently in enhancing quality of life.

Implications for Healthcare Providers

Menopause is a complex phenomenon that may cause a multitude of physical and psychological symptoms that vary considerably in severity, nature, frequency, and persistence. In addition to these internal biological factors, numerous external dynamics interact with the hormonal environment of midlife women. These dynamics can include family and relationships, socioeconomic issues, cultural variations, general health and well-being, and the ability to adapt to changes associated with aging. These factors often determine women's toler-ance to their menopausal symptoms, so it is essen-tial that a thorough assessment of midlife women include questions relating not only to hormonal status but to their social and emotional well-being (Reddish, 2004). The unique and distinctive nature of the menopause experience further emphasizes the importance of conducting a comprehensive assessment of all interplaying factors in order to determine an individualized plan of care specific to each woman's situation. This comprehensive

understanding is fundamental to the success of an overall plan to manage menopause (Reddish, 2004).

Although an abundance of information about menopause is found in lay literature, women's mag-azines, television, newspapers, the Internet, and a vast array of advertising material, these sources vary considerably in accuracy and motive. Also, well-meaning family and friends can further add to mis-conceptions with descriptions of their menopause experiences. Women often have difficulty obtaining accurate information. Healthcare providers need to be well informed about evidence-based manage-ment options supported by the latest research find-ings. The wide assortment of treatment options can be confusing and overwhelming. Imparting up-to-date accurate information, removing mis-conceptions, and presenting all treatment options allows women to make informed decisions and take control of their own lives and health management (Reddish, 2004).

Healthcare providers should monitor women's response to treatment closely through follow-up visits. Because different treatment options are efficacious for some women but not others, healthcare providers need to work closely with their patients to determine which strategies work best for them. Treatment options may need to be tried and discarded before the strategy that works most effectively is found. Furthermore, healthcare providers need to be alert for possible factors that may interfere with treatment compliance (such as financial constraints, cultural barriers, com-plicated directions, bothersome side effects) and initiate corrective measures as needed.

Special Concerns of Age and Ethnicity

Menopause is a benchmark in the lives of middle-aged women. While it is a normal developmental stage, menopause gives women the opportunity to evaluate their health risks for diseases of aging—most notably, cardiovascular disease, osteoarthritis, osteo-porosis, and Alzheimer's disease—and to institute lifestyle changes to prevent disease and promote health. With women of the baby boomer genera-tion experiencing menopause in unprecedented numbers, healthcare providers are in prime posi-tion to counsel midlife women about healthy aging. Women who experience premature menopause or induced menopause are at higher risk for develop-ing the diseases of aging due to loss of the protective influence of estrogen over a longer period of time. The increased vulnerability of younger women to diseases of aging needs to be aggressively addressed with lifestyle changes and preventative modalities.

Attitudes toward menopause, frequency and severity of symptoms, use of hormonal therapy, and perceptions of the healthcare system vary widely across racial and ethnic groups. Differ-ences between women of various racial, ethnic, and sociocultural backgrounds will have implications for the way they experience menopause and for their future health and quality of life. It is impor-tant to note that a good deal of the current body of information about menopause is based on studies involving relatively healthy middle-class Cauca-sian women. Research studies, such as the SWAN study and others with multiple ethnic groups, have been invaluable in bringing to light ethnic differ-ences related to menopause. Attitudes toward the menopause experience as well as the experience of symptom frequency and severity differ across ethnic groups and can be influenced by such factors as socioeconomics, smoking, and acculturation. Assumptions cannot be made about the meno-pause experience of women from different ethnic groups living in Western countries. Healthcare pro-viders need to be culturally sensitive and mindful of cultural beliefs and practices that can influence the view of menopause held by women of various racial, ethnic, and cultural backgrounds.

Attention to the sensitive management of les-bians is often overlooked. Lesbians represent a varied group in race, ethnicity, education, age, and sexual practice. They may be celibate, sexually active with women, or bisexual. Many healthcare providers assume that all women they are caring for are heterosexual and frequently overlook the needs of lesbian patients or are insensitive to their sexual orientation. Consequently, lesbians tend to receive a lower quality of health care in the face of higher risk for certain chronic diseases, generalized anxiety disorders, mood disorders, and unhealthy risk factors such as smoking, alcohol consumption, and obesity. These factors can negatively influence menopausal transition. Healthcare providers need to provide sensitive, nonjudgmental care to lesbi-ans and remove barriers to accessing appropriate quality care.

Research Review

Does quality of life change over the course of the menopausal transition?

Avis, N., Colvin, A., Bromberger, J., Hess, R., Matthews, K., Ory, M., & Schocken, M. (2009). Change in health-related quality of life over the menopausal transition in a multi-ethnic cohort, of middle-aged women: Study of Women's Health Across the Nation. *Menopause:*

The Journal of the North American Menopause Society, 16(5), 860–869.

Health-related quality of life is an important outcome in the appraisal of both function and disease progression among healthy and ill pop-ulations. Health-related quality of life refers to aspects of life most likely to be affected by changes in health status. Thus, the purpose of this study was to examine changes in health-related quality of life over the course of the menopausal transition. The researchers hypothesized that symptoms associated with changes in the menopausal transition are associated with changes in health-related quality of life and these symptoms can explain associations between changes in menopause status and health-related quality of life.

This was a prospective longitudinal study of women, aged 42 to 52 years at baseline who were recruited at seven sites in the United States, in the multiethnic Study of Women's Health Across the Nation. Each site recruited one minority population (African-American, Chinese, Hispanic, or Japanese) and one white population from community-based samples. Women had to be between the ages of 42 to 52, have an intact uterus and at least one ovary, and not be currently using exogenous hormones. Study participants were either premenopausal or perimenopausal, and self-identified as one of the study's designated racial/ethnic groups. A total of 3,302 women participated in this study. Health-related quality of life was measured by five subscales of the Medical Outcomes Short-Form Health Survey: pain, role limitations due to physical health, role limitations due to emotional problems, social functioning, and vitality. The Medical Outcomes Short-Form Health Survey was administered to the study partici-

pants on six occasions over a 7-year period. The findings indicated that after adjustment for a wide range of variables, menopause status was independently related to physical limitations in role functioning but not to other domains of health-related quality of life. The odds of reduced physical functioning were greater at the early perimenopause, late perimenopause, and early postmenopause than at premenopause. Current and former users of hormone therapy were more likely to report poor physical functioning on all domains of health-related quality of life. Additional findings indicated that symptoms such as hot flashes, vaginal dryness, urine leakage, poor sleep and depression, perceived stress, and stressful life events were significantly related to declines in all of the domains of health-related quality of life. Significant racial/ethnic group differences were found in bodily pain and reduced social functioning domains. Findings suggested that African-American and Hispanic women reported more bodily pain and reduced social functioning than white women.

The findings of this study suggest that menopausal symptoms largely explain the changes in health-related quality of life over the menopausal transition. These results underscore the importance of symptom management in enhancing health-related quality of life though the menopause transition.

Chapter Summary Points

- The last century has seen a dramatic rise in the life expectancy of American women. Not only are women living longer but many are living a third to one-half of their lives beyond the menopause.
- Specific assumptions about menopause and the current state of knowledge of menopause have lead to the emergence of distinct conceptualizations which have shaped current attitudes and therapeutic approaches.

- The conceptualizations of menopause found in North American culture include biomedical, psychological/psychosocial, sociocultural, and feminist perspectives.
- The characteristic perimenopause, or transition to menopause, starts with menstrual irregularity at the approximate age of 47, followed by intermittent cycling that continues for about 4 years. Complete amenorrhea is achieved at approximately 51 to 52 years of age. Transition ends 12 months after the final menses.
- African-American and Latina women tend to experience menopause slightly earlier than the median age while Japanese-American and Chinese-American women tend to complete menopausal transition slightly later than the median age. Latina women tend to experience menopause approximately 6 months earlier than women of other ethnic groups.
- Hormonal and physiologic changes that occur at midlife and are associated with menopause may significantly increase women's risk for the development of cardiovascular disease, osteoarthritis, osteoporosis, and Alzheimer's disease.
- While menopause occurs in women, a similar condition of hormonal decline is thought to occur in men, referred to as andropause, male menopause, male climacteric, androgen deficiency, or partial androgen deficiency in the aging male (PADAM).
- The occurrence of menopause is indicated by a woman's age, changes in the menstrual cycle, and presence of menopausal symptoms.
- The classic symptoms of menopause include vasomotor reactivity, urogenital atrophy, and psychological distress.
- The experience of menopause is unique to each woman and several options are available to treat menopausal symptoms. Treatment approaches include lifestyle modification, nonprescription therapies, and prescription therapies.
- Menopause coincides with other major life events that signal transition toward aging. The added stress of menopausal symptoms to the demands of these life events can impair women's ability to adequately cope and can subsequently threaten quality of life.
- The unique and distinctive nature of the menopause experience further emphasizes the importance of a comprehensive assessment of all interplaying factors in order to determine an individualized plan of care specific to a woman's situation.
- Attitudes toward menopause, frequency and severity of symptoms, use of hormonal therapy, and perceptions of the healthcare system vary widely across racial and ethnic groups and have implications for the way these women experience menopause, their future health, and quality of life.

Critical Thinking Exercise

Case Study

Mrs. A. is married and has two sons, 24 and 21, and a daughter 18. Mrs. A. is a high school teacher and her husband is a sales manager. Their oldest son has just moved out of the home after finding a permanent job, the middle son is in his last year of college, and the daughter will be starting her freshman year. Mrs. A.'s elderly father is a widower who suffers from heart disease. He lives in an apartment attached to their home so she can care for him. Mrs. A. has been perimenopausal for 3 years. At age 46 she noticed that her periods became irregular and lengthened in duration with increasingly heavy flow and clots. Her heavy flow would last over a full week, and then eventually dwindle to a few weeks of staining, only to become heavy again by the next cycling. It seemed as if she was constantly wearing feminine protection products. When she turned 49, she began to experience hot flashes, especially in the summer. Hot flashes and night sweats became disruptive to her sleep. In the daytime she had difficulty concentrating on her work, was increasingly forgetful, and felt irritable and exhausted. Her last menstrual period occurred at age 50, to her relief, but her menopausal symptoms continue to plague her. Mrs. A. has a history of breast cancer and she fears many of the symptom remedies that are on the market. She is approximately 20 pounds overweight, and drinks several cups of coffee throughout the day. She noticed her desire for sex was diminishing, as well as her enjoyment and satisfaction. She has vaginal dryness and lack of arousal. She explained her difficulties to her husband, and although he understood that she was going through "the change," she could sense his disappointment and frustration in their declining sexual relationship. Mrs. A. feels useless and unattractive, and when she looks in the mirror she wonders where her life has gone.

Questions for Seminar Discussion

1. What physical, psychological/spiritual, socioeconomic, and family issues threaten Mrs. A.'s quality of life?
2. What issues and concerns are not readily apparent but could become problematic to Mrs. A. and her family?
3. What are Mrs. A.'s risks for developing comorbid conditions that could threaten her quality of life?
4. What strengths and weaknesses are present that factor into Mrs. A.'s ability to cope with her menopause and quality of life demands?
5. What areas do you need to assess in order to effectively develop an individualized plan to manage Mrs. A.'s menopausal transition?
6. What treatment options and interventions are available to help Mrs. A. resolve menopause symptoms that continue to plague her?
7. What types of referrals could be made that would help Mrs. A. improve her quality of life?

Internet Resources

American Congress of Obstetricians and Gynecologists: Menopause information for healthcare professionals, researchers, policymakers, and advocates. http://www.acog.org

Jacobs Institute of Women's Health: Menopause information for healthcare professionals, researchers, policymakers, consumers, and advocates. http://www.jiwh.org

National Women's Health Resource Center: Menopause information for consumers. http://www
.healthywomen.org

North American Menopause Society: Menopause information for healthcare professionals,
researchers, policymakers, consumers, and advocates. http://www.menopause.org

Office on Women's Health: Menopause information for healthcare professionals, researchers,
policymakers, consumers, and advocates. http://www.womenshealth.gov

Society for Women's Health Research: Menopause information for healthcare professionals,
researchers, policymakers, consumers, and advocates. http://www.womenshealthresearch.org

Women's Voices for Change: Menopause information for healthcare professionals, researchers, policymakers, consumers, and advocates. http://womensvoicesforchange.org/tag
/american-menopause-foundation

References

Abernethy, K. (2008). How the menopause affects the cardiovascular health of women. *Primary Health Care, 18*(6), 42–47.

Aiello, E., Yasui, Y., Tworoger, S., Ulrich, C., Irwin, M., Bowen, D., … McTiernan, A. (2004). Effect of a year-long, moderate intensity exercise intervention on the occurrence and severity of menopause symptoms in postmenopausal women. *Menopause: The Journal of the North American Menopause Society, 11*(4), 382–388.

Arias, E. (2014). United States life tables 2010. National Vital Statistics Reports, 63(7). Hyattsville, MD: National Center for Health Statistics. Retrieved from http://www.cdc.gov/nchs/data/nvsr/nvsr63/nvsr63_07.pdf

Asikainen, T., Kukkonen-Harjula, K., & Miilunpalo, S. (2004). Exercise for health for early postmenopausal women: A systematic review of randomized controlled trials. *Sports Medicine, 34*(11), 753–778.

Avis, N., Brockwell, S., & Colvin, A. (2005). A universal menopause syndrome? *The American Journal of Medicine, 118*(12B), 37S–46S.

Avis, N., Colvin, A., Bromberger, J., Hess, R., Matthews, K., Ory, M., & Schocken, M. (2009). Change in health-related quality of life over the menopausal transition in a multiethnic cohort of middle-aged women: Study of Women's Health Across the Nation. *Menopause: The Journal of the North American Menopause Society, 16*(5), 860–869.

Balk, J. (2003). Mind-body approaches to menopausal symptoms. *Alternative Therapies in Women's Health, 5*(2), 9–16.

Barile, L. (1997). Theories of menopause: Brief comparative synopsis. *Journal of Psychosocial Nursing, 35*(2), 36–39.

Berg, J., Larson, C., & Pasvogel, A. (2008). Menopausal symptom perception and severity: Results from a screening questionnaire. *Journal of Clinical Nursing, 17*(7), 940–948.

Brockie, J. (2008). Physiology and effects of menopause. *Nurse Prescribing, 6*(5), 202–207.

Bromberger, J., Kravitz, H., Matthews, K., Youk, A., Brown, C., & Feng, W. (2009). Predictors of first lifetime episodes of major depression in midlife women. *Psychological Medicine, 39*, 55–64.

Cimmino, M., & Parodi, M. (2005). Risk factors for arthritis. *Seminars in Arthritis and Rheumatism, 34* (6 Supp 2), 29–34.

Craig, M., & Murphy, D. (2009). Alzheimer's disease in women. *Best Practice & Research Clinical Obstetrics and Gynaecology, 23*, 53–61.

Daley, A., Stokes-Lampard, H., Mutrie, N., & MacArthur, C. (2007). Exercise for vasomotor menopausal symptoms. *Cochrane Database of Systematic Reviews*, Issue 4. Art. No. CD006108. doi: 10.1002/14651858.CD006108.pub2.

Deeks, A. (2004). Is this menopause? Women in midlife-psychosocial issues. *Australian Family Physician, 33*(11), 889–893.

de Melo, M., Soares, A., & Baragatti, A. (2013). Male hypogonadism or andropause: Integrative literature review study. *Journal of Nursing, 7*, 898–909.

Derry, P. (2004). Coping with distress during perimeno-pause. *Women & Therapy, 27*(3/4), 165–177.

Gallagher, J. (2007). Effects of early menopause on bone mineral density and fractures. *Menopause, 14*(3 Pt. 2), 567–571.

Geller, S., & Studee, L. (2005). Botanical and dietary supplements for menopausal symptoms: What works, what does not. *Journal of Women's Health, 14*(7), 634–649.

Ginsberg, T., & Cavalieri, T. (2008). Androgen deficiency in the aging male: The beginning, the middle, and the ongoing. *Clinical Geriatrics, 16*(4), 25–28.

Green, R., & Santoro, N. (2009). Menopausal symptoms and ethnicity: The study of women's health across the nation. *Women's Health, 5*(2), 127–133.

Gould, D. (2005). How to recognize and treat the andropause. *Practice Nurse, 30*(10), 12, 15, 17 passim.

Hash, V., Rubinow, D., & Schmidt, P. (2008). Can the menopausal transition trigger depression? *Contemporary OB/GYN, 53*(8), 28–33.

Holloway, D. (2008). Non-hormonal treatment options during the menopause. *Nurse Prescribing, 6*(11), 479–484.

Hunter, M. (2003). Cognitive behavioural interventions for premenstrual and menopausal symptoms. *Journal of Reproductive and Infant Psychology, 21*(3), 183–193.

Hunter, M., Coventry, S., Hamed, H., Fentiman, I., & Grunfeld, E. (2009). Evaluation of a group cognitive behavioural intervention for women suffering from menopausal symptoms following breast cancer treatment. *Psycho-Oncology 18*, 560–563. doi:10.1002/pon.1414

Leonard, B. (2004). Women's conditions occurring in men: Breast cancer, osteoporosis, male menopause, and eating disorders. *Nursing Clinics of North America, 39*, 379–393.

Li, S., Carlson, E., Snyder, D., & Holm, K. (1995). Perspectives on menopause. *Clinical Nurse Specialist, 9*(3), 145–148.

Lobo, R. (2007). Surgical menopause and cardiovascular risks. *Menopause, 14*(3 Pt. 2), 562–566.

Loprinzi, C., Wolf, S., Barton, D., & Laack, N. (2008). Symptom management in premenopausal patients with breast cancer. *The Lancet Oncology, 9*(10), 993–1001.

McAndrew, L., Napolitano, M., Albrecht, A., Farrell, N., Marcus, B., & Whiteley, J. (2009). When, why, and for whom there is a relationship between physical activity and menopause symptoms. *Maturitas, 64*, 119–125.

McKinlay, J., Travison, T., Araujo, A., & Kupelian, V. (2007). Male menopause—time for a decent burial? *Menopause: The Journal of the North American Menopause Society, 14*(6), 973–975.

Meyer, V. (2003). Medicalized menopause, U.S. style. *Health Care for Women International, 24*, 822–830.

Meyer, V. (2001). The medicalization of menopause: Critique and consequences. *International Journal of Health Services, 32*(4), 769–792.

Minarik, P. (2009). Sleep disturbance in midlife women. *Journal of Obstetric, Gynecologic, & Neonatal Nursing, 38*(3), 333–343.

Murkies, A. (2004). If not hormones, then what? *Australian Family Physician, 35*(11), 895–899.

National Institute of Arthritis and Musculoskeletal and Skin Diseases. (2013). Osteoarthritis. Retrieved from http://www.niams.nih.gov/Health_Info/Osteoarthritis/default.asp#2

North American Menopause Society. (2007). *Menopause practice* (3rd ed.). Cleveland, OH: Author.

North American Menopause Society. (2010). Estrogen and progestogen use in postmenopausal women: 2010 position statement of the North American Menopause Society. *Menopause: The Journal of the North American Menopause Society, 17*(2), 242–255.

North American Menopause Society. (2015). Five solutions for menopause symptoms. Retrieved from http://www.menopause.org/for-women/menopauseflashes/menopause-symptoms-and-treatments/five-solutions-for-menopause-symptoms

Peate, I. (2003). The male menopause: Possible causes, symptoms, and treatment. *British Journal of Nursing, 12*(2), 80–84.

Ravnikar, V., Santoro, N., & Utian, W. (2005). Managing menopause in the post hormone therapy era. *Patient Care, 39*(8), 26–42.

Reddish, S. (2004). Assessment of women in midlife. *Australian Family Physician, 33*(11), 883–887.

Santoro, N. (2004). What a SWAN can teach us about menopause. *Contemporary OB/GYN, 49*, 69–79.

Santoro, N. (2007). Women want to know: Predicting the final menses. *Sexuality, Reproduction & Menopause, 19*(5), 6–10.

Santoro, N., & Chervenak, J. (2004). The menopause transition. *Endocrinology and Metabolism Clinics of North America, 33*, 627–636.

Santoro, N., & Sutton-Tyrell, K. (2011). The SWAN song: Study of women's health across the nation's recurring themes. *Obstetrics and Gynecology Clinics of North America, 38*, 417–423.

Schutte-Rodin, S., Broch, L., Buysse, D., Dorsey, C., & Sateia, M. (2008). Clinical guidelines for the evaluation and management of chronic insomnia in adults. *Journal of Clinical Sleep Medicine, 4*(5), 487–504.

Shifren, J., & Gass, M., for the NAMS Recommendations for Clinical Care of Midlife Women Working Group. (2014). The North American Menopause Society recommendations for clinical care of midlife women. *Menopause: The Journal of the North American Menopause Society, 21*(10), 1–25.

SWAN: Study of Women's Health Across the Nation. (2003). SWAN highlights. Retrieved from http://www.swanstudy.org

Steffen, P. (2011). Spirituality and severity of menopausal symptoms in a sample of religious women. *Journal of Religious Health, 50,* 721–729.

Tunuguntla, H. (2005). Management of andropause: The male menopause. *Clinical Geriatrics, 13*(11), 27–34.

Vainiopää, K., & Topo, P. (2006). The construction of male menopause in Finnish popular magazines. *Critical Public Health, 16*(1), 19–34.

van der Mooren, M., & Kenemans, P. (2004). Postmenopausal hormone therapy: Impact on menopause-related symptoms, chronic disease, and quality of life. *Drugs, 64*(8), 821–836.

Varner, J. (2013). MANopause (Andropause). *The Alabama Nurse, 40*(1), 7–9.

von Mühlen, D., Morton, D., Von Mühlen, C., & Barrett-Connor, D. (2002). Postmenopausal estrogen and increased risk of clinical osteoarthritis at the hip, hand, and knee in older women. *Journal of Women's Health and Gender-Based Medicine, 11*(6), 511–518.

Whitcomb, B., Whiteman, M., Langenberg, P., Flaws, J., & Romani, W. (2007). Physical activity and risk of hot flashes among women in midlife. *Journal of Women's Health, 16*(1), 124–133.

Wiggins, D., & Dizon, D. (2008). Dyspareunia and vaginal dryness after breast cancer treatment. *Sexuality, Reproduction, & Menopause, 6*(3), 18–22.

Wilbur, J., Miller, A., McDevitt, J., Wang, E., & Miller, J. (2005). Menopausal status, moderate-intensity walking, and symptoms in midlife women. *Research and Theory for Nursing Practice: An International Journal, 19*(2), 163–180.

Cardiovascular Disease

Introduction

Although frequently considered a "man's disease," cardiovascular disease is the foremost cause of death and disability for women in the United States. Each year, more women die of cardiovascular disease than men. Misperceptions about the dangers of cardiovascular disease for women persist. This lack of understanding and awareness places women at a serious disadvantage both in recognizing cardiovascular disease as their greatest health threat and in obtaining adequate prevention and treatment measures. This chapter focuses on three prevalent cardiovascular conditions in

women: coronary heart disease, hypertension, and heart failure. In addition, the impact of these cardiovascular conditions on the quality of life of women is examined.

Incidence

The current statistics for the prevalence of cardiovascular disease in the United States are startling. In 2010, an estimated 83.6 million American adults, (approximately one in three) were diagnosed with one or more types of cardiovascular disease. Of this total, an estimated 42.9 million, or 34%, were women (Go et al., 2014). Cardiovascular disease is the leading cause of death for both men and women. In 2010, cardiovascular disease accounted for 787,650, or 31%, of all deaths, or one in every three deaths in the United States. Of this total, 400,332, or 50.8%, of the deaths were women. This statistic translates to more female lives lost yearly to cardiovascular disease than to breast cancer, lung cancer, or all forms of cancer combined (Go et al., 2014).

Cardiovascular disease disproportionately affects women of ethnic minorities. It is estimated that of the total women afflicted with cardiovascular disease in this country, 32.4% are white, 48.9% are African-American, and 30.7% are Mexican-American females (Go et al., 2014). African-American women have the highest overall death rate due to cardiovascular disease than white, Hispanic/Latina, Native American/Alaskan native, and Asian/Pacific Islander females (Go et al., 2014).

The mortality statistics for African-American women in overall and specific cardiovascular diseases indicate that African-American women have a higher death rate as compared to African-American men in total cardiovascular diseases, coronary heart disease, myocardial infarction, hypertension, and heart failure (Lloyd-Jones et al., 2009). Similarly, except for coronary heart disease and myocardial infarction, white women have a higher death rate than white men in overall and specific cardiovascular diseases (Lloyd-Jones et al., 2009).

Ethnic Considerations

The reasons for disparity in incidence and mortality of cardiovascular disease in racial/ethnic minorities are complex and not clearly characterized. Nevertheless, differences in socioeconomic status, levels of education, lack of health insurance, access to health services, and engagement in high-risk behaviors such as smoking, sedentary activity, and poor nutrition likely contribute to disparities in morbidity and mortality among

white and minority women (Finkelstein, Khavjou, Mobley, Haney & Will, 2004). These factors will be further examined in this chapter.

Etiology and Risk Factors

Certain human traits, conditions, and behaviors can increase the likelihood of the development of cardiovascular disease in women. Those traits or conditions that cannot be altered, reduced, or changed are non-modifiable risk factors, whereas conditions or behaviors that can be altered, eliminated, or controlled are considered modifiable risk factors. Contributing risk factors are those that are associated with increasing the risk of developing cardiovascular disease; however, the significance and prevalence of these factors have yet to be determined. The risk factors for developing cardiovascular disease in women are summarized below.

Non-Modifiable Risk Factors

Increasing Age

As women age, their risk for developing cardiovascular disease increases. Women are more likely to develop cardiovascular disease after menopause when the cardioprotective effects of estrogen diminish. Moreover, women commonly develop heart disease about 10 to 15 years later than men. However, by age 70, women have about the same risk for heart disease as same-aged men. As women age, arteries become stiffer and thicker, and systolic blood pressure becomes elevated. These age-related changes play a role in plaque buildup in artery walls (Office on Women's Health, 2009).

Heredity

A family history of cardiovascular disease increases individual risk for developing heart disease. Women with close blood relatives who have had heart disease or stroke have a substantially increased risk of cardiovascular disease (Office on Women's Health, 2009).

Ethnicity

Ethnicity may also confer risk in that African-American women tend to be at higher risk for hypertension, heart disease, and stroke than white women. In addition, evidence suggests that racial and ethnic minorities are more likely to develop heart disease (Office on Women's Health, 2009).

Modifiable Risk Factors

Smoking

Smoking is the foremost cause of cardiovascular disease in women, and yet the single most preventable risk factor. Smoking contributes to an increased risk of coronary heart disease and stroke. When smoking is combined with any of the other risk factors, the risk for cardiovascular disease is greatly elevated. Smoking increases blood pressure as well as diminishes exercise tolerance and increases the propensity for blood to clot. Smoking lowers estrogen levels and decreases high density lipoprotein cholesterol (HDL-C), elevates low density lipoprotein cholesterol (LDL-C), and damages the endothelium of arteries, thus enhancing the development of atherosclerosis. Younger women who use oral contraceptives and smoke experience a greatly increased risk of coronary heart disease and stroke (Gill, 2015). Secondhand or passive smoke has also been found to significantly increase the risk of cardiovascular-related death and disability

Dyslipidemia

Postmenopausal women's cholesterol levels tend to be higher than those found in premenopausal women. Estrogen seems to have a protective effect on the lipid profile by increasing HDL-C and reducing vascular injury and atherosclerosis (Gill, 2015). The HDL-C has a beneficial effect and

tends to lower the risk of heart disease, whereas LDL-C increases risk of heart disease. Within a year of menopause, however, total cholesterol, LDL-C, and apolipoprotein B increase substantially in women across ethnicities and geography. Evidence suggests that in women, low HDL-C is a stronger predictor of cardiovascular disease than high LDL-C (Gill, 2015).

Hypertension

High blood pressure is a common risk factor and significantly elevates the risk of progressive atherosclerosis, stroke, heart disease, kidney failure, and congestive heart failure in women. High blood pressure increases the workload of the heart and makes the heart and arteries more vulnerable to injury. Women who are elderly, obese, have family history of hypertension, or are African-American are at greater risk for developing high blood pressure. African-American women generally have higher average blood pressure levels than white women, and are more likely to be diabetic and obese (Birchfield, 2003). High blood pressure combined with obesity, smoking, dyslipidemia, or diabetes significantly increases the risk for heart disease or stroke.

Physical Inactivity

Lack of physical activity increases the risk for heart disease and indirectly increases the risk of stroke. Physical inactivity can contribute to weight gain, high blood pressure, dyslipidemia, and diabetes. Approximately 60% of American women are sedentary (Birchfield, 2003). On average, women of all races are less physically active than men.

Obesity

Obesity has risen to epidemic proportions in America, where more than half of adult women are obese (Mather, 2004). Compounding the situation, women who are obese are more likely to be diabetic and sedentary. Central obesity, in which a greater concentration of fat is distributed in the upper region of the body, carries a higher risk for heart disease, as it is considered less metabolically active and more frequently related to increased insulin resistance (Birchfield, 2003). A body mass index (BMI) greater than or equal to 30 kg/m² and/ or waist circumference greater than 35 inches are associated with high risk for cardiovascular disease and hypertension (Hendley et al., 2011; National Heart, Lung, and Blood Institute [NHLBI], 2012). Obesity accentuates hypertension and dyslipidemia, and increases intravascular volume, cardiac output, and heart rate (Birchfield, 2003; Mather, 2004).

Diabetes

Diabetes is one of the most compelling risk factors of cardiovascular disease in women. It is a stronger predictor of cardiovascular disease in women than in men (Gill, 2015). Women who are diabetic are three to seven times more likely to develop cardiovascular disease than nondiabetic women (Birchfield, 2003). Diabetes contributes to high blood pressure, dyslipidemia, and obesity in women and significantly increases the risk of stroke, heart failure, renal disease, and atherosclerosis.

Metabolic Syndrome

The presence of metabolic syndrome further escalates the risk for cardiovascular disease in women. Metabolic syndrome in women is characterized by the presence of three or more of the following: abdominal obesity (waist circumference greater than 35 inches), glucose intolerance (fasting glucose greater than or equal to 110 mg/dl), blood pressure greater than or equal to 130/85 mmHg, elevated triglycerides (greater than or equal to 150 mg/dl), and low HDL-C (less than 50 mg/dl) (NHLBI, 2004).

Contributing Risk Factors

Hypertriglyceridemia

Triglyceride levels increase as women age, and excessive triglyceride levels amplify risk for heart disease. High triglyceride levels often accompany higher levels of total cholesterol and LDL-C, lower levels of HDL-C, and increased risk of diabetes. Research findings have suggested that low levels of HDL-C combined with high triglyceride levels seem to be stronger predictors of cardiovascular disease mortality in women as compared to men (Mather, 2004).

Excessive Alcohol Intake

High levels of alcohol consumption, that is, greater than one drink per day for women and one or two drinks per day for men, is associated with increased cardiovascular risk. Heavy alcohol use can contribute to hypertension and accounts for about one-third of all cases of nonischemic dilated cardiomyopathy. Heavy alcohol consumption is also a frequent cause of atrial fibrillation, and markedly increases the risk of stroke (O'Keefe, Bhatti, Bajwa, DiNicolantonio, & Lavie, 2010). In addition, excessive alcohol consumption can contribute to obesity, high triglycerides, irregular heart rhythm, heart failure, cancer, and other diseases (Office on Women's Health, 2009).

Individual Response to Stress

Stress can affect high blood pressure and cholesterol levels and promotes plaque buildup in the arteries. The chemicals released into the blood when the body is exposed to stress can negatively affect the coronary arteries and cause hypercoagulability of blood. Stress can also contribute to unhealthy behaviors such as smoking, physical inactivity, and overeating.

Degree of Risk of Cardiovascular Disease

Cardiovascular risk assessment was previously estimated using the Framingham Risk Score, a prediction algorithm for coronary heart disease.

The Framingham Risk score incorporated age, sex, diabetes, systolic and diastolic blood pressures, levels of total LDL-C and HDL-C, and smoking to estimate a 10-year risk for angina, myocardial infarction, or death due to coronary heart disease (DeFilippis et al., 2015). However, the applicability of Framingham Risk Scores to modern populations became questionable. Framingham-based scores were based on a homogeneous, geographically limited, white male–dominated cohort from a period when cardiovascular risk profiles and preventive pharmacotherapy were both less well-developed and less used than in modern cohorts. Evidence from multiple studies in diverse populations suggested that Framingham-based risk-scoring systems misclassified risk, particularly in women, and overestimated coronary heart disease risk (DeFilippis et al., 2015).

The American Heart Association (AHA) and the American College of Cardiology (ACC) developed an updated atherosclerotic cardiovascular disease (ASCVD) risk score to guide ASCVD risk-reducing therapy. This new risk score is derived from data from racially and geographically diverse prospective cohort studies as well as "applicable data" from the Framingham cohort studies. Using the same traditional risk factors as the original Framingham risk scores, the new risk scores offer separate equations for white and African-American men and women (DeFilippis, 2015).

Risk Reduction

Smoking Cessation

Although the prevalence of smoking has fallen dramatically in the last two decades, the rate of smoking cessation is less for women than men (Birchfield, 2003). Cigarette smoking is a significant preventable risk factor of cardiovascular disease, and smoking cessation reduces the risk (Luo, Rossouw, & Margolis, 2013). Disease risk declines within months of smoking cessation, and

risk will reach levels similar to persons who have never smoked within 3 to 5 years (Mather, 2004). Women who are nonsmokers yet are exposed to secondhand smoke at home or work will have increased disease risk by 25% to 30%. Women should be encouraged and assisted in smoking cessation efforts, and nonsmokers must be aided in avoiding exposure to secondhand smoke. Smokers should also be advised that switching to low tar and low nicotine cigarettes will not achieve desired risk reduction (Mather, 2004).

Cholesterol Reduction

Lipid screening is a cornerstone of preventive care. A complete lipid profile should be performed on women as a baseline by the age of 30. The profile consists of measuring total cholesterol, HDL-C, LDL-C, HDL:LDL cholesterol ratio, and triglyceride level. With lifestyle modification, LDL-C should be maintained at less than 100 mg/dl and HDL-C less than 50 mg/dl. Triglycerides should be less than 150 mg/dl (Mosca et al., 2007).

Evidence suggests that women should consume a diet that emphasizes intake of vegetables, fruits, and whole grains, includes low-fat dairy products, poultry, fish, legumes, nontropical vegetable oils, and nuts, and limits intake of sweets, sugar-sweetened beverages, and red meats. A reduction of saturated fats intake to 5% to 6% of calories, as well as a reduction in trans fatty acids, is also recommended (Eckel et al., 2014).

Lipid-lowering drugs may also be administered along with lifestyle modification in women with high risk. Statins are the drugs of choice for lowering LDL-C. Statin drugs that are currently prescribed include altorvastatin, lovastatin, simvastatin, pravastatin, fluvastatin, pitavastatin, and rosuvastatin (Stone et al., 2013). Common side effects of statin drugs include myalgia, headache, dizziness, nausea, stomach upset, constipation, diarrhea, flatulence, and rash.

Blood Pressure Control

Lifestyle modification is also recommended to achieve blood pressure control in women at risk for cardiovascular disease. Maintenance of optimal blood pressure less than 120/80 is encouraged through weight control, increased physical activity, alcohol moderation, sodium restriction, and consumption of a heart-healthy diet (Mosca et al., 2007). If lifestyle modifications alone produce inadequate control, where blood pressure is greater than or equal to 150/90, or greater than or equal to 140/90 in women with chronic kidney disease or diabetes, treatment with pharmacotherapy is recommended (James et al., 2014). An in-depth discussion of high blood pressure is presented later in this chapter.

Physical Activity

Women are recommended to engage in at least three to four sessions, 40 minutes each, of moderate-to-vigorous physical activity per week. Moderate physical activity may include brisk walking, jogging, or other aerobic exercise (Eckel et al., 2014). Women who need to facilitate weight reduction or sustain weight loss should engage in 60 to 90 minutes of moderate-intensity physical activity on most (preferably all) days of the week (Mosca et al., 2007).

Weight Reduction

Women should strive to maintain or achieve a BMI between 18.5 kg/m^2 and 24.9 kg/m^2 and a waist circumference less than or equal to 35 inches. Weight loss through an appropriate balance of physical activity, caloric intake, and formal behavioral programs is recommended to reduce risk (Mosca et al., 2007).

Diabetes Control

Women with diabetes need to utilize lifestyle modification and pharmacotherapy in order to consistently control blood sugar and maintain glycosolated hemoglobin levels (HbA1c) less than 7% without significant hypoglycemia (Mosca et al., 2007). Research findings have suggested that people with diabetes may not adequately understand their risk for cardiovascular disease (Birchfield, 2003). Thus, thoroughly educating diabetic women regarding the association between diabetes and cardiovascular disease and their serious risk for disease development is essential part of risk reduction efforts.

Metabolic Syndrome Control

Intensive lifestyle modification must be pursued in all women with metabolic syndrome. Concerted effort in weight reduction, increased physical activity, blood pressure and lipid control, and prevention or control of diabetes is necessary to reduce the effects of metabolic syndrome on risk for cardiovascular disease (NHLBI, 2004).

Reduced Alcohol Intake

Evidence suggests that light to moderate alcohol intake—that is, up to one drink per day for women and one or two drinks per day for men—is associated with decreased risks for total mortality, coronary artery disease, diabetes mellitus, congestive heart failure, and stroke (O'Keefe et al., 2010). However, alcohol consumption by nondrinkers or increased alcohol consumption in those who drink is not recommended for risk reduction for cardiovascular disease. Women need to be cautious about their intake of alcohol since even light to moderate alcohol intake is associated with increased risk for breast cancer (O'Keefe et al., 2010).

Stress Management

Lifestyle modification that includes stress management techniques can be effective in modifying women's response to stress and reducing cardiovascular risk. Modifications that include following a low-fat diet, exercise, practicing relaxation techniques such as yoga, deep breathing, imagery, and meditation, and group support have been successful in reducing stress and promoting a healthy lifestyle (Koertge et al., 2003).

Gender Similarities and Differences

Over the years, the perception of cardiovascular disease as a "man's disease" has contributed to a general misunderstanding of cardiovascular disease in women by women, healthcare providers, and society (O'Keefe-McCarthy, 2008). Women may lack understanding of their risk for developing cardiovascular disease and this lack of awareness may lead to ineffective recognition of signs and symptoms and uncertainty concerning when to seek treatment for cardiovascular disease (Mosca, Mochari-Greenberger, Dolor, Newby & Robb, 2010; O'Keefe-McCarthy, 2008). The classic hallmarks used to diagnose and treat cardiovascular diseases emerged mainly from research that focused on white middle-aged men (Albarran, Clarke, & Crawford, 2007). It is becoming increasingly evident that these hallmarks cannot be applied to women, because women often experience cardiovascular disease differently than men. Gender differences in symptom presentation, treatment, and outcomes of cardiovascular disease are likely attributed to dissimilarity in anatomy, physiology, and gender roles.

Female hearts tend to be smaller and lighter than male hearts, and have smaller coronary arteries. Resting heart rate tends to be higher and have greater fluctuations in females as compared to males, and females are apt to have less pronounced wave amplitude on a resting electrocardiogram. Breast tissue in women can interfere with the accuracy of imaging in diagnostic tests such as echocardiogram and radioisotope testing (Nicholson, 2007). First major cardiovascular events often occur in men in the middle years and in women approximately ten years later. This difference is believed to be associated with a reduction in cardioprotective effects of estrogen experienced by women after menopause (Nicholson, 2007). Moreover, men tend to exhibit three-vessel disease and left main disease more frequently, as compared to women, who tend to initially present with normal coronary vessels or mild disease. However, because women are frequently older than men when disease develops, women also tend to have a greater number of comorbid health conditions and cardiovascular risk factors (Dey et al., 2009).

Symptom presentation can differ between men and women. Whereas chest pain as a symptom for coronary heart disease is common to both genders, women are more likely to experience atypical symptoms such as jaw pain, nausea, and vomiting. Chest pain in women often radiates to the upper limbs, jaw, neck, stomach, and particularly to the back, as opposed to the squeezing chest pressure that radiates to the left arm typically experienced by men. Women frequently experience prodromal symptoms such as shortness of breath, tiredness, sleep disturbances, and indigestion that may be easily overlooked or attributed to other causes. The subtleness of symptoms, lack of awareness of coronary heart disease, and reluctance to assume a "sick role" may cause women to dismiss their symptoms and delay seeking treatment. Overall, the atypical nature of coronary symptoms in women may lead to misdiagnosis, fewer admissions to coronary care units, and suboptimal care (Albarran et al., 2007; Nicholson, 2007). Women are less likely to undergo stress testing and therapeutic modalities such as coronary angiography, percutaneous coronary intervention, thrombolysis, or coronary artery bypass graft and less likely to receive statins, beta blockers, or aspirin therapy as compared to men (Crilly, Bundred, Leckey, & Johnstone, 2008; Dey et al., 2009).

Diagnosis and Treatment of Specific Cardiovascular Diseases

Coronary Heart Disease

Coronary heart disease, also known as coronary artery disease, is the number one killer of women in America. The coronary arteries are the major focus of disease. When atherosclerotic plaque builds up in the coronary arteries, the arteries narrow and blood flow to the myocardium is reduced. When the coronary arteries are narrowed to the point that they are unable to supply the myocardium with adequate oxygenated blood, the heart muscle becomes ischemic and angina occurs. *Stable angina* refers to the condition that develops when the myocardial demand for oxygen exceeds the oxygen supply and tissue ischemia produces chest pain. The classic characteristic of stable angina is an episodic chest pain that is brought on by exertion or emotional stress and lasts approximately 5 to 15 minutes. The chest pain is usually relieved by rest or by nitroglycerin.

As atherosclerotic changes progress in the coronary arteries and plaques rupture to form clots, the episodes of angina become increasingly unpredictable with advancement to *unstable angina*. The characteristics of unstable angina include new-onset exertional angina, angina that increases in frequency or duration, angina at rest, or angina that does not respond to nitroglycerin. Women who develop unstable angina have an increased risk for adverse cardiac consequences such as myocardial infarction or death. Another type of angina is *variant angina*, also known as *Prinzmetal angina*, and is a serious indicator of severe atherosclerosis of at least one major coronary vessel. Variant angina is thought to be caused by spasms of the coronary arteries. Anginal pain occurs primarily at rest and can be triggered by smoking. If atherosclerotic plaque ruptures in a coronary artery

and forms a thrombus that completely blocks the flow of blood to the myocardium, the ischemic heart tissue deprived of its blood supply will die. This results in a myocardial infarction, which is also known as a "heart attack."

Acute coronary syndrome is an inclusive designation of the spectrum of thrombotic coronary artery conditions that are consistent with acute myocardial ischemia. Acute coronary syndrome encompasses unstable angina, non-ST elevation myocardial infarction (NSTEMI), and ST elevation myocardial infarction (STEMI) (Coven, 2015).

DIAGNOSIS OF ACUTE CORONARY SYNDROME

The diagnosis of acute coronary syndrome can be especially challenging in women because symptom presentation is often atypical and offers a less recognizable clinical picture to healthcare providers (Dey et al., 2009). Subsequently, women with coronary syndrome are more likely to be sent home from the emergency department without further evaluation (Achar et al., 2005). A comprehensive systematic approach to assessing acute coronary syndrome is essential. The initial assessment will entail a focused history that includes analysis of risk factors, a thorough physical examination, electrocardiogram, diagnostic imaging modalities, and serum cardiac marker determination (Coven, 2015).

Symptoms of acute coronary syndrome may present as chest pain, referred pain, nausea, vomiting, dyspnea, diaphoresis, and lightheadedness. In some cases, chest pain may be absent and sudden dyspnea may be evident instead. The chest pain is characteristically substernal and is described as a squeezing, burning, or heavy pressure sensation across the precordium. Pain may radiate to the neck, shoulder, jaw, back, upper abdomen, or either arm. The physical examination of a woman with chest pain is frequently normal. However, mitral regurgitation murmur, hypotension, pulmonary crackles, a new third (S_3) or fourth (S_4) heart sound, or new jugular venous distension might be detected. On an electrocardiogram, transient ST-segment elevation or T-wave inversion may be noted. Serum cardiac markers may show elevated cardiac troponin T or I, or elevated creatine kinase (CK-MB) (Achar et al., 2005; Coven, 2015). Further diagnostic testing should include chest x-ray, echocardiogram, myocardial perfusion imaging, cardiac angiography, and computed tomography including CT coronary angiography and CT coronary artery calcium scoring (Coven, 2015).

TREATMENT OF CORONARY HEART DISEASE

The treatment of coronary heart disease is multifocal in approach and consists of numerous modalities that are tailored to individual needs. Treatment regimens are selected according to personal choice, presence of comorbidities, and location and severity of atherosclerotic plaque buildup in the coronary arteries.

Treatment of stable angina encompasses lifestyle modifications, pharmacologic therapy, and, when indicated, invasive therapies that increase patency of the coronary arteries. Lifestyle modifications include those measures to reduce cardiac risk that have been previously discussed: smoking cessation, blood pressure control, lipid management, dietary changes, weight management, diabetes control, and increased physical activity (Fraker & Fihn, 2007).

Pharmacological therapy is aimed at decreasing myocardial oxygen demand, increasing coronary artery blood flow, and reducing myocardial ischemia. Pharmacological therapy includes antiplatelet agents, nitrates, beta blockers, and calcium channel blockers. Antiplatelet agents such as clopidogrel, ticlopidine, prasugrel, ticagrelor, or aspirin are given to reduce platelet aggregation and decrease the risk of arterial thrombi formation (Coven, 2015). Although generally well tolerated, gastrointestinal upset, bleeding, dizziness, headache, and tinnitus (from aspirin) may be possible adverse effects of antiplatelet agents. Nitrates are given to produce relaxation of vascular smooth muscle and enhance coronary artery vasodilatation (Coven, 2015). This, in turn, reduces myocardial oxygen demand and increases blood flow to myocardial tissue. Nitrates may be administered via oral, sublingual, transdermal, translingual, submucosal, or intravenous routes. Nitrates are usually well tolerated; however, adverse effects may include headache, dizziness, hypotension, tachycardia, vertigo, faintness, gastrointestinal upset, and dermatitis (from topical application). Beta adrenergic receptor antagonists (beta blockers) are given to reduce cardiac workload by blocking the influence of the sympathetic nervous system on heart tissue (Coven, 2015). Beta blockers decrease blood pressure, heart rate, and myocardial contractility. Adverse effects of beta blockers include gastrointestinal upset, bradycardia, dysrhythmias, fatigue, cool extremities, and reduced exercise tolerance. Calcium channel blockers also reduce cardiac energy consumption and enhance the dilation of coronary arteries, which augments the delivery of oxygen to myocardial cells. Adverse effects of calcium channel blockers may include ankle edema, headache, dizziness, flushing, syncope, palpitations, and bradycardia.

Treatment for acute coronary syndrome encompasses the same lifestyle modifications and drug therapy previously discussed for stable angina with the inclusion of morphine for chest pain unresponsive to nitroglycerin, and angiotensin converting enzyme (ACE) inhibitors for patients who develop myocardial infarction. Morphine is known to cause hypotension, nausea, constipation, and respiratory depression. Women may develop a dry cough, tachycardia, gastrointestinal upset, and rash from ACE inhibitors as well as orthostatic hypotension when taken concurrently with diuretics.

When symptoms are suggestive of a myocardial infarction, early initiation of fibrinolytic therapy can be effective in reducing the severity of damage to the heart muscle or aborting damage altogether. Fibrinolytic therapy is administered intravenously to dissolve the clot that blocks the flow of blood through the coronary artery and restore blood flow to the heart muscle. The time of onset of symptoms to initiating fibrinolytic therapy is an important predictor of the size of myocardial infarction and patient outcomes. The efficacy of therapy in dissolving a clot lessens with the passage of time. Fibrinolytic therapy initiated within the first 2 hours (particularly the first hour) can occasionally terminate myocardial infarction and dramatically diminish mortality.

Antithrombotic therapy with anticoagulants may be indicated in some women with acute coronary syndrome. During the acute inpatient phase of care, women may receive heparin (nonfractionated or low molecular weight), hirudin, or fondaparinux to decrease risk of blood clotting. Wafarin in combination with aspirin may be given to post-myocardial infarction patients treated primarily with a noninvasive approach. Triple anticoagulation with warfarin, aspirin, and clopidogrel may be administered under specific indications such as atrial fibrillation, mechanical prosthetic valve, or left ventricular thrombus, in which risk of blood clot formation is severely high. Triple anticoagulation therapy should be administered for the minimum doses and time necessary to achieve protection due to the high risk of bleeding that may result from the therapy (Anderson et al., 2009).

Evidence has suggested that women derive the same beneficial effects as men from treatment with aspirin, clopidogrel, beta blockers, ACE inhibitors, anticoagulants, and statins. However, women tend to be given antiplatelet and anticoagulant therapy less frequently than men, with higher rates of dosing errors and bleeding episodes than men. Healthcare providers need to closely monitor women's dosages of medication to reduce risk of complications (Anderson et al., 2009).

In addition to conservative therapy of medication and lifestyle modification, a variety of revascularization procedures are available to reduce plaque buildup and improve blood flow through the coronary arteries. Revascularization procedures are considered for women who do not adequately respond to medical management or who may be at high risk for a major cardiac event as indicated by noninvasive testing. Prior to undergoing a revascularization procedure, coronary angiography is usually performed to determine risk stratification and extent of coronary stenoses, provide prognostic information, and direct management of therapeutic care (Anderson et al., 2009). The type of revascularization procedure selected is determined by various factors that present a comprehensive picture of the woman's cardiac condition—namely, extent, distribution, and severity of disease, left ventricular function, presence of comorbidities, risk of complications, effect on quality of life, and personal choice. The percutaneous cardiac intervention (PCI) procedures include percutaneous transluminal coronary angioplasty (PTCA), laser angioplasty, stent insertion, and athrectomy. Percutaneous procedures are recommended for women who have normal or mildly depressed left ventricular function, and focal blockage involving one or more vessels. Coronary artery bypass graft (CABG) involves open heart surgery in which narrowed or blocked coronary arteries are bypassed using sections of veins or arteries taken from elsewhere in the patient's body.

Coronary angiography and revascularization procedures can significantly reduce risk and provide an important avenue for prognostication (Anderson et al., 2009). Angiographic success and late outcomes after PCI for women with acute coronary syndrome have improved and are generally similar to men. However, current research suggests that early complications associated with angiography and PCI tend to occur more frequently in women.

Women who underwent CABG tended to have poorer outcomes than men, but recent research findings point to a more favorable outlook for women who have this procedure (Anderson et al., 2009).

Women with heart disease and their families should work closely with a healthcare team for aggressive management of treatment and reduction of risk factors. Women should be educated about medications, measures for risk reduction, and scheduling of timely follow-up appointments. Low-risk women who received conservative treatment or revascularization should return for follow-up visits with their healthcare providers in 2 to 6 weeks, and higher-risk women should return within 14 days. Women should be monitored closely for treatment compliance and referred as appropriate for cardiac rehabilitation and secondary prevention programs. Optimizing women's compliance with prescribed therapeutic regimens and recommended lifestyle modifications is essential to reduce the risk of recurrent cardiovascular events (Anderson et al., 2009).

Hypertension

Hypertension, or high blood pressure, is a common form of cardiovascular disease among women in America. Across all race and sex groups, the prevalence of hypertension increases with age. The systolic blood pressure levels in women are lower than in men during early adulthood. After the sixth decade of life, the systolic blood pressure levels in women become higher than in men. On the other hand, diastolic blood pressure tends to be marginally lower in women than in men regardless of age. Hypertension tends to be less common among women than men during early adulthood. However, the incidence of hypertension increases more rapidly in women after the fifth decade of life. Consequently, women older than 60 years have higher rates of hypertension compared with men. The highest prevalence rates of hypertension occur in elderly African-American women. More than 75% of African-American women older than 75 years of age have hypertension (Pemu & Ofili, 2008).

Several causal factors for hypertension have been identified. The presence of positive family history of hypertension; obesity (especially intra-abdominal and upper body obesity); smoking; dyslipidemia; excessive sodium; inadequate intake of potassium, fruits, and vegetables; excessive alcohol consumption; physical inactivity; or diabetes can significantly increase the likelihood of developing hypertension. In turn, women with hypertension have increased risk for developing stroke, myocardial infarction, heart failure, renal failure, progressive atherosclerosis, retinopathy, and dementia.

Diagnosis of Hypertension

The Joint National Committee on Prevention, Detection, Evaluation, and Treatment of High Blood Pressure (JNC7) has defined hypertension as a sustained systolic blood pressure greater than or equal to 140 mmHg and diastolic blood pressure greater than or equal to 90 mmHg. A diagnosis of hypertension is made when the average of two or more resting blood pressures obtained on at least two subsequent screening occasions is greater than or equal to 140/90 mmHg (NHLBI, 2004).

Hypertension is often asymptomatic and has been referred to as a "silent killer." Headaches, dizziness, fainting, spontaneous nosebleeds, or blurry vision may occur. When a diagnosis of hypertension is confirmed, women should be thoroughly assessed for lifestyle and any other cardiovascular risk factors or associated disorders that may identify the causes of hypertension, affect prognosis, and guide treatment. In addition, women should undergo a thorough medical history, physical exam, and diagnostic procedures to assess for the absence or presence of target organ damage and cardiovascular disease (NHLBI, 2004).

The JNC7 has presented a system of classification for hypertension for adults aged 18 and older. This

Table 13–1 HYPERTENSION CLASSIFICATIONS

Classification	Blood Pressure	Treatment Recommendations
Normal	Less than 120/80 mmHg	None
Prehypertension	120/80 – 139/89	Lifestyle modifications
Hypertension Stage 1	140/90 – 159/99	Lifestyle modifications and antihypertensive drug therapy
Hypertension Stage 2	Greater than or equal to 160/100	Lifestyle modifications and antihypertensive drug therapy

Modified from National Heart, Lung, and Blood Institute. (2004). *The seventh report of the Joint National Committee on Prevention, Detection, Evaluation, and Treatment of High Blood Pressure (JNC VII)*. (NIH Publication No. 04-5230). Washington, DC: Department of Health and Human Services.

classification system is presented in **Table 13–1**. The purpose of the classification system is to guide healthcare providers in prescribing appropriate treatment and follow-up care for patients with hypertension. It is most significant to note that the JNC7 has updated the classification system with the addition of the designation of prehypertension. This level identifies individuals with blood pressure that ranges between 120/80 to 139/89. Although not a disease category, the prehypertension grouping identifies individuals who are at high risk for developing hypertension. Thus, both patients and healthcare providers are alerted to the pending risk of disease development, and measures to prevent or delay the development of hypertension can be initiated. Individuals with prehypertension are not candidates for drug therapy to reduce their blood pressure and are advised to practice lifestyle modifications to reduce the risk of developing hypertension in the future (NHLBI, 2004).

TREATMENT OF HYPERTENSION

Treatment of hypertension begins with the adoption of healthy lifestyle behaviors. In addition to reduction of blood pressure, lifestyle modifications can prevent or delay the development of

hypertension, enhance effectiveness of antihypertensive drug therapy, and reduce the risk of cardiovascular diseases. Healthy lifestyle behaviors similar to those recommended for cardiovascular disease risk reduction include weight reduction, dietary modification, reduction in sodium intake, physical activity, and smoking cessation. Weight loss of at least 10 pounds (4.5 kg) can substantially reduce blood pressure and/or prevent hypertension in a large majority of overweight individuals. Maintaining a BMI ranging from 18.5 to 24.9 is ideal (NHLBI, 2004). Efforts toward weight reduction and maintenance should include reduction of caloric intake combined with increased physical activity and proven behavioral programs to decrease recidivism.

Recommended dietary modification in managing blood pressure is adherence to a dietary pattern that emphasizes intake of vegetables, fruits, and whole grains; includes low-fat dairy products, poultry, fish, legumes, nontropical vegetable oils and nuts; and limits intake of sweets, sugar-sweetened beverages, and red meats. The Dietary Approaches to Stop Hypertension (DASH) eating plan, the USDA food pattern, or the AHA diet each fit this recommended dietary pattern. It is recommended that this dietary pattern be adapted to provide appropriate caloric requirements, personal and cultural food preferences, as well as nutrition therapy for other medical conditions (including diabetes mellitus). Dietary sodium intake should be no more than 2.4 grams per day (Eckel et al., 2014).

In addition to dietary modifications, physical activity modifications are recommended. Adults should engage in 2 hours and 30 minutes a week of moderate-intensity, or 1 hour and 15 minutes (75 minutes) a week of vigorous-intensity aerobic physical activity, or an equivalent combination of moderate- and vigorous-intensity aerobic physical activity. Episodes of aerobic activity of at least 10 minutes duration preferably should be spread throughout the week (Eckel et al., 2014). A reduction of alcohol consumption to one drink per day, and most importantly, cessation of smoking, is also recommended (NHLBI, 2004).

In 2014, the 8th Joint National Committee on Prevention, Detection, Evaluation, and Treatment of High Blood Pressure (JNC8) updated JNC7 pharmacologic treatment guidelines. For women aged 60 years or older, drug therapy should be initiated to lower blood pressure at systolic blood pressure (SBP) of 150 mm Hg or higher or diastolic blood pressure (DBP) of 90 mmHg or higher. Women of this age category should be treated to achieve a goal SBP lower than 150 mmHg and goal DBP lower than 90 mmHg (James et al., 2014). If pharmacologic treatment for high BP results in lower achieved SBP (eg, < 140 mmHg) and treatment is well tolerated and without adverse effects on health or quality of life, treatment will not need to be adjusted (James et al., 2014).

For women younger than 60 years of age, drug therapy should be initiated to lower blood pressure at DBP of 90 mmHg or higher and treat to a goal DBP of lower than 90 mmHg. Drug therapy should be initiated to lower blood pressure at SBP of 140 mmHg or higher and treat to a goal SBP of lower than 140 mmHg. For women aged 18 or older who have chronic kidney disease or diabetes, drug therapy should be initiated to lower blood pressure at SBP of 140 mmHg or higher or DBP of 90 mmHg or higher and treat to goal SBP of lower than 140 mmHg and goal DBP lower than 90 mmHg (James et al., 2014).

For non-African–American women, including those with diabetes, initial antihypertensive treatment should include a thiazide-type diuretic, calcium channel blocker (CCB), angiotensin-converting enzyme inhibitor (ACEI), or angiotensin receptor blocker (ARB). For African-American women, including those with diabetes, initial antihypertensive treatment should include a thiazide-type diuretic or CCB. For women aged 18 years or older with chronic kidney disease and hypertension, initial (or add-on) antihypertensive treatment should include an ACEI or ARB to improve kidney outcomes. This applies to all women with chronic kidney disease with hypertension regardless of race or diabetes status (James et al., 2014).

Women using drug therapy for treatment of high blood pressure should be closely monitored for adverse side effects. Adverse side effects that seriously impact on quality of life may lead to noncompliance with the drug regimen. Thiazide therapy may cause hypokalemia, since thiazides promote potassium loss from the body. Women will need to replenish lost potassium by consumption of potassium-rich foods or potassium supplements to maintain optimal blood levels. Adverse effects of beta blockers, calcium channel blockers, and ACEIs have been previously discussed. Women who use ARBs may experience side effects similar to ACEIs but less severe and less frequent.

Once drug therapy has begun, close monitoring with monthly follow-up visits to the healthcare provider is essential until desired reduction in blood pressure has been achieved. Women with Stage 2 hypertension may require more frequent follow-up visits. Once the blood pressure goal has been reached and is stable, follow-up intervals may be reduced to every 3 to 6 months. Specific intervals for follow-up will be determined by factors such as the need for diagnostic tests and the presence of comorbidities and cardiovascular risk factors (NHLBI, 2004). Compliance with the treatment regimen and follow-up care is vital to achieving desired blood pressure control.

Heart Failure

Heart failure is a substantial problem and major public health concern in America. Heart failure develops primarily among the elderly, and with the population living longer, the incidence of the disease has increased significantly. The total direct and indirect costs of heart failure in the United States exceeds $30 billion (Yancy et al., 2013). The majority of individuals in the general population afflicted with heart failure are women—more specifically, elderly women. Yet, consistent with the perspective of heart failure being seen as "men's disease," research on heart failure has been conducted primarily with men. Women frequently present a clinical picture of heart failure that differs significantly from men (Jessup et al., 2009). Nevertheless, inadequate recognition of the disease as well as under- or overtreatment of heart failure based on male parameters occurs. A lack of sufficient female representation in clinical trials precludes drawing conclusions about safety and efficacy of heart failure treatment in women (Jessup et al., 2009). Evidence so far suggests differences in women's versus men's treatment outcomes that are associated with drug efficacy, survival benefits, and safety profile. In response to the existing gender disparity in evidence, extensive efforts have been mandated and are currently in progress to increase the representation of women in government-sponsored clinical trials (Jessup et al., 2009).

Heart failure is a complex disease that results from various cardiac disorders that impair the capability of the ventricle to fill with or eject blood. As a result, the heart fails to provide adequate perfusion to peripheral tissues and compensatory mechanisms are activated to meet tissue oxygen demand. The disease was previously referred to as congestive heart failure because of the possibility of fluid excess that can occur with the syndrome. Since fluid excess does not develop in all heart failure cases, the preferred designation of "heart failure" is considered more accurate. Heart failure develops primarily from coronary heart disease, hypertension, valvular disease, or dilated cardiomyopathy. The majority of those afflicted with heart failure have symptoms associated with dysfunction of the left ventricle. The continuum of dysfunction in heart failure can range from having normal-sized left ventricle and preserved capacity for blood ejection to severe left ventricular dilatation and/or markedly reduced capacity to eject blood. Heart failure is categorized into systolic and diastolic failure. In systolic failure, the ventricle, because of reduced myocardial contractility, has diminished capability to eject blood. In diastolic failure, the ventricle is unable to relax to appropriately fill with blood. Both systolic and diastolic failure can exist concurrently.

DIAGNOSIS OF HEART FAILURE

No one specific test can diagnose heart failure. Rather, the diagnosis of heart failure is made by careful assessment of the medical history and physical examination, and the clinical picture created by a comprehensive cardiac workup. This workup may include chest x-ray, blood and urine testing, electrocardiogram, echocardiogram, radionuclide ventriculography, noninvasive cardiac imaging, and coronary angiography as indicated.

The characteristic manifestations of left ventricular failure include fatigue, confusion, restlessness, and dyspnea upon exertion that can progress to dyspnea at rest as severity of dysfunction increases. Women may also develop orthopnea, nocturnal cough, and paroxysmal nocturnal dyspnea. Pulmonary congestion frequently leads to pulmonary edema, which is accompanied by crackles, wheezing, and frothy pink sputum. Tachycardia, heart murmurs, extra heart sounds (S_3 and S_4), and dysrhythmias may also develop. Failure of the right ventricle produces systemic manifestations, which include lower extremity edema that can ascend to the thighs and abdominal wall, hepatomegaly, weight gain, jugular venous distention, gastrointestinal upset, and frequent nocturnal urination.

In disease presentation, women tend to have more signs and symptoms than men, especially edema, exercise intolerance, S_3 heart sound, and jugular venous distension. Women also tend to have a greater number of hospitalizations, higher annual admission rate, and longer duration of hospital stay. In the continuum of heart failure syndrome, clinical severity varies substantially. The American College of Cardiology Foundation (ACCF) and the American Heart Association (AHA) staging system identifies those both at risk for heart failure as well as those symptomatic with heart failure with emphasis on both the development and progression of the disease (Yancy et al., 2013). The staging system is comprised of:

- Stage A: identifies individuals who are at high risk for heart failure but without structural heart disease or symptoms of heart failure.
- Stage B: identifies individuals at high risk for heart failure who have structural heart disease without signs or symptoms of heart failure.
- Stage C: identifies individuals with structural heart disease with prior or current symptoms of heart failure.
- Stage D: identifies individuals in refractory heart failure requiring specialized interventions (Yancy et al., 2013).

The staging system assists healthcare providers to identify women who are at risk for developing heart failure, and introduce therapeutic interventions prior to the appearance of left ventricular dysfunction or symptoms, to reduce morbidity and mortality of heart failure in the population. The staging system recognizes that both risk factors and abnormalities of cardiac structure are associated with heart failure. The stages of the system are progressive and inviolate, following a forward trajectory. Once a patient progresses to a higher stage, regression to an earlier stage of heart failure is not observed (Yancy et al., 2013).

TREATMENT OF HEART FAILURE

Treatment regimens for heart failure are determined by underlying etiology, precipitating factors, and stage of clinical severity. Women with underlying causes such as hypertension, cardiac ischemia, or valvular disease should be treated aggressively according to their respective guidelines to reduce the risk of heart failure occurring. Precipitating factors that can place additional stress on a weakened heart, such as anemia, volume overload, and decreased myocardial function should be sought and corrected as indicated (Yancy et al., 2013).

As is consistent with other cardiovascular diseases, lifestyle modifications play an important role in the treatment plan for heart failure. Cessation of smoking and avoidance of alcohol and illicit drug use must be encouraged. Management of lipid disorders, control of metabolic syndrome, and management of hypertension must be conscientiously achieved (Yancy et al., 2013).

Dietary restriction of sodium is essential in women with heart failure, especially with fluid retention. Sodium intake is generally limited to 2 g per day. Excessive sodium intake can increase fluid retention, edema, and blood pressure, and consequently increase the workload and oxygen requirements of the heart. Education about sodium content in foods and reading nutritional labels is indispensible in managing dietary intake of sodium. Exercise intolerance may be problematic, thus an individualized program of exercise training, starting with exercise testing, is also an essential aspect of treatment (Yancy et al., 2013). Although women are referred less frequently than men, cardiac rehabilitation, when possible, is beneficial in helping women build exercise tolerance (Daley et al., 2002).

Along with lifestyle modification, treatment of heart failure includes drug therapy. Cardiac drugs that are useful for treating various stages of heart failure include ACE inhibitors, ARBs, aldosterone blockers, beta blockers, hydralazine, and isosorbide dinitrate. When fluid retention is present, loop diuretics are usually given (Yancy et al., 2013). Close monitoring of serum potassium levels is needed with most drugs used for treatment of heart failure. Replenishment of potassium through supplementation and diet as needed is necessary with the use of loop diuretics (Yancy et al, 2013). Digoxin may be recommended for women with current or prior symptoms of heart failure and is useful in controlling atrial fibrillation. Serum digoxin levels should be monitored carefully, especially in the presence of decreased renal functioning or suspected noncompliance, since the risk of toxicity is increased. Symptoms of digoxin toxicity include nausea, bradycardia, visual disturbance, and cognitive dysfunction.

Other therapies may be recommended for some patients. The insertion of biventricular pacemakers in women in advanced stages of heart failure when indicated may improve symptoms, quality of life, exercise capacity, and pumping capacity of the left ventricle, as well as decrease hospitalizations (Yancy et al., 2013). Implantable defibrillators and extracorporeal or implantable left ventricular assist devices may also be used in some women as necessary. When heart failure has become refractory to standard treatment modalities (Stage D), few options remain and the appropriate level of care must be determined. These options may encompass compassionate end of life care and hospice. If suitable, extraordinary measures may be used that include heart transplant, chronic inotropes, permanent mechanical support, or experimental surgery or drugs (Yancy et al., 2013).

Close medical supervision and follow-up is an essential aspect of the treatment regimen for women with heart failure. Noncompliance with diet and medication can lead to the development of a profound clinical event that requires emergency care or hospitalization. Patient education along with close supervision by healthcare providers and family members can be effective in detecting subtle changes in symptoms or weight increases that may be early manifestations of clinical deterioration. Early detection may then provide the opportunity to initiate treatment that can prevent clinical decline (Yancy et al., 2013).

Quality of Life Issues Associated With Cardiovascular Disease

The quality of life of individuals with cardiovascular disease has become a priority research focus. The majority of studies that have addressed the subject have done so by comparing men with women. Not surprisingly, research findings have consistently indicated that women with cardiovascular disease have a poorer quality of life than their male counterparts (Brink, Karlson, & Hallberg, 2002; Ford et al., 2008; Garavalia et al., 2007; Urizar & Sears, 2006). Women's older age and greater number of comorbidities and risk factors likely contribute to the gender disparity in quality of life. Nonetheless, there is a scarcity of research that specifically addresses the quality of life issues of women with cardiovascular disease. In view of the physical and psychosocial differences that exist between men and women with respect to diagnosis, treatment, and outcomes of cardiovascular disease, the need for quality of life research that specifically focuses on women is essential and slowly forthcoming.

The quality of life issues that emerge in women with cardiovascular disease are multidimensional and encompass health and physical functioning, psychological and spiritual well-being, socioeconomic integrity, and family well-being. The lack of awareness of cardiovascular risk, the diagnosis of disease, the range of symptoms women experience with cardiovascular disease, and the aftereffects of medical and surgical interventions can impact profoundly across the various domains of quality of life.

Issues Affecting Health and Physical Functioning

Women's lack of awareness of cardiovascular disease can threaten their quality of life. Lack of awareness contributes to behaviors that increase risk for disease development, such as smoking, physical inactivity, poor dietary habits, obesity, and poor control of medical conditions such as hypertension and diabetes (Mosca et al., 2010). Lack of awareness often results in failure to recognize symptoms of cardiovascular disease and delay in seeking treatment (Mosca et al., 2010; O'Keefe-McCarthy, 2008). Lack of awareness may also be a factor in developing cardiovascular disease with a higher degree of severity, greater degree of debilitation, and greater risk of mortality.

Women with cardiovascular disease often experience symptom burden. The type and severity of symptoms are varied and, as previously discussed, are influenced by the nature of cardiovascular disease that has developed, as well as the presence of comorbid conditions. Moreover, the atypical manner of symptom presentation in women can lead to misdiagnosis and undertreatment by healthcare providers. Symptoms and comorbid conditions are significantly associated with poor quality of life and greater functional disability (Sherman et al., 2003). Chest pain in particular has been associated with poorer functioning on health-related quality of life outcomes in women (Sherman et al., 2003).

Women are more likely than men to face greater morbidity and mortality within the first year of recovery following a major cardiac event such as myocardial infarction. Women are at greater risk for decreased exercise and physical functioning

capacity, reinfarction, and death (Benz Scott, Ben-Or, & Allen, 2002). Cardiac rehabilitation is an effective approach for decreasing symptoms, improving functional capabilities, and enhancing quality of life (Shifren, 2003). Cardiac rehabilitation programs are long-term programs that involve strict medication adherence, lifestyle modification, physician-prescribed exercise regimens, education, and counseling. The purpose of cardiac rehabilitation is to facilitate patients' return to energetic and fruitful lives within the constraints of their disease for as long as possible. Specifically, cardiac rehabilitation endeavors to reduce the risk of sudden death, alleviate angina, prevent progression of underlying disease, and restore patients to the best possible level of physical, psychosocial, and vocational performance (Benz Scott et al., 2002). Cardiac rehabilitation is particularly recommended for women with recent acute coronary syndrome or revascularization intervention, new onset or chronic angina, or current/prior symptoms of heart failure or left ventricular ejection fraction of less than 40% (Mosca et al., 2007). Evidence suggests that women have positive outcomes in cardiac rehabilitation in rates similar to men. In fact, some studies have indicated that women who have completed cardiac rehabilitation show better improvements in exercise capacity and in prerehabilitation to postrehabilitation quality of life (Benz Scott et al., 2002).

Nonparticipation and nonadherence with respect to cardiac rehabilitation can adversely impact women's health and functioning over the long term (Shifren, 2003). Women, especially African-American women, are significantly less likely to participate in and to complete cardiac rehabilitation than men. Moreover, physician referral patterns, program characteristics, and patient-centered factors may influence women's participation in, adherence to, and completion of cardiac rehabilitation programs (Benz Scott et al., 2002). These factors include lack of physician referral, unsafe setting for exercising, location and accessibility of programs, lack of transportation, lack of awareness of the need for cardiac rehabilitation, presence of comorbid conditions, perception of exercise as tiring or painful, already participating in a home exercise routine, lack of health insurance coverage, and caregiver role pressures (Benz Scott et al., 2002; Grace et al., 2009; Shifren, 2003).

Women are less likely than men to be referred to cardiac rehabilitation. It is unknown why this gender bias exists. The literature hints that perhaps older age of female cardiac patients, the presence of more comorbidities in women, and differences in underlying diagnoses might influence the provider's referral patterns toward eligible women, but nothing conclusive has been determined. Although clinical guidelines have been developed that clearly designate appropriate referral practices that include women, it is unclear why healthcare providers do not increase their referrals of eligible women to cardiac rehabilitation programs. Evidence suggests that many physicians may not be aware that guidelines exist, may disagree with the content of the guidelines, may elect to ignore the guidelines in the provision of care, or may inconsistently follow the guidelines (Daley et al., 2002).

Program characteristics such as location of the rehabilitation program, accessibility, and safety of the setting may strongly influence women's adherence, participation, and ability to complete the program. Inconvenience of location and scheduling, poor accessibility, and lack of transportation to and from the program facilities can become substantial impediments. Lack of safety in the environment where they perform their exercises, inadequate monitoring, and lack of gender-specific staff support can also be off-putting to women (Benz Scott et al., 2002; Grace et al., 2009; Shifren, 2003). Rehabilitation programs that are conveniently located, easily accessible, provide close supportive monitoring and encouragement, and engage significant family members are more likely to promote program adherence

and completion among female attendees (Benz Scott et al., 2002).

Several patient-centered factors can reduce the likelihood of women's participation and completion of cardiac rehabilitation. Women who are older, widowed, less educated, who do not perceive the necessity for rehabilitation, or find exercising to be difficult or painful are less likely to be compliant with or complete their rehabilitation (Benz Scott et al., 2002). Women are more likely to have comorbidities such as diabetes, urinary incontinence, or osteoporosis that can dissuade them from exercise for fear of injury or accidents (Grace et al., 2009). Women are more likely to have inadequate health insurance coverage that limits their ability to pay for costly programs (Shifren, 2003). Women face more time demands due to caregiver, household, and employment responsibilities, and this may leave little time for them to manage their own health problems. They are often primary caregivers for grandchildren or ailing spouses and this creates role pressures that may hinder their ability to adhere to or complete rehabilitation (Grace et al., 2009; Shifren, 2003). Women with personality traits such as poor self-motivation, low self-efficacy, or poor self-esteem might find it difficult to participate in and complete cardiac rehabilitation programs (Grace et al., 2009, Shifren, 2003).

Women who are eligible for cardiac rehabilitation should be referred by their physicians according to clinical practice guidelines. Care should be taken to consider the type of program that would best fit individual needs, with particular attention to location, accessibility, scheduling, transportation, and cost. Programs that are tailored to meet the needs of women can better address their specific concerns and have a positive influence on program outcomes (Davidson et al., 2008). Once referred and enrolled in cardiac rehabilitation, women are likely to have better success at adherence to and completion of the program when they receive close supportive monitoring, gender-specific education and counseling, and encouragement from physicians, staff, and family members. These considerations are particularly important to lower the barriers that impede women from attaining successful outcomes with cardiac rehabilitation that ultimately enhance quality of life.

Issues Affecting Psychological and Spiritual Functioning

PSYCHOLOGICAL FUNCTIONING

Cardiovascular disease can have a considerable impact on women's psychological well-being. Initially, a major cardiac event can cause concerns about survival of a life-threatening occurrence, and later, issues about the social and psychological impact of impaired health can emerge (Plach, Napholz, & Kelber, 2003). Women at midlife and beyond already experience psychosocial pressures related to various lifestage demands such as menopause, multiple role and caregiver responsibilities, and the emergence of comorbidities, which may increase the likelihood of women's vulnerability to psychosocial distress and poor quality of life (Plach et al., 2003). The occurrence of a major cardiac event, along with issues of less than optimal treatment, often results in substantial emotional distress, depression, poor psychological adjustment, and subsequently poor quality of life. Factors that contribute to depression and poor psychological well-being in women include impaired physical functioning, having comorbid conditions such as diabetes, perceptions of disease severity, social isolation, having decreased social support, and perceived loss of control over their illness (Helgeson, 2003; Murphy et al., 2008). Women tend to experience depression more frequently and have poorer psychological adjustment and well-being post cardiac events than men (Kamm-Steigelman, Kimble, Dunbar, Sowell, & Bairan, 2006, Plach et al., 2003). Furthermore, cardiovascular disease and depression are highly comorbid and research

supports the premise that depression may be a cause, as well as a consequence, of heart disease that increases mortality and generates additional disease (Keyes, 2004).

Following a cardiac event, depression and distress usually diminish over time in patterns consistent with normal bereavement and adjustment for the majority of women. However, many women experience persistent or worsening of depression and distress over time (Murphy et al., 2008). Attention to the emotional impact of cardiovascular disease on women should not be minimized in the process of treating the physical consequences of the disease. Psychological management is particularly important to women's medical outcomes, especially considering the risks that depression may pose to morbidity and mortality. Thus, early screening for depression is important for identifying women at risk and initiating interventions to minimize depression and enhance psychological well-being (Plach et al., 2003). Assessing the presence of positive coping behaviors will help women to identify their available strengths and resources for managing depression and effecting psychological adjustment. Social support and participation in common activities that bring strength and comfort are simple and cost-effective strategies that tap the day-to-day resources present in women's lives. Social support provided by family, friends, and healthcare providers, and participation in comforting activities that are religious or spiritual are particularly effective in helping women cope with depression and maintain an acceptable quality of life (Kamm-Steigelman et al., 2006). Furthermore, women should be educated about the signs and symptoms of depression and encouraged to seek early treatment when necessary. Women and their families should also be educated about the physical and psychological recovery process following a major cardiac event in order to be flexible in their expectations and plan strategies to share household tasks and other responsibilities (Plach et al., 3003).

Spirituality

Religious and spiritual practices have been shown to have positive effects on health. Certain religious and spiritual practices may mediate stressors by inducing the relaxation response, which can, in turn, reduce muscle tension, decrease heart rate and blood pressure, and increase oxygenation, among other physiologic effects. Evidence suggests that spirituality and religiosity are associated with lower blood pressure and less hypertension, better lipid profiles consisting of lower LDL-C and higher HDL-C, and better immune function. Research findings have also indicated associations between non-explicit spiritual meditation (such as Zen, yoga, and transcendental meditation) and lower cardiovascular risks, lower levels of physiologic activation (such as lower blood pressure and pulse, lower endocrine activity, and lower body metabolism), and increased cerebral blood flow (Etnyre et al., 2006).

Issues Affecting Socioeconomic Integrity

Women with cardiovascular disease often experience socioeconomic issues that can seriously impact quality of life. In comparison to men, women encompass a disproportionate segment of those with limited financial means (Shaw et al., 2008). Women with limited financial resources tend to lack adequate health insurance and have a higher risk status, greater risk factor burden, and more functional disability. They are less likely to participate in cardiac rehabilitation and are likely to underutilize drug therapy or revascularization measures. Consequently, medical management is frequently ineffective and healthcare needs are often unmet, placing women with limited financial means at higher risk for poor cardiovascular outcomes and mortality (Shaw et al., 2008).

Another socioeconomic implication for women with cardiovascular disease encompasses employment and social issues. As discussed earlier, women tend to develop heart disease approximately a decade later than men, and tend to have a greater degree of severity and more comorbid conditions. This implies that women at older age may be less likely to return to work following a cardiac event, or they may have already been retired and living within a fixed income. Women who do work, particularly if they are of limited financial means, may experience more sick days and diminished productivity, which can further restrict income and lead to job strain. This can accelerate cardiovascular disease risk (Shaw et al., 2008). There is a greater tendency for women at this age to be unmarried or widowed and experience shrinking social networks due to loss of spouse or friends. Poor physical functioning and debilitation may further limit or prevent participation in social activities. Social isolation can occur, which may further restrict social networks and access to social support.

Social support is an essential resource that can considerably influence the socioeconomic quality of life of women with cardiovascular disease. Eligible women should be referred to cardiac rehabilitation and encouraged to adhere to and complete the program. Cardiac rehabilitation can provide a necessary source of social support through counseling, support groups, and socializing with other individuals with similar needs and experiences. Women should be closely assessed for socioeconomic constraints and measures made available to overcome financial and social barriers that may hinder them from receiving effective care. Family support, religious and spiritual activities, work, play, hobbies, support groups, and social relationships can assist women in maintaining a network of support that can improve coping with heart disease and effectively enhance quality of life (Kamm-Steigelman et al., 2006). Women should be assisted in recognizing social support resources and encouraged to utilize these resources in the self-management of cardiovascular disease and improvement of quality of life.

Issues Affecting Family Well-Being

Cardiovascular disease can have a significant impact on women's roles and relationships within the family and this can subsequently influence quality of life. Women traditionally are engaged in multiple household and relational roles with spouse and family members, including functioning as caregiver for grandchildren or ailing spouse. After a cardiac event, many women have to adjust to changes in their roles as spouses, parents, and caregivers by allowing others to assume the many housekeeping and caregiver responsibilities they have previously maintained. Often, the necessary role transitions can be difficult for women to effect. For some women, changes in their functional status may adversely affect their satisfaction with family members and family-related activities (Husser & Roberto, 2009). Women may refuse to accept help with household and caregiver responsibilities in order to maintain independence, autonomy, and belief in their own capabilities (Roberto, Gigliotti, & Husser, 2005). They may have increased worry about how their spouses and family members are coping with role changes (Emslie, 2005). Women might minimize their symptoms in order to be less of a burden to their family members. Moreover, women tend to put their family responsibilities before their personal health needs in order to reduce family disruption, and may be reluctant to make necessary lifestyle modifications (Emslie, 2005). Such behaviors may lead to treatment noncompliance and place women at risk for poor physical outcomes and inadequate quality of life.

In response to a cardiac event, family members often alter their relationships with women by becoming closer, more attentive, cherishing, and protective (Husser & Roberto, 2009). Many women may find these changes satisfying. However, some women might view such behavior changes as controlling, domineering, or overprotective (Husser & Roberto, 2009).

Accepting family assistance with mixed emotions may generate tension that could interfere with women's ability to manage their health. Refusing family help may result in concealing health problems that may eventually erode the family's willingness and ability to provide assistance in the event that further health problems develop (Roberto et al., 2005). Women need to reconcile their care needs, their willingness to accept help, the actions of family members, and past experiences and relationships with primary support persons in order to create a harmonious and beneficial relationship that supports their health condition (Roberto et al., 2005).

Implications for Healthcare Providers

Healthcare providers need to be cognizant of the gender differences that are related to cardiovascular disease in order to improve disease prevention, treatment, and quality of life outcomes in women. Although the last decade has seen an upswing in research that has focused specifically on women with cardiovascular disease, lack of awareness of women's gender-specific needs concerning disease prevention, diagnosis, treatment, rehabilitation, and quality of life persists. It is essential that nurses and other healthcare providers examine the growing body of evidence that focuses on women with cardiovascular disease and better delineates provision of effective care. Healthcare providers need to understand the physical, psychological, socioeconomic, and cultural factors that can impede women from seeking and receiving timely treatment, gaining effective symptom management, adhering to treatment recommendations and rehabilitation, and managing an acceptable quality of life. Patient education, aggressive risk reduction measures, accurate symptom recognition, and gender-sensitive treatment options should be implemented and continued for as long as needed to reduce morbidity and mortality of heart disease and better maintain women's well-being.

Social support is an essential aspect of care for women with cardiovascular disease. Support from friends and family assists women in adjusting to the demands of cardiovascular disease and maintaining an acceptable quality of life. The home and family milieu should be closely scrutinized and an accurate assessment of women's role demands and family support resources should be obtained, as well as a clear understanding of how the support role is negotiated between women and their family members. Tangible support (such as financial assistance, transportation, housekeeping, and grocery shopping) can help reduce the physical burden of household responsibilities, and emotional and informational support can facilitate coping and adjustment, and reduce stress and anxiety. Tangible and intangible support, particularly from adult children, can be strongly influential in enhancing women's participation in and completion of cardiac rehabilitation (Benz Scott et al., 2002).

Special Concerns of Age and Ethnicity

Although the mortality rate rises steadily as women age, cardiovascular disease threatens adult women across the spectrum of ages. Over one third of the women of the United States have two or more cardiovascular disease risk factors (Hayes et al., 2006). Age differences exist in the clustering of risk factors. For example, younger women tend to be smokers, while older women are more likely to have hypertension, diabetes, high cholesterol, and be physically inactive (Hayes et al., 2006). Older women are more likely to be diagnosed with chronic diseases than younger women because older women interface more frequently with the healthcare system and tend to be screened for chronic conditions due to the increased pervasiveness of these conditions in the elderly. Thus, with

older women, a greater emphasis should be placed on treating and controlling existing conditions along with promoting healthy lifestyle choices to avoid further disease development and maintain an acceptable quality of life (Hayes et al., 2006). On the other hand, younger women are less likely to have chronic conditions, but they should still be encouraged to make healthy lifestyle choices, especially before such conditions develop (Hayes et al., 2006).

Although the leading cause of death among all racial and ethnic groups is cardiovascular disease, African-Americans suffer the most and are more likely to die from the disease (Kamble & Boyd, 2008). African-American women have greater prevalence of cardiovascular disease in comparison to white women, as well as higher mortality (CDC, 2013; Rosenfeld, 2006). African-American women are more likely to be obese, have higher rates of hypertension, greater diabetes prevalence rates, higher rates of elevated blood cholesterol, and a higher calculated degree of coronary heart disease risk (Finkelstein et al., 2004; Kamble & Boyd, 2008). Furthermore, African-American women are less likely to receive appropriate preventive therapies and coronary revascularization procedures (Kamble & Boyd, 2008; Rosenfeld, 2006). Racial and ethnic disparities in cardiovascular disease risk and treatment are associated with a number of factors. African-American women who are economically disadvantaged and have lower levels of education may have inadequate or no health insurance, inadequate access to quality health care, and limited ability to make informed choices or challenge physicians to offer available treatment options (Kamble & Boyd, 2008). African-American women living at the low income strata may be more likely to engage in unhealthy behaviors, be unable to afford healthy foods, or may live in depressed areas where it is unsafe to participate in outdoor physical activity (Hayes et al., 2006; Kamble & Boyd, 2008). Strategies for lifestyle modification and reduction of risk factors in African-American women should be addressed through prevention, early recognition, and treatment. Interventions need to be grounded in education and improvements in the community-wide social environment. Efforts to improve healthcare access, support access, and help African-American women negotiate the system are essential. In particular, enhancing cultural competency, cultural diversity, and cultural sensitivity of healthcare providers must not be overlooked (Kamble & Boyd, 2008).

Research Review

What is the role of spirituality in the self-management and spirituality practices among older women?

Harvey, I. (2008). Assessing self-management and spirituality practices among older women. *American Journal of Health Behavior, 32*(2), 157–168.

The purpose of this study was to explore how older women use spirituality to manage their chronic illness. This study aimed to delineate whether ethnicity differed in the use of spirituality to manage chronic illness. A complementary, cross-sectional design was used. The quantitative component used a random sampling of 482 older women, aged 65 to 96, drawn from the Medicare enrollment file of Allegheny County, Pennsylvania. The sample was stratified by race and disease, and included community-dwelling independent white and African-American adult women with no obvious indication of cognitive impairment, diagnosed with either ischemic heart disease or osteoarthritis. The qualitative component used in-depth interview data from a purposively selected subgroup (n=24; 11 were African-American and 13 were white) from the original sample. Data for the quantitative component were collected during four separate interviews over a 3-year period. The interviews were composed of structured and semistructured questions, and included the completion of a structured questionnaire to identify core self-management behaviors for either heart disease or osteoarthritis. In-depth ethnological interviews were conducted with the 24 women in the qualitative subgroup during the third data collection period. Quantitative data were analyzed using descriptive statistics, t test, chi square, and logistic regression analysis. Narrative analysis was used to evaluate qualitative data.

The quantitative findings revealed that the African-American women were younger, less likely to be married, and had lower educational attainment than the white women. African-American women were more likely to report higher levels of spirituality than the white women. The white women were significantly more physically active and consistently maintained exercise levels. The findings also revealed that, for the African-American women, the higher the perceived level of spirituality, the more likely these women were to engage in physical activity.

The qualitative findings revealed respondents' descriptions of behavioral practices with respect to general issues of self-management for promoting health and recovering from illness, and their fundamental spiritual philosophies that help them manage their illnesses. Four main themes within self-management were identified: the union of traditional medicine and spiritual practices, health-promoting spiritual activities, prayer as a pain manager, and spirituality as a coping mechanism.

The findings suggested that spirituality can be a substantial source of coping and support in managing chronic illness such as cardiovascular disease in older women. Strong spiritual connections may enhance the older women's sense of satisfaction with life and enable them to adjust to disability and illness. Spirituality may also provide women with insights into optimizing the resources of chronic disease self-management practices for reducing the risk for cardiovascular disease through diet and exercise.

Chapter Summary Points

- Cardiovascular disease is the leading cause of death for women in the United States, with more female lives lost yearly to cardiovascular disease than to breast cancer, lung cancer, or all forms of cancer combined.
- African-American women are noted to have the highest overall death rate due to cardiovascular disease than white, Hispanic/Latina, Native American/Alaskan native, and Asian/Pacific Islander females.
- Non-modifiable risk factors for cardiovascular disease cannot be altered and include increasing age, heredity, and previous history of heart disease.
- Modifiable and contributing risk factors for cardiovascular disease can be eliminated or controlled, and include smoking, dyslipidemia, hypertension, physical inactivity, obesity, diabetes, metabolic syndrome, hypertriglyceridemia, and individual response to stress.
- Screening for risk factors followed by education in risk factor reduction is essential. Women are likely to initiate preventive health behaviors when they perceive that they are at higher risk for developing cardiovascular disease, and clinical efforts should be focused on risk factor reduction and modification.
- The hallmarks of diagnosis and treatment of cardiovascular disease are based on evidence derived from male-focused research that cannot be applied to women because women experience cardiovascular disease differently than men.
- Differences in symptom presentation, treatment, and outcomes of cardiovascular disease in women as compared to men are attributed to dissimilarity in anatomy, physiology, and gender roles.
- Women's lack of awareness of their risk for developing cardiovascular disease subsequently leads to ineffective recognition of signs and symptoms, and uncertainty concerning when to seek treatment for cardiovascular disease.
- Treatment of cardiovascular disease generally encompasses lifestyle modifications, pharmacologic therapy, and, when indicated, revascularization procedures.
- The quality of life issues that emerge in women with cardiovascular disease are multidimensional and encompass health and physical functioning, psychological and spiritual well-being, socioeconomic integrity, and family well-being.

- Social support is an essential aspect of care for women with cardiovascular disease and assists women to adjust to the demands of disease and maintain an acceptable quality of life.
- Cardiac rehabilitation is an effective approach for decreasing symptoms, improving functional capabilities, and enhancing quality of life.
- Healthcare providers should implement patient education, aggressive risk reduction measures, accurate symptom recognition, gender-sensitive treatment options, and cardiac rehabilitation for as long as needed to reduce the morbidity and mortality of heart disease in women and better maintain women's well-being.

Critical Thinking Exercise

Case Study

Mrs. R. is a 79-year-old woman who is retired. Her husband is 84 and has Alzheimer's disease. Mrs. R. is her husband's main caregiver. She has two adult sons, one of whom lives in her community, both married with young children. Mrs. R. has a history of high cholesterol and obesity, has never smoked, and has a family history of heart disease in which her father and older brother were diagnosed at middle age with coronary heart disease and subsequently both died of heart attacks before the age of 60. Mrs. R. attributes their early deaths to the fact that they smoked heavily and were male.

Mrs. R. experiences a substantial amount of stress in the daily care of her husband. His level of dementia requires that he be constantly supervised for the maintenance of hygiene, toileting, and safety. Mrs. R. also does the cooking, house cleaning, and grocery shopping and has little time for anything else. She awakens frequently at night to help her husband to the bathroom and to make sure he does not wander about the house. Mrs. R. refuses to consider nursing home placement for Mr. R., insisting that he would feel lost and abandoned, and would not receive proper care. Her family offers to help with caring for Mr. R., household chores, and grocery shopping but she often refuses assistance since she does not want to burden them with her responsibilities. Mrs. R. frequently feels angry and depressed that her husband's dementia has changed their lives and prevents them from socializing, traveling, and enjoying their retirement like they had planned.

Mrs. R. experiences occasional vague symptoms of indigestion accompanied by shortness of breath and back pain and attributes them to her age. One day Mrs. R.'s shortness of breath and back pain worsened to the point where she could not get out of bed. Her son called the emergency paramedics and she was transported to the emergency room where she was admitted to the coronary care unit with a diagnosis of myocardial infarction. During her hospitalization, adult day care was arranged for her husband as well as a home health attendant at night. Mrs. R. recovered and returned home on heart medications and a regimen that included weight loss, sodium restriction, low-fat diet, and exercise. Mrs. R. was referred to a cardiac rehabilitation program in her community; however, she was unsure if she would participate since she "didn't have time for it" and was not "an athletic woman."

Questions for Seminar Discussion

1. What factors place Mrs. R. at high risk for cardiovascular disease?
2. How did lack of awareness of cardiovascular disease risk impact Mrs. R. in the development of her cardiac event?
3. What lifestyle modifications can reduce the risk of cardiovascular disease for Mrs. R?
4. What strategies can remove the barriers to risk reduction present in Mrs. R.'s life?
5. Discuss the physical, psychological/spiritual, socioeconomic, and family issues that diminish Mrs. R.'s quality of life.
6. What resources of social support are available to help Mrs. R. manage her illness and improve her quality of life?
7. Discuss the importance of cardiac rehabilitation to Mrs. R.'s disease management, survival, and quality of life.
8. What strategies could effectively enhance Mrs. R.'s participation in and completion of her cardiac rehabilitation program?

Internet Resources

The American Heart Association: information and resources for patients, family, and professionals http://americanheart.org

Go Red For Women: an American Heart Association sponsored website offering information and support for women to reduce risk of cardiovascular disease http://www.goredforwomen.org

Mended Hearts, Inc.: information and support for patients, spouses, family members, friends, and health professionals http://www.mendedhearts.org

National Heart, Lung, and Blood Institute: information for health professionals and the general public about cardiovascular disease and related lung and blood disorders http://www.nhlbi.nih.gov

WomenHeart: The National Coalition for Women with Heart Disease: a nonprofit patient advocacy group that provides information and support for women with heart disease and their spouses, family members, friends, and health professionals http://www.womenheart.org

References

Achar, S., Kundu, S., & Norcross, W. (2005). Diagnosis of acute coronary syndrome. *American Family Physician*, *72*(1), 119–126.

Albarran, J., Clarke, B., & Crawford, J. (2007). 'It was not chest pain really, I can't explain it!' An exploratory study on the nature of symptoms experienced by women during their myocardial infarction. *Journal of Clinical Nursing, 16*, 1292–1301.

Anderson, J., Adams, C., Antman, E., Bridges, C., Califf, D., Casey, D., ... Wright, S. (2009). ACC/AHA 2007 guidelines for management of patients with unstable angina /non ST-elevation myocardial infarction executive summary: A report of the American College of Cardiology /American Heart Association task force on practice guidelines. *Journal of the American College of Cardiology, 50*, 652–726.

Benz Scott, L., Ben-Or, K., & Allen, J. (2002). Why are women missing from outpatient cardiac rehabilitation programs? A review of multilevel factors affecting referral, enrollment, and completion. *Journal of Women's Health, 11*(9), 773–791.

Birchfield, P. (2003). Identifying women at risk for coronary artery disease. *AAOHN Journal, 51*(1) 15–22.

Brink, E., Karlson, B., & Hallberg, L. (2002). Health experiences of first-time myocardial infarction: Factors influencing women's and men's health-related quality of life after five months. *Psychology, Health, & Medicine, 7*(1), 5–16.

Centers for Disease Control. (2013). Women and heart disease fact sheet. Retrieved from http://www.cdc.gov /dhdsp/data_statistics/fact_sheets/fs_women_heart.htm

Coven, D. (2015). Acute coronary syndrome. Retrieved from http://emedicine.medscape.com /article/1910735-overview

Crilly, M., Bundred, P., Leckey, L., & Johnstone, F. (2008). Gender bias in the clinical management of women with angina: Another look at the Yentl syndrome. *Journal of Women's Health, 17*(3), 331–342.

Daley, J., Sindone, A., Thompson, D., Hancock, K., Chang, E., & Davidson, P. (2002). Barriers to participation in and adherence to cardiac rehabilitation programs: A critical literature review. *Progress in Cardiovascular Nursing, 17*(1), 8–17.

Davidson, P., DiGiacomo, M., Zecchin, R., Clarke, M., Glenn, P., Lamb, K., ... Daly, J. (2008). A cardiac rehabilitation program to improve psychosocial outcomes of women with heart disease. *Journal of Women's Health, 17*(1), 123–134.

DeFilippis, A., Young, R., Carrubba, C., McEvoy, J., Budoff, M., Blumenthal R., ... Blaha, M. (2015). An analysis of calibration and discrimination among multiple cardiovascular risk scores in a modern multiethnic cohort. *Annals of Internal Medicine, 162*, 266–275.

Dey, S., Flather, M., Devlin, G., Brieger, D., Gurfinkel, E., Steg, P., ... Eagle, K. A. (2009). Sex-related differences in the presentation, treatment, and outcomes among patients with acute coronary syndromes: The Global Registry of Acute Coronary Events. *Heart, 95*, 20–26.

Eckel, R., Jakicic, J., Ard, J., Hubbard, V., de Jesus, J., Lee, I., ... Yanovski, S. (2014). AHA/ACC guideline on lifestyle management to reduce cardiovascular risk: A report of the American College of Cardiology American/Heart Association Task Force on Practice Guidelines. *Circulation. 129*(25 Suppl 2), S76–99.

Emslie, C. (2005). Women, men, and coronary heart disease: A review of the qualitative literature. *Journal of Advanced Nursing, 51*(4), 382–395.

Etnyre, A., Rauschhuber, M., Gilliland, I., Cook, J., Mahon, M., Allwein, D., ... Jones, M. (2006). Cardiovascular risk among older Hispanic women. *AAOHN Journal, 54*(3), 120-128.

Finkelstein, E., Khavjou, O., Mobley, L., Haney, D., & Will, J. (2004). Racial/ethnic disparities in coronary heart disease risk factors among WISEWOMAN enrollees. *Journal of Women's Health, 13*(5), 503–518.

Ford, E., Mokdad, A., Chaoyang, L., McGuire, L., Strine, T., Okoro, C., ... Zack, M. (2008). Gender differences in coronary heart disease and health-related quality of life: Findings from 10 states from the 2004 behavioral risk factor surveillance system. *Journal of Women's Health, 17*(5), 757–768.

Fraker, T., & Fihn, S. (2007). 2007 chronic angina focused update of the ACC/AHA 2002 guidelines for the management of patients with chronic stable angina. *Circulation, 116*, 2762–2772.

Garavalia, L., Decker, C., Reid, K., Lichtman, J., Perashar, S., Vaccarino, V., ... Spertus, J. (2007). Does health status differ between men and women in early recovery after myocardial infarction? *Journal of Women's Health, 16*(1), 93–101.

Gill, S. (2015). Cardiovascular risk factors and disease in women. *Medical Clinics of North America, 99*, 535–552.

Go, A., Mozaffarian, D., Roger, V., Benjamin, E., Berry, J., Blaha, M., ... Turner, M.B; on behalf of the American Heart Association Statistics Committee and Stroke Statistics Subcommittee. (2014). Heart disease and stroke statistics—2014 update: A report from the American Heart Association. *Circulation, 129*, e28–e292.

Grace, S., Gravely-Witte, S., Kayaniyil, S., Brual, J., Suskin, N., & Stewart, D. (2009). A multisite examination of sex differences in cardiac rehabilitation barriers by participation status. *Journal of Women's Health, 18*(2), 209–216.

Harvey, I. (2008). Assessing self-management and spirituality practices among older women. *American Journal of Health Behavior, 32*(2), 157–168.

Hayes, D., Denny, C., Keenan, N., Croft, J., Sundaram, A., & Greenlund, K. (2006). Racial/ethnic and socioeconomic differences in multiple risk factors for heart disease and stroke in women: Behavioral risk factor surveillance system, 2003. *Journal of Women's Health, 15*(9), 1000–1008.

Helgeson, V. (2003). Cognitive adaptation, psychological adjustment, and disease progression among angioplasty patients: 4 years later. *Health Psychology, 22*(1), 30–38.

Hendley, Y., Zhao, L., Coverson, D., Din-Dzietham, R., Morris, A., Quyyumi, A., … Vaccarino, V. (2011). Differences in weight perception among blacks and whites. *Journal of Women's Health, 20*(12), 1805–1811.

Husser, E., & Roberto, K. (2009). Older women with cardiovascular disease: Perceptions of initial experiences and long-term influences on daily life. *Journal of Women and Aging, 21*, 3–18.

James, P., Oparil, S., Carter, B., Cushman, W., Dennison-Himmelfarb, C., Handler, J., … Ortiz, E. (2014). *JAMA: Journal of the American Medical Association, 311*(5), 507–520.

Jessup, M., Abraham, W., Casey, D., Feldman, A., Francis, G., Ganiats, T., … Yancy, C. (2009). 2009 focused update incorporated into the ACC/AHA 2005 guidelines for the diagnosis and management of heart failure in adults: A report of the American College of Cardiology /American Heart Association task force on practice guidelines. *Circulation, 119*, e391–e479. Retrieved from http://circ.ahajournals.org

Kamble, S., & Boyd, A. (2008). Health disparities and social determinants of health among African American women undergoing percutaneous coronary interventions. *Journal of Cultural Diversity, 15*(3), 132–142.

Kamm-Steigelmann, L., Kimble, L., Dunbar, S., Sowell, R., & Bairan, A. (2006). Religion, relationships, and mental health in midlife women following acute myocardial infarction. *Issues in Mental Health Nursing, 27*, 141–159.

Keyes, C. (2004). The nexus of cardiovascular disease and depression revisited: The complete mental health perspective and the moderating role of age and gender. *Aging and Mental Health, 8*(3), 266–274.

Koertge, J., Weidner, G., Elliot-Eller, M., Sherwitz, L., Merritt-Worden, T., Marlin, R., … Ornish, D. (2003). Improvement in medical risk factors and quality of life in women and men with acute coronary artery disease in the Multicenter Lifestyle Demonstration Project. *American Journal of Cardiology, 91*, 1316-1322.

Lloyd-Jones, D., Adams, R., Carnethon, M., DeSimone, G., Ferguson, T., Flegal, K., … Hong, Y. (2009). Heart disease and stroke statistics-2009 update: A report from the American Heart Association statistics committee and stroke statistics sub-committee. *Circulation, 119*, e21–e181.

Luo, J., Rossouw, J., & Margolis, K. (2013). Smoking cessation, weight change, and coronary heart disease among postmenopausal women with and without diabetes. *JAMA: Journal of the American Medical Association, 310*(1), 94–96.

Mather, S. (2004). Intervening to prevent heart disease in women. *Patient Care, 38*(4), 11–16.

Mosca, L., Banka, C., Benjamin, E., Berra, K., Bushnell, C., Dolor, R., … Wenger, N. (2007). Evidence-based guidelines for cardiovascular disease prevention in women: 2007 update. *Journal of the American College of Cardiology, 49*, 1230–1250.

Mosca, L., Mochari-Greenberger, H., Dolor, R., Newby, L., Robb, K. (2010). Twelve-year follow-up of American women's awareness of cardiovascular disease risk and barriers to heart health. *Circulation: Cardiovascular Quality and Outcomes, 3*, 120–127.

Murphy, B., Elliot, P., Worcester, M., Higgins, R., LeGrande, M., Roberts, S., & Goble, A. (2008). Trajectories and predictors of anxiety and depression in women during the 12 months following an acute cardiac event. *British Journal of Health Psychology, 13*, 135–153.

National Heart, Lung, and Blood Institute. (2004). *The seventh report of the Joint National Committee on Prevention, Detection, Evaluation, and Treatment of High Blood Pressure (JNCVII).* (NIH Publication No. 04-5230). Washington, DC: Department of Health and Human Services.

National Heart, Lung, and Blood Institute. (2012). How Are overweight and obesity diagnosed? Retrieved from http://www.nhlbi.nih.gov/health/health-topics/topics /obe/diagnosis

Nicholson, C. (2007). Cardiovascular disease in women. *Nursing Standard, 21*(38), 43–47.

Office on Women's Health. (2009). Heart disease: Know your risk. Retrieved from http://womenshealth.gov /heart-health-stroke/heart-disease-risk-factors/index .html

O'Keefe, J., Bhatti, S., Bajwa, A., DiNicolantonio, J., & Lavie, C. (2010). Alcohol and cardiovascular health: The dose makes the poison…or the remedy. *Mayo Clinic Proceedings, 89*(3), 382–393.

O'Keefe-McCarthy, S. (2008). Women's experience of cardiac pain: A review of the literature. *Canadian Journal of Cardiovascular Nursing, 18*(3), 18–25.

Pemu, P., & Ofili, E. (2008). Hypertension in women: Part 1. *Journal of Clinical Hypertension, 10*(5),406–410.

Plach, S., Napholz, L., & Kelber, S. (2003). Depression during early recovery from heart surgery among early, middle-age, midlife, and elderly women. *Health Care for Women International, 24*, 327–339.

Roberto, K., Gigliotti, C., & Husser, E. (2005). Older women's experiences with multiple health conditions: Daily challenges and care practices. *Health Care for Women International, 26*, 672–692.

Rosenfeld, A. (2006). State of the heart: Building science to improve women's cardiovascular health. *American Journal of Critical Care, 15*(6), 556–566.

Shaw, L., Bairey Merz, C., Bittner, V., Kip, K., Johnson, B., Reis, S., ... WISE Investigators. (2008). Importance of socioeconomic status as a predictor of cardiovascular outcome and costs of care in women with suspected myocardial ischemia. Results from the National Institutes of Health, National Heart, Lung, and Blood Institute sponsored Women's Ischemia Syndrome Evaluation (WISE). *Journal of Women's Health, 17*(7), 1081–1092.

Sherman, A., Shumaker, S., Kancler, C., Zheng, B., Reboussin, D., Legault, C., ... Herrington, D. (2003).

Baseline health-related quality of life in postmenopausal women with coronary heart disease: The estrogen replacement and atherosclerosis (ERA) trial. *Journal of Women's Health, 12*(4), 351–361.

Shifren, K. (2003). Women with heart disease: Can the common-sense model of illness help? *Health Care for Women International, 24*, 355–368.

Stone, N., Robinson, J., Lichtenstein, A., Merz, N., Blum, C., Eckel, R., ... Wilson, P. (2013). 2013 ACC/AHA Guideline on the treatment of blood cholesterol to reduce atherosclerotic cardiovascular risk in adults: A report of the American College of Cardiology/American Heart Association Task Force on Practice Guidelines. *Circulation, 129*(suppl 2), S1–S45.

Urizar, G., & Sears, S. (2006). Psychosocial and cultural influences on cardiovascular health and quality of life among Hispanic cardiac patients in South Florida. *Journal of Behavioral Medicine, 29*(3), 255–268.

Yancy, C., Jessup, M., Bozkurt, B., Butler, J., Casey, D., Drazner, M., ... Wilkoff, B. (2013). 2013 ACCF/AHA guideline for the management of heart failure: a report of the American College of Cardiology Foundation /American Heart Association Task Force on Practice Guidelines. *Circulation, 128*, e240–e327.

Stroke

Introduction

Stroke, also known as brain attack, is the leading cause of functional disability in women in the United States and presents a formidable public health challenge. The morbidity and disability resulting from stroke presents a substantial physical, psychosocial, and socioeconomic burden on patients, families, employers, payers, as well as the healthcare system. Although stroke is a condition that can occur across age and gender, the prevalence of stroke is greater in women than in men, and incidence steadily increases from middle age onward. Lack of awareness of stroke risk and warning signs is a major public health problem that often leads to fatal and disabling delays in receiving effective time-sensitive treatment. This chapter explores the issues of older women who experience stroke. The significant impact of stroke on women's quality of life is also discussed.

Incidence

An estimated 6.6 million individuals over the age of 20 have had a stroke in this country. Each year, approximately 795,000 people experience new or recurrent stroke. Of this number, approximately 610,000 are first attacks, and 185,000 are recurrent attacks. Each year, 55,650 more women than men suffer a stroke. The lifetime risk of stroke is higher in women than in men. The lifetime risk of stroke among individuals 55 to 75 years of age is 1 in 5 for women (20% to 21%) and approximately 1 in 6 for men (14% to 17%). In younger and middle-aged groups, age-specific incidence rates are substantially lower in women than in men. However, these differences narrow so that in the oldest age groups, the incidence rates in women are approximately equal to or even higher than in men. It is estimated that, on average, someone in the United States has a stroke every 40 seconds (Mozaffarian et al., 2015).

The risk of first-ever stroke among African-Americans is almost twice that of white Americans. In the 45–84 year old age group, the incidence of stroke is 4.9 per 1,000 in African-American women as opposed to 2.3 per 1,000 white women. There is an increased incidence of stroke among Hispanic Americans as compared to non-Hispanic whites. Specifically, Mexican-Americans tend to have a higher incidence of intracerebral hemorrhage and subarachnoid hemorrhage as compared to non-Hispanic whites, as well as higher incidence of ischemic stroke and transient ischemic attack at younger ages (Roger et al., 2011). Furthermore, Native Americans (including both American Indian and Alaskan Natives) have the highest rate of risk factors for cardiovascular disease and the highest prevalence of stroke in noninstitutionalized adults (Trimble & Morgenstern, 2008).

It is estimated that every 4 minutes, someone dies from a stroke. More women than men die from stroke each year. Women account for approximately 60% of stroke deaths in this country (Mozaffarian et al., 2015). A greater decline in death rate from stroke has been seen in men as compared to women, especially among individuals aged 65 and older, as compared to younger ages. The stroke mortality rate among African-American women is notably higher as compared to white women, Hispanic women, Asian/Pacific Islander women, and Native American/Alaskan Native women (Roger et al., 2011).

Substantial geographic disparities in stroke mortality exist in the United States, with higher rates of mortality occurring in what has been defined as the "stroke belt" of the county. This region encompasses the eight southern states North Carolina, South Carolina, Georgia, Tennessee, Mississippi, Alabama, Louisiana, and Arkansas. The average stroke mortality rate is approximately 20% higher in the stroke belt than in the rest of the nation. Even within the stroke belt, the region along the coastal plains of North Carolina, South Carolina, and Georgia has a higher stroke mortality rate than the remainder of the belt. The average stroke mortality rate for this region is approximately 40% higher than the rest of the nation (Mozaffarian et al., 2015).

Ethnic Considerations

Women of racial and ethnic minorities have notably higher incidence of stroke of all types and higher stroke mortality rates than white women. Although a large proportion of the U.S. population has multiple risk factors for heart disease and stroke, the prevalence of risk factors is greatest among ethnic minorities and those of lower socioeconomic status. In particular, African-American and Hispanic women are more likely to be diabetic, physically inactive, overweight, and obese than white women (Christian, Rosamond, White, & Mosca, 2007; Goldstein et al., 2011). Factors that contribute to the disparities in stroke incidence and mortality rate in women of racial and ethnic minorities may be attributed to differences in socioeconomic status, levels of education, health literacy, stroke awareness, health insurance coverage, access to health services, and engagement in high-risk behaviors such as smoking, sedentary activity, and poor nutrition (Christian et al., 2007; Hayes et al., 2006).

Etiology and Risk Factors

A stroke can be caused by a blockage occurring in blood vessels leading to or within the brain or a rupture of blood vessels in or around the brain.

Atherosclerotic disease of extracerebral or intracerebral vessels causes narrowing of the vessels and impedes the circulation of blood to the brain. Ischemic stroke will then occur when the cerebral vessel is blocked by a clot or embolism, causing cerebral infarction. Hemorrhagic stroke is caused by an intracerebral or subarachnoid hemorrhage brought about by ruptured vessels or cerebral aneurysm. Approximately 87% of all strokes are ischemic, 10% are due to intracerebral hemorrhage, and 3% are attributed to subarachnoid hemorrhage (Bushnell et al., 2014).

Non-modifiable and modifiable factors that increase the risk of stroke in women are summarized below.

Non-Modifiable Risk Factors

INCREASING AGE

The risk for stroke increases as women age. The cumulative effects of aging on the cardiovascular system and the progressive nature of stroke risk factors over time considerably increase the risk for ischemic stroke and intracerebral hemorrhage (Meschia et al., 2014). Evidence suggests that the combined risk for fatal and nonfatal stroke has increased in women by 10%. Furthermore, an increased risk of stroke has been noted in younger individuals, with an increase in the proportion of stroke in individuals between 20 and 54 years of age (Meschia et al., 2014). Strokes that occur in younger individuals can potentially cause greater lifetime impairment and disability. It is estimated that middle-aged adults have a 1 in 6 or more lifetime risk of stroke (Meschia et al., 2014).

HEREDITY

A family history of stroke may increase the risk of stroke in women. Women with stroke are more likely to have a parental history of stroke than men. The increased risk of stroke associated with positive family history may be influenced by a variety of mechanisms that include genetic heritability of stroke risk

factors, inheritance of susceptibility to such risk factors, familial sharing of cultural/environmental and lifestyle risk factors, and interaction between genetic and environmental factors (Meschia et al., 2014).

RACE

African-Americans and some Hispanic Americans have a higher risk of stroke and higher mortality rates as compared to white individuals. It is unclear whether these racial differences are environmental, genetic, or a combination of these factors. The higher incidence and mortality rates of strokes in African-Americans may be associated with the greater prevalence of prehypertension, hypertension, obesity, and diabetes among African-Americans (Meschia et al., 2014). However, the higher prevalence of these risk factors may not explain all of the excess risk. Evidence suggests that race/ethnic differences may be the result of social determinants such as neighborhood characteristics, geography, language, access to and use of health care, and nativity (Meschia et al., 2014).

Modifiable Risk Factors

HYPERTENSION

Hypertension is a foremost risk factor for all types of stroke. A strong, continuous, independent, predictive, and etiologically significant relationship exists between hypertension and stroke. Consequently, the higher the blood pressure, the greater the risk of stroke, and the risk of stroke rises progressively with increasing blood pressure (Meschia et al., 2014). Although hypertension is the risk factor for which more treatment options exist, approximately two-thirds of all hypertension remains undetected or inadequately treated (Romero, 2007).

DIET AND NUTRITION

Evidence suggests that several aspects of diet influence the pathogenesis of hypertension, which is a major risk factor of ischemic stroke. Dietary risk factors that are causally associated with elevated BP include excessive salt intake, low potassium intake, excessive weight, high alcohol consumption, and suboptimal dietary pattern. African-Americans are especially sensitive to the blood pressure-raising effects of high salt intake, low potassium intake, and suboptimal diet. From this perspective, dietary changes have the potential to substantially reduce racial disparities in hypertension and stroke (Meschia et al., 2014).

CIGARETTE SMOKING

Cigarette smoking is a potent risk factor for stroke, most notably ischemic stroke and subarachnoid hemorrhage. Research findings suggest that cigarette smoking nearly doubles the risk of ischemic stroke among older age groups and ethnically diverse younger women, and is also associated with a two- to fourfold increase in risk for subarachnoid hemorrhage. Data regarding smoking and the risk for intracerebral hemorrhage is inconclusive (Meschia et al., 2014). Smoking is thought to increase stroke risk through acute effects on the risk of thrombus generation in atherosclerotic arteries and through chronic effects related to increased atherosclerosis. Evidence further suggests that exposure to environmental tobacco smoke (passive or secondhand smoke) creates a substantial risk for stroke, approaching nearly double that of active smoking (Meschia et al., 2014).

DIABETES

An independent risk factor for stroke, the presence of diabetes more than doubles the risk of stroke. The risk for stroke created by diabetes is associated with the increased susceptibility to atherosclerosis and the increased prevalence of risk factors for atherosclerosis, namely hypertension and abnormal blood lipids. Approximately 20% of individuals with diabetes will die of stroke (Meschia et al., 2014).

DYSLIPIDEMIA

Numerous research studies have established a relationship between higher total cholesterol levels and increased risk for ischemic stroke. Studies have also suggested an association between lower cholesterol levels and higher risk of hemorrhagic stroke. Evidence suggests that higher levels of high density lipoprotein cholesterol (HDL-C) are associated with reduced risk of ischemic stroke; however, research findings regarding the association between elevated triglyceride level and risk for ischemic stroke have been inconsistent (Meschia et al., 2014).

ATRIAL FIBRILLATION

Atrial fibrillation, the most persistent cardiac dysrhythmia in the elderly, is an independent risk factor for ischemic stroke. Atrial fibrillation conveys a four- to fivefold increase in risk due to embolism of stasis-induced thrombi that form on the walls of the left atrium. Embolism of stasis-induced thrombi accounts for approximately 10% of all ischemic strokes (Meschia et al., 2014). Atrial fibrillation is often asymptomatic and is frequently undetected clinically. This suggests that the stroke risk attributed to atrial fibrillation may be significantly underestimated (Roger et al., 2011).

PHYSICAL INACTIVITY

Physical inactivity increases the risk for stroke as well as numerous adverse health effects, including increased risk of total mortality and cardiovascular morbidity and mortality. Active women have a 25% to 30% lower risk of stroke or death than least active women (Meschia et al., 2014).

OBESITY

Being overweight or obese is associated with stroke, as well as with hypertension, heart disease, and diabetes mellitus. Since 1980, the prevalence of obesity in this country has doubled for adults and tripled for children. Women are classified as overweight with a body mass index (BMI) of 25 to 29 kg/m^2 and obese with BMI greater than 29 kg/m^2. Women with central obesity have a waist circumference greater than 35 inches or 88 cm. The waist-to-hip ratio can also be an indicator of abdominal obesity. Evidence suggests that for every 0.01 increase in waist-to-hip ratio, there is a 5% increase in risk of cardiovascular disease. In the BMI range of 25 to 50 kg/m^2, each 5 kg/m^2 increase in BMI is associated with a 40% increase in risk of stroke mortality (Meschia et al., 2014).

ALCOHOL CONSUMPTION

Heavy alcohol consumption is associated with increased risk for stroke. However, light to moderate alcohol consumption seems to have a protective effect. Heavy alcohol consumption for women is defined as consuming more than three drinks any single day and consuming more than seven drinks per week. A standard drink is defined as one 12-ounce bottle of beer or wine cooler, one 5-ounce glass of table wine, or 1.5 ounces of 80-proof distilled spirits (National Institute on Alcohol Abuse and Alcoholism [NIAAA], 2015). Heavy alcohol consumption can lead to hypertension, hypercoagulability, reduced cerebral blood flow, and increased risk of atrial fibrillation. On the other hand, light to moderate alcohol consumption is associated with increased levels of HDL cholesterol, reduced platelet aggregation, decreased fibrinogen concentrations, and enhanced insulin sensitivity and glucose metabolism. Studies have shown that women who were light drinkers had lower risk of stroke, whereas women who consumed 30 g of alcohol or more per day had a 40% higher risk of stroke (Meschia et al., 2014).

SLEEP APNEA

Sleep apnea has been identified as an independent risk factor for stroke. Sleep apnea is defined according to the apnea-hypopnea index (AHI), which describes the number of cessations or reductions of airflow per hour observed during sleep. An AHI greater than or equal to 5 per hour is indicative of sleep apnea. An increasing AHI indicates increasing severity of sleep apnea. Evidence suggests that an AHI greater than or equal to 20 events per hour increases the risk of stroke threefold. Evidence also suggests that the stroke risk associated with sleep apnea is somewhat greater for men than women (Meschia et al., 2014).

Degree of Risk of Stroke

It is vital to identify women who are at increased risk for stroke in order to counsel patients and select appropriate risk reduction strategies. The goals of risk assessment include identification of persons at elevated risk who might be unaware of their risk, assessment of risk in the presence of one or more risk factors, measurement of risk that can be tracked and lowered by suitable modifications, guidance of appropriate use of further diagnostic testing, and estimation of quantitative risk for selecting treatments or stratification in clinical trials. A number of risk assessment tools have been developed for use in screening and in selection of treatment for primary stroke prevention (Goldstein et al., 2011). A widely used risk assessment tool is the Framingham Stroke Risk Profile (FSRP). The FSRP uses clinical information consisting of age, systolic blood pressure, presence of diabetes, cigarette smoking, and history of cardiovascular disease and EKG abnormalities. FSP scores can be calculated to estimate sex-specific, 10-year cumulative stroke risk (Meschia et al., 2014).

Despite widespread use, the FSRP and other assessment tools have limited validity when used among persons of different age ranges and ethnic/minority groups since such use has not been adequately studied. Further research is needed to validate the use of assessment tools across age, sex, and racial/ethnic groups, as well as to determine if the addition of recently identified risk factors adds to the predictive accuracy of the tool. Further research is also needed to determine the effectiveness of a risk assessment tool in improving primary stroke prevention (Meschia et al., 2014).

Risk Reduction

Research has revealed that although knowledge of stroke warning symptoms and risk factors has modestly increased in this country between 1995 and 2005, overall a serious lack of awareness of stroke symptoms and risk factors remains, especially among the elderly, ethnic minorities, and individuals with lower educational attainment (Roger et al., 2011). These findings emphasize the need for efforts toward primary prevention of stroke. It is vital that screening for risk factors and adequate education in risk factor reduction be provided. Awareness of higher risk can initiate preventive health behaviors among women (Mather, 2004). Risk factor reduction and modification should be a priority of clinical focus.

An essential part of risk reduction and stroke prevention is the treatment of conditions that increase stroke risk. The treatment of hypertension, diabetes, and dyslipidemia effectively reduces the risk of stroke (Roger et al., 2011). Active screening for atrial fibrillation in patients over age 65 and treatment with anticoagulation therapy or antiplatelet therapy as appropriate is recommended to reduce the risk of stroke. Active screening for sleep apnea is recommended. More research is needed, however, since it is unknown if treatment of sleep apnea is effective for primary prevention of stroke (Meschia et al., 2014).

Smoking cessation has a formidable effect on stroke risk reduction and is also part of standard care for patients with stroke. Smoking cessation should be encouraged for both primary and secondary prevention. The use of multimodal strategies that include counseling, nicotine replacement, and oral smoking cessation medications is recommended (Meschia et al., 2014).

Weight reduction efficiently decreases the risk of stroke. The effects of weight loss in risk reduction may be mediated by improved control in other risk factors since weight reduction can reduce blood pressure, improve control of diabetes, and reduce risk of cardiovascular disease. Maintenance of BMI between 18.5 to 24 kg/m^2 and waist circumference of less than 35 inches is the recommended target for weight reduction to reduce stroke risk (Meschia et al., 2014). Dietary recommendations for reducing stroke risk include consuming a diet that is rich in fruits, vegetables, and low-fat dairy products, and is low in sodium, saturated fats, and total fats. Heavy alcohol intake should be avoided. Reasonable intake of alcohol for women who choose to consume alcohol should be no more than one drink per day (Meschia et al., 2014).

Increased levels of physical activity are positively associated with reduced stroke risk (Roger et al., 2011). The protective benefits of physical activity are influential through its effects in lowering blood pressure and in controlling other cardiovascular risk factors such as diabetes and obesity. Healthy women should perform moderate-to-vigorous-intensity aerobic physical activity at least 40 minutes per day, 3 to 4 days per week (Meschia et al., 2014).

Gender Similarities and Differences

Stroke was once considered primarily a disease of men, and consequently the burden of stroke was often underestimated in women. Since the early 1980s, perception of stroke in women has changed significantly and stroke is currently emerging as a major public health problem for women as well. Elderly women are the fastest growing segment of the American population and face an increased likelihood of stroke as well as the greatest risk of disability after stroke (Petrea et al., 2009). Research findings suggest that women have a higher lifetime risk for stroke than men, and women with stroke are apt to be older than men. These findings are likely associated with women's greater longevity (Petrea et al., 2009).

Etiology of acute ischemic stroke was found to differ in women as compared to men. Women are more likely to develop stroke from cardioembolism related to atrial fibrillation, while men are more likely to develop acute ischemic stroke from large and small vessel occlusive disease, especially of the internal carotid artery (Förster et al., 2009). Risk factor profiles of women with stroke have shown higher incidence of atrial fibrillation and hypertension, while men with stroke have shown higher incidence of coronary artery disease, dyslipidemia, diabetes, carotid stenosis, and history of tobacco smoking (Smith, Murphy, Santos, Philips, & Wilde, 2009). Research findings have suggested that lipids are less aggressively treated and antithrombotics are less commonly used in women, with women less likely than men to be on aspirin or statin drugs at the time of stroke (Smith et al., 2009; Stuart-Shor, Wellenius, DelloIacono, & Mittleman, 2009). This disparity is especially disturbing since data has shown that aspirin is an efficacious measure for primary stroke prevention in women but not men (Petrea et al., 2009). In addition to reduced use of antithrombotics, women are less likely than men to receive other stroke care interventions such as carotid endarterectomy, diagnostic testing, and treatment with thrombolytic agents (Kapral et al., 2006; Reid et al., 2008).

Evidence suggests that women and men do not differ significantly in the prevalence of traditional stroke symptoms (Lisabeth, Brown, Hughes, Majersik, & Morgenstern, 2009; Stuart-Shor et al., 2009). However, women may be more likely than men to experience nonspecific "somatic" symptoms as well as nontraditional stroke symptoms—in particular, altered mental status (Lisabeth et al., 2009; Stuart-Shor et al., 2009). Gender differences in presentation of prodromal stroke symptoms (traditional or somatic symptoms occurring prior to 24 hours of hospital admission) have been noted, with men more likely than women to experience weakness or clumsiness (Stuart-Shor et al., 2009). In addition, women are more likely than men to delay seeking treatment for stroke symptoms. The delay in hospital arrival can be as much as three times greater in women than men (Mandelzweig, Goldbourt, Boyko, & Tanne, 2006).

Diagnosis and Treatment of Stroke

Diagnosing Stroke

When an artery in the brain is occluded by atherosclerotic plaque, thrombus, or embolus, a core area of brain tissue is subjected to profound ischemia, which triggers a complex chain of cellular changes that result in tissue infarction. Tissue on the periphery of the main site of infarction is known as ischemic penumbra. Ischemic penumbra is an area of sublethal ischemia in which tissue can remain viable for several hours. Brain tissue within the ischemic penumbra may recover if prompt restoration of cerebral circulation is accomplished within a therapeutic time window.

The diagnosis of stroke in women is established from a comprehensive clinical assessment that begins with the health history and physical examination. A variety of diagnostic tests are used to examine the brain and detect areas of injury. It is essential that differentiation between ischemic stroke and hemorrhagic stroke is made so that early aggressive reperfusion therapy can be initiated in eligible women with ischemic stroke. Imaging tests such as computerized tomography scan or magnetic resonance imaging are used for acute evaluation. Prompt acquisition and imaging results will determine treatment (Summers et al., 2009).

In addition to imaging, diagnostic evaluation of stroke will also include a variety of tests to determine other conditions that may have contributed to the stroke. Cardiac workup is performed to rule out cardiogenic emboli. Cerebral angiography will reveal the condition of the cerebral vasculature and determine the location and extent of arterial occlusion. Duplex sonography with Doppler imaging will evaluate the presence and extent of carotid artery stenosis. Although no laboratory tests will confirm the presence of stroke, comprehensive metabolic panel, blood count, coagulation studies, and urinalysis will provide an evaluation of women's baseline status and a framework for anticoagulation as a therapeutic option.

Symptoms of stroke usually correspond to the area of the brain in which function has been disrupted by occluded cerebral circulation.

The five major categories of stroke symptoms include:

- Numbness or weakness of the face, arm, or leg, especially on one side of the body.
- Confusion or trouble speaking or understanding.
- Trouble seeing in one or both eyes.
- Difficulty walking, dizziness, loss of balance or coordination.
- Severe headache with no known cause.

The areas of the brain supplied by the major cerebral and cerebellar arteries are known as *arterial territories*. Specific groups of symptoms often manifest according to the affected artery and the corresponding arterial territory damage. These symptom groupings are known as *stroke syndromes* and are summarized in **Table 14–1**.

Table 14–1 STROKE SYNDROMES: AFFECTED ARTERIES AND ASSOCIATED SYMPTOM GROUPINGS

Strokes of the Middle Cerebral Artery	Strokes of the Anterior Cerebral Artery	Strokes of the Posterior Cerebral Artery	Strokes of the Internal Carotid Artery	Strokes of the Basilar Artery and Branches
Contralateral hemiparesis, hemianesthesia, hemianopsia with eye deviation to opposite side	Contralateral hemianesthesia, hemiparesis leg > arm	Contralateral homonymous hemianopsia	Contralateral hemiparesis	Hemiparesis or quadriparesis
Aphasia	Mutism	Alexia without agraphia	Aphasia (if dominant hemisphere)	Ataxia, clumsiness
Unilateral neglect or inattention	Acute confusional state	Cortical blindness with denial of deficit	Sensory deficits	Dysphagia, dysarthria,
Blindness	Eye deviation to affected side	Oculomotor apraxia, optic ataxia, simultagnosia	Visual field cuts, ipsilateral decreased visual acuity	Dizziness, nystagmus, diplopia, dysconjugate gaze

Table 14–1 STROKE SYNDROMES: AFFECTED ARTERIES AND ASSOCIATED SYMPTOM GROUPINGS (*continued*)

Strokes of the Middle Cerebral Artery	Strokes of the Anterior Cerebral Artery	Strokes of the Posterior Cerebral Artery	Strokes of the Internal Carotid Artery	Strokes of the Basilar Artery and Branches
Apraxia (if non-dominant hemisphere)	Urinary incontinence		Cranial nerve deficits	Bilateral motor and sensory deficits
	Abulia (absence of willpower or initiative to make decisions)			Vertigo

Transient ischemic attacks (TIAs) frequently precede ischemic strokes. Approximately 15% of all strokes are heralded by TIAs, and the prevalence of TIA increases as women age (Roger et al., 2011). TIAs produce temporary neurological deficits that resolve without residual effect in minutes to hours following the event. Ischemia is produced by a brief interruption of cerebral blood flow in an arterial territory. The interruption of blood flow may be related to microemboli that break off atherosclerotic plaque, to vasospasm, or to hypotension. A wide range of focal neurological deficits may occur in a TIA. Global deficits such as confusion or lethargy are not characteristic of TIA. Symptoms that are likely to occur in a TIA are presented in **Table 14–2**.

TIAs are a significant warning sign of impending stroke, especially in women with history of aortic stenosis. The 90-day stroke risk after a first-ever TIA is as much as 20%. Approximately one-half of all individuals who experience TIA fail to report the occurrence to a healthcare provider (Roger et al., 2011).

Hemorrhagic stroke due to an intracranial bleed evolves rapidly and often presents no warning signs. Women tend to lose consciousness and develop severe neurological impairment. Signs and symptoms of hemorrhagic stroke may be focal signs that are associated with the specific location

Table 14–2 SIGNS AND SYMPTOMS OF TRANSIENT ISCHEMIC ATTACKS

Motor Deficits	Sensory Deficits	Visual Deficits	Speech Deficits
Ataxia	Hemianesthesia	Diplopia	Aphasia
Unilateral/bilateral weakness	Sensory deficits in face or extremities	Unilateral/bilateral blindness	Dysarthria
Hemiparesis	Vertigo	Blurred vision	
Dysphagia	Dizziness	Tunnel vision	
Localized motor deficits in face or extremities	Tinnitus		

of the intracerebral bleed or they may be indicative of increased intracranial pressure and tentorial herniation. Signs and symptoms of hemorrhagic stroke are presented in **Box 14–1.**

Treatment of Stroke

Treatment for stroke is indicated mainly by the type and extent of stroke as well as resulting neurologic dysfunction. The initial treatment of acute ischemic stroke is thrombolytic therapy with administration of tissue plasminogen activator (t-PA). Intravenous or intra-arterial t-PA therapy is administered to achieve lysis of the clot blocking cerebral circulation and restore blood flow to the ischemic penumbra. Although t-PA therapy does not affect the infarcted necrotic brain tissue, reinfusion of the ischemic penumbra can reduce the extent of damage caused by the stroke. For t-PA therapy to be effective, it must be administered to the patient within 3 hours of the onset of stroke symptoms. Research has shown that patients with ischemic stroke who were treated within 3 hours of the start of stroke symptoms had a significantly higher likelihood of having favorable clinical outcomes after 3 months (Jaunch et al., 2013). Use of t-PA therapy does pose an increased risk of intracerebral hemorrhage; however, the benefits

of t-PA therapy generally outweigh the associated risk when properly administered.

Antiplatelet therapy is a cornerstone of medical treatment for ischemic stroke. The goal of antiplatelet therapy is to hinder platelet adhesion and aggregation. Common pharmacologic agents used for antiplatelet therapy include aspirin and clopidogrel. A major limitation of antiplatelet therapy is an increased risk of bleeding. Women receiving antiplatelet therapy should be closely monitored for signs of bruising, hemorrhage, and liver disease.

Anticoagulant therapy is frequently used to prevent the progression of TIAs or ischemic strokes. Intravenous or subcutaneous anticoagulation is initiated with subsequent progression to oral anticoagulant therapy with warfarin. Women with cardioembolic stroke associated with atrial fibrillation are commonly treated with warfarin therapy. Since anticoagulation therapy can increase risk of bleeding, women should be closely monitored for bruising, nosebleeds, bleeding gums, and blood in the urine and stool.

Women who have atherosclerotic disease in selected vessels may be treated with surgical options. Surgical options are selected based on location of the stenotic or occluded vessel, degree of occlusion, and ease of access to specialized facilities and surgical expertise. Women who have carotid

Box 14–1: Clinical Manifestations of Hemorrhagic Stroke

- Focal neurological deficits similar to ischemic stroke
- Decreased level of consciousness
- Headache (seen with subarachnoid hemorrhage)
- Neck pain
- Nausea
- Vomiting
- Photophobia
- Pupillary changes

artery stenosis with more than 70% occlusion may be offered carotid endarterectomy. Carotid endarterectomy involves removal of atherosclerotic plaque buildup from the carotid artery in the neck, which improves arterial circulation to the brain and decreases stroke risk. Endovascular procedures such as percutaneous angioplasty with or without intervascular stenting are effective alternatives offered to women for whom carotid endarterectomy poses an unacceptable surgical risk.

An extracranial–intracranial bypass procedure may be performed to bypass a blocked artery in the brain or to achieve revascularization in the treatment of cerebral aneurysms. The procedure involves a craniotomy, during which anastamosis of blood vessels (commonly the superficial temporal artery to the middle cerebral artery) is achieved to circumvent a blocked artery and improve overall circulation to the area.

Women who have cerebral aneurysms are at high risk for intracerebral hemorrhage. Cerebral aneurysms may be repaired surgically via craniotomy with use of surgical clips, or non-surgically with use of endovascular procedures such as coiling or stenting. The management of intracerebral hemorrhage involves measures to relieve the intracranial pressure caused by accumulation of blood clots. An increasingly worsening neurological condition with significant elevation of intracranial pressure may require evacuation of blood clots via craniotomy.

Quality of Life Issues Associated With Stroke

The quality of life of persons with stroke has emerged as a primary area of research interest, especially in view of the increasing awareness of gender influences in functional outcomes of stroke. Stroke can cause a significant decrease in quality of life, even among those who have no disability afterward (Dhamoon et al., 2010). Women with stroke are more likely than men to have poorer health-related quality of life and poorer health outcomes (Feigin et al., 2010; Kuroda, Tadashi, & Sakai, 2006). Research findings suggest that women tend to suffer greater disability in activities of daily living following stroke. In association with women's greater life expectancy, stroke that occurs later in life when health and ability to function independently are already compromised multiplies the level of disability observed in stroke survivors. Furthermore, women with stroke are more likely to suffer from anxiety and depression, less likely to be married, and more likely to be institutionalized than men (Kelly-Hayes et al., 2003; Petrea et al., 2009).

The quality of life issues that emerge in women with stroke are multidimensional and comprise health and physical functioning, psychological and spiritual well-being, socioeconomic integrity, and family well-being. Lack of awareness of stroke risk, the range of symptoms women experience with stroke, and the aftermath of neurological disability can impact profoundly across the various domains of quality of life.

Issues Affecting Health and Physical Functioning

A common outcome of stroke is disability, which can detrimentally affect quality of life. The disability that can result from stroke frequently leads to disruption as well as dependence in managing activities of daily living, even if the stroke was not severe (Western, 2007). The types and degrees of disability that follow a stroke are determined by which area of the brain is damaged. The disabilities associated with stroke are described below.

PARALYSIS

Paralysis is a common disability resulting from stroke. Paralysis usually appears on the side of the body opposite to the side of the brain that experienced damage. Paralysis may affect the face, an arm, a leg, or the entire side of the body. In the affected side spasticity may occur, causing an abnormal increase in muscle tone that can be painful and cause severe joint problems and contractures.

PARESTHESIA AND NUMBNESS

Stroke survivors may lose the ability to feel touch, pain, temperature, or position. Some experience pain, numbness, or odd sensations of tingling or prickling in paralyzed or weakened limbs. Loss of urinary continence and/or bowel control is fairly common immediately following a stroke and often results from a combination of sensory and motor deficits. Permanent incontinence following a stroke, however, is uncommon.

APHASIA

Approximately 25% of stroke survivors experience language impairment that involves the ability to speak, write, and understand spoken and written language. Research has shown that women with ischemic stroke are more likely to have aphasia than men (Beal, 2010).

ONE-SIDED NEGLECT AND VISUAL IMPAIRMENT

Some stroke survivors may develop one-sided neglect. In this perceptual disorder, the stroke survivor does not recognize one entire side of their world, and are unable to look past the middle of their range of vision to focus on people or things on the left or right. The individual may not acknowledge the existence of people talking on one side of their midline. In patients with aphasia, the right side of the body and visual field is lost. When visual neglect occurs, it is often associated with blindness in the right halves of both eyes, known as *homonymous hemianopsia.*

IMPAIRED MEMORY, LEARNING, AWARENESS

Stroke can damage the areas of the brain that govern memory, learning, and awareness. Stroke survivors may have dramatically shortened attention spans or may lose their ability to make plans, comprehend meaning, learn new tasks, or engage in other complex mental activities.

EMOTIONAL DISTURBANCES

Stroke survivors often feel fear, anxiety, frustration, anger, sadness, and a sense of grief for losses of physical and mental function. The physical effects of brain damage are likely responsible for some of the emotional disturbances and personality changes stroke survivors suffer. Clinical depression is commonly experienced by stroke survivors.

The conventional pathway of care for patients with stroke commonly involves hospital admission in which they receive acute care, followed by a variable period of rehabilitation aimed at restoring as much functional ability as possible. Rehabilitation helps stroke survivors relearn skills that were lost, and learn new ways of performing functional activities to compensate for disabilities consequent to the stroke. Stroke rehabilitation requires organized care provided by multidisciplinary teams of physicians, nurses, and therapists who exclusively manage stroke patients, the goal of which is to minimize post-stroke preventable complications and enhance independence in functional activities (Brewer & Williams, 2010). Therapy begins in the acute care setting after the stabilization of the patient's medical condition, often within 24 to 48 hours after the stroke. Research has indicated that stroke survivors who receive organized in-patient care in dedicated stroke units are more likely to survive, return home, and regain independence than patients who receive traditional care in general inpatient medical units (Brewer & Williams, 2010). Early hospital discharge with community based in-home rehabilitation is an alternative to rehabilitation in specialized inpatient stroke units that may be offered to certain stroke survivors (Winkel, Ekdahl, & Gard, 2008).

Depending on the extent of disability, stroke survivors may be discharged home with or without informal or family care providers, or to a long-term care facility. Women who experience no significant neurological disability are able to return home and live independently or with minimal support.

In-home or community-based rehabilitation may be offered as needed. Women with moderate disability may be able to return home but will likely require ongoing assistance with functional activities and supervision to maintain safety. In-home or community-based rehabilitative therapy may be continued. Women with disabilities that necessitate placement in long-term care facilities will require complex nursing care as well as extensive rehabilitative therapy.

Research has suggested that the negative impact on the health and physical functioning domain of quality of life is due to loss of mobility, dependence on others, limitations in performing household tasks, decreased stamina, and difficulty or inability to drive and engage in leisure activities (Tariah, Hersch, & Ostwald, 2006). Long-term rehabilitation that focuses on meeting the physical, occupational, and psychosocial needs of stroke survivors is an essential part of recovery to improve functional outcomes and enhance quality of life.

Issues Affecting Psychological and Spiritual Functioning

PSYCHOLOGICAL FUNCTIONING

Depression and anxiety commonly occur following stroke (Bergersen, Frøslie, Sunnerhagen, & Schanke, 2010). Depression is more likely to develop in women who have had strokes in the frontal portion of the brain. Two schools of thought explain why significant or prolonged bouts of depression develop following a stroke. One theory holds that, as previously mentioned, depression results from the brain injury or chemical imbalances that occur from the stroke. The second theory holds that depression may develop in response to coping with poststroke sequelae such as hemiplegia, poor balance, visual difficulties, and aphasia. Incidence of depression in stroke survivors may range from 20% to 50% (Robinson-Smith, 2004). Factors that appear to increase the risk of depression in stroke survivors include advanced

age, younger age, living alone, lack of social support, and increased degree of functional impairment. Depression can occur in the acute phase of stroke and has been noted to last for as long as 5 years afterward (Bergersen et al., 2010; Huang et al., 2010). It is also common for some stroke survivors to become obsessed with the possibility of stroke recurrence to the point of being unable to function on a day-to-day basis. While fear of stroke recurrence may be unavoidable, it is important to recovery that the fear be kept under control.

Depression in stroke survivors is a crucial matter, because depression affects the motivation that is needed for improving functional independence after stroke (Robinson-Smith, 2004). Depressed individuals may lack concern for others and may avoid family and friends, leading to social isolation. Many stroke survivors become withdrawn, inactive, and experience sleep and eating disturbances, irritability, and inability to focus or concentrate. They may lose interest in activities they previously enjoyed and struggle with feelings of guilt, worthlessness, isolation, and fear. Controlling depression is an essential step toward improving the chances of recovery.

The medical management of depression, particularly clinical depression, involves pharmacological therapy as well as some form of counseling. Antidepressant medications such as selective serotonin uptake inhibitors (SSRIs) are often prescribed. Counseling can be an effective treatment for depressed stroke survivors as long as they have the expressive language abilities and verbal comprehension to participate. Women with aphasia pose an exceptional challenge for counseling. They require individualized approaches by counselors, psychotherapists, or neuropsychologists who understand the specific nature of the communication disorder. The counselor should understand the frustration, anxiety, struggle, and word-finding problems found in aphasia so that appropriate psychological inferences can be made. When these approaches are not followed, counseling may worsen the depression.

Social support is essential to the recovery of women who have had a stroke and in maintaining an acceptable quality of life. Social support enhances the coping ability of stroke survivors and their ability to adapt to daily life events (Huang et al., 2010). Social support spans a number of domains including emotional support, informational support, tangible support, affectionate support, and social companionship (Hilari & Northcott, 2006). Social support, notably in the form of emotional support, has been associated with reduced levels of depression and improved functional recovery especially during the first 6 months following stroke. Additionally, social support, mainly in the forms of companionship, tangible support, and informational support, has been positively associated with life satisfaction, well-being, and improved quality of life (Hilari & Northcott, 2006; Huang et al., 2010).

The enhancement of social support toward management of depression and anxiety should be a priority in treatment and rehabilitation of stroke survivors. Family participation in the treatment of depression is essential. It is important that supportive ties with family and friends be maintained, especially since stroke survivors are at risk for social isolation and withdrawal from social contacts. Emotional and affectionate support from family and friends that imparts encouragement and positive, constructive attitudes is indispensable in helping to improve the self-esteem and self-concept of the stroke survivor. Healthcare professionals and social services can provide informational and tangible support through family and patient education, behavioral assistance, and material aid.

Spirituality

The life-changing event of a stroke may cause a spiritual crisis in which an individual may no longer find hope and purpose in life. Once this hope is clouded, both by contextual and personal changes, progress in rehabilitation may be hampered (Donica, 2008). Efforts for recovery and rehabilitation

should address the spiritual needs of stroke survivors and enhance spiritual connectedness as appropriate. Spirituality can impart meaning and purpose within the life of stroke survivors, as well as impact motivation, health, and well-being (Donica, 2008; Johnstone & Yoon, 2009). Spiritual connectedness can influence the ability of stroke survivors to cope after a stroke event and can impart stroke survivors with encouragement, a sense of hope, and a way to improve confidence after stroke. Spiritual connectedness enables stroke survivors to reach back to family spiritual life experience and link past to present. Prayer, the most common form of religious coping, often becomes a basic part of recovery. Prayer allows a connection to God or a higher power, and can be a source of strength, comfort, and of being unburdened (Giaquinto, Spiridigliozzi, & Caracciolo, 2007; Lamb, Buchanan, Godfrey, Harrison, & Oakley, 2008). Family, friends, and healthcare providers should encourage continuation of spiritual activities and religious practices that were a part of the stroke survivor's routine before the stroke. Interventions to accentuate spiritual connectedness should be ongoing.

Issues Affecting Socioeconomic Integrity

Without a doubt, stroke is a costly disease from individual, family, and societal perspectives. It is a leading cause of death and disability in this country and worldwide. In the United States, the estimated total direct and indirect costs for stroke are $34 billion (Centers for Disease Control and Prevention [CDC], 2015). Direct medical costs of stroke—approximately 67% of total costs—include hospital inpatient stays, hospital outpatient or office-based provider visits, emergency room visits, rehabilitation, prescribed medications, and home/nursing home care. Indirect costs—approximately 33% of total costs—are caused by lost productivity resulting from morbidity and mortality (DiCarlo, 2009). The lifetime cost of ischemic stroke is estimated to be $140,048. This includes inpatient care, rehabilitation, and follow-up care necessary for lasting deficits (Roger et al., 2011). The trajectory of direct and indirect costs during the 45-year period between 2005 and 2050 is estimated to produce an enormous economic burden of $1.52 trillion for non-Hispanic whites, $313 billion for Hispanics, and $379 billion for African-Americans (Roger et al., 2011).

A substantial share of direct medical costs for stroke is hospital and rehabilitation charges. Approximately 70% of post-stroke costs in the first year are attributed to inpatient hospital costs (Roger et al., 2011). Nursing home utilization also creates a significant financial burden both on the healthcare system and on stroke survivors and their families. Approximately 22% of patients surviving 1 year after stroke reside in a nursing home, and that number can increase to more than 50% when stroke is severe ("Societal Burden," 2009). It is estimated that 31% of stroke survivors require outpatient rehabilitation and 15% to 30% of stroke survivors remain permanently disabled. Women are especially vulnerable to disability and seem less likely than men to regain independence after stroke (Roger et al., 2011). A substantial portion of the expenses for long-term or home-based care are borne by stroke survivors and their families. Moreover, informal care, such as assistance imparted by family or friends that is not part of formal community support services, represents a significant hidden cost to society (Brewer & Williams, 2010). Efforts to reduce skyrocketing costs of stroke care and improve patient outcomes are multifaceted and include primary prevention and treatment of risk factors, admission to dedicated stroke units with a multidisciplinary approach, adherence to guidelines for acute phase management, early rehabilitation, use of telemedicine programs to facilitate improved delivery of acute stroke care, and availability of acute-phase treatments such as thrombolysis for eligible patients (Demaerschalk, Hwang, & Leung, 2010; DiCarlo, 2009).

Many working-age women in their 40s, 50s, and 60s develop strokes. As a result, stroke imposes substantial costs to employers that include higher healthcare claims, lost productivity, absenteeism, workplace accommodation, and increased use of human resource services ("Societal Burden," 2009). Stroke survivors and their families face lost productivity, absenteeism, lost wages, premature retirement due to disability, and worries about affordability of health care.

Stroke prevention is an essential step in helping to reduce excess direct and indirect medical costs. Workplace wellness programs that focus on reduction of stroke risk factors can substantially reduce aggregate costs of workplace absenteeism, health plan expenditures, workman's compensation, or disability plan expenses ("Societal Burden," 2009).

Issues Affecting Family Well-Being

Stroke is a major source of disruption for women and their families. Women with stroke encounter extensive physical, psychological, and social changes, crisis and loss, and altered roles (Kvigne, Kirkevold, & Gjengedal, 2004). Women tend to view their experience of stroke and disability differently than men. Evidence suggests that elderly women with stroke struggle to continue life in familiar ways and preserve the self. The struggle is associated with valued roles closely tied to their identity as mothers, wives, grandmothers, and housewives (Kvigne et al., 2004). Women with stroke are frequently challenged in the performance of basic activities of life, household duties, and traditional as well as nontraditional role responsibilities linked to their central position in the family structure, such as wife, mother, caregiver, or breadwinner. Shifting of role responsibilities often occurs. Women with stroke often have difficulty in enacting these roles or do not receive support to maintain their roles on new terms, which threatens well-being, dignity, and self-esteem (Kivigne et al., 2004).

The disabilities associated with stroke affect the entire family system (Bluvol & Ford-Gilboe, 2004). Stroke survivors frequently face significant functional disability, cognitive impairments, incontinence, and speech difficulties in the aftermath of stroke. When disabilities last indefinitely, stroke survivors will have need of lifelong caregiver assistance. Although formal in-home assistance such as home care services may be used, families are challenged with a multitude of stressors arising from coordination of medical services and arranging round-the-clock care of their loved ones (Saban, Sherwood, DeVon, & Hynes, 2010). Spouses and family members who are employed must frequently juggle their daily caregiving responsibilities and job demands, and may be less available to the stroke survivor, producing role overload, strain, and greater caregiver burden (Bluvol & Ford-Gilboe, 2004). Families must adjust to the physical, emotional, and psychological consequences of stroke, which frequently restrain their social roles and activities (Bluvol & Ford-Gilboe, 2004). Furthermore, family members often must manage grief associated with the changed relationship with their loved ones who have suffered stroke. Evidence has consistently documented that family caregivers are at risk for developing depression, anxiety, sleep disturbance, health problems, and poor quality of life (Saban et al., 2010).

Family quality of life can be enhanced through efforts directed toward decreasing the negative consequences stroke has on family functioning and relational harmony within the family structure. Efforts should include individual and family teaching, counseling, and education as well as provision of social support (Mattila, Leino, Paavilainen, & Åstedt-Kurki, 2009). Monitoring of the psychosocial functioning of spouses and other family members is important not only in the beginning of caregiving but over the long term as well. Spouses and family members benefit greatly from information and training specific to the caregiving role and access to support services and programs that will

help to improve quality of life (Visser-Meily et al., 2009; White, Poissant, Coté-Leblanc, & Wood-Dauphinee, 2006).

Implications for Healthcare Providers

The experience of stroke differs between women and men. Although once thought primarily a disease of men, the emergence of stroke as a major public health concern of women challenges healthcare providers to discard misconceptions of stroke in women in order to reduce the disparities that exist in treatment, rehabilitation, and quality of life. More gender-specific research is needed that will eliminate treatment decisions based on male-focused research findings and determine effective evidence-based treatment and rehabilitative guidelines that will better meet the needs of women who have suffered a stroke.

Prevention of stroke is essential to reducing the economic and societal burden of stroke. Public awareness of warning signs and risk factors for stroke is generally lacking, especially among persons 65 years of age and older, those with lower income and educational attainment, and those of African-American and Hispanic ethnicity (Roger et al., 2011). Healthcare providers need to improve public awareness of stroke risk factors and warning signs through patient education.

Healthcare providers should promote implementation of practical interventions for risk factor modification and drug therapy for people at risk for a first or recurrent stroke. Proactive reduction and treatment of stroke risk factors and warning signs are essential. Lifestyle modification that includes weight management, cessation of smoking, control of hypertension, diabetes, and dyslipidemia, and increased physical activity should be the cornerstone of health maintenance plans, especially for women at high risk for stroke. The quality of preventive care is directly associated with adherence of healthcare providers, patients, disease management programs, and workplace wellness projects to evidence-based recommendations ("Societal Burden," 2009).

Healthcare providers need to be cognizant of distinctive aspects of stroke in women that may increase the tendency for poorer patient outcomes. These aspects include the tendency to delay seeking treatment for stroke symptoms, the tendency to exhibit nontraditional and nonspecific somatic symptoms of stroke, and the likelihood of being prescribed less aggressive risk reduction therapies and stroke treatment measures. Healthcare providers need to be consistent and timely with providing preventive therapies as well as achieving early recognition of stroke. Aggressive treatment and rehabilitation according to evidence-based guidelines are imperative.

Social support in its varied domains: emotional, affectionate, tangible, informational, and social companionship plays a major role in stroke rehabilitation, recovery, and ultimately, quality of life. Social support is instrumental in strengthening the coping abilities of women with stroke and their families, and enhancing their quality of life. Healthcare providers should assess the supportive needs of patients and their families and facilitate access to resources of support as needed. Although provision of support may be facilitated by healthcare providers, this is not indicative that such support has been perceived by patients and families as helpful or effective. Ongoing evaluation of the efficacy of social support throughout the trajectory of rehabilitation and recovery is essential.

Special Concerns of Age and Ethnicity

In consideration of stroke as a major disabling condition, the risk of stroke incidence nearly doubles in each consecutive decade after 55 years of age, and a major proportion of stroke incidence occurs after age 65 (Roger et al., 2011). In the United States, the percentage of women in the population increases steadily with age. Approximately 67% of the population 85 years and older are women (Howden & Meyer, 2011). Since the lifespan of women exceeds that of men by an average of about 10 years, the risk of stroke increases for women at a time when they face the increased presence of comorbidities. Women of older age are more likely to have chronic health problems such as heart disease that may compound the amount of disability they experience with stroke. They are more likely to be without a spouse, have lower levels of educational attainment, limited financial resources, and decreased networks of social support that already challenge quality of life. Furthermore, women of older age with stroke are likely to experience functional limitations that can increase the likelihood of nursing home placement. Consequently, healthcare providers need to be cognizant of the vulnerability of women of older age to stroke and their greater risk for disability and institutionalization (Kelly-Hayes et al., 2003).

Women who are African-American, Hispanic, and Native American have higher risk for stroke, higher stroke occurrence at an earlier age, and for some, the likelihood of more severe strokes, as well as a poorer quality of life than non-Hispanic white women. As previously noted, the higher prevalence of risk factors, overall lower socioeconomic status, and healthcare system challenges for minority patients contribute to stroke disparities (Trimble & Morgenstern, 2008). The burden of stroke is especially devastating for minority women in terms of mortality, lost productivity, and disability. Healthcare providers need to further their efforts in reducing the health disparities among minority women who face the challenges of stroke. There is a need for healthcare providers to exhibit sensitivity to the difficulties minority women experience in negotiating a complicated healthcare system by reducing social, economic, geographic, cultural and language barriers that prevent access to care (Trimble & Morgenstern, 2008).

Healthcare providers must be proactive in recognizing and reducing risk factors in minority women, especially hypertension. Targeting high-risk minority women with programs to heighten awareness of stroke risk factors and symptoms is a fundamental step toward risk reduction.

Healthcare providers need to interact with cultural sensitivity and cultural competence. They need to establish better rapport with minority patients through understanding patient concerns within the cultural framework that defines their behaviors and decision making (Trimble & Morgenstern, 2008).

Research Review

What is the stroke literacy among a predominantly African-American urban population with a high proportion of its population living under the federal poverty level?

Willey, J., Williams, O., & Boden-Albala, B. (2009). Stroke literacy in Central Harlem: A high risk stroke population. *Neurology, 73,* 1950–1956.

The purpose of this study was to evaluate the knowledge of stroke symptoms and risk factors in a predominantly African-American urban population, a high proportion of which was living under the federal poverty level. The study sought to delineate whether any differences in stroke literacy existed based on race/ethnicity or gender. A cross-sectional survey design was used. Ten community-based sites in central Harlem were identified between 2005 and 2006 for administration of a stroke knowledge survey. Trained volunteers administered in-person questionnaires containing structured closed-ended questions that focused on stroke symptoms and risk factors. A sample size of 1,023 respondents completed the survey. The mean age of the respondents was 51.6 years, with a range between 13 and 94 years. Sixty eight percent of the respondents were women. African-American respondents comprised 65.7% of the sample, 16% were

Hispanic, 14% were classified as other racial/ethnic group members, and 4.3% were white. Data were analyzed with descriptive statistics, comparative statistics, and univariate and multivariate analyses.

The findings revealed that significant deficiencies in stroke literacy were present in this high-risk cohort, especially when compared with national findings. Of the four subgroups of respondents, Hispanics had the lowest overall stroke literacy, followed by the subgroup of other racial/ethnic groups, African-Americans, and whites. The findings also suggested that women in this cohort were less deficient in stroke literacy than men.

The differences in health literacy that were found by race/ethnicity and gender have important implications for public health. Increasing the awareness of stroke risk factors and symptoms is an important step toward stroke prevention. Prevention remains the most effective strategy for reducing morbidity and mortality linked with stroke. Innovative educational campaigns that are culturally tailored and sustainable are needed in high-risk communities to promote stroke prevention. Patients who are stroke-literate may be more proactive in risk factor control or symptom identification and reporting. This is an area worth further research.

Chapter Summary Points

- Stroke, also known as brain attack, is the leading cause of functional disability in women in the United States and presents a formidable public health challenge.
- An estimated 7 million individuals over the age of 20 have had a stroke in this country. Of this amount, 4.2 million are women and 2.8 million are men.
- Each year, 55,650 more women than men suffer a stroke. Women aged 45 to 54 are more than twice as likely as men to have had a stroke, and have greater than fourfold likelihood of having had a stroke as compared to women aged 35 to 44.
- Women of racial and ethnic minorities have notably higher incidence of stroke of all types and higher stroke mortality rates than white women. The prevalence of stroke risk factors is greatest among ethnic minorities and those of lower socioeconomic status.
- A stroke can be caused by a blockage occurring in blood vessels leading to or within the brain or a rupture of blood vessels in or around the brain.
- Nonmodifiable factors that increase the risk of stroke in women include increasing age, heredity, and race. Modifiable risk factors include hypertension, diabetes, atrial fibrillation, obesity, smoking, dyslipidemia, postmenopausal hormone therapy, physical inactivity, and excessive alcohol consumption.
- Elderly women are the fastest growing segment of the American population and face an increased likelihood of stroke as well as the greatest risk of disability after stroke.
- Not only are women more likely to delay seeking treatment for stroke symptoms, they are also more likely to exhibit somatic or nontraditional stroke symptoms, and are likely to be treated less aggressively than men.
- Treatment for stroke is indicated mainly by the type and extent of stroke as well as resulting neurologic dysfunction. Treatment encompasses thrombolytic, pharmacological, and surgical options.
- Women with stroke are more likely than men to have poorer health-related quality of life and poorer health outcomes.
- Stroke places substantial physical, psychosocial, and economic burdens on patients, families, society, and the healthcare system
- Healthcare providers need to be consistent and timely with providing preventive therapies as well as achieving early recognition of stroke. Aggressive treatment and rehabilitation according to evidence-based guidelines are imperative.
- Long-term rehabilitation that focuses on meeting the physical, occupational, and psychosocial needs of stroke survivors is an essential part of recovery to improve functional outcomes and enhance quality of life.
- Healthcare providers should assess the supportive needs of patients and their families as well as facilitate access to resources of social support as needed.
- Healthcare providers must be proactive in recognizing and reducing risk factors in minority women. Targeting high-risk minority women with programs to heighten awareness of stroke risk factors and symptoms is a fundamental step toward risk reduction.

Critical Thinking Exercise

Case Study

Ms. J. is a 65-year-old African-American woman who is moderately obese. She is divorced with no children, had an older sister who died a year ago from heart failure, and has a younger sister who is in good health. Ms. J. has a history of hypertension and atrial fibrillation, both of which have been controlled with medication. One evening she experienced mild headache and fatigue while cooking dinner. After supper, while watching television Ms. J. discovered she had a difficult time focusing her vision on the television screen. She attributed her blurry vision to her headache and fatigue and went to bed. The following morning her headache was worse and when she attempted to get out of bed, her left arm felt heavy and tingled with a "pins-and-needles" sensation. Ms. J. recalled the ladies in her church saying that unusual feelings in the left arm might mean a person was having a heart attack. Fearful, she telephoned her 58-year-old sister, Anna, for help. Ms. J. told Anna she felt unwell and thought she might be having a heart attack. Anna rushed over and found that Ms. J. was having trouble standing on her left leg and noticed that only one side of her mouth moved when Ms. J. talked. Anna telephoned 911 and Ms. J. was transported to the emergency department of a local hospital. Diagnostic tests revealed that Ms. J. had a right ischemic stroke. She was hospitalized for a week on a dedicated stroke unit and discharged with orders for outpatient rehabilitation and physical therapy.

Ms. J. had pronounced left-sided weakness in her arm and leg and drooping of the left side of her face as a result of the stroke. Her speech, vision, and swallowing were not affected. Ms. J. was recently retired from her occupation as a hotel housekeeper and received a modest pension and social security. She had been earning some extra money by babysitting her grand-niece but was unable to continue that due to the stroke. Her disability made it impossible for her to take care of her basic activities of daily living alone and she had to move in with Anna and her daughter.

Anna and her daughter became the in-home caregivers of Ms. J. and had to juggle their work responsibilities to provide adequate care. They saw to it that Ms. J. attended her clinic appointments, rehabilitation, and physical therapy. At times, Ms. J. felt like she was a burden on her sister and niece and was reluctant to inconvenience them any more than necessary. Ms. J. refused to attend social events. She was embarrassed by the drooping appearance of her face and felt she looked deformed. She refused to have friends visit because she did not want her deformity and weakness to be seen by others. Her sadness and depression deepened. Anna mentioned her sister's depression to the rehabilitation therapists, and counseling sessions were arranged for Ms. J. Knowing how important church was to Ms. J. prior to the stroke, Anna asked their pastor to visit. At first Ms. J. was reluctant to see the pastor but then allowed the visit, during which they prayed together and Ms. J. shared her sadness and disappointment associated with having had a stroke. The pastor mentioned that her friends at church missed her and wanted to visit with her. Ms. J. again reluctantly agreed and stated they could come at their own risk since she would not be responsible for scaring them to death with her ugly face. Her friends began to visit regularly and, soon Ms. J. started to feel more positive about her appearance and the relationships she had with her friends. Over time, therapy helped Ms. J. regain strength in her arm and leg so that she was able to advance from walking with a walker to walking with a cane. Ms. J. also regained the ability to perform basic activities of daily living by herself. Ms. J. continued to reside with her sister and felt proud when she was finally able to contribute to the upkeep of the family with light household chores and meal preparation. Ms. J. also returned to being an active member of her church.

Questions for Seminar Discussion

1. What risk factors placed Ms. J. at high risk for stroke? Discuss modifiable and non-modifiable risk factors and strategies for risk reduction.
2. How did her level of awareness of stroke symptoms impact Ms. J. in receiving timely treatment?
3. Discuss the physical, psychological/spiritual, socioeconomic, and family issues that influence Ms. J.'s quality of life.
4. What issues and concerns were not readily apparent but might become problematic to Ms. J. and her family?
5. What strengths and weaknesses are present that factor into the ability of Ms. J. and her family to manage illness and quality of life demands?
6. Discuss resources that are available to help Ms. J. manage her illness and improve her quality of life.
7. Discuss the importance of a multidisciplinary approach to Ms. J.'s stroke management, rehabilitation, and quality of life.
8. How might comorbid conditions affect Ms. J.'s stroke management, rehabilitation, and quality of life?
9. What strategies could effectively enhance Ms. J.'s compliance with her treatment and rehabilitation program?

Internet Resources

The American Stroke Association: information and resources for patients, family, and professionals. http://www.strokeassociation.org

The Hazel K. Goddess Fund for Stroke Research in Women: information and resources for patients, family, and professionals. http://www.thegoddessfund.org

Mayo Clinic: information and resources for patients, family, and professionals. http://www.mayoclinic.org/diseases-conditions/stroke/home/ovc-20117264

National Aphasia Association: information and resources for patients, family, and professionals. http://www.aphasia.org/

National Institute for Neurological Disorders and Stroke: information and resources for patients, family, and professionals. http://www.ninds.nih.gov/disorders/stroke/stroke.htm

The National Stroke Association: information and resources for patients, family, and professionals. http://www.stroke.org

PubMed Health: information and resources for patients, family, and professionals http://www.ncbi.nlm.nih.gov/pubmedhealth/PMH0001740/#adam_000726.disease.support-groups

The Stroke Network: an online support network for stroke survivors and stroke caregivers. http://www.strokenetwork.net

References

Beal. C. (2010). Gender and stroke symptoms: A review of current literature. *Journal of Neuroscience Nursing, 42*(2), 80–87.

Bergersen, H., Frøslie, K., Sunnerhagen, K., & Schanke A. (2010). Anxiety, depression, and psychological well-being 2–5 years poststroke. *Journal of Stroke and Cardiovascular Diseases, 19*(5), 364–369.

Brewer, L., & Williams, D. (2010). A review of early supported discharge after stroke. *Reviews in Clinical Gerontology, 20*, 327–337.

Bluvol, A., & Ford-Gilboe, M. (2004). Hope, health, and quality of life in families of stroke survivors. *Journal of Advanced Nursing, 48*(4), 322–332.

Bushnell, C., McCullough, L., Awad, I., Chireau, M., Fedder, W., Furie, K., … Walters, M., on behalf of the American Heart Association Stroke Council, Council on Cardiovascular and Stroke Nursing, Council on Clinical Cardiology, Council on Epidemiology and Prevention, and Council for High Blood Pressure Research. (2014). Guidelines for the prevention of stroke in women: A statement for healthcare professionals from the American Heart Association/American Stroke Association. *Stroke, 45*, 1545–1588.

Centers for Disease Control and Prevention (2015). Stroke frequently asked questions (FAQs). Retrieved from http://www.cdc.gov/stroke/faqs.htm#8

Christian, A., Rosamond, W., White, A., & Mosca, L. (2007). Nine-year trends and racial and ethnic disparities in women's awareness of heart disease and stroke: An American Heart Association national study. *Journal of Women's Health, 16*(1), 68–81.

Demaerschalk, B., Hwang, H., & Leung, G. (2010). Cost analysis of stroke centers, telestroke, and rt-PA. *The American Journal of Managed Care, 16*(7), 537–543.

Dhamoon, M., Moon, Y., Paik, M., Boden-Albala, B., Rundek, Y., Sacco, R., & Elkind, M. (2010). Quality of life declines after first ischemic stroke: The Northern Manhattan study. *Neurology, 75*, 328–334.

DiCarlo, A. (2009). Human and economic burden of stroke. *Age and Ageing, 38*, 4–5.

Donica, D. (2008). Spirituality and occupational therapy: The application of the psychospiritual integration frame of reference. *Physical and Occupational Therapy in Geriatrics, 27*(2), 107–121.

Feigin, V., Barker-Collo, S., Parag, V., Senior, H., Lawes, C., Ratnasabapathy, Y., & Glen, E. (2010). Auckland stroke outcomes study: Part 1: Gender, stroke types, ethnicity, and functional outcomes 5 year poststroke. *Neurology, 75*, 1597–1607.

Förster, A., Gass, A., Kern, R., Wolf, M., Ottomeyer, C., Zohsel, K., Hennerici, M., & Szabo, K. (2009). Gender differences in acute ischemic stroke: Etiology, stroke patterns, and response to thrombolysis. *Stroke, 40*, 2428–2432.

Giaquinto, S., Spiridigliozzi, C., & Caracciolo, B. (2007). Can faith protect from emotional distress after stroke? *Stroke, 38*, 993–997.

Goldstein, L., Bushnell, C., Adams, R., Appel, L., Braun, L., Chaturvedi, S., … Pearson, T. on behalf of the American Heart Association Stroke Council, Council on Cardiovascular Nursing, Council on Epidemiology and Prevention, Council on High Blood Pressure Research, Council on Peripheral Vascular Disease, and Interdisciplinary Council on Quality Care and Outcomes Research. (2011). Guidelines for the primary prevention of stroke: A guideline for healthcare professionals from the American Heart Association/American Stroke Association. *Stroke, 42*, 1–68.

Hayes, D., Denny, C., Kenan, N., Croft, J., Sundaram, A., & Greenlund, K. (2006). Racial/ethnic and socioeconomic differences in multiple risk factors for heart disease and stroke in women: Behavioral risk factor surveillance system, 2003. *Journal of Women's Health, 15*(9), 1000–1008.

Hilari, K., & Northcott, S. (2006). Social support in people with chronic aphasia. *Aphasiology, 20*(1), 17–36.

Howden, L., & Meyer, J. (2011). 2010 Census briefs. Age and sex composition: 2010. Retrieved from http://www.census.gov/prod/cen2010/briefs/c2010br-03.pdf

Huang, C., Hsu, M., Hsu, S., Cheng, P., Lin, S., & Chuang, C. (2010). Mediating roles of social support on poststroke depression and quality of life in patients with ischemic stroke. *Journal of Clinical Nursing, 19,* 2752–2762.

Jauch, E., Saver, J., Adams, H., Bruno, A., Connors, J., Demaerschalk, B., … Yonas, H. on behalf of the American Heart Association Stroke Council, Council on Cardiovascular Nursing, Council on Peripheral Vascular Disease, and Council on Clinical Cardiology. (2013). Guidelines for the early management of patients with acute ischemic stroke: A guideline for healthcare professionals from the American Heart Association/American Stroke Association. *Stroke, 44,* 870–947.

Johnstone, B., & Yoon, D. (2009). Relationships between the Brief Multidimensional Measure of Religiousness/Spirituality and health outcomes for a heterogeneous rehabilitation population. *Rehabilitation Psychology, 54*(4), 422–431.

Kapral, M., Devon, J., Winter, A., Wang, J., Peters, A., & Bondy, S. (2006). Gender differences in stroke care decision-making. *Medical Care, 44*(1), 70–80.

Kelly-Hayes, M., Beiser, A., Kase, C., Scaramucci, A., D'Agostino, R., & Wolf, P. (2003). The influence of gender and age on disability following ischemic stroke: The Framingham Study. *Journal of Stroke and Cerebrovascular Diseases, 12*(3), 119–126.

Kuroda, A., Tadashi, K., & Sakai, F. (2006). Gender differences in health-related quality of life among stroke patients. *Geriatrics and Gerontology International, 6,* 165–173.

Kvigne, K., Kirkevold, M., & Gjengedal, E. (2004). Fighting back-Struggling to continue life and preserve the self following a stroke. *Health Care for Women International, 25,* 370–387.

Lamb, M., Buchanan, D., Godfrey, C., Harrison, M., & Oakley, P. (2008). The psychosocial spiritual experience of elderly individuals recovering from stroke: A systematic review. *International Journal of Evidence Based Healthcare, 6,* 173–205.

Lisabeth, L., Brown, D., Hughes, R., Majersik, J., & Morgenstern, L. (2009). Acute stroke symptoms: Comparing women and men. *Stroke, 40,* 2031–2036.

Mandelzweig, L., Goldbourt, U., Boyko, V., & Tanne, D. (2006). Perceptual, social, and behavioral factors associated with delays in seeking medical care in patients with symptoms of acute stroke. *Stroke, 37,* 1248–1253.

Mattila, E., Leino, K., Paavilainen, E., & Åstedt-Kurki, P. (2009). Nursing intervention studies on patient and family members: A systematic literature review. *Scandinavian Journal of Caring Sciences, 23,* 611–622.

Mather, S. (2004). Intervening to prevent heart disease in women. *Patient Care, 38*(4), 11–16.

Meschia, J., Bushnell, C., Boden-Albala, B., Braun, L., Bravata, D., Chaturvedi, S., … Wilson, J., on behalf of the American Heart Association Stroke Council, Council on Cardiovascular and Stroke Nursing, Council on Clinical Cardiology, Council on Functional Genomics and Translational Biology, and Council on Hypertension. (2014). Guidelines for the primary prevention of stroke: A statement for healthcare professionals from the American Heart Association/American Stroke Association. *Stroke, 45,* 3754–3832.

Mozaffarian, D., Benjamin, E., Go, A., Arnett, D., Blaha, M., Cushman, M., … Turner, M., on behalf of the American Heart Association Statistics Committee and Stroke Statistics Subcommittee. (2015). Heart disease and stroke statistics—2015 update: A report from the American Heart Association. *Circulation, 131,* e29–e322.

National Institute on Alcohol Abuse and Alcoholism. (2015). Overview of alcohol consumption. Retrieved from http://www.niaaa.nih.gov/alcohol-health/overview-alcohol-consumption

Petrea, R., Beiser, A., Seshadri, S., Kelly-Hayes, M., Kase, C., & Wolf, P. (2009). Gender differences in stroke incidence and poststroke disability in the Framingham Heart Study. *Stroke, 40,* 1032–1037.

Reid, J., Dai, D., Gubitz, G., Kapral, M., Christian, C., & Philips, S. (2008). Gender differences in stroke examined in a 10-year cohort of patients admitted to a Canadian teaching hospital. *Stroke, 39,* 1090–1095.

Robinson-Smith, G. (2004). Verbal indicators of depression in conversations with stroke survivors. *Perspectives in Psychiatric Care, 40*(2), 61–69.

Roger, V., Go, A., Lloyd-Jones, D., Adams, R., Berry, J., Brown, T., … Wylie-Rosett, J. on behalf of the American Heart Association Statistics Committee and Stroke Statistics Subcommittee. (2011). Heart disease and stroke statistics 2011 update: A report from the American Heart Association. *Circulation, 123,* e000–e000. Retrieved from http://circ.ahajournals.org

Romero, J. (2007). Prevention of ischemic stroke: Overview of traditional risk factors. *Current Drug Targets, 8,* 794–801.

Saban, K., Sherwood, P., DeVon, H., & Hynes, D. (2010). Measures of psychological stress and physical health in family caregivers of stroke survivors: A literature review. *Journal of Neuroscience Nursing, 42*(3), 128–138.

Smith, D., Murphy, P., Santos, P., Philips, M., & Wilde, M. (2009). Gender differences in the Colorado Stroke Registry. *Stroke, 40,* 1078–1081.

The societal burden of stroke: A major cause of morbidity and disability. (2009, August). *American Health & Drug Benefits, 2*(suppl 7), S174–S179.

Summers, D., Leonard, A., Wentworth, D., Saver, J., Simpson, J., Spilker, J., … Mitchell, P., on behalf of the American Heart Association Council on Cardiovascular Nursing and the Stroke Council. (2009). Comprehensive overview of nursing and interdisciplinary care of the acute ischemic stroke patient. *Stroke, 40*, 2911–2944.

Stuart-Shor, E., Wellenius, G., DelloIacono, D., & Mittleman, M. (2009). Gender differences in presenting and prodromal stroke symptoms. *Stroke, 40*, 1121–1126.

Tariah, H., Hersch, G., & Ostwald, S. (2006). Factors associated with quality of life: Perspectives of stroke survivors. *Physical & Occupational Therapy in Geriatrics, 25*(2), 33–50.

Trimble, B., & Morgenstern, L. (2008). Stroke in minorities. *Neurologic Clinics, 26*, 1177–1190.

Visser-Meily, A., Post, M., van de Port, I., Maas, C., Forstberg-Wärleby, G., & Lindeman, E. (2009). Psychosocial functioning of spouses and patients with stroke from initial inpatient rehabilitation to 3 years poststroke: Course and relations with coping strategies. *Stroke, 40*, 1399–1404.

Western, H. (2007). Altered living: Coping, hope, and quality of life after stroke. *British Journal of Nursing, 16*(20), 1266–1270.

White, C., Poissant, L., Coté-Leblanc, G., & Wood-Dauphinee, S. (2006). Long-term caregiving after stroke: The impact on caregivers' quality of life. *Journal of Neuroscience Nursing, 38*(5), 354–360.

Willey, J., Williams, O., & Boden-Albala, B. (2009). Stroke literacy in Central Harlem: A high-risk stroke population. *Neurology, 73*, 1950–1956.

Winkel, A., Ekdahl, C., & Gard, G. (2008). Early discharge to therapy-based rehabilitation at home in patients with stroke: A systematic review. *Physical Therapy Reviews, 13*(3), 167–187.

Musculoskeletal Disorders

Introduction

Musculoskeletal disorders are the leading causes of disability in this country and encompass a variety of conditions that affect the muscles, joints, bones, and connective tissues of the body. Musculoskeletal disorders present physical encumbrances that include pain, deformity, immobility and psychological stress, as well as substantial economic burdens on the individual, the community, and the healthcare system. A variety of musculoskeletal conditions affect women at higher rates than men. This chapter focuses on the musculoskeletal conditions that are most prevalent in older women:

osteoarthritis and osteoporosis. The significant impact that osteoarthritis and osteoporosis have on women's quality of life is also discussed.

Incidence

Osteoarthritis

Osteoarthritis, also known as degenerative joint disease, is the most frequently occurring noninflammatory arthritic condition and a leading cause of disability. Approximately 13.9% or 27 million adults aged 25 or older in this country are affected with osteoarthritis. Moreover, 33.6% or 12.4 million of those affected are over the age of 65. The average annual prevalence of adults with osteoarthritis in the ambulatory health system was estimated to be 3.5%, or 7.7 million (Centers for Disease Control and Prevention [CDC], 2014). Women have significantly higher prevalence of osteoarthritis than men, especially after age 50. Osteoarthritis prevalence increases with age and is higher among women than men in nearly every age group (CDC, 2014).

Osteoarthritis accounts for approximately 6% of all arthritis-related deaths per year. This statistic translates into approximately 500 deaths per year, and mortality rates have increased over the past decade (CDC, 2014). Individuals with osteoarthritis are at higher risk of death compared with the general population, especially if there is history of diabetes, cancer, or cardiovascular disease as well as the presence of walking disability (Nüesch et al., 2011). Osteoarthritis deaths are likely underestimated because deaths due to treatment, such as upper gastrointestinal bleeding associated with nonsteroidal anti-inflammatory drugs (NSAIDs), are not counted in the mortality statistic (CDC, 2014).

All races and ethnic groups are affected by osteoarthritis. It is estimated that 36 million white adults, 4.6 million black adults, 2.9 million Hispanic adults, and 1.4 million adults of other races have osteoarthritis. Evidence suggests that in comparison to white adults, a higher proportion of African-Americans, Hispanics, and other races have arthritis-attributable activity limitations, work limitations, and severe joint pain (Bolen et al., 2010).

Osteoporosis

Osteoporosis, or porous bone, is a major public health threat. Evidence suggests that an estimated 9% of adults over the age of 50 experience osteoporosis either at the neck of the femur or in the lumbar spine. About half of the older adults in the population experience low bone mass at the femur neck or lumbar spine, as opposed to 48% of older adults who experience normal bone density in this area

(Looker, Borrud, Dawson-Hughes, Shepherd, & Wright, 2012). Osteoporosis at either skeletal site is estimated to range from 3% to 7% in men and 7% to 35% in women. Prevalence of osteoporosis in men tends not to increase with age until 80 years of age and over (Looker et al., 2012). However, in women, osteoporosis prevalence tends to increase for each decade after age 50 years. Low bone mass prevalence at either skeletal site by age ranges from 32% to 60% in men and 54%–67% in women. The prevalence of low bone mass in men tends not to increase with age until aged 70 years, after which it increases progressively. The prevalence of low bone mass in women tends to increase until age 70 years, after which it tends to remain stable (Looker et al., 2012).

Evidence suggests that after adjustment for age differences between the racial and ethnic groups, the prevalence of osteoporosis or low bone mass prevalence at either the neck of the femur or lumbar spine differs by race and ethnicity in women. The age-adjusted prevalence of osteoporosis at either skeletal site is lower in non-Hispanic black women (9%) as compared to non-Hispanic white women (15%), and Mexican-American women (26%). The age-adjusted prevalence of low bone mass at either skeletal site is lower in non-Hispanic black women (44%) as compared to non-Hispanic white women (62%), and women of other races (72%) (Looker et al., 2012).

Ethnic Considerations

Osteoarthritis is a common illness that has a considerable impact on women of all racial and ethnic populations. Disparities are apparent in the incidence, severity, processes of care, and health outcomes related to osteoarthritis and osteoporosis among individuals of different racial and ethnic groups. Research findings indicate that there is greater prevalence of obesity, a substantial risk factor for osteoarthritis, among African-American, Hispanic, and Native American women. African-American women also tend to have higher bone mineral density than other ethnic groups (Wright, Riggs, Lisse, & Chen, 2008). Higher bone mineral density enhances breakdown of joint cartilage, which is integral to the development of osteoarthritis. Thus, obesity and higher bone mineral density likely explain the greater prevalence of osteoarthritis in African-American women, as well as poor joint health found in obese women from other ethnic groups (Wright et al., 2008).

Evidence suggests that the prevalence of obesity and higher bone mineral density of African-American women contributes to a lower incidence of osteoporosis as compared to white, Asian, Native American, and Hispanic women (Pothiawala, Evans, & Chapman-Novakofski, 2006). Differences, however, exist in the presence of dietary, biologic, and lifestyle risk factors that contribute to the development of osteoporosis. Although calcium intake is lower than recommended in women of all ages, it is disproportionately lower in African-American and Native American women and highest in white and Hispanic women. African-American women also have lower vitamin D status than white and Hispanic women. Additionally, white women are inclined to be more physically active than African-American and Hispanic women (Pothiawala et al., 2006).

Fracture rates among Mexican-American, African-American and Asian women are lower as compared to white women and this may be explained by differences in bone density and bone dimensions (Pothiawala et al., 2006). However, disparities exist in treatment and management of osteoporosis. African-American women tend to be undertreated and have poorer outcomes related to fractures, with increased mortality, prolonged hospital stays, and increased disability. Mexican-American women tend to receive less than adequate preventive counseling for osteoporosis. Minorities overall are apt to receive less screening, less lifestyle therapy, and less medication therapy for osteoporosis (Pothiawala et al., 2006).

Etiology and Risk Factors

Osteoarthritis

Osteoarthritis is a chronic condition characterized by deterioration of joint cartilage. Healthy joint cartilage cushions the ends of bones and facilitates smooth movement of the joints. In osteoarthritis, joint cartilage degenerates and softens, with resultant fibrillation and fissuring of the cartilage surface. The cartilage in due course wears through to expose underlying bone. Moreover, the deterioration of cartilage causes changes to underlying bone. The bone thickens and develops osteophytes (bony spurs), bone cysts, and microfractures, which eventually causes joint deformities and malalignment. Osteoarthritis may be localized or generalized throughout the body, and may involve joints unilaterally and asymmetrically.

Osteoarthritis can be categorized as primary (idiopathic) or secondary in origin. Primary osteoarthritis has no apparent cause and is associated with aging. Secondary osteoarthritis, by contrast, has an identifiable cause, and may be attributable to traumatic, congenital, metabolic, endocrine, neuropathic, and other medical causes. Non-modifiable and modifiable risk factors have been associated with osteoarthritis, and these are presented as follows.

Non-Modifiable Risk Factors

AGE

The risk of developing osteoarthritis increases with age. As women age and joints are subjected to ongoing wear and tear, the risk of developing osteoarthritis is amplified from joint usage over the years (National Institute of Arthritis, and Musculoskeletal and Skin Diseases [NIAMS], 2013).

GENDER

Women have higher rates of osteoarthritis as compared to men, especially after age 50

(NIAMS, 2013). Evidence suggests that osteoarthritis is linked to estrogen deficiency (Wright, et al., 2008). The sharp increase of osteoarthritis incidence among postmenopausal women may be associated with loss of the protective effects of estrogen on joint cartilage (NIAMS, 2013; Wright et al., 2008).

Heredity

It is thought that genetics plays a role in the development of osteoarthritis. Inherited abnormalities of the bones that influence the shape and stability of joints can increase the risk of osteoarthritis. Certain inherited traits, such as joint laxity, being bowlegged, or being double-jointed might also increase the risk of developing osteoarthritis. Research findings suggest that a defect in the gene responsible for manufacturing cartilage may be associated with increased risk for disease development. Women with a familial history of osteoarthritis have an increased risk for disease development, especially in osteoarthritis of the hands and hip (Arthritis Foundation, 2015; NIAMS, 2013).

Modifiable Risk Factors

Obesity

Increased body weight is a significant risk factor for osteoarthritis. Excessive weight can contribute to disease development and progression in hips and knees. Weight gain gradually increases stress on joints. For every pound of weight that is gained, three pounds of pressure is exerted on the knee joints and six pounds of pressure is exerted on the hip joints (CDC, 2014; Mayo Clinic, 2015).

Joint Injury or Overuse

The long-term repetitive use of joints can injure and intensify stress on the joints and can ultimately increase the risk of developing osteoarthritis in susceptible individuals. Activities and occupations that cause repetitive stress on knees, hips, and other joints may increase vulnerability to joint overuse. Joints that have been fractured or have had surgery are also susceptible to developing osteoarthritis in later years (Mayo Clinic, 2015; NIAMS, 2013).

Infections and Other Diseases

Many bacterial agents can infect joints and potentially cause the development of various forms of arthritis. In addition, having diabetes or other rheumatic diseases such as gout and rheumatoid arthritis can increase the risk of developing osteoarthritis (CDC, 2014; Mayo Clinic, 2015).

Osteoporosis

Osteoporosis, or *porous bone*, is the most common bone disease in women. The disease is characterized by low bone mass and structural deterioration of bone tissue. This condition leads to bone fragility and elevated risk of fractures, particularly of the hip, spine, and wrist. The process of bone resorption figures into the development of osteoporosis. During one's lifetime, old bone is removed (resorption) and new bone is added to the skeleton (formation). In childhood and teenage years, bone formation occurs faster than bone resorption, resulting in bones that are larger, heavier, and denser. The process will continue in this vein until about age 30 when peak bone mass, consisting of maximum bone density and strength, has been reached. Subsequently, bone resorption will slowly begin to surpass bone formation (National Institutes of Health Osteoporosis and Related Bone Diseases-National Resource Center [NIH], 2012).

Women experience bone loss fastest in the first few years following menopause and bone loss continues into the postmenopausal years. Estrogen deficiency of any cause increases the rate of bone resorption and plays a major role in the development of osteoporosis. Primary osteoporosis has no identifiable cause or attributable underlying illness. Secondary osteoporosis is attributable to an acquired or inherited abnormality or disease. Certain medications can cause osteoporosis by inducing hypogonadism or interfering with the metabolism of vitamin D. Non-modifiable and modifiable risk factors have been associated with osteoporosis and are presented below.

Non-Modifiable Risk Factors

GENDER

The risk of developing osteoporosis is greater in women than in men. Women have less bone tissue and tend to lose bone faster due to estrogen deficiency related to menopause (NIH, 2012).

AGE

The risk of osteoporosis increases with age. Resorption causes bones to become thinner and weaker as women age (NIH, 2012).

BODY SIZE

Women who are small and thin-boned tend to have a higher risk of developing osteoporosis (NIH, 2012).

ETHNICITY

The risk of developing osteoporosis is highest in Caucasian and Asian women. African-American and Hispanic women have lower but significant risk (NIH, 2012).

HEREDITY

Genetic factors that primarily affect the development of peak bone density are associated with increased risk of osteoporosis. A positive family history of osteoporosis, maternal hip fracture, slight stature, and low body mass increase osteoporosis risk (NIH, 2012).

Modifiable Risk Factors

HYPOGONADISM

Conditions associated with low levels of estrogen can increase the risk of osteoporosis development. Women who experience natural or surgical menopause, athletic amenorrhea, or anorexia nervosa are at increased risk for osteoporosis (NIH, 2012).

CALCIUM AND VITAMIN D DEFICIENCY

An inadequate supply of calcium over a lifetime is likely associated with low bone mass, rapid bone loss, and high fracture rates. Lack of vitamin D reduces calcium absorption and subsequently contributes to decreased bone density. Research findings suggest that vitamin D production decreases in the elderly, in people who are housebound, and in general during the winter (NIH, 2012).

PHYSICAL INACTIVITY

A sedentary lifestyle and prolonged periods of bed rest tend to weaken bone and increase the risk of osteoporosis development (NIH, 2012).

CIGARETTE SMOKING AND ALCOHOL CONSUMPTION

Nicotine from cigarette smoking contributes to osteoporosis risk by lowering levels of circulating estrogen. Women who smoke tend to go through menopause earlier and are likely to absorb less dietary calcium. Women who consume 2 to 3 ounces of alcohol per day are more prone to bone loss and fractures due to poor nutrition and increased risk for falls (NIH, 2012).

MEDICATIONS THAT PROMOTE BONE LOSS

Certain drugs used for long-term therapy can lead to loss of bone density and fractures. These drugs include glucocorticoids, certain antiseizure drugs such as phenytoin and barbiturates, gonadotro-pin-releasing hormone, aluminum-based antacids, certain cancer treatments, and thyroid hormone (NIH, 2012).

Degree of Risk of Osteoarthritis and Osteoporosis

Osteoarthritis

The degree of risk associated with osteoarthritis varies according to dimensions such as disease location, gender, ethnicity, occupation, and geographic area (Wright et al., 2008). Nonetheless, research findings confirm that the degree of risk for the development of osteoarthritis in women increases with age and body mass index (Wright et al., 2008). Thus, the greater the body mass index in postmenopausal women, the higher the odds of developing osteoarthritis. The role obesity plays in osteoarthritis formation may be explained by the tendency for higher bone density in obese individuals to increase subchondral bone stiffness and facilitate cartilage breakdown coupled with the increase of dynamic stress on the joints that leads to cartilage disruption (Wright et al., 2008).

Osteoporosis

Clinical evaluation for risk of osteoporosis should be done in all postmenopausal women in order to establish the necessity for bone mineral density testing. The more risk factors for osteoporosis that women have, the greater their risk of fractures. Although osteoporosis is preventable and treatable, the absence of warning signs prior to the development of a fracture often precludes timely diagnosis and initiation of effective therapy in the early stages of the disease (Cosman et al., 2014).

Risk assessment for osteoporosis-related fracture includes the clinical evaluation of non-modifiable

and modifiable risk factors previously discussed as well as the presence of medical conditions and diseases that may be secondary causes of osteoporosis. Bone mineral density is an essential component in the diagnosis and treatment of osteoporosis (Cosman et al., 2014). Bone mineral density is reported in terms of standard deviation (SD), calculated by comparing individual results with the average bone density of normal young healthy adults of the same sex (T-score) or the expected bone mineral density for the patient's age and sex (Z-score). Bone density decreases approximately 10% to 12% for each SD below normal, so risk for fracture doubles with each SD below normal bone density.

Bone density is only one indicator of fracture risk and it is important to also consider other risk factors for fractures. The Fracture Risk Assessment Tool (FRAX®) algorithm was developed by the World Health Organization (WHO) to evaluate fracture risk based on an integration of risk associated with clinical risk factors and bone mineral density at the femoral neck (World Health Organization Collaborating Center for Metabolic Bone Diseases [WHO], 2015). FRAX® models were developed from investigating population-based cohorts in the United States, Europe, Australia, and Asia. The FRAX® algorithm provides a 10-year probability for developing a hip fracture or major osteoporotic fracture in the spine, forearm, hip or shoulder. The FRAX® algorithm assists clinicians in identifying individuals at high risk for osteoporotic fractures and in deciding appropriate treatment. The FRAX® WHO Fracture Risk Assessment Tool may be accessed online at www .shef.ac.uk/FRAX/.

Risk Reduction

OSTEOARTHRITIS

The modification of certain lifestyle factors can have a positive effect on decreasing the risk of developing osteoarthritis, preventing joint damage, preventing or reducing pain, and improving function and activities (Bijlsma & Knahr, 2007). Overweight or obese women who do not have the disease can reduce the risk of developing osteoarthritis by losing weight (NIAMS, 2013). Weight loss reduces stress on weight-bearing joints such as hips, knees, back, and feet.

Participation in moderate regular physical activity plays an important role in strengthening muscles and bones, increasing flexibility and stamina, improving joint function, and maintaining weight control (NIAMS, 2013). Women should protect their joints by maintaining good posture, using proper body mechanics, and avoiding injury due to accidents or overuse. Avoiding repetitive stress on joints is especially important, which includes avoiding uninterrupted repetition of motion or activity, unnatural or awkward motions, overexertion, muscle fatigue, or incorrect posture. Pain should be recognized as a significant sign of joint overuse. Activity should be stopped before a painful state is reached. Balancing rest and activity is most favorable for joint health and an important preventative aid (NIAMS, 2013).

A number of nutritional factors are associated with reducing the risk of and progression of osteoarthritis. Maintaining a healthy diet that avoids obesity and being overweight, and facilitates weight control is necessary. Evidence suggests that a high intake of vitamins C, D, E, and beta carotene may slow the progression of osteoarthritis; however, further research is needed to support these claims (Bijlsma & Knahr, 2007; NIAMS, 2013).

Studies that have investigated the relationship between hormone replacement therapy and risk of osteoarthritis have produced conflicting results. Although osteoarthritis has been linked to estrogen deficiency, contrasting research findings suggest that the use of hormone replacement therapy may either increase or decrease the odds of developing osteoarthritis in postmenopausal women (Von Mühlen et al., 2002; Wright et al, 2008). Further research is needed to clarify the effects of hormone replacement therapy on osteoarthritis risk before definitive recommendations can be made.

Osteoporosis

Several interventions are available that will help women to reduce their risk of fracture. Adequate daily intake of calcium and vitamin D is essential for the acquisition of peak bone mass and maintenance of bone health. Adequate intake of dietary calcium recommended for women over 50 years of age is at least 1,200 mg per day, including supplements as needed. A calcium intake above 1,200 to 1,500 mg per day will likely not increase the potential for benefit and may increase the risk of developing kidney stones, cardiovascular disease, or stroke. Women above 50 years of age typically consume approximately 600 to 700 mg of calcium per day, thus calcium supplements should be used when dietary intake of calcium falls below recommended levels (Cosman et al., 2014). Adequate intake of vitamin D is essential for calcium absorption, bone health, muscle performance, balance, and reducing the risk for falls. The recommended daily intake of vitamin D to prevent risk of fracture for women 50 years of age and older is 800 to 1,000 international units (IU) (Cosman et al., 2014). Women who suffer from chronic illnesses that interfere with vitamin D absorption, who are housebound, or who have limited sun exposure are at risk for deficiency and may require higher dosages of vitamin D to maintain adequate serum levels. The principal dietary sources of vitamin D include vitamin D-fortified milk, cereals, egg yolks, saltwater fish, and liver. Vitamin D may also be found in most multivitamins and some calcium supplements (Cosman et al., 2014).

Weight-bearing and muscle-strengthening exercises play an important role in reducing the risk of falls and fractures. They can increase agility, strength, and bone density. Exercise is also beneficial for improving posture and balance, which can reduce the risk of falls. Lifelong physical activity is important for osteoporosis prevention and overall health, and benefits may be lost when exercise is stopped. Weight-bearing exercises are activities in which the bones and muscles work in opposition to gravity as the feet and legs bear the weight of the body. These exercises include walking, jogging, tai chi, stair climbing, dancing, and tennis. Muscle-strengthening exercises are exercises performed by moving a weight, one's body, or some other resistance against gravity, and include weight training, use of elastic exercise bands, or lifting one's own body weight. Prior to beginning an exercise program, women should be evaluated by their healthcare provider for safe recommendations (Cosman et al., 2014).

Preventing falls is a key strategy in reducing the risk of fractures. It is important that sensory deficits in vision and hearing be recognized and corrected. Neurological deficits need to be evaluated and treated. Medications should be reviewed for side effects that may adversely affect balance. Safety risks in the home environment should be recognized and corrected. Wearing undergarments with hip pad protectors may protect women who have high risk for falls or who previously had hip fractures (Cosman et al., 2014).

Tobacco and alcohol use can have detrimental effects on bone health. Smoking tobacco should be avoided. Women who smoke should be encouraged to stop and offered assistance with smoking cessation interventions (Cosman et al., 2014). While moderate intake of alcohol likely has no harmful effect on bone health, women should be advised that chronic heavy use of alcohol, particularly during adolescence and young adult years, can decrease bone density, dramatically compromise bone quality, and increase the risk of osteoporosis. The damaging effects of alcohol on bone cannot be reversed even if alcohol consumption is terminated. Women should avoid excessive intake of alcohol to reduce the risk of detrimental effects on bone health as well as decrease the risk for falls (Sampson, 2003).

Gender Similarities and Differences

Gender similarities and differences in osteoarthritis and osteoporosis are becoming apparent as findings from gender-based research come to light. It is well known that physical activity decreases the risk and progression of musculoskeletal diseases, as well as increases strength, physical functioning, and longevity (Pinn, 2006). Older men tend to be more active than older women and, among older men and women who are active, older men tend to have higher overall activity levels. Among adults aged 55 and older, men are more likely to engage in regular leisure-time physical activity than women (Pinn, 2006).

Women tend to have a greater risk than men of developing osteoarthritis of the knee or hip. Moreover, osteoarthritis of the knee tends to be significantly more severe in women than in men (CDC, 2014). Research findings suggest that the rate of loss of knee cartilage volume is significantly greater in women than in men (Hanna, et al., 2009). Women also tend to experience higher rates of arthritis-related functional limitations as well as arthritis-related disability. Women with arthritis-related disability also tend to experience a greater incidence of role limitations and life strain (Hootman, Sniezek, & Helmick, 2002).

The prevalence of osteoporotic fractures is greater in women, as are consequences of increased morbidity, increased healthcare costs, and risk of fragility fractures. Contributing factors to gender disparity in osteoporosis and fracture incidence include physiological differences in bone size, strength, and density (men's bones are bigger, stronger, and denser than women's). Men tend to have fewer falls, lose less bone during aging, and have a shorter life span than women (Geusens & Dinant, 2007; Orwig, Chan, & Magaziner, 2006). The most frequent cause of fractures in women is osteoporosis, which is mainly hypogonadal and age-associated. On the other hand, middle-aged and older men are more likely to develop osteoporosis from the influence of glucocorticoids used in the treatment of other conditions, alcohol abuse, and smoking. In addition, androgen ablation therapy for the treatment of prostate cancer in men accelerates bone loss (Geusens & Dinant, 2007).

Overall, there is an indication that osteoporosis and fracture risk tend to be underdiagnosed and undertreated in both genders, yet more so in men (Geusens & Dinant, 2007). Osteoporosis is a silent disease that is often diagnosed after a debilitating fracture. There is a lack of public and physician awareness of osteoporosis beyond it being a women's health issue pertaining only to older women (Johnson, McLeod, Kennedy, & McLeod, 2008). Women tend to have more frequent screening opportunities than men and more contact with health professionals who can recognize emerging problems at an earlier stage (Geusens & Dinant, 2007). The health literature and public health emphasis related to osteoporosis are more focused on women than on men, and very little attention has been paid to the prevention of osteoporosis in men, which undoubtedly contributes to decreased awareness of bone health in men (Johnson et al., 2008).

Diagnosis and Treatment of Osteoarthritis and Osteoporosis

Osteoarthritis

DIAGNOSIS OF OSTEOARTHRITIS

The diagnosis of osteoarthritis in women is established from a comprehensive clinical assessment that includes the health history, physical examination, and radiographic evidence. The health history often discloses familial history, prior joint trauma or deformity, and the patterns of symptoms such as pain, inflammation, and stiffness. A physical examination of all joints of the hands, arms, legs, feet, and spine is essential to identify affected areas, asymmetrical joint involvement, and further evidence that would differentiate osteoarthritis from other arthritic conditions. Laboratory tests and arthrocentesis (joint aspiration) may be done to determine a differential diagnosis. Radiographic evidence of osteoarthritis is obtained through x-rays and magnetic resonance imaging, and reveals diminished joint space, presence of osteophytes (bone spurs) and bone sclerosis, and abnormal separation of articular surfaces of the joints. Systemic symptoms such as fever and malaise are not found in osteoarthritis.

The symptoms of osteoarthritis begin to appear in the fourth or fifth decade of life, and by age 40 most women will have radiographic evidence of osteoarthritis in weight-bearing joints. Common symptoms of osteoarthritis include joint pain that appears during activity and is relieved by rest, and joint stiffness that develops after periods of inactivity or sleep but resolves when activity resumes. Typically, joint pain may be mild in the morning and increases in severity towards evening after the day's activity, and the duration of joint stiffness is usually no more than 30 minutes. Joint pain and stiffness may eventually cause a decline of coordination, posture, and walking.

Women with osteoarthritis of the hands commonly develop Heberden's nodes at the distal interphalangeal joints of the fingers or toes. Bouchard's nodes often develop in the proximal interphalangeal joints. Both types of nodes result from the formation of osteophytes (bone spurs) in the joints. Herberden's and Bouchards nodes are often accompanied by redness, tenderness, and swelling in the affected joints and can lead to significant deformity and limitation of joint mobility.

Women with osteoarthritis of the hip may experience groin, buttock, thigh, or knee pain. They may experience pain when standing or walking, which can result in limping. Pain may eventually occur when sitting or lying down. With progression, women may experience significant difficulty lowering into or rising from a sitting position. Also, pain at night may disrupt sleep.

With osteoarthritis of the knee, women may experience pain upon movement, especially when going up or down stairs or rising from a chair. Audible grating or crunching sounds (crepitus) when moving the knee may also occur. Women may develop a varus deformity of the knee, which causes an inward deviation of the lower leg toward the midline of the body.

Osteoarthritis of the feet is caused by injury, sprains, fractures, and abnormal foot mechanics that can result from having high arches or flat fleet. Osteoarthritis commonly targets the ankle, the three joints of the hindfoot, the midfoot, or the great toe. Women who develop osteoarthritis of the feet may experience pain, stiffness, bony protrusions, swelling, reduced range of motion, and difficulty walking.

Osteoarthritis of the spine is a common cause of lower back pain in women. It may cause a deterioration of the spinal discs leading to bony overgrowth. In advanced osteoarthritis, nerve root compression and stenosis of the spinal canal may develop and can lead to diffuse pain, stiffness, numbness and tingling in the neck, shoulder, arm, lower back, buttocks, and legs.

TREATMENT OF OSTEOARTHRITIS

The goals of treatment for osteoarthritis are to relieve pain and control symptoms, improve joint mobility, and slow disease progression. The treatment plan will include a combination of pharmacologic therapy, rehabilitative interventions, and surgical options, if necessary.

Pharmacologic therapy is commonly used to relieve pain, ease symptoms, and slow the progression of the disease. Analgesics are widely used to relieve mild to moderate pain without relieving inflammation or swelling. Acetaminophen is commonly prescribed for women with mild

to moderate pain and tends to have few, if any, side effects. Acetaminophen should be used cautiously by women with conditions of the liver or kidney due to the risk of permanent liver or kidney damage that can result from prolonged use or high dosages of the drug taken over a short period.

Topical analgesics may also be used to relieve pain. These are available over the counter and can be used in combination with oral analgesics. Topical analgesics contain a variety of active ingredients that include salicylates, capsaicin, and counterirritants such as camphor, oil of wintergreen, eucalyptus oil, or menthol. The topical analgesic is applied directly over the painful area and should be discontinued if skin irritation develops. Topical analgesics should never be used in combination with heat treatments, as this can cause serious burns.

For moderate to severe pain, nonsteroidal anti-inflammatory drugs (NSAIDs) may be prescribed. Although osteoarthritis is not an inflammatory disease, pain relief from NSAIDs can be obtained with lower doses of the drugs. There is a significant risk for the development of adverse gastrointestinal side effects, especially in elderly women and those with a history peptic ulcers, gastrointestinal bleeding, use of oral corticosteroids, use of anticoagulants, smoking, and alcohol intake. Women taking NSAIDs should be monitored closely for peptic ulcers, gastrointestinal irritation, and bleeding. NSAIDs such as ibuprofen, low-dose naproxen, and diclofenac are commonly prescribed and should be taken with food to reduce the risk of stomach irritation. Misoprostol or other stomach protective drugs such as omeprazole or sucralfate may be given concurrently with NSAIDs to reduce the risk of gastrointestinal irritation. Celecoxib may be given to women with moderate to severe pain who are at great risk for adverse gastrointestinal events. Celecoxib is a cyclo-oxygenase-2 (COX-2) selective NSAID that has fewer gastrointestinal side effects than nonselective NSAIDs (Lo & Meadows, 2006).

Intra-articular injection of corticosteroids is a short-term treatment of moderate to severe osteoarthritis pain. This provides temporary pain relief for a period of several weeks to several months. Injections of corticosteroids into the same joint must be limited to no more than two to four treatments per year, because too many can cause accelerated deterioration of articular cartilage and weakening of surrounding tendons and ligaments (NIAMS, 2013). Osteoarthritis of the knee may be treated with intra-articular injections of hyaluronan. Hyaluronan injections are also known as viscosupplementation. Hyaluronan supplements the natural lubricating and shock absorbing mechanisms of synovial fluid, resulting in pain relief and improved joint mobility. Hyaluronan therapy may be administered in a series of three to five injections (NIAMS, 2013).

Rehabilitative interventions encompass a wide variety of therapies aimed at the whole person as well as the affected joints. These interventions should be tailored to a woman's needs, lifestyle, and health. Rehabilitative interventions include exercise, weight control, rest and relief from joint stress, pain relief techniques, and complementary and alternative therapies.

Exercise is essential in maintaining flexibility, improving joint range of motion, controlling weight, improving cardiovascular function, and promoting general physical fitness. Exercise should include muscle strengthening activities to strengthen muscle groups that support affected joints. Aerobic exercise such as walking, swimming, or water aerobics will help improve cardiovascular function, overall fitness, and weight control. Range of motion activities will help sustain joint flexibility, and agility exercises will help to maintain daily living skills (NIAMS, 2013).

Keeping to a healthy diet or participating in a weight reduction program is essential in the prevention of obesity, the reduction of stress on weight-bearing joints, slowing the progression of osteoarthritis, pain reduction, and maintenance

and improvement of joint function (Bijlsma & Knahr, 2006). Weight loss and control is facilitated by leading an active lifestyle.

Rest and relief from joint stress are important for preserving joint function and reducing the wear and tear on involved joints. Rest from repetitive activities, avoidance of injury or trauma, and use of braces, splints, aids, and assistive devices work to decrease the mechanical impact of activities on involved joints, provide extra support to joints, and keep joints in proper alignment. Splints and braces that immobilize joints are used only for limited periods of time because joints and muscles must then be exercised to prevent stiffness and weakness (NIAMS, 2013).

Nonpharmacological modalities for pain relief are often prescribed. Heat and cold therapy can be applied in various ways. Heat increases blood flow to the joints and eases pain, stiffness, and muscle spasms. Heat can be applied by using warm towels, hot packs, or warm bath or shower. The application of cold can reduce inflammation, relieve pain, or numb an area of soreness. Cold can be applied by using cold packs in the form of bags of ice or ice packs. Transcutaneous electrical nerve stimulation (TENS) may relieve pain by blocking transmission of pain sensation to the brain and by modifying pain perception. Massage of painful muscles surrounding affected joints, by a trained therapist, can increase blood flow and warmth to a stressed area (NIAMS, 2013).

Complementary and alternative therapies may be adjunctive to the treatment of osteoarthritis but should not replace pharmacological and nonpharmacological modalities. Research investigating the effectiveness of acupuncture in reducing pain and improving function in osteoarthritis has shown promise. Additionally, evidence is growing that supports the positive influence of vitamins D, C, E, and beta carotene on symptom reduction and slowing of disease progression. Glucosamine and chondroitin sulfate are two nutritional supplements that have shown potential for reducing pain of osteoarthritis; however, no conclusive results have yet been obtained (Mayo Clinic, 2015; NIAMS, 2013.)

Surgery is an alternative, especially if severe joint damage, extreme pain, or very limited range of motion is present. Surgical procedures are available to relieve severe pain, restore joint function, and prevent or correct joint deformity. The surgical procedures most commonly performed are presented in **Table 15–1**.

An essential part of an effective treatment plan for osteoarthritis is patient education and support through participation in patient education programs, arthritis self-management programs, and arthritis support groups. These programs help women understand about osteoarthritis, learn self-care, reduce pain while remaining active, cope physically, mentally, and emotionally with

the disease, and build confidence in the ability to live active, independent lives. Women who participate in these programs are more likely to have positive outcomes and enjoy a better quality of life (Bijlsma & Knahr, 2006; NIAMS, 2013).

Osteoporosis

DIAGNOSIS OF OSTEOPOROSIS

Osteoporosis is diagnosed by measurement of bone mineral density. Women who are diagnosed with osteoporosis are those who are at risk for the disease and who incur fragility fractures—that is, fractures that occur with little or no force or trauma (Cosman et al., 2014).

Bone mineral density is measured by dual-energy x-ray absorptiometry (DXA) measurement of the hip or spine. This measurement can

Table 15–1 SURGICAL PROCEDURES USED IN THE TREATMENT OF OSTEOARTHRITIS

Surgical Procedure	Description
Arthroscopy	A small fiberoptic scope is inserted into the joint to assess the extent of damage. Tissue samples may be taken. Procedure includes removal of loose cartilage, repair of torn cartilage, smoothing rough articular surface, and removal of diseased synovial tissue. Common sites of arthroscopy are knee, hip, shoulder, elbow, and wrist.
Arthrodesis	Two bones of the joint are fused to form one bone. This procedure results in loss of joint mobility but may be useful in relieving severe pain and gaining joint stability. Common sites of arthrodesis are the cervical and lumbar spine, fingers, wrists, and ankles.
Osteotomy	Bone is surgically incised in order to redistribute joint stress onto healthier areas of cartilage, or achieve bone realignment. Common sites of osteotomy are proximal tibia, distal femur, and the intertrochanter area of the hip.
Arthroplasty	The articular surfaces of the joint are reconstructed or replaced with man-made components. This procedure is recommended for women over 50 or those with severe disease progression. Common sites of arthroplasty are hips and knees; however, joints of the shoulders, elbows, hands, and feet may also be replaced. Replaced joints commonly last between 20 to 30 years.

establish or confirm a diagnosis of osteoporosis, predict future fracture risk, and monitor disease progression through serial assessments. Bone mineral density is expressed in absolute terms of grams of mineral per square centimeter scanned (g/cm^2) and also by comparing the woman's obtained score to the expected bone mineral density for the woman's age and sex (Z-score), or to the expected bone mineral density of "young normal" adults of the same sex (T-score). The difference between the patient's obtained score and the normative score is calculated as standard deviations (SDs) above or below the mean. The equivalent of 1 SD equals 10% to 15% of the bone mineral density value expressed in g/cm^2 (Cosman et al., 2014).

The WHO has developed diagnostic classifications of bone mineral density appropriate for postmenopausal women and men over age 50, based on DXA measurements at the spine, hip, or forearm, as listed here.

- Normal – Bone mineral density is within 1 SD of a young normal adult (T-score > –1.0).
- Low bone mass – Bone mineral density is between 1.0 and 2.5 SD below that of a young normal adult (T-score between –1.0 and –2.5).
- Osteoporosis – Bone mineral density is 2.5 SD or more below that of a young normal adult (T-score below –2.5).
- Severe osteoporosis – Bone mineral density is 2.5 SD or more below that of a young normal adult and the presence of one or more fragility fractures (Cosman et al., 2014).

The WHO bone mineral density diagnostic classifications should not be applied to premenopausal women, men under 50 years of age, or children. For those groups, ethnic or race adjusted Z-scores should be used for diagnostic purposes (Cosman et al., 2014).

Other densitometric technologies are available that measure bone mass and predict fracture risk. The peripheral dual energy x-ray absorptiometry

(pDXA) measures bone density of forearm, finger, or heel. The measurements obtained from pDXA devices can assess vertebral and overall fracture risk in postmenopausal women, but there is insufficient evidence to support fracture risk in men. The pDXA is not used to monitor bone density after treatment (Cosman et al., 2014). Quantitative computed tomography (QCT) measures volumetric trabecular and cortical bone density at the spine and hip. Similar density measurements can be obtained at the forearm or tibia with the peripheral QCT (pQCT). Bone density measurements made by CT-based absorptiometry can be predictive of fractures in postmenopausal women; however, there is little evidence to support fracture prediction in men (Cosman et al., 2014). Quantitative ultrasound densitometry (QUS) measures speed of sound and broadband ultrasound attenuation at peripheral skeletal sites. QUS can predict fractures in postmenopausal women, notably of vertebral, hip, and overall fracture risk. It can also predict hip and nonvertebral fractures in men aged 65 and older. There is no radiation exposure with the QUS (Cosman et al., 2014).

TREATMENT OF OSTEOPOROSIS

Postmenopausal women should be considered for treatment of osteoporosis if they present with a hip or vertebral fracture, or their bone mineral density indicates osteoporosis or severe osteoporosis. In addition, postmenopausal women with low bone mass and a 10-year probability of hip fracture greater than or equal to 3%, or 10-year probability of a major osteoporosis-related fracture greater than or equal to 20% (based on U.S. adapted FRAX® algorithm) should also be considered for treatment (Cosman et al., 2014).

Pharmacologic therapy is an option for the prevention and/or treatment of postmenopausal osteoporosis. FDA-approved pharmacologic therapy has been shown to decrease fracture risk in women who have had fragility fractures and osteoporosis or have osteoporosis as indicated by DXA measurement. Evidence suggests that pharmacologic therapy may also reduce fracture risk in women with osteopenia. Nevertheless, healthcare providers should assess the potential risks and benefits of drug therapy in individual women when determining a treatment plan (Cosman et al., 2014). Drugs that are prescribed for the prevention and treatment of osteoporosis are presented in **Table 15–2**.

Nonpharmacological modalities that focus on proper nutrition, exercise, and rehabilitation are essential to reduce disability, improve physical function, and decrease the risk of subsequent falls. A balanced diet rich in calcium, minerals, and vitamin D is important in maintaining bone health. Calcium and vitamin D supplements, as previously discussed in the risk reduction section, are an integral part of treatment. A rehabilitative program that includes weight-bearing and muscle-strengthening exercises, postural training, balance training, progressive resistance training, and stretching activities should be prescribed based on the initial condition of the individual. Such activities can increase muscle strength, improve coordination, enhance balance, and foster bone health. Women should be instructed to follow principles of safe movement before undertaking exercise.

Women who sustain hip fractures are generally treated with surgical repair to achieve the best possible functional results. Surgical options may even be considered for the very elderly with multiple comorbidities, unless they were not ambulatory prior to the fracture (Stone & Lyles, 2006). An organized program of rehabilitation therapy in the postoperative period is essential for regaining mobility, and the setting for rehabilitation is determined according to individual needs. It is frequently determined by prefracture functional levels and social support, and may include the home, rehabilitation facility, or nursing home (Stone & Lyles, 2006).

Women who suffer vertebral fractures require effective pain management. This may be achieved by a variety of pharmacological, physical, and behavioral strategies. Caution must be taken with the use of analgesics that produce side effects such as sedation or disorientation, which can increase the risk of falls. The use of orthoses such as back braces, corsets, or postural training devices may be helpful in reducing pain by aligning vertebrae and decreasing stress on the fracture sites. Careful use of orthoses is recommended because long-term bracing can lead to muscle weakness and additional deconditioning (Cosman et al., 2014). Women who are unresponsive to the conservative approaches to pain management may be candidates for percutaneous interventional radiological procedures such as kyphoplasty or vertebroplasty. Both procedures involve placement of bone cement within the collapsed vertebral body. The end result is mechanical stabilization and marked reduction of pain. Patients who undergo kyphoplasty or vertebroplasty tend to have successful outcomes, with low rates of complications and notable improvement of quality of life (Diel et al., 2009; Wilhelm, 2009).

Quality of Life Issues Associated With Osteoarthritis and Osteoporosis

Osteoarthritis and osteoporosis are prevalent musculoskeletal disorders that disproportionately affect women, most notably in the postmenopausal years. The impact of osteoarthritis and osteoporosis on disability and healthcare expenditure is enormous, and disease burden and its effect on quality of life have evolved into major public health concerns. Quality of life issues and concerns associated with osteoarthritis and osteoporosis are multidimensional, encompassing health and physical functioning, psychological and spiritual well-being, socioeconomic integrity, and family well-being. The likelihood of the existence of comorbid conditions among postmenopausal women with osteoarthritis

Table 15–2 Pharmacologic Therapy for the Prevention and Treatment of Osteoporosis

Drugs	Common Side Effects	Care Recommendations
Biphosphonates: Alendronate sodium (Fosamax) Ibandronate sodium (Boniva) Risendronate sodium (Actonel)	*Oral administration*: gastrointestinal problems such as difficulty swallowing, inflammation of the esophagus or stomach, diarrhea, constipation, flatulence, gastric ulcer, abdominal, muscle, joint, or back pain *Intravenous administration*: flu-like symptoms, fever, muscle pain, joint pain, headache (may last for 2–3 days following infusion)	Drug should be taken first thing in the morning on an empty stomach, with 8 ounces of plain water. No food, drink, or other medications should be taken for 30–60 minutes, depending on which drug is taken. Individual must remain upright for this period of time. Antacids or calcium may be taken 2 hours after biphosphonates. Depending on the medication, oral drugs may be taken daily, weekly, or monthly. IV biphosphonates are administered by the healthcare provider yearly or every 3 months, depending on the drug.
Calcitonin (Miacalcin, Fortical)	*Nasal administration*: rhinitis, nasal irritation *Subcutaneous administration*: allergic reaction, flushing of the face and hands, frequent urination, nausea, skin rash	Approved for use by women who are at least 5 years post-menopausal. May have pain-relieving effect on osteoporotic fractures.
Teriparatide (Forteo)	*Injectable administration*: headache, nausea, dizziness, leg cramps	Acts by stimulating new bone formation. May be used up to 24 months and if other treatments are ineffective or not tolerated. Drug is given by daily subcutaneous injection at home. Not given to women with unexplained elevation in alkaline phosphatase, Paget's disease, or previous bone irradiation.
Raloxifene (Evista)	*Oral administration*: hot flashes, blood clots in the veins, leg cramps, joint pain, sinus inflammation	Not to be used by women with history of thrombophlebitis or women taking hormone replacement therapy.
Estrogen Therapy /Hormone Therapy	*Administered in various forms (oral, skin patch, cream, ring, spray gel)*: vaginal bleeding, spotting, breast tenderness, bloating, cramps, weight changes, hypertension, nausea, vomiting, headache, vaginal yeast infections, mood disturbances, gallbladder disease	May increase the risk of cancers of the breast, ovarian, or uterine lining. Non-estrogen medications should be carefully considered before resorting to estrogen therapy. Must not be used in combination with raloxifene.

Modified from Cosman, F., de Beur, S., LeBoff, M., Lewiecki, E., Tanner, B., Randall, S., & Lindsay, R. (2014). Clinician's guide to prevention and treatment of osteoporosis. *Osteoporosis International*, *25*, 2359–2381.

or osteoporosis can further impact across the various domains of quality of life.

Issues Affecting Health and Physical Functioning

The symptom burden of osteoarthritis has far-reaching effects on health and physical functioning. Pain and stiffness cause considerable reduction in function, loss of mobility, dependence, and disability, which can significantly diminish quality of life (Ağlamis, Toraman, & Yaman, 2009). The severity of pain is associated with a greater degree of disability in performing activities of daily living (Moskowitz, 2009). Pain can limit the performance of simple activities such as showering, grooming, dressing, and walking as well as more strenuous activities such as house cleaning, shopping, cooking, or driving (Baird, Yehle, & Schmeiser, 2007). Furthermore, functional deficits can extend beyond the immediate location of the joint pain. For example, women with pain and stiffness of the hands may experience difficulties in performing activities that involve both upper and lower extremities (Moskowitz, 2009). The outcomes of chronic and progressive pain include decreased mobility, activity restriction, disability, and limited independence. Although intensity and persistence of symptoms vary from person to person, older women frequently find their level of symptoms to be incapacitating (Baird et al., 2007). Consequently, diminished physical functioning in older women will presage increased dependency in activities of daily living, increased use of healthcare resources, increased use of nursing homes, and increased mortality (Bayliss, Ellis, & Steiner, 2007).

The various treatment interventions for osteoarthritis that were previously discussed can be effective in obtaining reduction of symptom burden, increase in functional status, and improvement of quality of life. Treatment should be individualized according to specific need, with particular awareness of the risks and benefits of each modality. Surgical treatment should be considered only after nonsurgical treatment has been unsuccessful (Sarzi-Puttini et al., 2005).

Self-management is an essential approach that can facilitate maintaining a satisfactory quality of life in women with osteoarthritis. Self-management is the substantial responsibility that individuals take to manage the symptoms, treatment, physical and psychosocial consequences, and lifestyle changes intrinsic for living with a chronic condition such as osteoarthritis (Barlow, Wright, Sheasby, Turner, & Hainsworth, 2002). Successful self-management, in conjunction with and under the guidance of physicians and other healthcare providers, requires monitoring one's illness while incorporating cognitive, behavioral, and emotional responses needed to maintain quality of life (Barlow et al., 2002). Acknowledgment of the crucial role that self-management plays in achieving successful outcomes with osteoarthritis has led to the development of multicomponent patient-centered arthritis self-management programs that can help individuals develop necessary skills. Arthritis self-management programs are typically community based and use a group approach. Most programs are run by health professional group leaders, but programs run by lay group leaders are also available, and comparisons made between health professional- and lay-run programs have shown no differences in outcomes (Barlow et al., 2002).

The purpose of arthritis self-management programs is to help people understand their disease, reduce pain while remaining active, cope physically, emotionally, and mentally, have greater control over the disease, and build confidence in their ability to live an active, independent life (NIAMS, 2013). Arthritis self-management programs directly target interventions that are aimed at increasing individuals' involvement and control in their treatment and its effect on their lives (Newman, Steed, & Mulligan, 2004). A growing body of evidence indicates that, when compared to standard care, self-management approaches can be more effective in improving health and functioning, increasing knowledge, enhancing performance of self-management behaviors, and increasing self-efficacy (Barlow et al., 2002).

The fractures that result from osteoporosis can have a devastating effect on health and functioning. The quality of life of women is reduced as a result of any osteoporotic fracture, and morbidity and mortality are increased (Lewiecki, 2009). The most common and disabling osteoporotic fractures are hip fractures and vertebral fractures. Hip fractures lead to significant morbidity and disability, and many women do not return to the level of functioning they had prior to the fracture (Boonen & Singer, 2008). The negative effects of hip fracture are often prolonged, and a substantial number of women require assistance with walking and essential activities of daily living up to a year or longer following the fracture (Boonen & Singer, 2008). Vertebral fractures also increase mortality and can cause severe back pain, reduced pulmonary function, decreased height, and kyphosis, which can restrict movement and increase the risk of falls and further fractures (Lewiecki, 2009). The negative impact on activities of daily living and restrictions to mobility resulting from vertebral fractures can frequently persist for a year or longer (Boonen & Singer, 2008).

Osteoporosis imposes a tremendous burden on society and on the quality of life of affected women. Interventions that will maximize bone mass and identify disorders that diminish peak bone mass are vital for reducing the risk of developing osteoporosis. The identification of at-risk women prior to the onset of fractures will help them gain greater benefits from treatment (Stone & Lyles, 2006).

When considering strategies to maximize the quality of life of women with osteoporosis, prevention of osteoporotic fractures must be emphasized. The occurrence of fragility fractures in postmenopausal women is one of the most compelling risk factors for future fractures and thus should be interpreted as an indicator of osteoporosis. Interventions to decrease fracture risk should be initiated as soon as possible to prevent future fractures (Boonen & Singer, 2008). Fall prevention is an integral factor in reducing the impact of osteoporosis. Interventions should be implemented to help women improve reaction times so they can break a fall. Pharmacological therapies to improve muscle strength can be another option. In addition, rearrangement of the home environment is important in decreasing the risk of falls. Level flooring, non-skid surfaces, wide doorways to accommodate assistive devices, grab bars, and nighttime lighting in hallways and bathrooms can help improve home safety and reduce the incidence of falls (Stone & Lyles, 2006).

Rehabilitation therapy to increase functional ability and muscle strength is beneficial for women who experience osteoporotic fractures. Therapy should include exercise programs that focus on increasing muscle strength and flexibility, and enhancing posture. Rehabilitation therapy can provide pain relief, preserve physical independence, improve general health and well-being, and enhance quality of life (Hale & Goehring, 2003; Stone & Lyles, 2006).

Issues Affecting Psychological and Spiritual Functioning

PSYCHOLOGICAL FUNCTIONING

The physical symptoms of osteoarthritis often create a psychological burden on the quality of life of women. The pain and disability produced by osteoarthritis can lead to psychological distress. Women may experience anxiety, depression, helplessness, low self-efficacy, fatigue, and sleep disturbance. The presence of obesity, which is common in osteoarthritis, is associated with increased pain as well as increased psychological distress (Devos-Comby, Cronan, & Roesch, 2006; Somers, Keefe, Godiwala, & Hoyler, 2009).

The symptom burden of osteoarthritis can lead to activity limitations and depression, which subsequently contributes to increased social isolation (Machado, Gignac, & Badley, 2008). Social isolation can limit or diminish access to social support resources, and lack of access to social support can consequently hamper women's ability to cope effectively with the illness demands of osteoarthritis (Luger, Cotter, & Sherman, 2009). In addition, the personality traits of optimism and pessimism can influence adaptation to osteoarthritis. Individuals who are optimistic tend to anticipate positive outcomes and those who are pessimistic tend to anticipate negative outcomes. Of the two traits, pessimism likely exerts a greater influence on physical and mental health outcomes. Thus, women with osteoarthritis who are pessimistic are vulnerable for poorer physical and psychological well-being (Luger et al., 2009). In particular, women with higher pessimism may also experience lower social support as well as higher social strain. *Social strain* refers to the negative interactions with others that can cause hurt or unpleasant affect. The stress of social strain may also influence higher levels of distress and depressive symptoms (Luger et al., 2009).

When considering the interrelationship of the physical symptoms of osteoarthritis with psychological functioning, it follows logically that a reduction in pain and disability would have a positive effect on psychological well-being. Interventions aimed at modifying women's coping strategies are particularly essential (Savelkoul, de Witte, & Post, 2003). Arthritis self-management programs are ideally suited to meet the physical and psychosocial needs of women with osteoarthritis. Along with exercise and patient education, self-management programs can provide evidence-based psychological interventions that enhance self-efficacy, improve coping skills, increase access to social support, and expand social skills to improve social relationships (Devos-Comby et al., 2006; Luger et al., 2009).

Bearing in mind the negative influence that pessimism may exert on physical and mental health outcomes, women with osteoarthritis should be encouraged to adopt a "good-health attitude." This positive attitude would entail focusing on abilities instead of disabilities, and strengths instead of weaknesses. To attain and preserve a good-health attitude, women should be encouraged to break down activities into small, manageable tasks and develop strategies to minimize and manage stress. Rest should be balanced with activity, and a support system of family, friends, and healthcare professionals should be developed and maintained (NIAMS, 2013). Women should be advised as to the essential necessity of maintaining a good-health mindset and its value toward improving quality of life.

The pain, physical deformity, and disability produced by osteoporotic fractures can have dramatic impact on the psychological functioning of women. Women with serious disease and vertebral deformity are particularly vulnerable to major psychological difficulties (Gold, 2001). Affective and cognitive changes frequently occur, especially immediately following a fracture event, and may comprise fear, anxiety, depression, and lower self-esteem (Andersen, 2007; de Oliveira Ferreira, 2009). Depression has been repeatedly associated with lower bone density. The incidence of depression is particularly problematic in women who suffer osteoporotic hip fracture, in that depression and poor cognition have been repeatedly associated with poor recovery (Orwig et al., 2006, Shyu et al., 2009). During the first year following hip fracture, women who have had poor prefracture functional ability and have low emotional and social support will be at higher risk for developing depression (Shyu et al., 2009).

Although pharmacologic therapy may be an option for treating osteoporosis-related anxiety and depression, the changing pharmacodynamics of older women may decrease drug efficacy or toleration of drug therapy. Thus, nonpharmacologic interventions may be more suitable choices. Multidisciplinary interventions that provide exercise, patient education, and empowerment are likely to be effective in improving women's psychological functioning and self-management abilities (Hale & Goehring, 2003). Improvement of psychological functioning and self-management capabilities can assist women to retain control over their lives and impart a sense of competence, autonomy, and self-reliance that will enhance quality of life (Roberto, 2004).

SPIRITUALITY

Spirituality is viewed by many as an essential part of psychological well-being that helps women cope with chronic illness demands (Harvey, 2008). Spiritual practices serve as an inner resource and means to actively cope with symptom burden, as well as a source of comfort and strength. Spirituality may also assist women in finding meaning and purpose in living with osteoarthritis or osteoporosis, increase their self-esteem, shape their perspective toward having gratitude, provide social support through attendance at a church, temple, or mosque, and foster a greater sense of connection. Spiritual practices are associated with better health outcomes, increased engagement in physical activity, fewer depressive symptoms, improved self-confidence, and higher levels of energy in women with chronic illness such as osteoarthritis or osteoporosis (Harvey, 2008; McCauley, Tarpley, Haaz, & Bartlett, 2008; Roberto, Gigliotti, & Husser, 2005). Interested women should be encouraged to utilize spiritually-based strategies to enrich their psychological well-being and improve quality of life.

Issues Affecting Socioeconomic Integrity

The social and economic effects of osteoarthritis and osteoporosis on the quality of life of women are profound. The financial costs associated with either disease are considerable and can encompass hospitalizations, emergency room treatment, medications, outpatient treatment, and nursing home care. The total annual direct and indirect costs for women living with osteoarthritis are approximately $5,700 per person (CDC, 2014). The average total annual direct and indirect costs for women with nonvertebral, non-hip, osteoporotic fractures are approximately $13,387 per person. For women with nonvertebral, osteoporotic fractures of the hip, multiple sites, or femur, the average per-person costs are approximately $25,519, $20,137, and $19,403 respectively (Pike et al., 2010). As women advance in age and develop osteoarthritis or osteoporosis, as well as other comorbidities, the financial burden associated with disease management can be overwhelming, especially when women must manage financial constraint, fixed income, loss of wages, and inadequate or lack of health insurance. The disabilities associated with osteoarthritis and osteoporosis can reduce employment productivity, force unplanned retirement, or can eventually require major lifestyle adjustments and nursing home care. The financial burden of disease management can become a barrier to treatment compliance, which can influence poorer health outcomes and diminished quality of life (Andersen, 2007).

The social impact of osteoarthritis and osteoporosis on women is also substantial. Physical disability and depressive symptoms can lead to activity limitation that restricts participation in social activities such as community events, traveling, and visiting with family and friends (Machado et al., 2008; Silverman, Shen, Minshall, Xie, & Moses, 2007; Somers et al., 2009). The loss of employment either by retirement or disability further diminishes social interaction and compounds social isolation. As physical disability and anxiety limit the range of activities in which afflicted women participate, the ability to maintain and perform lifelong and important social roles may decline. Women who lack the physical ability to reciprocate in social relationships may find their nonfamilial relationships eventually diminishing. Social isolation can also reduce social support resources and, combined with anxiety and depression previously discussed, create severe stress that can negatively influence their abilities to cope with and adapt to disease demands.

Multidisciplinary referrals and self-management interventions are important strategies in assisting women to manage the socioeconomic issues that threaten their quality of life. Physical and occupational therapy can help women improve strength, enhance mobility, and modify lifestyle to safely continue participation in valued relationships and activities. Social workers can help vulnerable women to recognize and access sources of social support, and can also provide a framework for effective coping that enables women to improve interpersonal interactions and minimize stress in their lives. Self-management interventions can help women improve functionality, enhance coping abilities, provide social interaction, and enhance treatment compliance. Counseling, patient education, and maintaining supportive healthcare provider-patient relationships are also essential in maintaining social and economic integrity while managing the illness demands of osteoarthritis and osteoporosis.

Issues Affecting Family Well-Being

The burden of osteoarthritis or osteoporosis can considerably impact on family well-being. As is similar with other chronic diseases, the psychological distress, depression, and physical disability of osteoarthritis and osteoporosis frequently interfere with women's ability to perform social roles within the family. Many women find themselves unable to do things for their families that they were previously able to do, such as household chores, caring for grandchildren, grocery shopping, and preparing holiday meals (Roberto, 2004). The decline in the ability to carry out role responsibilities frequently necessitates transferring responsibilities to other family members and shifting from the position of family "caregiver" to that of "care receiver." Husbands/partners or adult children often assume

the caregiver role, which requires adjustment and renegotiation of role responsibilities, or restructuring of the spousal/partner relationship (Roberto et al., 2005; Roberto, Gold, & Yorgason, 2004). The changes in family dynamics can lead to stress and tension on family relationships, especially if the expectations regarding care arrangements held by women and their family members are dissimilar (Roberto et al., 2005).

Families provide a valuable source of assistance and support for women who must manage their health conditions within the context of their daily lives. For the most part, family members react and respond to the development of the disease and supply assistance and care as needed, and may frequently help women navigate the healthcare system. Family may also facilitate women's compliance with their therapeutic regimen by activities such as meal preparation and transportation to medical appointments. Nonetheless, although support is motivated by good intentions, family involvement should be balanced in accordance with what women may actually need or desire (Roberto et al., 2005).

Implications for Healthcare Providers

There is a misconception held by many older adults that osteoarthritis is an inevitable outcome of aging about which nothing can be done (Baird et al., 2007), and this can lead to underdiagnosis, undertreatment, and underutilization of self-management resources. Likewise, the mistaken belief that osteoporosis is an unavoidable result of aging is also prevalent (Andersen, 2007). The insidious nature of osteoporosis frequently allows the disease to remain hidden until a fragility fracture occurs. Even then, opportunities to diagnose osteoporosis in older women can be overlooked in the healthcare system. Vertebral fractures observed incidentally on chest x-rays are often disregarded instead of evaluated for treatment; and after hip or other fragility fractures women are not always routinely referred for osteoporosis assessment (Andersen, 2007). What is more, a majority of older women with hip fractures frequently do not receive adequate treatment (Andersen, 2007). These practices can impede effective prevention, diagnosis, and treatment of osteoarthritis and osteoporosis as well as diminish the quality of life of afflicted women. Increased efforts need to be directed toward disease prevention, recognition of at risk women, and proactive treatment strategies.

Self-management is an essential aspect of the treatment plan that can facilitate the achievement of clinical outcomes. Self-management requires not only adherence to treatment guidelines but incorporation of the psychological and social management of living with a chronic illness (Newman, Steed, & Mulligan, 2004). Optimum self-management may be difficult to achieve. Obstacles to self-management can detrimentally influence compliance to treatment guidelines, psychological adjustment, health outcomes, mortality, and quality of life. Healthcare providers need to be cognizant of the various factors that can hinder self-management, such as inadequate social support, difficulties with time management, troubled emotional state, low self-efficacy, conflicting personal health beliefs, physical limitations, lack of knowledge about the medical condition, and the presence of comorbid diseases (Bayliss, et al., 2007). The presence of multiple comorbid conditions is frequently associated with high levels of morbidity, diminished physical functioning, depression, low self-efficacy, and diminished social well-being that negatively influence quality of life outcomes (Bayliss, et al., 2007). Even so, many of the obstacles to effective self-management can be overcome by self-management interventions such as identification and treatment of depression, provision of specific patient education, enhancement of physical functioning through physical therapy, manual aids, and other supports, resolution of conflicting

and compounding effects of symptoms and treatments of comorbid conditions, and striving for collaborative care choices within the individual's financial capabilities (Bayliss et al., 2007).

The literature concerning osteoarthritis and osteoporosis is abundant with evidence that supports effective methodologies for prevention, treatment, and restoration of physical functioning. Although existing literature also recognizes the psychological, social, and economic impact of osteoarthritis and osteoporosis on women, there is a noticeable lack of current inquiry that explores specific approaches to successfully meet these challenges. Additional research is needed in this area.

Special Concerns of Age and Ethnicity

Osteoarthritis and osteoporosis are chronic diseases, the incidence of which increases substantially with age. Whereas the disabilities associated with these conditions mostly appear in older women, the risk factors that often lead to these conditions appear years earlier. Younger women with risk factors for either osteoarthritis or osteoporosis should be educated regarding preventive measures. For example, younger women who are obese or engage in activities that injure or overuse joints need to lose weight, exercise regularly, and modify activities to protect their joints. Younger women also need to enrich their diets with calcium and vitamin D, and avoid smoking and excess alcohol intake. Education and preventive care of younger women can significantly reduce future incidence of osteoarthritis and osteoporosis.

African-American, Hispanic, and Native American women have an increased risk of osteoarthritis as compared to white women. The greater prevalence of obesity and physical inactivity found among ethnic women likely contributes to the greater incidence. Furthermore, the disabling effects of osteoarthritis disproportionately affect racial and ethnic minorities. The reasons for racial and ethnic disparities in arthritis-related limitations may be attributed to differences in healthcare access, use of available healthcare services, treatment disparities, and the influence of cultural beliefs and language barriers (Bolen et al., 2005; Odutola & Ward, 2005).

However, the risk of osteoporosis in older African-American women is lower than that of older white, Hispanic, Native American, and Asian women. Even so, disparities in health care likely influence poorer health outcomes for women of ethnic minorities who develop osteoporosis and fragility fractures (Pothiwala et al., 2006). Healthcare providers need to be particularly vigilant in identifying at-risk minority women, and institute prevention strategies early. Widespread awareness and screening programs are essential, especially patient and healthcare provider education regarding disease prevention and maintenance of joint and bone health (Pothiwala et al., 2006). Furthermore, healthcare providers need to be cognizant of the disparities that can influence poorer health outcomes and quality of life in women of ethnic minorities and be prepared to mobilize efforts to overcome barriers to adequate care and treatment.

Research Review

What are the experiences of women living with osteoarthritis in environments where they receive assistance with basic living skills?

Baird, C., Yehle, K., & Schmeiser, D. (2007). Experiences of women with osteoarthritis in assisted living facilities. *Clinical Nurse Specialist, 21*(6), 276–284.

The purpose of this study was to examine emic (personally meaningful) experiences in order to explore what older women who live with decreased independence believe about their arthritis symptoms. It was purported that recognition of the challenges, strengths, and etiologies of symptoms of older women with osteoarthritis may lead to improved health and quality of life, and improved independent living.

A qualitative methodological approach was chosen for this study. An emergent design rooted in a naturalistic and phenomenological inquiry framework was used to address the research problem. The context-specific setting for the study was assisted living facilities. No a priori theory was used in order to preclude the formation of premature conclusions, and thus data were allowed to unfold unhampered by preconceived notions regarding the findings. A purposive sample of 23 women, aged 73–94 (mean age of 85 years) who lived in eight assisted living facilities in a suburban area of a Midwestern city participated in the study. The women were able to give a rich description about their experiences with osteoarthritis. Audiotaped interviews lasting 1 to 3 hours were conducted, following a semistructured interview guide. Transcriptions were analyzed by deconstruction and reconstruction. Procedures to assure trustworthiness of the findings to readers were followed.

The study findings revealed two major themes, *Restricting* and *Constricting*. *Restricting* reflected women feeling limited in what they usually did as a result of osteoarthritis and thus actively restricting their lives so as not to exacerbate their symptoms. The intermediate categories that led to the theme of *Restricting* were *Not doing because of disability*, and *Not doing by choice. Not doing because of disability* indicated that the women were unable to do or had difficulty doing activities of daily living, instrumental activities of daily living, or were unable to move normally. *Not doing by choice* referred to women determining what increased their pain and symptoms so they could stop doing those things. The theme of *Constricting* referred to women feeling constrained by their environment. The intermediate categories that led to the theme of *Constricting* were *Limiting ability to move without assistive devices* and *Living within confining spaces*. *Limiting ability to move without assistive devices* referred to feeling that having to use assistive devices constricted the possibilities for the women. *Living within confining spaces* indicated the constriction of living within the boundaries of their environment that included limited ability to leave and interact with community and limited range of activities.

The findings of this study are significant in that they present aspects of living with osteoarthritis that had not been previously described. The findings suggest opportunities for intervening to improve the quality of life of older women with osteoarthritis. Practice implications in the assisted living facility setting included advancing methods and procedures for regular assessments that determine changes in function and etiologies of those changes, and increased use of nonpharmacologic pain interventions. Interventions to increase muscle strength and stability of residents, reduce barriers to increased independence, facilitate increased social interaction, and increase functional self-efficacy were also recommended.

Chapter Summary Points

- Osteoarthritis and osteoporosis are prevalent musculoskeletal disorders that disproportionately affect women, most notably in the postmenopausal years.
- The disabling effects of osteoarthritis and osteoporosis disproportionately affect women of racial and ethnic minorities. Disparities are apparent in the incidence, severity, processes of care, and health outcomes.
- Disparities may be attributed to differences in dietary, biologic, and lifestyle factors as well as healthcare access, use of available healthcare services, treatment differences, and the influence of cultural beliefs and language barriers.
- Nonmodifiable risk factors for osteoarthritis comprise increasing age, gender, and heredity. Modifiable risk factors consist of obesity and joint injury/overuse.
- Non-modifiable risk factors for osteoporosis comprise gender, age, body size, ethnicity, and heredity. Modifiable risk factors consist of hypogonadism, calcium and vitamin D deficiency, physical inactivity, cigarette smoking and alcohol consumption, and medications that promote bone loss.
- Although osteoporosis is preventable and treatable, the absence of warning signs prior to the development of a fracture often precludes timely diagnosis and initiation of effective therapy in the early stages of the disease.

- Lifestyle modification can have a positive effect on decreasing the risk of developing osteoarthritis or osteoporosis.
- Gender similarities and differences in osteoarthritis and osteoporosis are becoming apparent as findings from gender-based research come to light.
- The treatment plan for either osteoarthritis or osteoporosis will include a combination of pharmacologic and nonpharmacologic therapies, rehabilitative interventions, and surgical options, if necessary.
- Quality of life issues and concerns associated with osteoarthritis and osteoporosis are multidimensional and encompass health and physical functioning, psychological and spiritual well-being, socioeconomic integrity, and family well-being.
- The likelihood of the existence of comorbid conditions among postmenopausal women with osteoarthritis or osteoporosis can further impact across the various domains of quality of life.
- Common misconceptions held by many older adults view osteoarthritis and osteoporosis as inevitable outcomes of aging about which nothing can be done. These misconceptions frequently lead to underdiagnosis, undertreatment, and underutilization of self-management resources.
- Concerted efforts need to be directed toward disease prevention, recognition of at risk women, and proactive treatment strategies.

Critical Thinking Exercise

Case Study

Mrs. T. is a 72-year-old woman who was recently widowed. She emigrated from Hong Kong over 20 years ago with her husband and daughter. Mrs. T. lives in the upstairs apartment of a two-family home. Her daughter is divorced and lives in the lower apartment with her young child. Mrs. T. is retired and babysits for her 2-year-old grandchild while her daughter works. Mrs. T. lives on social security and a small retirement pension. She receives Medicare. Although Mrs. T. has been treated for a mild case of heart failure and is maintained on a diuretic, she prefers to use Chinese herbs for her other healthcare needs. She went through menopause at the age of 51 and has never taken hormone replacement therapy. Mrs. T. is 5 feet tall, weighs about 100 lbs, and has smoked a pack of cigarettes per day since the age of 21. Mrs. T. admits to being physically inactive except for doing the housework and occasionally taking her grandchild for a walk to the playground in a stroller. Mrs. T. enjoys socializing with other Chinese women at the Chinese Senior Citizens Center in the neighborhood and goes on outings or plays mahjong with them three afternoons a week. Recently, after viewing some family photographs, Mrs. T.'s daughter commented that lately her mother looks like she's gotten shorter and stoop shouldered. Mrs. T. replied that it's probably because she's "getting old."

Mrs. T. recently developed a sharp pain in the lower back that occurs when she bends over to pick up her grandchild. She attributes the pain to the aches and pains of getting old. One morning her daughter found Mrs. T. lying on the bathroom floor. She had apparently fallen when she got up to go to the bathroom in the middle of the night. Mrs. T. was hospitalized with a broken hip, which was subsequently repaired with surgery. During her hospitalization, Mrs. T. underwent dual-energy x-ray absorptiometry (DXA) measurement of bone mineral density and was found to have a T-score below –2.5. Mrs. T. was started on biphosphonate therapy with calcium and vitamin D supplements. When recovered from her hip surgery, Mrs. T. was discharged to a rehabilitation facility. After 8 weeks of rehabilitation, Mrs. T. was able to walk with a cane and discharged to her home. Mrs. T. was not strong enough to continue babysitting for her granddaughter, and her daughter was able to make other child care arrangements with a day care center in the neighborhood. Mrs. T. was saddened that she did not feel well enough to do the things she had been able to do before she broke her hip.

Questions for Seminar Discussion

1. What factors placed Mrs. T. at high risk for osteoporosis and fragility fractures?
2. How did lack of awareness of osteoporosis risk impact Mrs. T. in the development of fragility fractures?
3. What lifestyle modifications should be done to reduce the risk of fractures for Mrs. T.?
4. What strategies can enhance Mrs. T.'s bone health?
5. Discuss the physical, psychological/spiritual, socioeconomic, and family issues that influence Mrs. T.'s quality of life.
6. What resources are available to help Mrs. T. manage her illness and improve her quality of life?
7. Discuss the importance of a multidisciplinary approach to Mrs. T.'s disease management, survival, and quality of life.
8. How might disease comorbidities affect Mrs. T.'s disease management and quality of life?
9. What strategies could effectively enhance Mrs. T.'s compliance with her treatment and rehabilitation program?

Internet Resources

The American College of Rheumatology: information and resources for physicians, health professionals, and students. http://www.rheumatology.org

The Arthritis Foundation: information and resources for patients, family, and health professionals. http://www.arthritis.org

National Center for Chronic Disease Prevention and Health Promotion: information and resources for patients, family, and health professionals. http://www.cdc.gov/arthritis/basics/osteoarthritis.htm

National Institutes of Health Osteoporosis and Related Bone Diseases-National Resource Center: information and resources for patients, family, and health professionals. http://www.niams.nih.gov/bone

National Osteoporosis Foundation: information and resources for patients, family, and health professionals. http://nof.org

The National Women's Health Information Center-U.S. Department of Health and Human Services Office of Women's Health: information and resources for patients, family, and health professionals. http://www.womenshealth.gov

References

Ağlamis B., Toraman, N., & Yaman, H. (2009). Change of quality of life due to exercise training in knee osteoarthritis: SF-36 and WOMAC. *Journal of Back and Musculoskeletal Rehabilitation, 22*, 43–48.

Andersen, S. (2007). Osteoporosis in the older woman. *Clinical Obstetrics and Gynecology, 50*(3), 752–766.

Arthritis Foundation (2015). Osteoarthritis causes. Retrieved from http://www.arthritis.org/about-arthritis/types/osteoarthritis/causes.php

Baird, C., Yehle, K., & Schmeiser, D. (2007). Experiences of women with osteoarthritis in assisted living facilities. *Clinical Nurse Specialist, 21*(6), 276–284.

Barlow, J., Wright, C., Sheasby, J., Turner, A., & Hainsworth, J. (2002). Self-management approaches for people with chronic conditions: A review. *Patient Education and Counseling, 48*(2), 177–187.

Bayliss, E., Ellis, J., & Steiner, J. (2007). Barriers to self-management and quality of life outcomes in seniors with multimorbidities. *Annals of Family Medicine, 5*(5), 395–402.

Bijlsma, J., & Knahr, K. (2007). Strategies for the prevention and management of osteoarthritis of the hip and knee. *Best Practice and Research Clinical Rheumatology, 21*(1), 59–76.

Bolen, J., Schieb, L., Hootman, J., Helmick, C., Theis, K., Murphy, L., & Langmaid, G. (2010). Differences in the prevalence and impact of arthritis among racial/ethnic groups in the United States, National Health Interview Survey, 2002, 2003, and 2006. *Preventing Chronic Diseases, 7*(3), A64.

Boonen, S., & Singer, A. (2008). Osteoporosis management: Impact of fracture type on cost and quality of life in patients at risk for fracture I. *Current Medical Research and Opinion, 24*(6), 1781–1788.

Centers for Disease Control and Prevention. (2013). Risk factors. Retrieved from http://www.cdc.gov/arthritis/basics/risk_factors.htm

Centers for Disease Control and Prevention. (2014). Osteoarthritis. Retrieved from http://www.cdc.gov/arthritis/basics/osteoarthritis.htm

Cimmino, M., & Parodi, M. (2005). Risk factors for arthritis. *Seminars in Arthritis and Rheumatism, 34* (6 Supp 2), 29–34.

Cosman, F., de Beur, S., LeBoff, M., Lewiecki, E., Tanner, B., Randall, S., & Lindsay, R. (2014). Clinician's guide to prevention and treatment of osteoporosis. *Osteoporosis International, 25*, 2359–2381.

De Oliveira Ferreira, N., Arthuso, M., da Silva, R., Orcesi Pedro, A., Pinto Neto, A., & Costa-Paiva, L. (2009). Quality of life in women with postmenopausal osteoporosis: Correlation between QUALEFFO 41 and SF-36. *Maturitas, 62*, 85–90.

Devos-Comby, L., Cronan, T., & Roesch, S. (2006). Do exercise and self-management interventions benefit patients with osteoarthritis of the knee? A metaanalytic review. *The Journal of Rheumatology, 33*, 744–756.

Diel, P., Merky, D., Röder, C., Popp, A., Malgorzata, P., & Heini, P. (2009). Safety and efficacy of vertebroplasty: Early results of a prospective one-year case series of osteoporosis patients in an academic high-volume center. *Indian Journal of Orthopaedics, 43*(3), 226–233.

Geusens, P., & Dinant, G. (2007). Integrating a gender dimension into osteoporosis and fracture risk research. *Gender Medicine, 4*(Suppl. B), S147–S161.

Hale, L., & Goehring, M. (2003). A multidisciplinary approach to managing osteoporosis. *Annals of Long-Term Care, 11*(6), 40–47.

Hanna, F., Teichtahl, A., Wluka, A., Wang, Y., Urquhart, D., English, D., ... Cicuttini, F. (2009). Women have increased rates of cartilage loss and progression of cartilage defects at the knee than men: A gender study of adults without clinical knee osteoarthritis. *Menopause: The Journal of the North American Menopause Society, 16*(4), 666–670.

Harvey, I. (2008). Assessing self-management and spirituality practices among older women. *American Journal of Health Behavior, 32*(2), 157–168.

Hootman, J., Bolen, J., Helmick, C., & Langmaid, G. (2006). Prevalence of doctor-diagnosed arthritis and arthritis-attributable activity limitation – United States, 2003–2005. *MMWR Weekly, 55*(40), 1089–1092.

Johnson, C. S., McLeod, W., Kennedy, L., & McLeod, K. (2008). Osteoporosis health beliefs among younger and older men and women. *Health Education and Behavior, 35*(5), 721–733.

Leppert P., & Piepert J. (2004). *Primary care for women* (2nd ed.). Philadelphia: Lippincott, Williams, & Wilkins.

Lewiecki, E. (2009). Current and emerging pharmacologic therapies for the management of postmenopausal osteoporosis. *Journal of Women's Health, 18*(10), 1615–1626.

Lo, V., & Meadows, S. (2006). When should COX-2 selective NSAIDs be used for osteoarthritis and rheumatoid arthritis? *The Journal of Family Practice, 55*(3), 260–262.

Looker, A., Borrud, G., Dawson-Hughes, B., Shepherd, J., & Wright, N. (2012). Osteoporosis or low bone mass at the femur neck or lumbar spine in older adults: United States, 2005–2008. Retrieved from http://www.cdc.gov/nchs/data/databriefs/db93.pdf

Luger, T., Cotter, K., & Sherman, A. (2009). It's all how you view it: Pessimism, social relations, and life satisfaction in older adults with osteoarthritis. *Aging and Mental Health, 13*(5), 635–647.

Machado, G., Gignac, M., & Badley, E. (2008). Participation restrictions among older adults with osteoarthritis: A mediated model of physical symptoms, activity limitations, and depression. *Arthritis & Rheumatism, 59*(1), 129–135.

Maetzel, A., Li, L., Pencharz, J., Tomlinson, F., & Bombardier, C. (2004). The economic burden associated with osteoarthritis, rheumatoid arthritis, and hypertension. *Annals of Rheumatic Diseases, 63*(4), 395–401.

Mayo Clinic. (2015). Osteoarthritis. Retrieved from http://www.mayoclinic.org/diseases-conditions/osteoarthritis/basics/definition/con-20014749

McCauley, J., Tarpley, M., Haaz, S., & Bartlett, S. (2008). Daily spiritual experiences of older adults with and without arthritis and the relationship to health outcomes. *Arthritis and Rheumatism, 59*(1), 122–128.

Moskowitz, R. (2009). The burden of osteoarthritis: Clinical and quality of life issues. *The American Journal of Managed Care, 15*(8), S223–S229.

National Institute of Arthritis and Musculoskeletal and Skin Diseases. (2013). Osteoarthritis. Retrieved from http://www.niams.nih.gov/Health_Info/Osteoarthritis/default.asp#2

National Institutes of Health Osteoporosis and Related Bone Diseases-National Resource Center. (2012). Osteoporosis overview. Retrieved from http://www.niams.nih.gov/Health_Info/Bone/Osteoporosis/overview.asp

Nüesch, E., Dieppe, P., Reichenbach, S., Williams, S., Iff, S., & Jüni, P. (2011). All cause and disease specific mortality in patients with knee or hip osteoarthritis: Population based cohort study. *British Medical Journal, 342*(7798), 638.

Newman, S., Steed, L., & Mulligan, K. (2004). Self-management interventions for chronic illness. *The Lancet, 364*, 1523–1537.

Odutola, J., & Ward, M. (2005). Ethnic and socioeconomic disparities in health among patients with rheumatic diseases. *Current Opinion in Rheumatology, 17*, 147–152.

Orwig, D., Chan, J., & Magaziner, J. (2006). Hip fracture and its consequences: Differences between men and women. *Orthopedic Clinics of North America, 37*, 611–622.

Pike, C., Birnbaum, H., Schiller, M., Sharma, H., Burge, R., & Edgell, E. (2010). Direct and indirect costs of non-vertebral fracture patients with osteoporosis in the US. *Pharmacoeconomics, 28*(5), 395–409.

Pinn, V. (2006). Past and future: Sex and gender in health research, the aging experience, and implications for musculoskeletal health. *Orthopedic Clinics of North America, 37*, 513–521.

Pothiawala, P., Evans, E., & Chapman-Novakofski, K. (2006). Ethnic variation in risk for osteoporosis among women: A review of biological and behavioral factors. *Journal of Women's Health, 15*(6), 709–719.

Roberto, K. (2004). Care practices and quality of life of rural older women with osteoporosis. *Journal of the American Medical Women's Association, 59*(4), 295–301.

Roberto, K., Gold, D., & Yorgason, J. (2004). The influence of osteoporosis on the marital relationship of older couples. *The Journal of Applied Gerontology*, *23*(4), 443–456.

Roberto, K., Gigliotti, C., & Husser, E. (2005). Older women's experiences with multiple health conditions: Daily challenges and care practices. *Health Care for Women International*, *26*, 672–692.

Sampson, H.W. (2003). Alcohol and other factors affecting osteoporosis risk in women. *National Institute on Alcohol Abuse and Alcoholism*. Retrieved from http://pubs.niaaa.nih.gov/publications/arh26-4/292-298.htm

Sarzi-Puttini, P., Cimmino, M., Scarpa, R., Caporali, R., Parazzini, F., Zaninelli, A., ... Canesi, B. (2005). Osteoarthritis: An overview of the disease and its treatment strategies. *Seminars in Arthritis and Rheumatism*, *35*(Suppl 1), 1–10.

Savelkoul, M., de Witte, L., & Post, M. (2003). Stimulating active coping in patients with rheumatic diseases: A systematic review of controlled group intervention studies. *Patient Education and Counseling*, *50*, 133–143.

Shyu, Y., Cheng, H., Teng, H., Chen, M., Wu, C., & Tsai, W. (2009). Older people with hip fracture: Depression in the postoperative first year. *Journal of Advanced Nursing*, *65*(12), 2514–2522.

Silverman, S., Shen, W., Minshall, M., Xie, S., & Moses, K. (2007). Prevalence of depressive symptoms in postmenopausal women with low bone mineral density and/or prevalent vertebral fracture: Results from the Multiple Outcomes of Raloxifene Evaluation (MORE) Study. *The Journal of Rheumatology*, *34*(1), 140–144.

Somers, T., Keefe, F., Godiwala, N., & Hoyler, G. (2009). Psychosocial factors and the pain experience of osteoarthritis patients: New findings and new directions. *Current Opinion in Rheumatology*, *21*, 501–506.

Stone, L., & Lyles, K. (2006). Osteoporosis in later life. *Generations*, *30*(3), 65–70.

Von Mühlen, D., Morton, D., Von Mühlen, C., & Barrett-Connor, D. (2002). Postmenopausal estrogen and increased risk of clinical osteoarthritis at the hip, hand, and knee in older women. *Journal of Women's Health and Gender-Based Medicine*, *11*(6), 511–518.

Wilhelm, K. (2009). Kyphoplasty: Better or worse than vertebroplasty? *The Neuroradiology Journal*, *22* (Suppl. 1), 149.

World Health Organization Collaborating Center for Metabolic Bone Diseases. (2015). FRAX®: WHO fracture risk assessment tool. Retrieved from http://www.shef.ac.uk/FRAX/

Wright, N., Riggs, G., Lisse, J., & Chen, Z. (2008). Self-reported osteoarthritis, ethnicity, body mass index, and other associated risk factors in postmenopausal women—Results from the Women's Health Initiative. *Journal of the American Geriatrics Society*, *56*, 1736–1743.

Alzheimer's Disease

Introduction

Alzheimer's disease is a significant health issue in aging women. As the population ages and life expectancy lengthens, the incidence and prevalence of Alzheimer's disease will inevitably increase. Although Alzheimer's disease affects men and women similarly, women are more likely to develop the disease, owing to having a longer life span than men. Furthermore, family caregivers of Alzheimer's patients are predominantly women. Alzheimer's disease is a common cause of dementia and is characterized by a subtle onset and slow progression over years. Along its trajectory, Alzheimer's disease produces a progressive decline or loss of memory, cognitive abilities, emotional control, and social behaviors. Alzheimer's disease is devastating not only to those afflicted, but can be emotionally, socially, and financially devastating to family members who provide care and support. This chapter explores the issues of women with Alzheimer's disease and women who are caregivers of those afflicted with the disease. The significant impact of Alzheimer's disease on women's quality of life is also discussed.

Incidence

Alzheimer's disease has emerged as a significant societal and healthcare problem, as its incidence increases with aging and longevity. It is estimated that 5.3 million Americans have Alzheimer's disease.

Of this number, 5.1 million people are aged 65 and older, of which 3.2 million are women and 1.9 million are men. The remaining 200,000 are younger than 65 and have early-onset Alzheimer's disease (Alzheimer's Association, 2015b). It is estimated that 473,000 people 65 years of age or older will have been diagnosed with the disease in 2015. Currently, one in nine individuals aged 65 and older (11%) have Alzheimer's disease and 32% of people aged 85 or older are similarly afflicted. It is also estimated that 14% of people 75 years of age or older in the United States are afflicted with dementia, and 81% of people who have Alzheimer's disease are 75 years of age or older (Alzheimer's Association, 2015a). Moreover, the number of people in this country aged 65 and older is increasing, particularly the number of oldest-old. Consequently, the annual number of new cases of Alzheimer's and other dementias is projected to double by 2050. In addition, by 2050, the number of people age 65 and older with Alzheimer's disease may more than triple, from 5 million to an estimated 16 million, barring development of medical breakthroughs to prevent, slow, or arrest the disease (Alzheimer's Association, 2014).

Because the risk for developing Alzheimer's disease increases with age, by age 90 approximately 33% of women and 23% of men will have developed Alzheimer's disease (Geis & Lessick, 2009). At age 65, the lifetime risk for Alzheimer's disease is estimated to be 20% in women as compared to 17% in men. This translates into a lifetime risk at age 65 of approximately 1 in 6 women and nearly 1 in 11 men (Alzheimer's Association, 2015a).

As the underlying cause of death for 72,432 people, Alzheimer's disease is the seventh leading cause of death in the United States and the fifth leading cause of death for adults aged 65 and older. The death rate of individuals with Alzheimer's disease rises dramatically with age. Survival after diagnosis can range from 4 to 8 years for people 65 or older, yet some live as long as 20 years with Alzheimer's disease. Median survival time tends to decrease with age and is longer for women (Alzheimer's Association, 2015a; Mehta, et al., 2008). It was estimated that in 2010, 600,000 people age 65 and older died with Alzheimer's disease, meaning they died after developing Alzheimer's disease. Of this number, 400,000 were estimated to be age 85 and older and 200,000 were estimated to be age 65 to 84. Moreover, it was estimated that in 2015, 700,000 people in the United States age 65 or older would die with Alzheimer's disease (Alzheimer's Association, 2015a).

Underreporting of deaths by Alzheimer's disease, both in nursing homes and local communities, has been documented, suggesting that the death rate attributable to the disease could be higher. One likely explanation points to the fact that *how* death results from Alzheimer's disease creates ambiguity about the underlying cause of death. Severe complications often arise in Alzheimer's patients, such as immobility, loss of ability to swallow, and malnutrition. These complications increase the risk of pneumonia, which is a frequent cause of death among the elderly with Alzheimer's disease. The underlying cause of death, whether caused *by* Alzheimer's disease or from complications that develop *because of* Alzheimer's disease, can be indistinct (Alzheimer's Association, 2014).

Disparities in the prevalence of Alzheimer's disease among racial and ethnic minorities have been noted. Available research indicates that older African-Americans are about two times as likely to develop Alzheimer's disease and other dementias as older white adults. It is also estimated that older Hispanics are at least one and one-half times more likely than older white adults to develop Alzheimer's disease and other dementias (Alzheimer's Association, 2015a). Research also suggests that African-American and Hispanic adults with Alzheimer's disease live longer after diagnosis as compared to white adults with Alzheimer's disease, while no difference in length of survival was noted between Asian Americans, Native Americans and whites with Alzheimer's disease. Hispanic women with Alzheimer's disease appear to have a stronger mortality advantage than Hispanic men with Alzheimer's disease (Mehta et al., 2008).

Ethnic Considerations

The increased incidence and prevalence of Alzheimer's disease in racial and ethnic populations are associated with a number of factors. Research findings indicate that the first-degree relatives of African-Americans with Alzheimer's disease have a higher cumulative risk for disease development as compared to the first-degree relatives of whites with Alzheimer's disease. Research has also suggested that African-Americans and Caribbean Hispanics have an increased risk of Alzheimer's disease associated with the ApoE epsilon 4 genotype (Gies & Lessick, 2009). In addition to this, a higher risk for Alzheimer's disease as well as earlier disease onset may be seen in African-American and Hispanic adults as compared to non-Hispanic white adults. This is likely attributed to a higher rate of risk factors associated with the disease, such as hypertension, diabetes, and other metabolic abnormalities occurring in the minorities, as compared to their non-Hispanic white counterparts (Alzheimer's Association, 2015a; Griffith & Lopez, 2009). In addition to increased disease risk and earlier onset, African-American and Hispanic adults are frequently diagnosed at later stages of the disease, with many experiencing a delay of up to 7 years before having their symptoms evaluated. Along with delayed diagnosis, African-Americans and Hispanics often experience a delay in initiation of pharmacotherapy. Delay in diagnosis and initiation of treatment may result in greater cognitive impairment at the time of diagnosis and the greater likelihood of patients being unresponsive to therapy because of being in advanced stages of the disease (Griffith & Lopez, 2009).

A number of barriers likely contribute to delayed diagnosis and treatment of Alzheimer's disease in African-Americans and Hispanics. In some African-American and Hispanic communities, the early symptoms of Alzheimer's disease, such as memory loss and functional decline, are likely to be interpreted as signs of normal aging. Uncertainty about the severity of the problem, reluctance to upset the patient, embarrassment, shame, guilt, and cultural barriers among family caregivers also contribute to delays in seeking medical care for symptomatic patients. In addition to these factors, the likelihood of lack of formal education, low income, and lack of health insurance can also impede early diagnosis and treatment among African-American and Hispanic populations (Griffith & Lopez, 2009).

Etiology and Risk Factors

Alzheimer's disease is an irreversible progressive brain disorder in which increasing numbers of brain cells deteriorate and die. In a healthy adult brain, 100 billion nerve cells function to transmit information in the form of chemical signals from neuron to neuron across junctions called synapses. Different strengths and patterns of signals move constantly through the brain cells and create the cellular basis of memories, thoughts, and skills (Alzheimer's Association, 2014). The brain of a person with Alzheimer's disease develops amyloid plaques and neurofibrillary tangles. Plaques are dense deposits of protein and cellular material that form outside and around the neurons. It is not clear whether the plaques cause the disease or are a by-product of the disease process. Neurofibrillary tangles are insoluble twisted fibers that build up inside neurons. A form of protein called *tau* is the main component of tangles. In healthy neurons, tau proteins help stabilize the structure of the cell. In brains affected by Alzheimer's disease, the tau protein is chemically altered and cannot hold the structure together. Information transmission at the synaptic junctions begins to fail as neurons collapse and the brain cells die. Brains that have advanced Alzheimer's disease demonstrate dramatic reduction in size from cell loss and widespread debris from dead and dying neurons (Alzheimer's Association, 2014).

Alzheimer's disease manifests in two forms, early-onset (also known as familial disease) and late-onset disease. Early-onset disease develops before age 60, progresses faster than late-onset disease, and affects about 5% of the people with Alzheimer's disease. Late-onset disease is the most common and typically develops after age 65.

The cause of Alzheimer's disease is not yet known; however, most experts agree that a number of factors contribute to the development of the disease rather than a single cause. The most common risk factor for Alzheimer's disease is advancing age; however, Alzheimer's disease is not a normal part of aging. Numerous risk factors have been linked to Alzheimer's disease. These factors are presented as below.

Heredity

Early-onset disease is linked to mutations in three genes: amyloid precursor protein (APP) on chromosome 21, presenilin 1 (PSEN 1) on chromosome 14, and presenilin 2 (PSEN 2) on chromosome 1. The presence of gene mutation leads to overproduction of amyloid beta peptides, which influences the production of amyloid plaques. The genes are inherited in an autosomal dominant fashion. Only one mutation in any of these genes is required for disease development. Thus, the presence of a first-degree relative (parent or sibling) with Alzheimer's disease will likely increase the risk of early-onset disease development significantly (Gies & Lessick, 2009).

The genetic influences of late-onset disease are less clear, but a combination of gene mutation, lifestyle, and environmental factors are believed to be involved. The apolipoprotein (ApoE) gene has been observed to triple the risk of developing late-onset disease. A variant of ApoE, epsilon 4 allele (Apoee4), is carried by 40%–70% of late-onset Alzheimer's patients and confers significant risk of disease development. However, Apoee4 is not a definitive predictor of Alzheimer's disease since persons without this allele may develop the disease and persons with the allele may not develop the disease (Gies & Lessick, 2009; Godfrey & El-Badri, 2009).

Nearly all persons with Down's syndrome (trisomy 21) develop neuropathological changes associated with Alzheimer's disease after the age of 40, and more than 50% exhibit cognitive decline. This is thought to be due to the overexpression of APP on chromosome 21 in people with Down's syndrome that results in the overproduction of beta-amyloid in their brains (Gies & Lessick, 2009).

Environmental Factors

Certain environmental factors are believed to act on a predisposing genetic background to increase the risk of developing late-onset disease. Research has suggested that traumatic brain injury presents a potential risk factor but the mechanisms underlying this association are unclear. A direct relationship exists between inflammation-mediated diseases and conditions and the risk of developing Alzheimer's disease, especially in women. These conditions include hypertension, hyperlipidemia, diabetes, and metabolic syndrome. Elevated homocysteine levels combined with higher risk for cardiovascular disease and stroke may also increase the risk for Alzheimer's disease (Godfrey & El-Badri, 2009). Increased risk for Alzheimer's disease has also been linked to reduced thyroid stimulating hormone level, exposure to pesticides, and history of major depressive episodes (Scalco & van Reekum, 2006). Women who exhibit mild cognitive impairment (MCI) whereby they experience a phenomenon of rapid forgetting but are otherwise cognitively and functionally normal are at high risk for developing Alzheimer's disease. Approximately 10%–15% of women per year who have MCI will develop Alzheimer's disease (Godfrey, 2006).

Lifestyle factors such as physical inactivity, smoking, and excessive use of alcohol significantly increase the risk for developing Alzheimer's disease. Excess body weight, especially morbid obesity in which the body mass index exceeds 30 during midlife can triple the risk of disease development, whereas body mass index of 25–29 doubles the risk (Godfrey & El-Badri, 2009).

Degree of Risk of Alzheimer's Disease

The degree of risk for the development of Alzheimer's disease in women increases with advancing age and is compounded by family history and the presence of other risk factors. The first step in identifying risk is to obtain a comprehensive history. Ideally, a three–generation family history can help to identify possible inherited patterns and risk of Alzheimer's disease that could necessitate referral to genetics specialists. Genetics referral would be needed if the family history revealed early onset disease in first-degree relatives and a pattern of autosomal dominant inheritance. No genetics referral would be necessary if the history revealed random cases of Alzheimer's disease in relatives older than 65 years of age (Gies & Lessick, 2009).

Research has been conducted on tests to identify early markers of Alzheimer's disease or characteristics that could predict those who are likely to acquire the disease. Currently no tests have enough evidence that supports their safety and predictive ability to allow widespread use in the general population. Nonetheless, neuropsychologic and cognitive tests are frequently used with individuals at high risk for Alzheimer's disease and those who report cognitive or memory problems. Neuropsychologic tests, which consist primarily of tests of verbal and episodic memory, have been useful in detecting Alzheimer's disease, discriminating

between those with mild disease and normal controls, and in predicting disease after up to 5 years of follow-up (Scalco & van Reekum, 2006).

A consistent assessment tool that tracks cognitive changes over time is the Mini-Mental State Examination (MMSE). This measure tests orientation, registration, attention and calculation, language, and recall. Declining scores on the MMSE will denote cognitive decline, and the measure is useful in identifying most but not all women with early disease. Some women who are highly educated can obtain perfect scores on the MMSE even in the presence of persistent memory decline, and should be referred for specialty evaluation (Gies & Lessick, 2009).

Neuroimaging procedures such as magnetic resonance imaging, positron emission tomography, and single proton emission computed tomography can detect cerebral changes that occur with MCI. These changes include hippocampal and entorhinal cortex atrophy and reduced blood flow and glucose metabolism in the temporoparietal and posterior cingulated areas, and are considered well-established risk factors for subsequent development of Alzheimer's disease in the MCI population. These neuroimaging findings, however, are not specific enough to be used as predictors of Alzheimer's disease in the general population. Long-term prospective follow-up studies need to be conducted in order to establish the early marker and predictive merit of neuroimaging in Alzheimer's disease.

Risk Reduction

Risk factor reduction and modification may have a role in the prevention of Alzheimer's disease. A growing body of evidence indicates that the health of the brain, which is the most highly vascular organ of the body, is closely associated with the health of the cardiovascular system. Thus, reduction of cardiovascular risk factors such as hyperlipidemia, hypertension, type 2 diabetes, smoking, obesity, and physical inactivity may help to avoid or delay cognitive decline (Alzheimer's Association, 2014). Research has investigated a variety of therapies for the treatment and prevention of Alzheimer's disease, such as nerve growth factors, nonsteroidal anti-inflammatory drugs, cholesterol-lowering agents, beta-amyloid vaccination, gingko biloba, antioxidants, and antihypertensive agents. Results have thus far been inconclusive (Gies & Lessick, 2009). Research has also investigated the influence of estrogen therapy on the prevention and treatment of Alzheimer's disease but results have been equivocal. Findings have suggested that estrogen therapy given to women at the time of menopause may delay or reduce the risk of developing Alzheimer's disease but does not have clinical benefits as a treatment for the disease (Craig & Murphy, 2009).

Research findings suggest that consumption of a low-fat, high-fiber, nutrient-rich heart-healthy diet may be beneficial in reducing risk, as well as physical exercise and frequent participation in stimulating cognitive activities such as doing puzzles and reading newspapers (Gies & Lessick, 2009; Scalco & van Reekum, 2006).

Gender Similarities and Differences

More women than men develop Alzheimer's disease and other dementias. Nearly two-thirds of people who have Alzheimer's disease in the United States are women. Women are at higher risk for developing Alzheimer's disease than men. This disparity is primarily explained by the fact that women live longer than men, giving women more time to develop the disease. Since the overall death rate is higher for men than women, the outcome is that less men than women are alive with and without Alzheimer's disease (Alzheimer's Association, 2015a; Gies & Lessick, 2009). Although studies investigating the age-specific incidence of Alzheimer's disease have shown no significant

difference between women and men regarding disease development (Alzheimer's Association, 2014), a school of thought purports that women have a significantly higher risk for developing Alzheimer's disease that exceeds the risk accounted for by their greater life expectancy. It is posited that cessation of ovarian function and estrogen production contribute to the cascade of pathological processes that lead to disease development in women. Current understanding of the biological actions of estrogen on the structure and function of the brain supports this theory (Craig & Murphy, 2009).

Although midlife onset of hypertension and hypercholesteremia in both men and women predicts a higher risk of developing Alzheimer's disease later in life, research findings have indicated that the greater prevalence of vascular risk factors such as hypertension, hyperlipidemia, and diabetes in women above the age of 75 substantially increases their risk of developing Alzheimer's disease as compared to similarly-aged men. Midlife obesity likely increases the risk of subsequent development of Alzheimer's disease in women to a greater extent than in men. In addition, Apoee4 genotype status appears to have greater deleterious effect on gross hipocampal pathology and memory performance in women as compared with men (Azad, Al Bugami, & Loy-English, 2007).

Gender-related differences exist in brain structure and function. Men tend to have larger brain size, higher neuron count, and greater neuron density as compared to women. Men and women also differ in patterns of cerebral blood flow and cerebral glucose metabolism. These biological differences may explain gender differences in cognitive reserve, with men maintaining greater cognitive reserve than women. Having less cognitive reserve is thought to underlie women's higher susceptibility to functional cerebral damage in Alzheimer's disease as compared to men (Perneczky, Drzezga, Diehl-Schmid, Li, & Kurz, 2007). In Alzheimer's disease, men's greater cognitive reserve likely enables them to compensate for functional brain damage to a greater degree than women. Women's lesser cognitive reserve probably explains why cognitive symptoms of neurodegeneration tend to be more severe in women when both genders exhibit the same level of cerebral pathology (Perneczky et al., 2007).

Some study findings have indicated that women with Alzheimer's disease likely experience greater language deficits than similarly afflicted men, especially in naming and word recognition skills, but other studies have obtained conflicting results. Proponents of gender differences in language function in Alzheimer's patients believe that discrepancy in language function may be influenced by differing patterns of neural organization or the influence of sex hormones on the brain. Further research is needed to shed more light on cognitive differences between male and female Alzheimer's patients (Ott & Cahn-Weiner, 2003).

Research findings have also revealed gender differences in behavioral disturbances occurring in patients with Alzheimer's disease. Women with Alzheimer's disease tend to exhibit more reclusiveness, emotional lability, inappropriate laughter or crying; they tend to refuse help and have a greater prevalence of depression and delusions. On the other hand, men with Alzheimer's tend to exhibit more apathy, wandering, abusiveness, physical, verbal, and sexual aggression, social impropriety, and vegetative changes such as excessive eating and sleeping (Ott & Cahn-Weiner, 2003).

Diagnosing Alzheimer's Disease

Alzheimer's disease is intrinsically fatal and the available treatments do little to change the progression of the disease. However, early diagnosis is essential so that therapy can be initiated to slow the inevitable cognitive and behavioral decline.

The formation of amyloid plaques and neurofibrillary tangles in the cerebral cortex and hippocampus of the brain is thought to lead to the progression of symptoms that occur in Alzheimer's disease. These pathological changes worsen over time and hinder normal brain function. In the early stages of Alzheimer's disease cognitive impairment manifests as short-term memory loss, which is often poorly recognized or overlooked by close family members. As the disease progresses, impaired judgment, confusion, disorientation, impaired language, and mutism may develop. In advanced stages of the disease, behavioral and functional changes such as depression, agitation, restlessness, aggression, apathy, withdrawal, hallucinations, incontinence, and inability to carry out activities of daily living can occur. In the terminal stage, women become bedridden, lose control of bodily functions, no longer respond to their environment, and become entirely dependent on others for nourishment, hygiene, and other necessities. They become susceptible to a variety of illnesses and infections, and death eventually results from general exhaustion, malnutrition, and pneumonia (Gies & Lessick, 2009). Progression from diagnosis to death takes about 10 to 12 years but this depends on the speed at which the disease progresses from stage to stage and length of survival in the terminal stage. The presence of comorbid conditions such as heart disease, stroke, infections, or fractures as well as the quality of care and support that the individual receives can influence speed of disease progression. The stages of Alzheimer's disease, symptoms characteristic of each stage, and approximate duration of each stage are presented in **Table 16–1**.

Currently, a definitive diagnosis of Alzheimer's disease is made when the presence of amyloid plaques and intraneuronal neurofibrillary tangles are confirmed by autopsy examination of the brain. The process of making a clinical diagnosis is based on recognition of a pattern of cognitive deficit, with prominent memory symptoms from the beginning, normal balance, gait, and movements at early stages, and neuroimaging that reveals no abnormalities other than shrinking of

Table 16–1 STAGES AND SYMPTOMS OF ALZHEIMER'S DISEASE

Stage of Alzheimer's Disease	Characteristic Symptoms	Duration of Stage
1: Normal	Free of subjective and objective complaints regarding memory function, and free of personality, mood, and behavior changes.	
2: Benign Aged Forgetfulness	Subjective awareness that memory is not functioning like it used to. Changes attributed to advancing age. Can no longer recall names as they could 5 or 10 years ago or recall where items such as keys or sunglasses were placed. Also difficulty with concentration and finding the correct word while speaking.	
3. Mild Cognitive Impairment	Difficulty in learning and making new memories. Decreased ability to remember names when introduced to new people or retain material when reading or watching television. Inability to learn or master new skills. Repeats queries, frequently misplaces valuable objects, and shows decreased ability to plan and organize. Decline in work performance and increased difficulties in performing activities of daily living. Deficits noticed by family and associates. Professionally active patients are usually forced to retire.	Approximately 7 years. Diagnosis is usually made midway through this stage, most notably when deficits become evident to family or friends. By the end of this stage a confident diagnosis of early-stage Alzheimer's disease can be made in most but not all patients.
4: Mild Disease	Memory deficits are more evident. Patients may not recall many major events and unable to accurately recall the day of the week, the month, or the season. However, patients can recall their address, head of state, or outdoor weather conditions. Decline in mathematical skills causes difficulty with balancing a checkbook or paying bills. Reduced capacity to perform complex tasks such as food shopping or meal preparation. Reduced emotional responsiveness leads to social withdrawal and dependence on others when unable to cope with a new situation.	Approximately 2 years.
5: Moderate Disease	Memory deficit progresses to involve not only current events but major events from the past. Unable to recall current address, telephone number, year, or current president. Unable to recall the school from which they graduated. Severe arithmetic deficit: unable to count backward from 40 by 4s or from 20 by 2s. Severe cognitive deficit increases risk for accident or injury if left alone.	Approximately 1–1½ years.

Table 16–1 STAGES AND SYMPTOMS OF ALZHEIMER'S DISEASE (*continued*)

Stage of Alzheimer's Disease	Characteristic Symptoms	Duration of Stage
6: Moderately Severe Disease	Loss of ability to perform basic activities of daily living. Unable to select and put clothing on properly. Unable to bathe independently or carry out toileting and other hygiene activities. Urinary and bowel incontinence occur. Remembers own name but confuses names of close family members. Cannot count backwards from 10 by 1s. Speech is difficult to understand due to stuttering and neologisms (made-up words). Personality changes and behavior disturbances include delusions, hallucinations, suspiciousness, compulsiveness, and repetitive behavior.	Approximately 2–2 ½ years.
7: Severe (End-Stage) Disease	Requires continuous assistance with basic activities. Speech is severely impaired, language limited to a few understandable words until ability to speak is lost. Increased difficulty walking until confined to wheelchair or bed. Eventually unable to sit independently or smile. At the final stage, is unable to hold up head independently and develops prolonged contractions in the extremities.	Approximately 5 years. Intensive nursing and medical care may extend survival in this stage for several years.

the hippocampus. Additionally, treatable conditions that produce dementia, such as depression, hypothyroidism, or vitamin B12 deficiency will be ruled out. After ruling out all other disorders causing dementia, the conclusion is made that the symptoms are most likely the result of Alzheimer's disease. When the evaluation is performed by experienced specialists, correlations between the clinical diagnosis of probable Alzheimer's disease and definitive autopsy results are highly accurate. In rare cases, either Alzheimer's disease has an unusual course that mimics other forms of dementia or it coexists with other neurodegenerative conditions.

Treatment

Although there is no cure for Alzheimer's disease, the goals of treatment are to slow the progression of symptoms, maintain cognitive ability at the highest level possible, and control neuropsychological symptoms. Pharmacological therapy is the mainstay of treatment and includes drug therapy for cognitive symptoms as well as behavioral and psychiatric symptoms. In addition, nonpharmacological approaches are also available to augment symptom control.

Cholinesterase Inhibitors

Cholinesterase inhibitors are drugs that block the enzyme cholinesterase, which breaks down acetylcholine. Acetylcholine is a neurotransmitter that is vital for a functioning memory system. Cholinesterase inhibitors enhance the amount of acetylcholine in nerve cells that are still functioning, which allows them to partially compensate for deficits created by the nerve cells that die from the Alzheimer's disease process. As a result, cholinesterase inhibitors will lessen symptoms and slow the clinical (but not biological) progression of Alzheimer's disease.

Cholinesterase inhibitors have been approved by the U.S. Food and Drug Administration (FDA) for treatment of cognitive symptoms such as memory loss, confusion, and problems with thinking and reasoning. These drugs are donezepil, rivastigmine, and galantamin (Alzheimer's Association, 2015b). In addition to inhibiting cholinesterase, galantamine acts directly on acetylcholine receptors to increase their response to acetylcholine. Treatment with cholinesterase inhibitors continues through the course of the disease until the end stages, at which time they are usually withdrawn, since the drugs will no longer have an effect. Side effects of cholinesterase therapy include nausea, vomiting, diarrhea, anorexia, weight loss, dizziness, insomnia, and urinary incontinence. To mitigate the unpleasant side effects, drug dosages are often increased slowly, given at night with food, or women may be switched to a different cholinesterase inhibitor that is better tolerated. If nausea and vomiting are the major side effects, antiemetic drugs may be given for relief. Cholinesterase inhibitors may be contraindicated in women who have active peptic ulcer disease, unstable asthma, chronic obstructive pulmonary disease, or heart disease. Cholinesterase inhibitors must be used with caution if women take heart medications such as digoxin or beta-blockers, or if there is a history of blackouts or seizures. Because of adverse reactions with anesthesia, women who need to undergo surgery must discontinue the cholinesterase inhibitor about 2 weeks prior to surgery and slowly resume the drug after recovery.

Memantine

Memantine has been approved by the FDA for treatment of moderate to severe Alzheimer's disease. This drug helps to improve memory, attention, reason, language, and the ability to perform simple tasks (Alzheimer's Association, 2015b). Memantine controls the action of glutamate. Glutamate is a neurotransmitter, which is secreted by nerve cells and is also involved with learning and memory

function. Memantine blocks excessive glutamate that could damage nerve cells. Women with mild to moderate disease as well as advanced disease may show moderate improvement after taking memantine. Side effects of memantine include headache, dizziness, constipation, and confusion. Memantine may be taken concurrently with donezepril, which is the only cholinesterase inhibitor approved to treat all stages of Alzheimer's disease, including moderate to severe (Alzheimer's Association, 2015b).

Antidepressant, Anxiolytic, and Antipsychotic Drugs

The first-line treatment of neuropsychiatric symptoms is a behavioral approach, which focuses on recognizing and avoiding factors that trigger neuropsychiatric symptoms. When behavioral approaches are not effective in reducing neuropsychiatric symptoms, drug therapy can be prescribed. Prior to resorting to antidepressants and antipsychotic drugs, treatable conditions that may cause neuropsychiatric symptoms must be ruled out by a comprehensive physical exam. These conditions may include side effects of prescription medications taken for other health conditions, physical discomforts caused by conditions such as urinary retention, constipation, infections, or uncorrected vision or hearing problems.

Antidepressants may be prescribed for Alzheimer's patients with symptoms of agitation associated with low mood, irritability, or depressed appetite. Antidepressants most frequently given are citalopram, fluoxetine, paroxeine, sertraline, and trazodone (Alzheimer's Association, 2015b). These drugs are usually well tolerated and have few possible side effects. Side effects may include abdominal cramps, diarrhea, constipation, nausea, and rare vomiting.

Anxiolytics such as lorazepam and oxazepam may be given for relief of anxiety, agitation, verbally disruptive behavior, and resistance (Alzheimer's Association, 2015b). These drugs have sedative properties and are usually given in the evening. This can be especially helpful in reducing episodes of late-day confusion, or "sundowning," which involves periods of increased confusion, agitation, anxiety, and disorientation that begin at dusk and continue throughout the night. Side effects of these drugs may include drowsiness, depression, lethargy, apathy, fatigue, nausea, constipation, diarrhea, dry mouth, and headache.

Women with Alzheimer's disease who develop delusions and paranoia may be prescribed antipsychotic drugs. The use of antipsychotic drugs in patients with Alzheimer's disease needs to be done with extreme caution, as evidence suggests that the risk of stroke and death may be increased with the use of antipsychotic drugs in the older adult with dementia. Governmental warnings, guidance from oversight bodies, and research evidence form the basis of the following recommendations for indications of use of antipsychotic medications in individuals with dementia only under one of the following conditions (Alzheimer's Association, 2015b):

- The behavioral symptoms are due to psychosis or mania.
- The symptoms place the individual or others in danger.

- The individual is experiencing inconsolable or persistent distress, a significant decline in function, or substantial difficulty receiving needed care.

Antipsychotic drugs must be given in the minimum dosage to patients with Alzheimer's disease, for the minimum amount of time possible. These drugs should never be used to sedate or restrain patients with dementia, and patients receiving antipsychotic medications must be carefully monitored for adverse side effects (Alzheimer's Association, 2015b). Antipsychotic drugs can trigger extrapyramidal symptoms such as acute muscle stiffening, restlessness, and involuntary movements of facial muscles and the hands. Metabolic abnormalities such as insulin resistance, type 2 diabetes, and hyperlipidemia can also occur (Gauthier et al., 2010). Although antipsychotics are the most frequently used medications for agitation, some patients with dementia may be prescribed a seizure medication/mood stabilizer, such as carbamazepine (Alzheimer's Association, 2015b).

A summary of the various drugs prescribed for neuropsychiatric symptoms of Alzheimer's disease is presented in **Table 16–2**.

Table 16–2 Drugs Prescribed for Treatment of Neuropsychiatric Symptoms of Alzheimer's Disease

Antidepressants	Anxiolytics	Antipsychotics
Citalopram (Celexa)	Lorazepam (Ativan)	Aripiprazole (Abilify)
Fluoxetine (Prozac)	Oxazepam (Serax)	Clozapine (Clozaril)
Paroxetine (Paxil)		Haloperidol (Haldol)
Sertraline (Zoloft)		Olanzapine (Zyprexa)
Trazodone (Desyrel)		Quetiapine (Seroquel)
		Risperidone (Risperdal)
		Ziprasidone (Geodon)

Antioxidants

Antioxidants are able to neutralize free radicals, which are toxic by-products of metabolic reactions in the body. Free radicals increase greatly during inflammation. Increased production of free radicals is thought to be linked with the cellular damage and neurodegeneration associated with the development of Alzheimer's disease. Evidence suggests that high doses of vitamin E might slow functional decline in individuals with mild-to-moderate Alzheimer's disease (Alzheimer's Association, 2015b). Although the results of this evidence are encouraging, more research is needed before changes to clinical practice should be considered. Risks associated with taking vitamin E include increased risk of bleeding as well as adverse interaction with drugs prescribed to lower cholesterol or prevent blood clots. Vitamin E may also slightly increase risk of death (Alzheimer's Association, 2015b).

Nonpharmacological Interventions

Various evidence-based psychological therapies have shown efficacy in reducing neuropsychiatric symptoms. Interventions such as music therapy, sensory stimulation, relaxation training, Learning Theory approaches, massage therapy, simulated presence therapy (use of audio or video tapes of family members), contingent reinforcement, and use of reminiscence groups have been used with varying degrees of success in decreasing problem behavior. A key to effective use of behavioral interventions is that selected interventions must be individualized to the needs of the patient (Gauthier et al., 2010).

Quality of Life Issues Associated With Alzheimer's Disease

Alzheimer's disease is the most common cause of dementia in elderly women. Alzheimer's disease damages the cognitive, functional, and social abilities of aged women, which in turn can significantly diminish quality of life (Huang, Chang, Tang, Chiu, & Weng, 2008). The burden of care for afflicted individuals falls mainly on family and friends, and the majority of informal caregivers are female family members and friends (Alzheimer's Association, 2015a). The disease burden associated with Alzheimer's disease emerges as a double-edged sword for both patients and caregivers. The enormous healthcare expenditure derived from disease chronicity and severity as well as the effects of disease burden on the quality of life of patients and their informal caregivers have evolved into major societal and public health concerns of paramount importance, especially in view of the predicted surge of the disease with the aging of the population (Alzheimer's Association, 2015a).

The quality of life issues throughout the trajectory of Alzheimer's disease are commonly multidimensional and can encompass health and physical functioning, psychological and spiritual well-being, socioeconomic integrity, and family well-being. However, being able to accurately determine the quality of life of individuals with Alzheimer's disease is challenging because the subjective perceptions of quality of life of patients often differ when compared to that of informal caregivers and professionals (Conde-Sala, Garre-Olmo, Turró-Garriga, López-Pousa, & Vilalta-Franch, 2009). The declining cognitive function that occurs with the advancement of Alzheimer's disease limits the individual's ability to accurately or validly appraise their quality of life (Huang et al., 2008). Patients tend to perceive a better quality of life as compared to the perceptions of the patients' quality of life made by their informal caregivers (Conde-Sala et al., 2009; Hoe, Katona, Orrell, & Livingston, 2007). Various factors may influence the discrepancy between patient and caregiver perception, such as the patient's mood status, neuropsychiatric symptoms, whether they take cholinesterase inhibitors, and whether patients live at home or in

24-hour care settings (Hoe et al., 2007). Healthcare providers should carefully weigh appraisals of quality of life from the patient and informal caregiver as well as various influential factors when assessing the quality of life of Alzheimer's patients.

Issues Affecting Health and Physical Functioning

Alzheimer's disease often begins with decreasing facility of cognitive function and ends with total loss of ability to maintain physical functioning and perform activities of daily living unassisted (VandeWeerd, Paveza, & Fulmer, 2006). The cognitive decline that women experience in Alzheimer's disease can increase the risk for falls and accidents that can lead to physical injuries and dysfunction. Women with Alzheimer's disease are also at increased risk for abuse and neglect by caregivers that can result in disease mismanagement, physical injuries, and malnourishment (VandeWeerd et al., 2006).

Women with Alzheimer's disease are likely to have other chronic diseases common to the aged, such as heart disease or diabetes. Declining cognitive function will likely interfere with self-management of comorbid conditions such that treatment regimens are not followed, symptoms are not recognized, and follow-up appointments with healthcare providers are forgotten. Cognitive decline creates a barrier to self-management that often leads to illness complications that can compound dependency in activities of daily living, increase use of healthcare resources, increase use of nursing homes, and increase mortality (Bayliss, Ellis, & Steiner, 2007). Toward the end stage of the disease, poor appetite, lack of interest in food, difficulty swallowing, and increased immobility will frequently lead to constipation, malnourishment, skin breakdown, increased rate of infection, and pneumonia. The domino effect of the cognitive decline of Alzheimer's disease clearly can impact the health and physical functioning domain of quality of life.

Early initiation of pharmacological therapy and nonpharmacological interventions will help to slow neuronal degeneration and control behavioral symptoms such as agitation, depression, and sleep disorders. Slowing disease progression and controlling behavior symptoms will help to maximize physical function and reduce risk of accidents, falls, and physical injuries. Caregivers need to supervise patients closely in taking prescription and over-the-counter drugs for treatment of Alzheimer's disease and other chronic conditions. As cognitive decline progresses, patients can take incorrect dosages, forget to take their medications, or sequester pills in the mouth and later spit them out unobserved. Caregivers should ascertain that medications were taken by the patient correctly as prescribed. Patients should be monitored for medication side effects that could be detrimental to physical functioning. Nonpharmacological interventions can help to decrease behavioral symptoms and in turn reduce recourse to drugs for behavior control and their subsequent adverse effects.

Caregivers need to create a safe, secure environment in the home that will minimize the risk of falls and accidents. Some strategies include removing obstacles, household clutter, and scatter rugs, making sure floors are not slippery, installing handrails and grab bars in the bathroom, providing adequate lighting in living areas (especially at night), removing locks on inside doors, and locking doors and cabinets to bar access to dangerous areas and substances. To reduce the possibility of wandering, motion detectors may be used, and door alarms and deadbolt locks should be installed on entrance doors. Preparing the home for the safe care of Alzheimer's patients should also include being prepared for various kinds of emergencies. Caregivers should keep an updated list of emergency phone numbers and addresses for local police and fire departments, hospitals, poison control help lines, and emergency family contacts. Fire extinguishers and smoke alarms should be installed and checked regularly. Although some of these measures may not be applicable to every household, caregivers need to weigh their usefulness for ensuring safety against limiting a patient's independence.

Issues Affecting Psychological and Spiritual Functioning

Psychological Functoning

The neurodegeneration and subsequent symptoms that occur with Alzheimer's disease will create a substantial psychological burden on the quality of life of women. Neuropsychiatric symptoms are present in all stages of the disease such that symptoms will likely manifest in almost all women at some point during the course of the disease (Gauthier et al., 2010). The neuropsychiatric symptoms may exhibit as mood alterations such as depression, anxiety, euphoria, and disinhibition; psychotic manifestations such as delusions and hallucinations; various symptoms with motor manifestations such as apathy, agitation, wandering, and aggressiveness; and sleep or appetite disturbances (Spalletta et al., 2010).

As the disease progresses, the neuropsychiatric symptoms and intellectual impairment will increase in severity. Cognitive decline and progressive disability in performing activities of daily living will lead to increased dependency on others. In addition, the worsening neuropsychiatric symptoms, intellectual impairment, and functional impairment contribute not only to patient distress but to informal caregiver distress as well (Gauthier et al., 2010). Caregivers often experience depression, social isolation, relational difficulties, and sleep disturbance (Rodriguez et al., 2003).

Neuropsychiatric symptoms are as clinically relevant as the cognitive and functional impairments caused by Alzheimer's disease. They represent an indication of disease progression and strongly determine the patient's daily function and the treatment choices of the healthcare provider. Neuropsychiatric symptoms add to distress in the patient and caregiver and are a major contributor

to their suffering and diminished quality of life, leading to caregiver burnout and patient institutionalization (Gauthier et al., 2010).

Numerous nonpharmacological interventions may be used for management of neuropsychiatric symptoms; however, there is no single treatment that works for all patients or in all situations. Alzheimer's disease commonly causes women to lose the ability to understand their needs or make them known to caregivers. As a result, neuropsychiatric symptoms are frequently an expression of unmet physical or psychological needs, such as hunger, thirst, pain, sex, distress, or fear of endangerment. It is important for caregivers to determine what may be triggering neuropsychiatric symptoms and attempt to correct reversible factors before resorting to pharmacological interventions (Gauthier et al., 2010).

Sundowning is often triggered by environmental factors that reduce the patient's threshold for stress, such as understimulation or overstimulation, inconsistent routine, or provocation by others. Specific strategies aimed at modification of the environment have shown efficacy in reducing episodes of sundowning. These strategies include simplifying late afternoon and evening routines to allow for relaxation and adjustment, making the living area pleasant and comfortable, and using music, sound, and aromatherapy to enhance the environment and promote relaxation (Gauthier et al., 2010).

Education of caregivers in psychological management approaches for neuropsychiatric symptoms can be beneficial for both symptom control and reduction of caregiver distress. Research has suggested that psychoeducation and behavioral training for caregivers can have positive effects on caregiver distress and depression as well as equivalent benefits for the neuropsychiatric symptoms of care recipients (Gauthier et al., 2010).

Spirituality

Religion and spirituality play an essential role as a coping resource and in maintaining the quality of life of women with Alzheimer's disease and their caregivers. Spiritual care and support is as necessary as physical and emotional care and support (Stuckey, Post, Ollerton, FallCreek, & Whitehouse, 2002). Spiritual practices are a meaningful way to connect with personal faith, important memories, and present support. Common attributes of spirituality embrace belief systems, meaning and purpose of life, connectedness, and transcendence (Beuscher & Grando, 2009). The spiritual needs of persons with Alzheimer's disease include the need to feel connected, the need to be loved, and the need to have hope. Active engagement in spiritual beliefs, including traditional religious practices, is an important aspect of coping and fulfilling spiritual needs (Bell & Troxel, 2001; Beuscher & Grando, 2009). Women with Alzheimer's disease remain spiritual beings even deep into the progression of the disease (Stuckey et al., 2002). In the early stages of the disease, patients frequently draw from their spirituality and faith to find meaning and courage in facing the challenges of cognitive losses and to obtain relief from fears and anxiety (Beuscher & Beck, 2008). Practices such as daily prayer and reading bible verses enable patients to seek hope and reassurance in facing the burdens of the disease. Engagement in church activities offers a vital connection with other people and a sense of belonging and identity (Beuscher & Grando, 2009). Traditional religious services afford an abundance of cognitive-based expressions of faith such as reciting scripture and prayers, singing hymns, listening to homilies or sermons, and responsive reading. The multisensorial experience of traditional worship services can sustain feelings of connection and may be associated with a slower rate of cognitive decline. Memories may be triggered by religious symbols that hold meaning and importance in the lives of patients (Kaufman, Anaki, Binns, & Freedman, 2007; Stuckey et al., 2002).

Issues Affecting Socioeconomic Integrity

Alzheimer's disease poses great cost to patients and caregivers alike. The breadth of financial demands of Alzheimer's disease is extensive since it is the third most costly illness in the United States. In 2015, the healthcare costs for Alzheimer's disease were approximately $226 billion. Of this amount, an estimated $113 billion was attributed to Medicare payments, $41 billion to Medicaid payments, $44 billion to out of pocket payments, and $29 billion to other payment sources such as private insurance, health maintenance organizations, other managed care organizations, and uncompensated care (these payments were rounded and do not add up to the total cost) (Alzheimer's Association, 2015a). The total per-person healthcare and long-term care payments from these sources averaged $47,752 in 2014. In the course of the disease, many patients will receive long-term care services, such as home care, adult day centers, assisted living facilities, or nursing homes. The costs of these services are high (e.g. assisted living can average $42,000 annually and nursing home care can average $77,380 to $87,600 per year). Patients eventually deplete their financial assets and then must apply for Medicaid, which is the only public program that covers the costs of nursing home care that most Alzheimer's patients will require in the late stages of illness (Alzheimer's Association, 2015a). The magnitude of these expenses is enormous and the cost of care can be burdensome and use up a significant portion of a family's assets. In addition, the capacity of patients to make legal and financial decisions diminishes over time, thus it is essential that legal and financial planning be started as soon as a diagnosis of Alzheimer's disease is made. Legal counseling from an attorney specializing in elder care should be sought to prepare power of attorney, healthcare directives, wills, and living trusts. Early action and effective planning will help to ensure financial means for future care.

Various government-provided benefits such as Medicare, Medicaid, and Social Security disability as well as private health insurance plans may help defray the costs of health care for women with Alzheimer's disease. However, specific regulations and procedures can be complicated with respect to eligibility for benefits and obtaining coverage, especially concerning home health care and long-term care. Enlisting the assistance of a social worker or elder care attorney is recommended to help families navigate through complex financial processes.

Issues Affecting Family Well-Being

The burden of Alzheimer's disease has substantial influence on family well-being. The cognitive decline, psychological distress, depression, and eventual physical disability of Alzheimer's disease will ultimately interfere with women's ability to perform social roles within the family. Women with Alzheimer's disease lose the ability to perform activities and tasks for their families that they were previously able to do, such as household chores, caring for grandchildren, grocery shopping, and meal preparation. Moreover, they lose the ability to function in relational roles and manage their own finances, legal affairs, and activities of daily living. The decline in the ability to carry out role responsibilities will dictate the transference of responsibilities to other family members. Women with Alzheimer's disease will transition from the role of "caregiver" to the role of "care receiver." The caregiver role is frequently assumed by husbands/partners or adult children, and necessitates adjustment and renegotiation of role responsibilities, or restructuring of the spousal/partner relationship (Roberto, Gigliotti, & Husser, 2005). The changes in family dynamics subsequently bring about stress and tension on family relationships. Family members may come to feel increasingly separated from the parts of their lives that have been supported by and experienced with their loved one. Shared intimacy, goals, and social activities are no longer attainable as the disease progresses (Beeson, Horton-Deutsch, Farran, & Neundorfer, 2000).

The majority of family caregivers of patients with Alzheimer's disease are women who care for an afflicted parent/parent-in-law, spouse, grandparent, or other relative. Frequently, the caregiver resides in the same household as the person for whom they are providing care, and may have children or grandchildren also living in the home (Alzheimer's Association, 2014). Caring for the individual with Alzheimer's disease presents substantial challenges and afflicted individuals require increasing levels of supervision and personal care. Family caregivers can experience high levels of stress and negative impacts on their health, employment, income, and financial security (Alzheimer's Association, 2014). Worry and anger about the potential for genetic predisposition, and guilt among unaffected relatives can also contribute to high levels of family stress (Gies & Lessick, 2009). Some caregivers may refuse assistance from others and attempt to handle everything themselves. This may cause caregivers to become burned out, depressed, and resentful toward their loved ones with Alzheimer's disease. Often, other family members withdraw from interacting socially with afflicted family members and their caregivers because they do not understand the changes brought about by the disease and are afraid of the strange behavior exhibited by patients. Family members may also deny what is happening or may disagree with financial and care decisions, resulting in a divided family. It is essential that open communication be maintained among family members. Family meetings to discuss the caregiver role and responsibilities, problems, and feelings can help to ease tensions. Education about the disease, its symptoms, and the tasks of a caregiver can be helpful in breaking barriers. The inclusion of a professional counselor or clergy member at family meetings can also be effective in facilitating communication, understanding, and reduced stress.

Caring for a loved one with Alzheimer's disease increases the risk of the caregiver engaging in abusive behaviors. Elder mistreatment encompasses physical abuse or aggression, sexual abuse, psychological mistreatment or chronic verbal aggression, financial or material mistreatment, and neglect. The increased risk of elder mistreatment is likely related to high levels of internal and external stress. Internal stresses comprise burden of care, depression, and other caregiver emotional problems, whereas external stresses include being financially, emotionally, and housing-dependent on care recipients. The poor quality of the relationship between caregiver and care recipient, social isolation, poor coping mechanisms such as substance abuse, and increased level of dependence and vulnerability of care recipients are also factors likely to increase the risk of caregivers engaging in elder mistreatment (VandeWeerd et al., 2005).

Pharmacologic treatment, supportive psychotherapy, education groups, and respite services that reduce the number of hours per day spent providing care represent effective strategies that can reduce stress, social isolation, and caregiver depression (VandeWeerd et al., 2005). Referring family members to support groups and community service resources can assist families in managing stress and emotional, financial, and other issues (Geis & Lessick, 2009).

Spirituality is an important resource that facilitates coping with the burdens associated with caring for family members with Alzheimer's disease. Caregivers rely on spirituality for strength when coping with the caregiver situation. Research findings suggest that spiritual practices such as prayer, attending religious activities, and discussing spiritual matters with family and friends can play a critical role in the lives of caregivers to help them through the caregiving experience (Spurlock, 2005).

Implications for Healthcare Providers

When considering strategies to improve the quality of life for women with Alzheimer's disease, it is important to emphasize early diagnosis and subsequent early initiation of pharmacological and behavioral interventions to maximize cognitive function and slow progression of the disease. Early diagnosis is often challenging, particularly when persons have limited capacity to recognize their own symptoms and attribute cognitive decline to chronic illness or aging. Healthcare providers who have limited contact in brief office visits with their elderly patients, especially without a spouse or adult child present, may overlook the presence of early-stage Alzheimer's disease. Insufficient time, inadequate reimbursement for services, and uncertainty about the value of early diagnosis may also contribute to the failure of healthcare providers to routinely screen older adults for Alzheimer's disease (Cotter, 2006). Healthcare providers need to be aware of their own prejudices and misconceptions in order to impart care that is responsive to the holistic needs of patients with Alzheimer's disease. Their attitudes can greatly influence the quality of care they offer as well as the quality of life of their patients (Murray & Boyd, 2009).

Although current therapies have, at best, moderate effects on slowing disease progression, studies have consistently shown that active medical management of Alzheimer's disease can significantly improve quality of life through all stages of the disease for patients and their caregivers. Active management includes appropriate application of available treatment options, effective integration of coexisting conditions into the treatment plan, coordination of care among all healthcare providers involved in maximizing the quality of life of the patient, and use of supportive services inclusive of counseling, activity and support groups, and adult day center programs (Alzheimer's Association, 2014).

Special Concerns of Age and Ethnicity

Older women with Alzheimer's disease, especially those who are members of ethnic minorities, are at risk for health disparities. Health disparities are differences in health or in factors that can influence health among disadvantaged social groups, who consequently experience poorer health than those who belong to groups with more social advantages (Murray & Boyd, 2009). Co-occurring morbidities that are either newly developed or pre-existing multiply health disparities. The impact of additional health disparities that develop as a result of co-occurring diseases is great, not only in terms of increased out-of-pocket healthcare expenses and greater need for long-term care services, but also in contributing to a higher mortality rate. The risk of elderly women with Alzheimer's disease receiving inadequate care is great and they often fall through the gaps between psychiatric and medical services (Murray & Boyd, 2009).

Barriers to healthcare access and utilization can further increase health disparities of elderly women with Alzheimer's disease. Policies and programs that determine reimbursement for care and services dependent on their socioeconomic status can greatly affect options for care for diagnosed women. Medicare and Medicaid are available for eligible individuals to meet some long-term care needs; however, several limitations in these systems jeopardize healthcare utilization for many Alzheimer's patients. The harsh reality is that families pay for much of the costs of Alzheimer's care as well as bear the burden of caregiver costs from lost productivity (Murray & Boyd, 2009).

Inadequate knowledge among healthcare providers regarding prevalence, diagnosis, evaluation, and treatment of Alzheimer's disease also creates barriers to healthcare access and utilization. Healthcare providers also may lack knowledge of community-based care, especially in areas of adult day health care, alternatives to residential care, and the role of nutrition in the care of Alzheimer's patients. Inadequate preparation for an aging population is a reality in the healthcare professions. The need for a holistic and interdisciplinary approach to addressing the learning needs of healthcare providers is great (Murray & Boyd, 2009).

A diagnosis of Alzheimer's disease frequently carries with it a perceived stigma, which underlies many of the barriers for healthcare access and utilization. Perceived stigma among affected persons and their caregivers, as well as the belief that cognitive decline is a normal part of advancing age can lead to delayed diagnosis and treatment, and can make older adults reluctant to express their needs. Additionally, the ethnocultural background of affected individuals and their family members can be an influential factor that affects access to and utilization of services. Stigma and shame associated with Alzheimer's disease and belief that the disease is a part of normative aging are common among racial and ethnic groups in the United States. Other factors that create barriers to care among racial and ethnic minorities include poor health literacy about Alzheimer's disease, economic constraints, language barriers, preference for traditional services, and mistrust of healthcare providers. Since the cultural and ethnic beliefs and attitudes towards Alzheimer's disease are strong factors that influence access to care and services, it is essential that healthcare providers practice in a person-centered and culturally competent manner in the provision of appropriate care (Murray & Boyd, 2009).

Research Review

What is the meaning of living alone from the perspective of older women with Alzheimer's disease?

De Witt, L., Ploeg, J., & Black, M. (2010). Living alone with dementia: An interpretive phenomenological study with older women. *Journal of Advanced Nursing, 66*(8), 1698–1707.

An increasing international trend among the elderly in developed and developing countries is toward living alone. The safety of older people with dementia who live alone is a serious community care issue. The ethical dilemma centers on balancing concerns about safety with rights for independence. The risks and problems experienced by older women living alone have been investigated mostly through quantitative research. The purpose of this qualitative study was to understand the meaning of living alone from the perspective of older women with Alzheimer's disease or a related dementia.

A Heideggerian interpretive phenomenological design was used in this study. Participants were recruited in Ontario, Canada through community health and social services agencies or professional colleagues using purposive sampling. Inclusion criteria included having been diagnosed with mild to moderate Alzheimer's disease or a related dementia, having discussed their diagnosis with their physician, having lived alone in the community, having spent the night alone, being able to speak English, and being 55 years of age or older. Potential participants were screened for study eligibility with an eligibility questionnaire administered by the principal investigator by telephone. Eight women aged 58–87 were recruited for the study. All study participants were English-speaking white women of European descent. Marital status of the participants included two divorced, five widowed, and one separated from a previous partner. Five participants lived in houses, three lived in apartments. Six participants received assistance with medications, four participated in adult day care, five received assistance with bathing, three received meal delivery, and one received grocery delivery. Seven participants received informal support from adult children and one relied on a sibling. Fourteen face-to-face, audiotaped open-ended interviews were conducted and data collection was concluded when information redundancy was achieved. Iterative data collection and analysis was guided by van Manen's method. A framework of rigor for interpretive phenomenology was applied.

The study findings revealed that the theme of *holding back time* expressed the overall temporal meaning of living alone with dementia. The women sought to *hold back time* and continue to live alone. Pharmacological treatments to slow disease progression represented *stored time*. *Stored time* offered the opportunity to hold back future *dreaded time*, which was their own possibility of being worse. Holding back dreaded future time enabled the women to hold on to the present or the "now." Past experiences with other persons with dementia was a context for *holding on to now* and facing some risks of living alone with memory loss. The women acknowledged having *limited time* remaining for, and identified endpoints to, living alone.

The findings of the study showed that even though memory loss interfered with these older women's experiences of "ordinary" clock and calendar time, living alone was rich with the meaning of time. The future was a central temporal feature of living alone as the women sought to hold back time. They faced a feared and dreaded future with illness progression and the inevitable move away from home, and death.

The findings of this study lend insight into the viewpoint of women with dementia who live alone. Understanding the perspective of *holding on to now* enables nurses to counsel patients about risks of living alone and better assess their need for community health and social services. The study findings provide insight into the emotional impact that past experiences with others with dementia has on individuals. Nurses can advocate for health and social services that are sensitive to the potential emotional impact of mixing people with varied levels of dementia in the same program. Furthermore, the study findings give nurses insight into the importance of *stored time* that can be enhanced by early diagnosis and treatment and can give future patients the opportunity to participate in planning for their forthcoming living arrangements.

Chapter Summary Points

- Alzheimer's disease is an irreversible progressive brain disorder in which increasing numbers of brain cells deteriorate and die, resulting in an advancing decline or loss of memory, cognitive abilities, emotional control, and social behaviors.
- The risk for developing Alzheimer's disease increases with age so that by age 90, approximately 33% of women and 23% of men will have developed Alzheimer's disease.
- Older African Americans are about two times as likely to develop Alzheimer's disease and other dementias as older white adults, and older Hispanics are at least one and one-half times more likely than older white adults to develop Alzheimer's disease and other dementias.
- Alzheimer's disease manifests as early-onset disease, which develops before age 60, and affects about 5% of the people with the disease. Late-onset disease is the most common and typically develops after age 65.
- Women are more likely to develop Alzheimer's disease than men. This disparity is primarily explained by the fact that women tend to live longer than men, giving women more time to develop the disease.
- Alzheimer's disease is intrinsically fatal and the available treatments do little to change the progression of the disease. However, early diagnosis is essential so that therapy can be initiated to slow the inevitable cognitive and behavioral decline.
- Although there is no cure for Alzheimer's disease, the goals of treatment are to slow the progression of symptoms, maintain cognitive ability at the highest level possible, and control neuropsychological symptoms.
- Pharmacological therapy is the mainstay of treatment and includes drug therapy for cognitive symptoms as well as behavioral and psychiatric symptoms. In addition, nonpharmacological approaches are available to augment symptom control.
- The quality of life issues throughout the trajectory of Alzheimer's disease are commonly multidimensional. However, being able to accurately determine the quality of life of individuals with Alzheimer's disease is challenging because the subjective perceptions of quality of life of patients often differ when compared to that of informal caregivers and professionals.

- The burden of care for afflicted individuals falls mainly on family and friends, and the majority of informal caregivers are female family members and friends.
- The enormous health care expenditure derived from disease chronicity and severity as well as the effects of disease burden on the quality of life of patients and their informal caregivers have evolved into major societal and public health concerns of paramount importance, especially in view of the predicted surge of the disease with the aging of the population.
- Insufficient time, inadequate reimbursement for services, and uncertainty about the value of early diagnosis may contribute to the failure of health care providers to routinely screen older adults for Alzheimer's disease.
- The risk of elderly women with Alzheimer's disease receiving inadequate care is great, and they often fall through the gaps between psychiatric and medical services.
- A diagnosis of Alzheimer's disease frequently carries with it a perceived stigma, which underlies various barriers for healthcare access and utilization. Perceived stigma among affected persons and their caregivers, as well as the belief that cognitive decline is a normal part of advancing age, can lead to delayed diagnosis and treatment.

Critical Thinking Exercise

Case Study

Mrs. B. is an 80-year-old Hispanic woman who has a 20-year history of hypothyroidism that has been controlled with oral thyroid hormone replacement therapy. Mrs. B. lives alone in the home she shared with her husband of 52 years before his death 2 years earlier. Mrs. B. has two daughters who are married with families of their own and live in the same town as their mother. She enjoys participating in her needlecraft group and volunteering at her church. She also enjoys cooking holiday meals for her family. Mrs. B. takes care of her home, and does the cooking, cleaning, and grocery shopping. One day, Mrs. B. called Mary, her oldest daughter, and asked her to take her grocery shopping because she had misplaced the car keys. When Mary arrived and looked in the refrigerator to see what her mother needed at the grocery store, she found the car keys in the vegetable drawer. Mrs. B. shook her head and said she must be getting old. While Mary was in the kitchen she noticed a stack of unopened mail in a cupboard that turned out to be bills that had not been paid and were long overdue. When Mary inquired about the bills her mother stated that she forgot to pay them. Mary became concerned because her mother had always been organized in managing her finances and paying bills. Mrs. B. became upset and insisted she was just getting old and everyone forgets things when they get old.

Mary was uneasy and decided to call her sister Betty to discuss the situation of their mother's forgetfulness. Betty also became troubled when Mary told her about the misplaced keys and the unpaid bills. Betty related recent incidents where her mother forgot to pick up Betty's children from school twice when Betty had to work late. Betty agreed that their mother's behavior was unusual and she needed to be evaluated by her doctor, if only to make sure that mother's hypothyroidism was under control.

Mary accompanied her mother to the primary care physician, where she discovered that her mother had missed two previous appointments. The doctor performed a comprehensive physical examination, which was unremarkable. In response to Mary's report of her mother's forgetfulness, the physician administered a screening test for cognitive decline. Based on receiving positive results, the physician administered the MMSE to Mrs. B. The results indicated impaired cognition, suggesting a mild, slowly progressive dementia, which was likely Alzheimer's disease. The physician also ordered blood work and diagnostic tests, including an MRI, to rule out other causes of cognitive functional decline. Several days later Mrs. B. and her daughters returned to the doctor and learned that the laboratory values and diagnostic tests were within normal limits. The MRI revealed some brain atrophy. Mrs. B. was diagnosed with Alzheimer's disease because other causes of dementia were ruled out and diagnostic criteria were met. The doctor discussed the diagnosis with Mrs. B. and her daughters and recommended initiating treatment. Mrs. B. was started on donepezil with instructions to return for follow-up appointments to assess side effects and monitor tolerability. Mrs. B. tolerated the drug well with little to no side effects. On the advice of the doctor, Mrs. B. and her daughters met with an attorney who specialized in elder law to place Mrs. B.'s legal and financial affairs in order.

Over the next 3 years, Mrs. B. experienced a slow decline in cognition and independent functioning. She experienced behavioral changes such as agitation, wandering, and complaining that her husband was late returning from work. Eventually, Mrs. B. was unable to manage living alone and it was decided that she move in with Mary and her family. Mary's living situation afforded her more time to attend to her mother since her children were in college, whereas Betty's children were younger and needed more attention. Mrs. B. was started on memantine. The doctor referred Mary and Betty to an educational group to learn how to manage agitation and oppositional behavior. Mary managed most of the care for Mrs. B. since Medicare and supplemental health insurance provided limited coverage for Mrs. B.'s healthcare costs. Betty helped out when she could to give her sister much-needed respite. As Mrs. B.'s condition worsened, her care demanded most of Mary's time and attention and placed a great deal of stress on her marriage. Mary became depressed and exhausted.

Mrs. B. eventually needed to be placed in a nursing home. Mary and Betty enlisted the aid of a social worker to help them navigate through the process of nursing home placement. Over the next year, Mrs. B.'s physical and cognitive function steadily declined to the point where she was bedridden, totally dependent, and no longer able to interact meaningfully with her family members. Mrs. B.'s living will stated that she wanted no extreme medical measures, CPR, or feeding tube to be administered when she became incapacitated. She eventually developed pneumonia and died peacefully in her sleep.

Questions for Seminar Discussion

1. What early symptoms suggested that Mrs. B. might have Alzheimer's disease? Discuss the difficulties associated with early diagnosis and why early diagnosis of Alzheimer's disease is essential.

2. What overt physical, psychological/spiritual, socioeconomic, and family issues threatened the quality of life of Mrs. B. and her family?

3. What issues and concerns were not readily apparent but might become problematic to Mrs. B. and her family?

4. What strategies should be used to manage behavior symptoms and provide a safe and secure home environment for Mrs. B.?

5. What pitfalls exist in assessing quality of life in women with Alzheimer's disease? How should healthcare providers obtain a thorough assessment of the quality of life of Mrs. B. and her family?

6. What strengths and weaknesses are present that factor into the ability of Mrs. B. and her family to manage illness and quality of life demands?

7. What community resources are available that would help Mrs. B. and her family improve quality of life?

Internet Resources

Alzheimer's Association: information and resources for patients, family, and professionals. http://alz.org

Alzheimer's Disease.com: information and support for caregivers. www.AlzheimersDisease.com

Alzheimer's Foundation: information and resources for patients, family, and professionals. http://www.alzfdn.org

Medline Plus: information and resources for patients, family, and professionals. http://www.nlm.nih.gov/medlineplus/alzheimersdisease.html

National Institute on Aging: information and resources for patients, family, and professionals. http://www.nia.nih.gov/Alzheimers/AlzheimersInformation/GeneralInfo/

References

Alzheimer's Association. (2014). 2014 Alzheimer's disease facts and figures. Retrieved from http://www.alz.org/downloads/Facts_Figures_2014.pdf

Alzheimer's Association. (2015a). 2015 Alzheimer's disease facts and figures. Retrieved from https://www.alz.org/facts/downloads/facts_figures_2015.pdf

Alzheimer's Association. (2015b). Treatments for Alzheimer's disease. Retrieved from http://www.alz.org/alzheimers_disease_treatments.asp

Azad, N., Al Bugami, M., & Loy-English, I. (2007). Gender differences in dementia risk factors. *Gender Medicine*, *4*(2), 120–129.

Bayliss, E., Ellis, J., & Steiner, J. (2007). Barriers to self-management and quality of life outcomes in seniors with multimorbidities. *Annals of Family Medicine, 5*(5), 395–402.

Beeson, R., Horton-Deutsch, S., Farran, C., & Neundorfer, M. (2000). Loneliness and depression in caregivers of persons with Alzheimer's disease or related disorders. *Issues in Mental Health Nursing, 21*, 779–806.

Bell, V., & Troxel, D. (2001). Spirituality and the person with dementia: A view from the field. *Alzheimer's Care Quarterly, 2*(2), 31–45.

Beuscher, L., & Beck, C. (2008). A literature review of spirituality in coping with early-stage Alzheimer's disease. *Journal of Nursing and Healthcare of Chronic Illness, 17*, 5a, 88–97.

Beuscher, L., & Grando, V. (2009). Using spirituality to cope with early-stage Alzheimer's disease. *Western Journal of Nursing Research, 31*(5), 583–598.

Conde-Sala, J., Garre-Olmo, J., Turró-Garriga, O., López-Pousa, S., & Vilalta-Franch, J. (2009). Factors related to perceived quality of life in patients with Alzheimer's disease: The patient's perception compared with that of caregivers. *International Journal of Geriatric Psychiatry, 24*, 585–594.

Cotter, V. (2006). Alzheimer's disease: Issues and challenges in primary care. *Nursing Clinics of North America, 41*, 83–93.

Craig, M., & Murphy, D. (2009). Alzheimer's disease in women. *Best Practice & Research Clinical Obstetrics and Gynaecology, 23*, 53–61.

De Witt, L., Ploeg, J., & Black, M. (2010). Living alone with dementia: An interpretive phenomenological study with older women. *Journal of Advanced Nursing, 66*(8), 1698–1707.

Dharmarajan, T.S., & Gunturu, S. (2009). Alzheimer's disease: A health care burden of epidemic proportion. *American Health & Drug Benefits, 2*(1), 39–47.

Gauthier, S., Cummings, J., Ballard, C., Brodaty, H., Grossberg, G., Robert, P., & Lyketsos, C. (2010). Management of behavioral problems in Alzheimer's disease. *International Psychogeriatrics, 22*(3), 346–372.

Gies, C., & Lessick, M. (2009). Alzheimer's disease in women: A clinical and genetics perspective. *Nursing for Women's Health, 13*(4), 314–324.

Godfrey, J. (2006). Toward optimum health: Leon J. Thal discusses the latest in Alzheimer's disease in women. *Journal of Women's Health, 15*(6), 704–708.

Godfrey, J., & El-Badri, N. (2009). Toward optimal health: Advising aging women about dementia. *Journal of Women's Health, 18*(7), 929–933.

Griffith, P., & Lopez, O. (2009). Disparities in the diagnosis and treatment of Alzheimer's disease in African American and Hispanic patients: A call to action. *Generations: The Journal of the American Society of Aging, 33*(1), 37–46.

Hoe, J., Katona, C., Orrell, M., & Livingston, G. (2007). Quality of life in dementia: Care recipient and caregiver perceptions of quality of life in dementia: The LASER-AD study. *International Journal of Geriatric Psychiatry, 22*, 1031–1036.

Huang, H., Chang, M., Tang, J., Chiu, Y., & Weng, L. (2008). Determinants of the discrepancy in patient- and caregiver-rated quality of life for persons with dementia. *Journal of Clinical Nursing, 18*, 3107–3117.

Kaufman, Y., Anaki, D., Binns, M., & Freedman, M. (2007). Cognitive decline in Alzheimer's disease: Impact of spirituality, religiosity, and QOL. *Neurology, 68*, 1509–1514.

Mehta, K., Yaffe, K., Perez-Stable, E., Stewart, A., Barnes, D., Kurland, B., & Miller, B. (2008). Race/ethnic differences in Alzheimer's disease survival in US Alzheimer's Disease Centers. *Neurology, 70*(14), 1163–1170.

Murray, L., & Boyd, S. (2009). Protecting personhood and achieving quality of life for older adults with dementia in the U.S. health care system. *Journal of Aging and Health, 21*(2), 350–373.

Ott, B., & Cahn-Weiner, D. (2003). Gender differences in Alzheimer's disease. *Psychiatric Times, 20*(2), 46.

Perneczky, R., Drzezga, A., Diehl-Schmid, J., Li, Y., & Kurz, A. (2007). Gender differences in brain reserve: An ^{18}F-FDG PET study in Alzheimer's disease. *Journal of Neurology, 254*, 1395–1400.

Roberto, K., Gigliotti, C., & Husser, E. (2005). Older women's experiences with multiple health conditions: Daily challenges and care practices. *Health Care for Women International, 26*, 672–692.

Rodriguez, G., DeLeo, C., Girtler, N., Vitali, P., Grossi, E., & Nobili, F. (2003). Psychological and social aspects in management of Alzheimer's patients: An inquiry among caregivers. *Neurological Science, 24*, 329–335.

Scalco, M., & van Reekum, R. (2009). Prevention of Alzheimer's disease: Encouraging evidence. *Canadian Family Physician, 52*, 200–207.

Spalletta, G., Musico, M., Padovani, A., Rozzini, L., Perri, R., Fadda, L., … Palmer, K. (2010). *American Journal of Geriatric Psychiatry, 18*(11), 1026–1035.

Spurlock, W. (2005). Spiritual well-being and caregiver burden in Alzheimer's caregivers. *Geriatric Nursing, 26*(3), 154–161.

Stuckey, J., Post, S., Ollerton, S., FallCreek, S., & Whitehouse, P. (2002). Alzheimer's disease, religion, and the ethics of respect for spirituality: A community dialogue. *Alzheimer's Care Quarterly, 3*(3), 199–207.

VandeWeerd, C., Paveza, G., & Fulmer, T. (2006). Abuse and neglect in older adults with Alzheimer's disease. *Nursing Clinics of North America, 41*, 43–55.

Index

Note: Page numbers followed by *b*, *f*, or *t* indicate material in boxes, figures, or tables, respectively.